# Genetic Effects
# On Aging II

# Genetic Effects On Aging II

**David E. Harrison**

**Jackson Laboratory**
**Bar Harbor, Maine**

The Telford Press, Inc.
Caldwell, New Jersey

THE TELFORD PRESS, INC.

Post Office Box 287, Caldwell, New Jersey 07006


Genetic effects on aging II / [edited by] David E. Harrison.

        p. cm.

    Includes bibliographical references.

    ISBN 0-936923-31-8

     1. Aging—Genetic aspects.  I. Harrison, David E.

II. Title: Genetic effects on aging 2.

III. Title: Genetic efffects on aging two.

QP86.G395   1990

612.6'7—dc20                                    90-10747

                                                     CIP

CONTENTS

## Section 5    CHROMOSOME REGIONS AND MUTATIONS AFFECTING AGING

CONTRIBUTORS

Jonathan R. Archer
The Jackson Laboratory
Bar Harbor, ME 04609

Glenn C. Bewley
Department of Genetics
North Carolina State University
Raleigh, NC 27695-7614

Roderick T.Bronson
Tufts Veterinary Diagnostic
Laboratory
305 South St.
Jamaica Plain, MA 02130

W. Ted Brown
Division of Human Genetics
Department of Pediatrics
North Shore University Hospital
Manhasset, NY 11030

William A. Calder III
Department of Ecology and
Evolutionary Biology
The University of Arizona
Tucson, AZ 85721

Brian Charlesworth
Department of Ecology and
Evolution
The University of Chicago
1103 E. 57th St.
Chicago, IL 60637

Wen-Hsiu Chiang
Department of Chemistry
Illinois State University
Normal, IL 61761

Mark D. Crew
Department of Pathology, School
of Medicine
University of California
Los Angeles, CA 90025

Caleb E. Finch
Andrus Gerontology Center
University of Southern California
Los Angeles, CA 90089-0191

Paul A. Fitzpatrick
Department of Applied Biology
Massachusetts Institute of
Technology
Cambridge, MA 02139

K. Flurkey
Boston University School of
Medicine
80 E. Concord St.
Boston, MA 02118

Norma Foltz
Department of Zoology
University of Hawaii at Manoa
Honolulu, HI 96822

David B. Friedman
Department of Genetics
University of Washington
Seattle, WA 98195

Alan Garen
Department of Molecular
Biophysics and Biochemistry
Yale University
260 Whitney Avenue
New Haven, CT 06511

D.C. Gajdusek
Laboratory of Central Nervous
System Studies
National Institute of Neurological
Disorders and Stroke
National Institutes of Health
Bethesda, MD 20892

Rebecca S. Gelman
Division of Biostatistics
Dana-Farber Cancer Institute
44 Binney St.
Boston, MA 02115

**Joseph L. Graves, Jr.**
Department of Ecology and
Evolutionary Biology
School of Biological Sciences
University of California
Irvine, CA 92717

**Thomas Grigliatti**
Department of Zoology
University of British Columbia
Vancouver, British Columbia
Canada V6T 2A9

**Mao-Zhi Gu**
Department of Chemistry
Illinois State University
Normal, IL 61761

**D.C. Guiroy**
Laboratory of Central Nervous
System Studies
National Institute of Neurological
Disorders and Stroke
National Institutes of Health
Bethesda, MD 20892

**Jonathan L. Haines**
Neurogentics Unit
Research 3
Massachusetts General Hospital
Boston, MA 02114

**David E. Harrison**
The Jackson Laboratory
Bar Harbor, ME 04609

**Edward W. Hutchinson**
Institute for Behavioral Genetics
Campus Box 447
University of Colorado at
Boulder
Boulder, CO 80309-0447

**Donald K. Ingram**
Gerontology Research Center
National Institute on Aging
Francis Scott Key Medical Center
Baltimore, MD 21224

**Diane Janick-Buckner**
Department of Biochemistry and
Biophysics
Iowa State University
Ames, IA 50011

**Thomas E. Johnson**
Institute for Behavioral Genetics
Box 447
University of Colorado
Boulder, CO 80309

**Fred J. Kieras**
New York State Institute for
Basic Research in Developmental
Disabilities
Staten Island, NY 10314

**Thomas B.L. Kirkwood**
Laboratory of Mathematical
Biology
National Institute for Medical
Research
The Ridgeway, Mill Hill
London NW7 1AA, U.K.

**Steven G. Kohama**
Andrus Gerontology Center
University of Southern California
Los Angeles, CA 90089-0191

**Steven P. Lerner**
Animal & Veterinary Science
West Virginia University
Morgantown, WV 26506

**William J. MacKay**
Biological Department
St. Anselm College
Manchester, NH 03102

Gerald E. McClearn
Center for Developmental and
Health Genetics
The Pennsylvania State
University
University Park, PA 16802

George M. Martin
Departments of Pathology and
Genetics
University of Washington
Seattle, WA 98195

Richard A. Miller
Dept. of Pathology
Boston University School of
Medicine
Boston, MA  02118

James F. Nelson
Department of Obstetrics and
Gynecology
Center for the Study of
Reproduction
Center for Studies of Aging
McGill University
Montreal, Quebec, Canada
H3A 1A1

Arlan Richardson
Department of Chemistry
Illinois State University
Normal, IL 61761

Murray Richter
Department of Zoology
University of British Columbia
Vancouver, British Columbia
Canada V6T 2A9

Michael R. Rose
Department of Ecology and
Evolutionary Biology
School of Biological Sciences
University of California
Irvine, CA 92717

George S. Roth
Gerontology Research Center
Francis Scott Key Medical Center
Baltimore, MD 21224

Richard L. Russell
Department of Biological
Sciences
University of Pittsburgh
Pittsburgh, PA 15260

Renee I. Seppa
Department of Biological
Sciences
University of Pittsburgh
Pittsburgh, PA 15260

Jo Ellen Shoemaker
Department of Molecular Biology
and Biochemistry
University of California at Irvine
Irvine, CA 92717

George S. Smith
Department of Pathology
School of Medicine
University of California
Los Angeles, CA 90024-1732

Susan Waggoner
Department of Chemistry
Illinois State University
Normal, IL 61761

Roy L. Walford
Department of Pathology
School of Medicine
University of California
Los Angeles, CA  90024-1732

Carol M. Warner
Department of Biology
Northeastern University
Boston, MA 02115

**Ada L. M. Watson**
Division of Immunogenetics
Dana-Farber Cancer Institute
Boston, MA 02115

**Ian Whitehead**
Department of Zoology
University of British Columbia
Vancouver, British Columbia
Canada V6T 2A9

**R. Michael Williams**
Division of Immunogenetics
Dana-Farber Cancer Institute
Boston, MA 02115

**Edmond J. Yunis**
Division of Immunogenetics
Dana-Farber Cancer Institute
Boston, MA 02115

**Michael Zebrower**
New York State Institute for
Basic Research in Developmental
Disabilities
Staten Island, NY 10314

# 1

# INTRODUCTION AND PREDICTIONS

David E. Harrison

## INTRODUCTION

### Background and Objectives

The first *Genetic Effects on Aging* volume resulted from a conference held in 1976. The rapid rate of progress in this field since then required a new volume with a new approach. It is based on the fact that the combination of classical genetics and the powerful new tools of molecular genetics are greatly expanding our understanding of mammalian development. The same kinds of approaches should expand our understanding of aging processes; however, genetic studies of aging are only beginning in mammals. This volume provides background knowledge useful to those setting out to do genetic studies of aging in mammals, and raises vital questions: How many genes are important in mammalian aging? What are optimal methods for their study, both within a species and by comparing different species? To what degree are patterns of aging, and patterns of growth and development part of the same process? Do patterns of development predict subsequent patterns of growth and aging? Are there a few fundamental aging processes, or does every biological system age?

Although mammalian systems are emphasized in this volume, representatives of the advanced genetic studies in *Drosophila* and other model systems are also included. The purpose is to enrich and stimulate genetic studies of mammalian aging by suggesting and evaluating future possibilities. This approach resulted in lively discussions, demonstrating that the biology of aging has come of age. We welcome constructive critical thinking about what is required for the best science. I have summarized important issues raised in the discussions following the papers, trying to present all sides. The papers in this volume were peer reviewed, and in some cases disagreements between reviewer and author are summarized in the same fashion. Finally, two commentaries are given for issues that could not be contained in the discussion sections.

## Summary of Volume Contents

After the Introduction and Predictions for the future of research in mammalian aging, the *Evolutionary Genetics of Aging* is introduced by Kirkwood with his "Disposable Soma" theory. The following paper by Charlesworth describes a theory, developed from natural selection considerations, that predicted the results of selection for longevity in *Drosophila*. These results are summarized and extended in the next three papers. The success in *Drosophila* led to extensive discussions about the advisability of doing similar selection studies in mice, summarized in the commentary: Selection for Longer-lived Rodents.

The next section, *Aging Genetics in Nonmammals* includes work by Johnson *et. al.* on mutations in *C. elegans* that extend longevities and by Russell and Seppa, on testing aging in *C. elegans* mutants using biomarkers. Grigliatti *et. al.* discuss mutations in *Drosophila*, while Garen relates development and aging in this species. Calder describes studies of hummingbirds in the wild with surprisingly long lifespans.

The *Genetics of Aging Retardation* is introduced by Ingram, outlining genetic variability in behavioral aging. McClearn discusses biomarkers (which have the advantage of not harming the mouse) giving data on various confounding effects, while Richardson (paper by Waggoner *et. al.*) outlines how some, but not all, genes are affected at the level of transcription by dietary restriction. The commentary in this section appeared in *Growth Development and Aging* and gives ideas on how the beneficial effects of dietary restriction may have evolved.

*Strain and Mutant Effects on Neuroendocrine and Immune Aging* is introduced by the pathology of aging with Bronson's massive data summary and reference list on the occurrence rate of lesions in a large variety of different mouse and rat strains. This includes information that should be useful for all researchers using those strains, especially as it is taken from apparently healthy individuals. Bewley and Mackay describe effects of catalase mutants in *Drosophila*, while Nelson relates reproductive senescence to puberty and longevity in different mouse strains. Roth describes molecular genetic models of hormone and neurotransmitter changes during aging, and Miller reviews molecular changes in T cell populations with age.

*Chromosome Regions and Mutations Affecting Aging* continues in the immune system as Janick-Buckner and Warner described changes with age in MHC antigens on lymphocytes. Lerner and Finch discuss how neuroendocrine aging relates to reproductive senescence in females. Flurkey and Harrison describe how neuroendocrine mutations affect aging patterns, using mutant mice to determine how different biological systems interact during aging. Smith *et. al.* outline studies in the long-lived rodent, *Peromyscus*, which they are inbreeding, and Yunis (paper by Watson *et. al.*) reviews studies of genetics of aging using congenic, backcross and recombinant inbred lines of mice.

*Examples of Modern Mammalian Genetics* were discussed by Nadeau, Birkenmeier, and Eicher, of The Jackson Laboratory. Since their studies are detailed elsewhere, only the bibliographies suggested as useful by these authors are given in this volume.

*Progeroid Mutants and Alzheimer's disease* are introduced by Martin, who outlines how a wide variety of human mutations are potential models for particular aspects of aging. Brown *et al.* focus on the Hutchinson-Gilford and Werner progerias as models of premature aging. Guiroy and Gajdusek discuss the biochemistry of amyloid fibers in human dementias, while Haines *et al.* describe linkage analysis in familial Alzheimer's disease. The book ends with information about the sponsor, The Growth Publishing Company and its journal, *Growth, Development and aging*.

## PREDICTIONS

As modern techniques of molecular genetics are beginning to define the chemical controls of developmental processes, the same techniques will be applied to aging. Basic questions will be answered, and these answers will lead to treatments for deleterious aging processes. Gene therapies will test mechanisms of aging, initially in transgenic mice, with an obvious progression to precursor cells of the bone marrow and potential clinical use.

These areas of biomedical science illustrate something that rarely occurs in the history of science - basic and applied research have become the same thing. Presently, and for the next few decades, revolutionary advances in medicine will result from applying basic research in mammalian biology. Thus, our basic research has become applied medical research. As such, it can and should be funded not only by the NIH and NSF, but also by far more wealthy business sources. There are tremendous advances in human health to come, and very large amounts of money to be made.

### The 4 "M"s - Mapping, Mutations, Mice, Mechanisms

Currently there is a focus on mapping the human genome. Whether or not this becomes a huge federal initiative, it is an idea whose time has come, and is rapidly being accomplished. However, even after its DNA chemistry is defined, we still will not know what a gene does. To do this, it is necessary that the laboratory mouse genome be mapped at the same time as the human genome. Fortunately, this will not be difficult. The DNA chemistries of their genes are so similar that as soon as a sequence is cloned in one species, the homologous sequence can almost always be found in the other.

Methods for inducing specific mutations at each mapped sequence are being developed, and soon will be routine. These will be used to define how genes work by producing specific mutations. While some of these studies will be done on human cells in tissue culture, most of them will be done in laboratory mice, where there is a wealth of experience in defining mutations, and where interactions of tissues can be studied more realistically than in culture. Although this will require enormous amounts of work in many areas of mammalian biology, the mechanisms behind the effects of mutations will soon be understood, and how the genes operate will be defined.

The 4 "M"s outline how this will occur: *mapping* of the DNA sequences in man and *mouse*, induction of gene-specific *mutations*, so that the *mechanisms* of gene action can be traced. This work will require a fifth "m", *money*. Fortunately, it should be available, since the ability to transplant and control genes will offer enormous health benefits.

It is vital that the biology of aging be advanced as rapidly as possible, taking advantage the new knowledge. The other chapters in this book give the background needed to plan this advancement; here I will give examples of potential advances that should be important for the biology of aging.

## Potential New Clinical Treatments Using PSCs

While there have been almost unbelievable advances in the ability to insert new genes and turn them on in specific tissues, these have been in transgenic mice in which the new gene constructs are placed in fertilized ova. These studies illustrate the possibility of gene transplantation therapy, but are not directly relevant to clinical work in human beings.

More relevant will be gene transplantation into primitive immune and hemopoietic stem cells (PSCs). Recently it has become obvious that human gene transplantation *via* marrow cells will soon become clinically important. PSCs are an attractive tool, because they and their descendants have enormous proliferative capacity; one's own PSC would be removed from the bone marrow, genetically engineered to do what is needed, and returned, thus avoiding any ethical questions beyond the safety and effectiveness of the procedure. PSCs from mice have been good models for those in man, so the basic work can readily be done in mice.

Using gene transplantation, with PSCs as vehicles, curing single gene defects is only the beginning. Soon it should be possible to insert genes into PSCs to both turn on and to regulate the production of gene products at defined levels in differentiated cells descended from the genetically altered

PSCs. PSCs produce T and B cells normally, so it should eventually be possible to introduce genes that reverse losses in immune function with age, to cure cancers using genetically altered PSCs that make immune cells designed to eliminate the cancer cells, or to cure AIDS using altered PSCs whose T cells resist and remove the virus. Diabetes might be cured by PSCs engineered to produce descendants that supply insulin physiologically; this would offer a model for other endocrine adjustments, including those that might retard or reverse changes with age. If high HDL cholesterol cleans arteries, the mechanisms producing HDL cholesterol might be transferred to PSCs, so that their descendants would clean out arteries by increasing HDL:LDL proportions.

Hypothesized mechanisms of aging could be tested, with obvious clinical applications for those that effectively retarded aging rates in mice. For example, to test whether free radical damage causes aging, genes whose products reduce free radicals could be introduced *via* PSCs. If extracellular macromolecules age due to glycosylation or other mechanisms of crosslinking, PSCs could be engineered to produce macrophages that removed damaged molecules. Work with PSCs would be a model for work with other cell types, including precursors of brain neurons that might be introduced to repair neuronal damage resulting from age or disease.

## Potential for Assays of Aging

Another area of potential business support is in developing and using assays for aging in human beings. It is now possible to measure aging changes in individuals, to advise them whether they need to try to retard their personal aging rates, and whether their "interventions" are working. While developing interventions that retard aging in particular biological systems is only beginning, such interventions are sure to come, as the previous section illustrates. But well defined assays will be necessary to determine which interventions to use on each individual. We should start defining assays for aging now, by repeatedly testing individuals, and determining which assays best predict the effectiveness of interventions.

While there is no question of the need, there is the question of whether available assays are good enough, and, even more important, whether the interventions currently available would be useful. Two points give reason for optimism: First, interventions have been working, at least on the level of American society. In their talks at the 1988 Summer Institute in Research on Aging, Bernice Neugarten and Matilda Riley pointed out that life expectancies of US residents have been increasing steadily throughout the past 50 years, and that progress in this area does not seem to be slowing down. In addition, increasing percentages of elderly people can live independently. This suggests that interventions are useful, and that even now the rate of gain in health can be accelerated by objectively evaluating and recommending interventions.

Second, millions of Americans are currently spending large amounts of time and money on interventions that they hope will increase their "healthspans"- their periods of healthy life. These interventions may be changes in diet, exercise or other parts of their life-styles; increasingly they include high doses of micronutrients, and sometimes hormone or drug treatments. These interventions are being selected and used with no objective evidence that they are needed or useful.

This is dangerous, as there are large individual differences in genotype and environment, so that the same interventions will not be good for everyone. Our studies with mice have shown that a particular dietary restriction intervention effective for some individual genotypes was harmful for others. Therefore, testing is needed to determine whether an intervention is right for each individual. Furthermore, few specific, and no general, interventions have been proven to retard or reverse deleterious changes with age in human beings, because it has been too difficult to demonstrate whether aging changes have in fact been retarded or reversed. Longevity is the traditional assay for aging, but it is worthless in evaluating an individual.

In order to develop effective interventions, even using wonderful new techniques such as gene transplantation, we need objective measures to tell if a person needs an intervention, and whether it is effective. People who are now paying in both time and money for interventions should be happy to pay for objective tests of whether their interventions are needed and whether they are effective. Moreover, experience in evaluating interventions in many different people over time would help predict which interventions would be most effective.

## NROs, Nonprofit Research Organizations

The potential for future advances in human health is impressive; however, some of the most important advances in the biology of aging will be difficult, requiring complex new techniques. The rate that they occur will depend on funding. While the NIH and NSF are vital sources of support, they should be supplemented with business funding for projects that have real medical value. Two problems must be solved to maximize the rate that advances are made: 1. We need to attract business funding for applied research, to answer basic questions about mammalian aging, and yet plow back profits into further research. 2. We must allow the basic researcher to control the direction of the work, while attracting outside funds, in addition to those normally available for basic research.

The danger in getting business capital is that the best research ideas rarely come from the best fund raisers and business administrators; these are very different skills. Even when one person can do both, the pressure of every day business will distract from the long term basic research.

In order to maximize the rate of progress in biomedicine, a new type of organization should be developed: the NRO, nonprofit research organization. Its researchers would be eligible for NIA and NSF funds, but NROs would also raise investment money and try to make money for future research with all projects that were clinically relevant. Much of its researchers' shares in the profits would go to the NRO, to be plowed back into more research. The best researchers would generally find that it would be worth losing some potential to make money to avoid the business headaches and distractions, while maintaining control over the direction of their work.

NROs should include local medical researchers and hospitals, because the large payoffs will come from work in humans. Hospitals with young physicians who are not currently doing research would be the best partners; big medical schools with currently active research programs would not need NRO collaborations.

Of course NROs would be effective not only in the biology of aging, but in all areas of biomedical research that have obvious relevance to human health. However they are especially important in aging for two reasons. 1. The biology of aging is so broad that it cuts through many biological disciplines, and is criticized as "unfocused" to those not knowledgeable about aging. Thus it is not encouraged in conventional universities and medical schools, although they are pursuing the same objectives as NROs. A new sort of organization is needed to produce excellent research in the biology of aging. 2. The amount of support for research on aging must be as broad as possible, to avoid temporary cutoffs in funding. These waste years of work for researchers, because traditional funding sources are unreliable and research in aging is uniquely vulnerable to damage when funds are cut. Once an aged mouse or rat colony has been eliminated due to lack of funds, it takes 2 - 3 years before aged animals are again available.

## Hard Headed Dreamers

Currently, working to substantially increase the human healthspan is considered neither reasonable nor respectable. Yet the possibilities are there, as illustrated above. One of the great dreams of mankind has always been to increase the healthspan, to gain experience and wisdom but not pay for it by becoming physically frail and ill. Now is the time to turn this dream into real plans. Pooling the new tools of molecular genetics with the discipline of gerontology, now is the time for the hard headed dreamers who will finally make the dream a reality. May they find this book useful.

## ACKNOWLEDGEMENTS

Funding for the conference on which this book is based was provided by the National Institute on Aging. The Growth Publishing Company (a nonprofit corporation) sponsored the conference grant application and production of this volume. It demonstrates the recently broadened interests of this organization, as shown by the change in the name of its journal from Growth to *Growth, Development and Aging* (GDA). Some of the foregoing material was originally published in GDA, reprinted by permission.

# Section 1

## EVOLUTIONARY GENETICS OF AGING

# 2

# THE DISPOSABLE SOMA THEORY OF AGING

Thomas B.L. Kirkwood

## ABSTRACT

The disposable soma theory suggests that aging occurs because natural selection favors a strategy in which organisms invest fewer resources in the maintenance of somatic cells and tissues than are necessary for indefinite survival of the individual. This predicts that aging is due to the accumulation of unrepaired somatic defects. The evolutionary divergence of species' lifespans is explained by optimizing the investment in somatic maintenance to take account of differences between the levels of environmental mortality in different ecological niches. For example, in a hazardous niche there is likely to be less advantage in investing in a potentially long-lived soma. The disposable soma theory provides a direct connection between evolutionary and physiological approaches to the study of aging.

## INTRODUCTION

The chapter in this volume by Charlesworth describes theories on the evolution of aging suggested by Medawar (1952), Williams (1957) and Hamilton (1966). These theories explain aging in terms of different types of genes having general effects on survivorship at different ages. This chapter describes a more specific view, termed the disposable soma theory, which suggests not only why aging occurs evolutionarily, but also how it is caused physiologically (Kirkwood, 1977, 1981; Kirkwood and Holliday, 1979, 1986).

The disposable soma theory was first proposed (Kirkwood, 1977; Kirkwood and Holliday, 1979) to provide evolutionary support for the error theory of aging, which attributes senescence to cumulative errors in the molecular processes of DNA replication, transcription and translation (see Kirkwood *et al.*, 1984; Holliday, 1986). Later, the theory was extended to suggest that aging is due to an accumulation of somatic defects resulting from insufficient investment in a broad range of processes of maintenance and repair, including proofreading the synthesis of macromolecules, DNA repair, protein turnover, detoxification, wound healing, cell renewal, and regeneration (Kirkwood 1981).

The theory is outlined here assuming (i) an iteroparous life history, *i.e.* that the organism is capable of repeated reproduction, and (ii) that there is a clear distinction between germ-line and somatic tissue. Aging is defined, following Maynard Smith (1962), as "the sum of those effects which render individuals as they grow older more susceptible to the various factors, intrinsic or extrinsic, which may cause death". The reason for concentrating on iteroparous species is that a life history which gives the opportunity for repeated reproduction could, in principle, extend indefinitely, so the question of why a species should have a well-defined maximum lifespan has particular interest. The theory may be extended, with modification, to semelparous species, and even to species capable of vegetative reproduction, but in these cases the concept of aging is less sharply defined (Kirkwood, 1981; Kirkwood and Cremer, 1982).

## EVOLUTION OF AGING THROUGH OPTIMIZING THE INVESTMENT IN SOMATIC MAINTENANCE

The idea that aging is linked to the failure of maintenance systems has a long history (for reviews, see Comfort, 1979; Kirkwood and Cremer, 1982). The outward signs of aging are consistent with wear and tear, and can be identified with the progressive accumulation of defects in artefacts such as buildings and automobiles. It is mistaken, however, to accept that biological wear and tear will inevitably bring about aging. Senescence is not evident in all living organisms. There are many microorganisms, plants, and even some simple animals, which have regenerative powers that appear to allow their indefinite survival (Comfort, 1979). There is no fundamental reason why organisms, which are open thermodynamic systems, should not continuously utilize energy from their environment to combat the intrinsic tendency of an ordered system to decay into a disordered state.

An organism may be regarded as an entity which takes up energy, primarily in the form of nutrients, from its environment, and ultimately converts this energy into progeny. The law of natural selection asserts that those organisms (strictly, the genes which determine the phenotypes of the organisms) which are most efficient in this process are the ones most likely to survive (Townsend and Calow, 1981). Of the energy taken in, however, only a fraction is allocated directly to reproduction, the rest being divided among activities such as growth, foraging, and defense, as well as, in particular, the maintenance and repair of the soma. The greater the fraction of energy allocated to one particular activity, the less is available for the others. It is possible to select for an increased total intake of energy. However, this does not avoid the problem of how best to divide the resources currently available.

The problem of optimal allocation of resources is a central issue in life-history theory, particular attention having been paid to the costs of reproduction (Calow 1977, 1979; Stearns, 1976, 1977; Sibly and Calow, 1986; Partridge and Harvey, 1988). Here we concentrate on the costs of *maintenance* and on its trade- offs with other functions. Too little investment in somatic maintenance and the organism may die before it can effectively reproduce; too great an investment and the organism will mature late and reproduce only slowly. The question is: does there exist a level of investment in somatic maintenance which is optimal, and if so, is this more or less than the minimum required to keep the organism in a physiological steady state by repairing damage as fast as it arises? That such a level exists, at least in theory, was implied by the assertion made earlier that there is no fundamental biological reason why a complex organism should be unable to maintain its physiological integrity indefinitely.

To answer these questions requires that the effects of varying the level of investment in somatic maintenance on survivorship and fecundity as functions of age can be determined. Once these are known, the net effect on the intrinsic rate of natural increase, $r$, can be determined from the equation

$$\int e^{-rx} \, l(x;s) \, m(x;s) \, dx = 1$$

where $l(x;s)$ and $m(x;s)$ are the mean survivorship and fecundity at age $x$, given a level of investment $s$ in somatic maintenance. The optimum level of investment in somatic maintenance will be that which maximises $r$, subject to appropriate constraints.

At present, experimental data are not yet available to permit these trade-offs to be evaluated in detail for real organisms. Nevertheless, some insight can be gained with plausible models. A simple model described by Kirkwood and Holliday (1986) serves to illustrate the main conclusions.

A convenient representation of the survivorship function, $l(x;s)$ can be derived from the observation that, among several species, adult mortality is fairly well approximated by the Gompertz-Makeham equation

$$\mu_x = \mu_0 e^{\beta x} + \gamma$$

where $\mu_x$ is the age-specific mortality rate at age $x$ and the parameters $\mu_0$, $\beta$ and $\gamma$ represent "basal vulnerability", "actuarial aging rate" and age-independent environmental mortality, respectively (see Sacher, 1978; Kirkwood, 1985). The possibilities of periodic (*e.g.* seasonal) effects on mortality and of non-Gompertzian mortality curves (*e.g.* for species where growth is indeterminate and adult mortality initially declines due to increasing body size) are not considered here.

If $s$ is defined on a scale between zero and one so that s=0 corresponds to no investment in maintenance and s=1 corresponds to the maximum which is physiologically possible, after allowing for other essential activities, then $\beta$, and probably also $\mu_0$, will be decreasing functions of $s$. To be consistent with the assertion that it is possible, at least in principle, to prevent damage from accumulating by investing enough in maintenance, it is assumed that $\beta$ reaches zero for some intermediate level of repair s = s' (0 <s'<1). $\mu_0$, on the other hand, can be expected to decrease steadily across the entire range from s=0 to s=1. Finally, it may be noted that, although for computing the intrinsic rate of natural increase it is not necessary to know the distribution of mortality across the age range prior to reproductive maturity, the overall dependence on $s$ of survivorship to the end of the juvenile period must be specified.

For reproductive rate $m(x;s)$ the primary parameters affected by s will be age at first reproduction a, likely in general to be increased by raising s, and the peak reproductive rate f, likely to be decreased by raising $s$. For an organism with s < s', $i.e.$ one with $\beta > 0$, accumulation of somatic damage is likely to take its toll on reproductive rate as age increases and needs also to be allowed for in the model.

Arbitrary functions giving plausible dependences of $\mu_0$, $\beta$, a and f on s can be assumed as follows: $\mu_0 = \mu_{min}/s$ , $\beta = \beta_0(s'/s-1)$ for s <s', a = $a_0/(1-s)$ and f = $f_{max}(1-s)$. It is additionally assumed that juvenile survivorship can be represented by survival of a fraction $s$ to adulthood, with the Gompertz-Makeham equation applying thereafter, and that reproduction begins at peak rate $f$ at age $a$, with an age-related decline at the same Gompertzian rate as survivorship for $\beta>0$. With these assumptions the survivorship and fecundity functions are

$$l(x;s) = s \exp\left[-(e^{\beta x}-e^{\beta a})\, \mu_0/\beta-\gamma(x-a)\right]$$
and
$$m(x;s) = f \exp\left[-(e^{\beta x} - e^{\beta a})\mu_0/\beta\right] \quad x>a$$

*with the dependence of* $\mu_0$, $\beta$, a and f *on s as above.*

The net effects on $l(x;s)$ and $m(x;s)$ of varying s are shown in Figure 1. When these effects are combined together to give the dependence of r on s, the result is as in Figure 2.

The model shows that an optimum level of investment in somatic maintenance does exist, and furthermore, that the optimum value of s, s = s$^*$, is *less* than the minimum, s = s', above which the actuarial ageing rate is assumed to

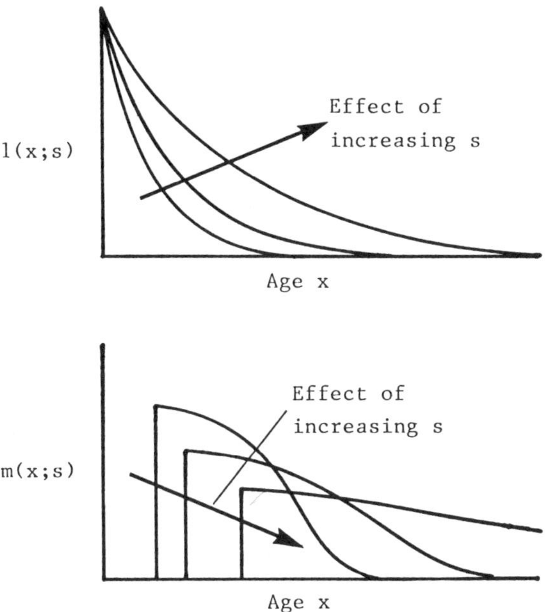



**Figure 1**. Effects on survivorship *l(x;s)* and fecundity *m(x;s)* of  varying the investment s in somatic maintenance.

be zero. These results do not depend critically on the particular model illustrated above and have been found to hold quite generally. The fact that $s^*$ < s′ can be understood intuitively as follows. Since no species is immune to purely random mortality exacted by the environment, there is no advantage to be gained from investing in potential somatic immortality when in practice the return from this investment cannot be realized. This means that even though it may be physiologically possible to set the level of investment in somatic maintenance high enough that damage can be prevented from accumulating, it is not to an iteroparous species' advantage to do so. Instead, it is preferable only to invest sufficient resources in maintenance to ensure that the soma remains viable through its normal expectation of life in the wild, and to use any extra resources to increase reproduction.

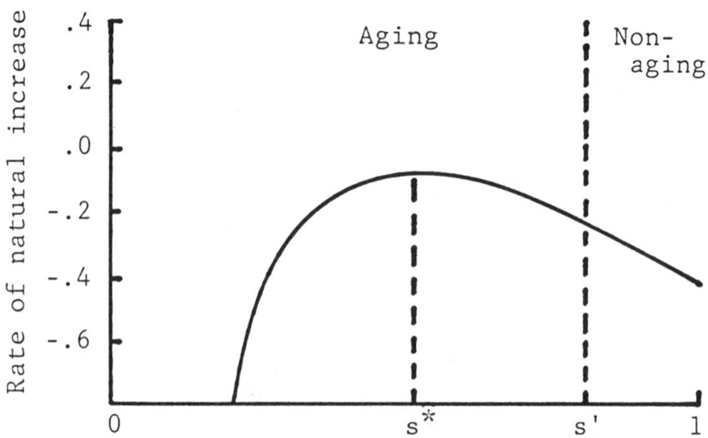


**Figure 2.** Effect on intrinsic rate of natural increase r of varying the investment s in somatic maintenance. [Parameter values: $s' = 0.8$, $\mu_{min} = 0.005$, $\beta_0 = 0.5$, $a_0 = 2$, $f_{max} = 10$, $\gamma = 0.38$; see text for definitions].

This view of the evolution of aging was termed the disposable soma theory for its obvious analogy with the manufacture of disposable goods, where little is invested in their long-term durability.

## DIVERGENCE OF SPECIES' LIFESPANS

For any theory of the evolution of aging, an important secondary problem is to account for the divergence of species' lifespans. For the disposable soma theory, the question is how the optimum investment in somatic maintenance and longevity is expected to vary from one ecological niche to another.

The key factor in determining the optimum level of investment in somatic maintenance is the level of environmental mortality to which individuals are exposed. If the level of environmental mortality is high, the individual can expect to survive only a short time and there is little point in investing heavily in somatic maintenance. In consequence, even if the organism is removed to a protected environment, senescence will occur early and maximum longevity will be short. Conversely, if the level of environmental mortality is reduced,

**Table 1.** Effect of varying environmental mortality $\gamma$ on the optimum level of investment $s^*$ in somatic maintenance, and associated effects on fecundity and longevity.[a,b]

| $\gamma$ | $f_{max}$ | $s^*$ | Longevity |
|---|---|---|---|
| $0.51(40\%)$[c] | 18.6 | 0.46 | 8[d] |
| 0.22 (20%) | 7.0 | 0.54 | 12 |
| 0.11 (10%) | 2.9 | 0.65 | 28 |
| 0.05 (5%) | 1.5 | 0.74 | 57 |

[a] Parameter values $s' = 0.8$, $\mu_{min} = 0.005$, $\beta_0 = 0.5$, $a_0 = 2$.

[b] It is assumed that with reduction in $\gamma$ a compensatory adjustment in $f_{max}$ occurs so that after reaching the new optimum the population stabilizes with r=0.

[c] Figures in brackets show equivalent % mortality per year.

[d] 99th percentile of lifespan distribution.

survivorship in the natural environment will be enhanced and there may be advantage to be gained from investing more heavily in somatic maintenance so that the organism does not die of senescence before it has realized its potential for a longer life.

This argument can be formalized within the mathematical framework of the life-history model described above, where environmental mortality is represented through the parameter $\gamma$ of the Gompertz-Makeham equation. If it is assumed an adaptation leads to a reduction in $\gamma$, a compensatory change in one or more of the parameters $\mu_{min}$, $\beta_0$, $a_0$ or $f_{max}$ is likely to follow. This may occur either through population density effects, to preserve a long-term stable population size, or as a direct physiological trade-off. For example, evolution of a larger brain may at the same time bring about a reduction both in $\gamma$ and in $f_{max}$. Introducing these variations into the model, while leaving the other parameters fixed, brings about a resulting change in the optimum value of *s*, with corresponding effects on longevity (Table 1).

The disposable soma theory therefore predicts a strong positive correlation of the level of environmental mortality with fecundity and a negative correlation with longevity, these effects having evolved through selection to vary the investment in somatic maintenance.

## RELATIONSHIP TO OTHER THEORIES ON THE EVOLUTION OF AGING

As noted earlier, the disposable soma theory originated from studies of specific cellular and molecular theories of aging, the objective being to provide these theories with evolutionary support (Kirkwood, 1977). For this reason the disposable theory has a stronger emphasis on *mechanisms* of aging than the more general theories that preceded it, although like these other theories, the disposable soma theory recognizes that for an organism which reproduces more than once in its lifetime, events which occur late in the lifespan, whether good or bad, are of lesser significance than events which occur early (Haldane, 1941; Medawar, 1952; Williams, 1957; Hamilton, 1966; Charlesworth, 1980).

The disposable soma theory has its closest connections with Williams' (1957) pleiotropic genes theory, in which aging is seen as the late deleterious by-product of genes which are beneficial to the organism during the earlier and biologically more important stages of its lifespan. Williams was not specific about the nature of these genes, citing only as a hypothetical example a mutation arising that has a favorable effect on the calcification of bone in the developmental period but which expresses itself in a subsequent somatic environment in the calcification of the connective tissue of the arteries. The disposable soma theory, in contrast, is based on a phenotypic model incorporating specific physiological trade-offs. It is, of course, necessary that these trade-offs can be related to genes whose evolution in the postulated way makes sense in terms of population genetics, but this is straightforward. The genes in question are the genes which regulate somatic maintenance and repair. We know these genes exist and in some cases, for example DNA repair genes (Sedgwick, 1986), we know something of their molecular biology. The trade-offs result either from the direct costs in energy and/or time of a mutation which elevates the level of a particular maintenance activity, for example proofreading the synthesis of macromolecules (see Kirkwood *et al.*, 1986), or from the indirect costs which may be associated with organizational constraints to make repair possible (see Kirkwood, 1981). That the total cost of somatic maintenance is considerable is readily apparent if one considers the number and variety of processes whose primary function is to maintain viability of the organism.

It is interesting to compare the predictions of the disposable soma theory with those of the pleiotropic genes theory. Nine testable deductions were drawn by Williams' (1957) from his theory: 1). Senescence should be found wherever the conditions specified in the theory are met, and should not be found where these conditions are absent; 2). Low adult death rates should be associated with low rates of senescence, and high adult death rates with high rates of senescence; 3). Senescence should be more rapid in those organisms that do not increase markedly in fecundity after maturity than in those that do show such an increase; 4). Where there is a sex difference, the sex with the higher mortality rate and lesser rate of increase in fecundity should undergo the more rapid senescence; 5). Senescence should always be a generalized deterioration, and never due largely to changes in a single system; 6). There should be little or no post-reproductive period in the normal life-cycle of any species; 7). The time of reproductive maturation should mark the onset of senescence; 8). Rapid individual development should be correlated with rapid senescence; 9). Successful selection for increased longevity should result in decreased vigor in youth. These predictions carry over with little or no modification to the disposable soma theory. In relation to 7), the disposable soma theory is not specific about the relative timing of reproductive maturation and the onset of senescence, which will depend on the interplay between the effects of varying the investment in somatic maintenance on the schedules of mortality and fecundity. Generally, it might be expected that the accumulation of defects responsible for senescence will begin early in development, possibly as soon as the differentiation of soma from germ-line, but the effects of this accumulation will show only gradually. In addition, the disposable soma theory also predicts the physiological nature of the mechanisms by which aging is brought about and by which differences in longevity are produced, namely, increasing maintenance of the soma at some expense of reproductive effort. These predictions are directly testable at the molecular and cellular level.

## CONCLUSIONS

The disposable soma theory provides a link between evolutionary studies on aging and the broad front of gerontological research which over the years has seen many specific types of damage suggested as the cause of senescence (Sacher, 1980). The theory provides an explanation of aging which is directly consistent with the apparent wear and tear nature of the process, and which lends support to the damage hypotheses as a class, but which suggests that no single form of damage is likely to account fully for senescence in all the diverse forms of organism in which it occurs. Certain universal types of damage, such as those affecting DNA replication and gene expression, may however play a more critical role in regulating the duration of life than others.

One obvious way to test the disposable soma theory is through comparative study of the efficiency of different systems for somatic maintenance. Studies on the efficiency of DNA excision repair following ultraviolet irradiation have already revealed that there are correlations with mammalian longevity (Hart and Setlow, 1974; Francis *et al.*, 1981; Treton and Courtois, 1982; Hall *et al.*, 1984). Further studies of this type may be made either between species of different longevities, or within a single species between populations having different lifespans, for example as a result of selection for increased lifespan. By careful comparative analysis of different systems of somatic maintenance, particularly those which are vital but costly, it may be possible to identify systems whose efficiency correlates most strongly with longevity. The identification of maintenance systems whose efficiencies are correlated with longevity would not, of course, *prove* a cause-and-effect relationship. However, such correlations will be valuable in selecting primary targets for more direct genetic analyses, for example, using transgenic animals.

## REFERENCES


CALOW, P. (1977) Ecology, evolution and energetics: a study in metabolic adaptation. *Advances in Ecological Research* **10**: 1-62

CALOW, P. (1979) The cost of reproduction - a physiological approach. *Biological Reviews* **54**: 23-40

CHARLESWORTH, B. (1980) *Evolution in Age-structured Populations*. Cambridge: Cambridge University Press.

COMFORT, A. (1979) *The Biology of Senescence*, 3rd edition. Edinburgh: Churchill Livingstone.

FRANCIS, A. A., Lee, W. H. and Regan, J. D. (1981) The relationship of DNA excision repair of ultraviolet-induced lesions to the maximum life-span of mammals. *Mechanisms of Ageing and Development* **16**: 181-189

HALDANE, J. B. S. (1941) *New Paths in Genetics*. London: Allen and Unwin.

HALL, K. Y., Hart, R. W., Bernischke, A. K. and Walford, R. L. (1984) Correlation between ultraviolet-induced DNA repair in primary lymphocytes and fibroblasts and species maximum achievable lifespan. *Mechanisms of Ageing and Development* **24**: 163-173

HAMILTON, W. D. (1966) The moulding of senescence by natural selection. *Journal of Theoretical Biology* **12**: 12-45

HART, R. W. and Setlow, R. B. (1974) Correlation between deoxyribonucleic acid excision repair and lifespan in a number of mammalian species. *Proc. Natl. Acad. Sci. USA* **71**: 2169-2173

HOLLIDAY, R. (1986) *Genes, Proteins and Cellular Ageing*. Philadelphia: Van Nostrand Reinhold.

KIRKWOOD, T. B. L. (1977) Evolution of ageing. *Nature* **270**: 301-304

KIRKWOOD, T. B. L. (1981) Repair and its evolution: survival versus reproduction. **In:** *Physiological Ecology: an Evolutionary Approach to Resource Use*. Ed. C.R. Townsend and P. Calow, pp.165-189. Oxford: Blackwell Scientific Publications

KIRKWOOD, T. B. L. (1985) Comparative and evolutionary aspects of longevity. **In:** *Handbook of the Biology of Aging*. Ed. C.E. Finch and E.L. Schneider, pp. 27-44. New York: Van Nostrand Reinhold

KIRKWOOD, T. B. L. and Cremer, T. (1982) Cytogerontology since 1881: a reappraisal of August Weismann and a review of modern progress. *Human Genetics* **60**: 101-121

KIRKWOOD, T. B. L. and Holliday, R. (1979) The evolution of ageing and longevity. *Proceedings of the Royal Society* **B205**; 531-546

KIRKWOOD, T. B. L. and Holliday, R. (1985) Ageing as a consequence of natural selection. **In:** *The Biology of Human Ageing*. Ed. K.J. Collins and A.H. Bittles, pp. 1-16. Cambridge: Cambridge University Press.

KIRKWOOD, T. B. L., Rosenberger, R. F and Galas, D. J. (1986) *Accuracy in Molecular Processes: Its Control and Relevance to Living Systems*. London: Chapman and Hall.

MAYNARD SMITH, J. (1962) Review lectures on senescence. I. The causes of ageing. *Proceedings of the Royal Society* **B157**: 115-127

MEDAWAR, P. B. (1952) *An Unsolved Problem in Biology*. London: H.K. Lewis. [Reprinted in Medawar, P.B. 1981. Uniqueness of the Individual. New York: Dover.]

PARTRIDGE, L. and Harvey, P. H. (1988) The ecological context of life history evolution. *Science* **214**: 1449-1455

SACHER, G. A. (1980) Theory in gerontology. Part I. *Ann. Rev. Geront. Geriat.* **1**: 3-25

SEDGWICK, S. G. (1986) Stability and change through DNA repair. In: *Accuracy in Molecular Processes: Its Control and Relevance to Living Systems* (Eds T. B. L. Kirkwood, R. F. Rosenberger and D. J. Galas), pp. 233-289. London: Chapman and Hall.

SIBLY, R. and Calow, P. (1986) *Physiological Ecology of Animals: An Evolutionary Approach.* Oxford: Blackwell Scientific Publications.

STEARNS, S. C. (1976) Life-history tactics: a review of the ideas. *Quarterly Review of Biology* **51**: 3-47

STEARNS, S. C. (1977) The evolution of life history traits: a critique of the theory and a review of the data. *Ann. Rev. Ecol. Systematics* **8**: 145-171

TOWNSEND, C. R. and Calow, P. (1981) *Physiological Ecology: an Evolutionary Approach to Resource Use.* Oxford: Blackwell Scientific Publications.

TRETON, J. A. and Coutois, Y. (1982) Correlation between DNA excision repair and mammalian lifespan in lens epithelial cells. *Cell Biology International Reports* **6**:

WILLIAMS, G. C. (1957) Pleiotropy, natural selection and the evolution of senescence. *Evolution* **11**: 398-411

## DISCUSSION

1. In answer to a question about whether the longevities of species in the wild (where, after all, they evolved) supported his theory, Kirkwood answered that generally they do, but the data are patchy.

2. The basic assumption that energy input needs to be related to survival and reproduction was questioned by pointing out that repair rates in bacteria are very much above rates necessary to avoid error catastrophes. Kirkwood answered that bacteria contain the germ line and the soma in the same cell. As to whether energy is a limiting resource, he argued that starvation is a common cause of death in most species.

3. The theory predicts that generally there should not be combinations of genes that simultaneously increase longevity and fecundity, since energy input used for repair must reduce reproductive rates. Yet Roderick and Storer (*Science*, **134**: 48-9, 1961) reported strong correlations between mean litter size and mean life spans among 12 inbred strains of mice. Kirkwood pointed out that inbred strains were not naturally selected and so are not a valid model. Also, while certain gene combinations may confer general vigor these do not invalidate the concept of a general trade-off between survivorship and fecundity.

# 3

# NATURAL SELECTION AND LIFE HISTORY PATTERNS

Brian Charlesworth

## INTRODUCTION

The life history pattern typical of a species can be described in terms of variables such as the average mortality rate of individuals as a function of age, the timing of the age of first reproduction, the spacing of reproductive episodes during life, and the average reproductive success of individuals as a function of age. These characteristics are all of obvious relevance to Darwinian fitness, and have attracted considerable attention from ecologists and evolutionists (Fisher, 1930; Medawar 1946, 1952; Cole, 1954; Lack, 1954; Williams, 1957, 1966; Hamilton, 1966; Stearns, 1976, 1977; Charlesworth, 1980; Dingle and Hegmann, 1982; Lande, 1982; Sibly and Calow, 1986; Bell and Koufopanou, 1985; Partridge and Harvey, 1988). The general aim of work in this field has been to produce evolutionary models that are capable of explaining the patterns of life-histories observed in nature. Life-histories are astonishingly variable, even within a relatively homogeneous group of organisms such as eutherian mammals, where maximum life-spans in captivity range from a low of a few months for a small insectivore to a high of 80 years or more for humans (Comfort, 1979). Other aspects of the life history, such the age at first reproduction and the number of offspring per litter, show similar diversity within mammals (Harvey and Read, 1988).

It is thus clear that all aspects of the life history are susceptible to evolutionary modification, and we now possess a large body of theory based on genetic principles which provides a framework in which this diversity of life history patterns can be understood in terms of the different pressures of selection imposed by differences in ecology (Williams, 1957; Stearns, 1976, 1977; Charlesworth, 1980; Sibly and Calow, 1986; Partridge and Harvey, 1988). As will be discussed in more detail below, a key to this understanding has been the realization that the intensity of selection for modifying survival and reproduction at different ages is highly age-dependent, such that effects early in reproductive life generally have a higher impact on net fitness than effects later on (Haldane, 1941; Medawar, 1946, 1952; Williams, 1957;

Hamilton, 1966; Charlesworth, 1980, Chap. 5). Coupled with the fact that this age dependence is more strongly marked if extrinsic sources of mortality such as predation and disease are more intense, and if population growth is high, a good many features of life history diversity can be understood.

Despite this diversity of life-histories, we can observe an almost universal pattern: that of senescent decline in survival and reproductive performance with advancing age (Comfort, 1979; Finch and Schneider, 1985). This decline results from the deterioration of a multiplicity of different biological parameters with advancing age, and it would seem that no unitary proximate cause of senescence can be found (Finch and Schneider, 1985). At first sight, this run-down of originally near-perfect biological mechanisms appears to constitute a severe challenge for evolutionary theory, since natural selection, at least on a naive view, is supposed to promote increased fitness. But, as will be described in more detail below, this is exactly what is predicted from the evolutionary theories of aging, which state that senescence is a consequence of the greater selective premium on genes with favorable effects on survival or fecundity early in the life history (Medawar, 1946, 1952; Williams, 1957; Hamilton, 1966; Charlesworth, 1980). Regardless of the physiological details of the ways in which genes affecting survivorship or fecundity express their effects, this factor will lead to the evolution of a life history in which mortality increases and fecundity decreases with advancing age, provided that genetic variability with the appropriately age-specific effects is available for natural selection to utilize. From this perspective, senescence is an almost inevitable consequence of the operation of natural selection.

Of course, the intensity of the selective premium on high early performance varies considerably with ecological circumstances, as noted above, and this leads to considerable variation in the rate at which senescent decline is expected to occur. Such variation is clearly observable even within groups of closely related taxa. Nonetheless, in species in which there is a clear distinction between reproductive and somatic structures (including all multicellular, sexually reproducing species and species where asexual eggs are produced, but excluding multicellular species reproducing exclusively by budding or unicellular species), senescence is an evolutionary consequence of the facts that somatic structures are merely vehicles for the propagation of genes across the generations, and that maximization of the individual's genetic contribution does not coincide with maximization of the length of life. In nature, of course, extrinsic causes of mortality may be so high that it is difficult to detect any increase in mortality rates with age, and a decline in fecundity may only occur at ages so great that few individuals are present in the population. Nevertheless, the study of captive populations in which individuals are protected from extrinsic causes of death as far as possible yields evidence for senescent decline, even in groups such as fish where senescence is often postponed (Comfort, 1979). The importance of senescence for the present condition of humans in industrialized societies needs no comment. Senescence can also be detected in the wild in groups such as large mammals that are especially suitable for demographic study (Caughley, 1977). Lack of evidence for senescence in demographic studies of wild populations thus does not provide evidence against its near universality as a biological phenomenon in multicellular organisms. The evolution of senescence is one aspect of the general evolutionary problem of explaining life-histories and their diversity.

## MODELS OF LIFE HISTORY EVOLUTION

A full understanding of the evolutionary biology of life histories requires a theory of the dynamics of natural selection on age-specific survival and fecundity rates that is based firmly on the principles of population genetics. Much of my research effort over the past fifteen years has been devoted to the development of such a theory, and its integration with ecological and demographic knowledge (Charlesworth, 1980, 1984). Work by Hill (1974, 1977) and Lande (1982) has linked this theory with quantitative genetics approaches, so that we now have a theoretical understanding of the ways in which selection can mold life history variables, both at the level of changes in frequencies of single genes, and at the level of quantitatively varying characters that are controlled by many genes of relatively small effect. The main conclusions of these studies are as follows.

### How to Calculate Fitness

For the purposes of discussion, it is most convenient to describe life-histories in terms of discrete time-intervals, such that individuals of a given age $x$ have characteristic probabilities, $P(x)$, of survival to the next time-interval, when they will be aged $x+1$. Sex differences will be ignored for the purpose of this discussion. Fecundity at age $x$, $m(x)$, can be described by the expected number of daughters that a female aged $x$ will produce. Their chance of survival to the next time interval, when they are of age 1 and their surviving parents are age $x+1$, is $P(0)$, so that the effective fertility of females aged $x$ is $P(0)m(x)$. A genotype $i$ at a given locus will in general have its own set of life history characteristics *i.e.* a set of values of the probabilities of survival to age $x$ ($x=1,2...$), $l_i(x)=P_i(0)\,P_i\,(1)...P_i\,(x-1)$, and fecundities at age $x$, $m_i\,(x)$.

This representation is exact for species that reproduce at discrete time-intervals, such as annually breeding species of birds or mammals. It provides an approximate representation of the demography of continuously reproducing species such as man or *Drosophila*; the adequacy of the approximation can be made arbitrarily good by increasing the number of age-classes into which the life history is divided.

The Darwinian fitness of a genotype can, for most purposes, be equated to the intrinsic rate of increase of the life history, $r_i$, given by the real root of the Euler-Lotka equation

$$\sum_x e^{-r_i x}\, l_i(x)\, m_i(x) = 1 \qquad (1)$$

where the summation is taken over all ages $x$.

The intrinsic rate $r_i$ is the rate of population growth that would be attained by a population that consists entirely of individuals with the life history characteristics of the genotype in question. In the case of a heterozygote, which cannot form a true-breeding population, $r_i$ is the hypothetical rate of population growth that would be attained by a population, all of whose members have the life history characteristics of the heterozygote. Provided that selection is not too strong, and that sex differences in survival probabilities and fecundities can be neglected, this measure of fitness can be used to predict changes in the genetic composition of populations (Charlesworth, 1980). In particular, the rate of change in frequency of a rare mutant gene that modifies the life history is proportional to the difference in $r$ between carriers of the mutant and wild-type. Modifications to handle strong selection and sex differences are discussed by Charlesworth (1980, Chap.4). The theory is also easily extended to situations in which the overall population growth rate is held to approximately zero by density-dependent governing factors; the rate of increase of a mutant in this case is determined by the value of $r$ for the mutant, holding the density-dependent factors constant at the level that confers a zero rate of population growth for the wild-type population (Charlesworth, 1980, Chap. 4).

A general equation for fitness is available for the purpose of determining equilibrium frequencies; the genotypic fitness $w_i$ is given by

$$w_i = \sum_x e^{-rx}\, l_i(x)\, m_i(x) \qquad (2)$$

where $r$ is the rate of growth of the population as a whole (Charlesworth, 1980, Chap. 3). This has proved useful for the purpose of estimating the intensity of selection in human populations (Charlesworth and Charlesworth,

1973). If selection is weak, the relative values of the $w_i$ are similar to those of the $r_i$.

## Sensitivity of Fitness to Age-specific Changes in the Life History

The effect on Darwinian fitness of a small change in the probability of survival from age $x$ to $x + 1$ is measured by the partial derivative of $r$ with respect to the logarithm of $P(x)$, $\partial r / \partial \ln P(x)$. This is conveniently referred to as the sensitivity of $r$ to a change in survival at age $x$, and is given by the following equation, originally due to Hamilton (1966):

$$\partial r / \ln P(x) = \sum_{y=x+1} e^{-ry} \, l(y) \, m(y) \, / \, T \qquad (3)$$

where T is the generation time given by $T = \sum y e^{-ry} \, l(y) \, m(y)$.

The corresponding sensitivity of r with respect to a change in fecundity at age $x$ is

$$\partial r / \partial m(x) = e^{-rx} \, l(x) \, / T \qquad (4)$$

From the form of these equations, it is easily seen that an increase in survival of a given magnitude that is confined to a single age has a greater impact on fitness if it occurs early in reproductive life, rather than late (the timing of changes in pre-reproductive survival is irrelevant); a change in fecundity at a given age always has a greater impact, the earlier it occurs, unless the population is declining fairly rapidly in size. Furthermore, the magnitude of the effect of age is increased by a high rate of mortality and population growth (see Figure 5.1 of Charlesworth, 1980). It follows that natural selection places greater weight on early-acting genetic effects on fecundity or survival than on effects later in the life history, and that this effect is strongly dependent on the demographic environment imposed by extrinsic, ecological factors, such as the death rate due to predation. Using total differentials, equations (3) and (4) can be used to determine the net effect on fitness of simultaneous small changes in survival and fecundity at a collection of different ages (Charlesworth, 1980, p. 208), and they have played a central role in the development and testing of quantitative evolutionary models of optimal life-histories (reviewed by Charlesworth, 1980, Chap. 5; Sibly and Calow, 1986).

Such models assume that natural selection acts to maximise the intrinsic rate of increase of a population; the single locus genetic models described above provide the justification for this notion, since a mutant gene that perturbs the life history will be unable to invade the population if it is located at a maximum of $r$. Optimization models of life-histories proceed by assuming that there are constraints on the use of resources by individuals of a given age $x$. A favorite model has been the reproductive effort model, which assumes that resources allocated to increased survival at age $x$ will be drained away from fecundity at that age, so that $P(x)$ is a decreasing function of $m(x)$. If the form of this function is specified, so that $\partial P(x)/\partial m(x)$ is known, the optimal life history can be computed by taking the total derivative of $r$ with respect to $m(x)$ at each age, and equating it to zero *i.e.* by solving the system

$$\{\partial r/\partial m(x)\}\{1 + \partial m(x)/\partial \ln P(x)\} = 0 \quad (x=1,2,\ldots) \quad (5)$$

While these equations can in principle be used to calculate the form of the optimal life history, it cannot be said that there has been much success in practice in providing detailed predictions concerning the form of the life history that a given species would be expected to adopt (Sibly and Calow, 1986). Nevertheless, models of this kind have provided a useful framework within which the effects of differences in ecological circumstances on the evolution of differences in the allocation of resources between survival, growth and reproduction can be studied *e.g.* they predict lower reproductive effort in environments where adult survival is relatively high (Charlesworth, 1980, Chap. 5; Partridge and Harvey, 1988).

## Quantitative Genetic Models of Life History Evolution

In general, it is likely that genetic variation in life history traits in natural populations will normally be under the control of many loci, each with a relatively small effect in comparison with the total range of variability in the trait. Lande (1982), building on the work of Hill (1974, 1977), has developed such a theory for the case of weak, frequency-independent selection in density-independent environments. It is assumed that a given life history phenotype is described by a vector **z**, such that the components of **z** completely determine the values of $l(x)$ and $m(x)$. For example, under the reproductive effort model, the values of $m(x)$ for $x=1,2$ etc., would form the components of **z**. The vector **z** is assumed to follow a multi-variate normal distribution within a population, whose variance-covariance matrix is the sum of genetic and environmental components. The genetic component of this matrix can be further partitioned into a matrix **G** of variances and covariances of *breeding* *values* or *additive genetic values* (Falconer, 1981, p.106) of the components of **z**, such that $g_{ij}$ is the genetic covariance in breeding value between $z_i$ and $z_j$ ($g_{ii}$ is the additive genetic variance in $z_i$). The matrix **G** can be estimated empirically from data on resemblances between relatives for the traits in question (Kempthorne, 1957; Becker, 1984).

The effect of natural selection on z is determined by the *selection gradient vector* $\nabla \bar{r}$, whose components are the derivatives of the mean intrinsic rate of increase of the population with respect to the respective components of the mean value of **z**, $\partial \bar{r} / \partial \bar{z}_i$. In practice, $\nabla \bar{r}$ can usually be approximated by the vector of derivatives of $r$ with respect to the $z_i$, evaluated at the population mean of **z**. Lande (1982) shows that the change from one time-interval to the next obeys the approximate equations

$$\nabla \bar{z}_i = \sum_j g_{ij} \, (\partial \bar{r} / \partial \bar{z}_j) \approx \sum_j g_{ij} (\partial r / \partial z_j)_{\bar{z}} \qquad (i = 1, 2, ..) \quad (6)$$

At equilibrium under selection alone, these expressions are all equated to zero. This has the interesting implication that either all the components of $\nabla \bar{r}$ are equal to zero or that the determinant of **G** is zero (Charlesworth, 1984, p.123). The latter condition is biologically most likely; if the components of **z** are chosen to be life history variables such as fecundity or survival (as in the above example), the derivatives of $r$ must be positive (see equations [3] and [4] above). Thus, if there is additive genetic variance in at least some of the $z_i$, so that some of the $g_{ii}$ are positive, the equilibrium version of equation (6) requires that there be some negative additive genetic covariances between the $z_i$, in order for the terms on the right-hand side to sum to zero. (This conclusion about equilibrium does not require that selection be frequency-independent.)

Hence, under rather general conditions, selection theory predicts that life history traits in equilibrium populations that exhibit additive genetic variance which is maintained by selection will be expected to show negative genetic covariances and correlations with some other additively variable life history traits. This has been known to specialists in animal improvement for a long time (Dickerson, 1955; Robertson, 1955). It is a consequence of the fact that selection exhausts additive genetic variance for net fitness, so that any remaining additive genetic variation in fitness-related traits must reflect the properties of genes whose beneficial effects on some traits are counter-balanced by deleterious effects on other characters (*antagonistic pleiotropy*: see below). Rose (1982, 1985) has provided some explicit models of how this can be achieved. To the extent that genetic variation in life history traits reflects non-equilibrium situations or the action of non-selective pressures, such as mutation, this conclusion is weakened (Charlesworth, 1987). Nevertheless, it suggests that most genetically variable components of the life history are often likely to show some evidence of negative genetic correlations with other traits, reflecting the physiological trade-offs between traits envisaged in the optimization models discussed above. Indeed, combining explicit models of such trade-offs with the quantitative genetic formulation of equation (6) shows that the optimization approach yields nearly identical solutions for the outcome of selection to those provided by quantitative genetics (Charlesworth, 1990).

## Evolutionary Explanations of Aging

This body of genetically-based theory has shed new light on the various evolutionary explanations of aging, originally proposed by Haldane (1941), Medawar (1946, 1952), Williams (1957) and Hamilton (1966). These theories may be divided into three categories (Charlesworth, 1980, p. 217; Rose, 1983).

### *Differential Rates of Gene Substitution*

This proposes that there is a higher rate of incorporation into the population of favorable genes that increase survival at earlier ages within the reproductive period, compared with genes that act later (Hamilton, 1966). This would have the effect of gradually raising survival at earlier ages compared with later on. An initially non-senescent population, in which survivorship is independent of age would gradually become converted into one which exhibits senescence, in the sense of exhibiting a decline in survivorship with advancing age. It seems, however, somewhat unlikely that this process could account for the pathological aspects of aging, which contribute largely to decline in survival in later life (Finch and Schneider, 1985).

### *Mutation-accumulation*

Deleterious alleles are maintained in populations at a large number of loci as a result of mutation pressure, and must contribute to a significant reduction in the average fitness of individuals in the population, compared with that of mutation-free individuals. Studies of *Drosophila*, for example, suggest that a typical gamete may have a probability near one of carrying a new mutation with a small, detrimental effect on fitness (Simmons and Crow, 1977); the probability must be considerably higher in mammals, with their much larger genomes. Medawar (1952) and Edney and Gill (1968) suggested that deleterious mutations with effects limited to later ages would equilibrate at higher frequencies than mutations with early-acting effects; taking into account the contributions of all loci, a lower mean survivorship would thus be expected for individuals of more advanced age. This theory has been placed on a quantitative basis by Charlesworth (1980, pp. 140-142, p. 218), using the population genetic results outlined above.

Many rare genes causing hereditary diseases with delayed ages of onset are well-known in human genetics, and their fitness effects can be calculated from equation (2) (Charlesworth and Charlesworth, 1973). The effects of these genes on fitness is, as expected from equations (3) and (4), highly dependent on the demographic environment; a gene with a deleterious effect on survival late in life will have a smaller selective disadvantage in a population with a low rate of mortality from other causes. Thus, individuals with Huntington's chorea suffered an estimated loss in fitness relative to normal individuals of about 15% in the US population of 1939-41, compared with a loss of 9% in the Taiwan population of 1906 (Charlesworth, 1980, p.151). Over the long-term, this increased net selection pressure would cause the frequencies of genes with delayed age of onset to equilibrate at lower frequencies in low-mortality populations, leading to an improvement in survivorship late in life compared with high-mortality populations with the same genetic make-up. This process is thus capable in principle of explaining the data on species differences in longevities referred to in the introduction.

A related process was proposed by Haldane (1941, pp. 192-194), who suggested that there might be significant selection for modifier genes which delay the age of onset of hereditary diseases. Medawar (1952) endorsed this as a probable major factor in the evolution of senescence. However, Charlesworth (1980, pp. 218-219) showed that the magnitude of the selective advantage of such a modifier is of the order of the rate of mutation at the locus it is modifying. This process is thus unlikely to be of much evolutionary significance.

*Antagonistic Pleiotropy*

Williams (1957) argued that it is likely that genes that increase survivorship or fecundity at one age or set of adjacent ages will have deleterious effects at other ages, since an increase in the efficiency of a physiological process that improves survival or fecundity will usually place a demand on resources that would otherwise be utilized in a different way or at a different time. From the principle that changes early in life have a larger effect on fitness than later changes, Williams proposed that selection will thus tend to cause the fixation of genes with positive early effects and negative later ones, rather than genes with the opposite pattern. An explicit physiological model of this kind of trade-off has been formulated in terms of repair and maintenance versus reproduction (Kirkwood, this volume). Genetic models of such antagonistic pleiotropy have been elaborated by Charlesworth (1980, pp. 208-209), Templeton (1980), Rose (1982, 1985), confirming the basic insight of Williams. As with the mutation-accumulation theory, the evolutionary pressure in favor of senescence will be greater in demographic environments where there is a high overall rate of mortality.

## EMPIRICAL TESTS OF THE THEORIES

Theories of life history evolution can be tested at several levels. The long-term effects of natural selection can be examined by comparison of different taxonomic groups that differ in their ecologies in a manner that is expected to produce characteristic differences in their life history patterns as an evolutionary response. Differences between populations of the same species inhabiting different types of environment can similarly be studied. The genetic response of laboratory populations of the same species to artificially created changes in their demographic environment can be analyzed. Finally, the values of quantitative genetic parameters of life history variation or the properties of individual genes affecting life-histories can be related to the assumptions of the different classes of model described above. All of these research strategies have been usefully applied to the problem of life history evolution. A general review is provided by Partridge and Harvey (1988).

### Interspecies Comparisons

Williams (1957) provided the first broad survey of species differences in life history characteristics, in relation to the theories of aging discussed above. He noted, for example, that birds tend to have longer maximum life-spans in captivity than mammals of comparable size, and interpreted this in terms of their greater protection against mortality due to predation in nature, resulting in a weakened pressure of selection in favor of early versus late survivorship and fecundity (see above). This observation has since been confirmed by later, more quantitative, comparisons of birds and mammals (Calder, 1985, this volume). Species where fecundity increases with age, such as many cold-blooded vertebrates, also tend to have high maximum life-spans compared with warm blooded vertebrates of comparable size (Williams, 1957; Comfort, 1979), and this is again a situation in which the decline with age in the sensitivity of fitness to changes in survival is reduced.

Similarly, the life-spans of vertebrate species are strongly positively correlated in an allometric fashion with their body weight and brain weights (Sacher, 1959, 1978). This may be interpreted in terms of the lower vulnerability of larger or more intelligent species to extrinsic sources of mortality, resulting in a diminished decline with age in the fitness sensitivities. There is no reason to believe that the allometric relations between life history characteristics and body size are inexorable consequences of physiological constraints. Unless there is a genetic correlation of close to one between a given trait and body size, and only body size is under selection, there is no reason to expect the trait simply to track changes in body size over the amount of evolutionary time that typically separates even closely related species (Zeng, 1988). It is much more likely that allometric relations of life history traits and body size reflect the effects of common ecological and demographic circumstances on the direction of selection pressures on these characters.

While these broad-brush comparisons reveal patterns which can be easily interpreted in terms of the general theory presented earlier in this chapter, they hardly constitute a critical test. There are many problems of inference involved in assessing the significance of such general comparisons, in particular the fact that related species share a common evolutionary history and hence do not necessarily constitute independent "data points" (Felsenstein, 1985; Harvey and Read, 1988). In addition, species differ with respect to so many different but inter-related characteristics that there is danger in making inferences concerning causation from correlations between life history traits and a variable that has been singled out on theoretical grounds as a likely cause of evolutionary responses.

Interest among comparative biologists has recently focussed on relating deviations of life history traits from the values predicted by their allometric relations with body size to ecological and demographic parameters, pooling groups of related species in order to minimize the problem of lack of evolutionary independence. In mammals, Harvey and Zammuto (1985) showed that age at first reproduction for mammalian species is an increasing function of longevity in the wild, once body size is corrected for. There is also a negative correlation between survival rate in the wild with litter size, and a positive correlation with inter-litter interval (Harvey *et al.*, unpublished). Curiously, no significant relation between maximum life-span and survival was detected in this study. In birds, Saether (1988) found a positive correlation between age at maturity, and a negative correlation of clutch size, with survival. These findings are in general accord with the predictions of evolutionary models based on the principles discussed in an earlier section.

## Intraspecies Comparisons

One way of overcoming the problem of the confounding of the effects of multiple differences when making comparisons is to compare different populations of the same species that have recently been exposed to different demographic circumstances, with respect to life history traits that might be expected to respond to such differences. Care must of course be taken to make the comparisons between the different populations on individuals raised in a common environment, in order to avoid purely environmental effects on the traits in question. Perhaps the most illuminating study of this kind is that of Law (1979), on populations of the grass *Poa annua*. He compared stable pastureland populations with populations from more temporary habitats, where adult mortality and population growth rates are likely to be high. He found that the former types of population exhibited higher survival rates after reaching maturity, and also engaged in two episodes of reproduction during their life, with the majority of their reproduction in their second year. Plants from the other populations tended to start reproduction earlier, had lower survival rates, and reproduced mainly in their first year. Other studies of this kind are reviewed by Law (1979) and Partridge and Harvey (1988).

## Selection Experiments

Rose (this volume) provides a thorough review of the results of selection experiments in *Drosophila*, for which most information is available, so that only a brief sketch will be given here. Two kinds of artificial selection experiments can be performed. One is to practice direct selection for changes in life history components at given ages, and to observe the rate of change of the selected trait and changes in potentially correlated traits. This was done for early and late fecundity of *D. melanogaster* females by Rose and Charlesworth (1981). Three generations of selection for early fecundity succeeded in increasing it, but there were no correlated responses in fecundity at later ages or in longevity. Selection for fecundity late in life did, however, produce a significant decrease in early fecundity, and an increase in longevity. As discussed by Rose and Charlesworth, there are problems in interpreting such experiments, due to the confounding role of genetic drift in small populations in creating genetic correlations (Falconer, 1977).

The alternative method is to select life history traits indirectly by creating situations in which either unusually old or unusually young individuals are used to propagate the stock. The former type of selection puts a premium on increased longevity and reproduction late in life, whereas the latter favors reproduction early in life. The advantage of these designs is that there is little labor involved compared with direct selection procedures, and much larger numbers of individuals can be maintained. This essentially eliminates the problem of genetic drift just referred to. Several experiments of the former kind have now been performed on random-bred laboratory populations of *Drosophila* (Rose, this volume). The consensus from these experiments is that longevity and late fecundity are increased significantly, whereas early fecundity declines, except when flies are raised at low densities.

The results of these experiments are consistent with the antagonistic pleiotropy model of aging, and with the pattern of genetic correlations for these traits described below. However, as pointed out by Charlesworth (1984), they are in themselves also consistent with the mutation accumulation model; selection for late reproduction of this kind means that early reproduction is irrelevant for the fitness of the flies, and so it is conceivable that the decline in early fecundity could have been due, at least in part, to the increase in frequency under mutation pressure of deleterious alleles reducing early fecundity. Indeed, the recent experiment of Mueller (1987) is consistent with this interpretation. He imposed a selective environment where late reproduction was unimportant, because flies were bred from during the first four days of adult life; this led to a decline in late fecundity with no change in early fecundity, over a period of 120 generations. This was interpreted as being due to the accumulation of deleterious mutations affecting the later part of the life history. The fact that $F_1$'s between replicate lines showed a smaller decline in late fecundity is circumstantial evidence in favor of this interpretation (Mueller, 1987). An alternative interpretation is that the early-selected flies, which had lower population densities, were more subject to inbreeding than the late ones. Thus, these experiments do not provide unequivocal support for mutation-accumulation. There is little evidence of this kind for vertebrates, although Reznick and Endler (1982) reported changes in reproductive effort in the expected direction between populations of guppies maintained in artificial streams with different levels of predation.

## Estimates of Genetic Parameters

The theories of life history evolution presented above are predicated on the existence of heritable variation in the relevant traits. A prediction of Medawar's mutation-accumulation theory is that the additive genetic variance in an age-specific fitness component, contributed by the segregation of deleterious mutations, should increase with age (Rose and Charlesworth 1980, 1981). This follows from the fact that this variance is proportional to the equilibrium frequencies of the allele frequencies concerned, and (as mentioned earlier) these frequencies are greater for genes whose effects are confined to later stages of the life-cycle. If senescence is caused, at least in part, by higher frequencies of alleles with deleterious effects confined to later ages, compared with the frequencies of deleterious alleles with effects on earlier ages, an increase in additive variance with age should occur. This increase should be of a similar magnitude to the decline in mean survival or fecundity with age.

This was tested by Rose and Charlesworth (1980, 1981), using age-specific fecundity as the component of fitness for a wild-derived laboratory population of the fruit-fly *Drosophila melanogaster*. Additive genetic variances were highly significant for each age. No significant change with age was detected for additive variance, although the environmental component of variance increased sharply as the flies aged, suggesting a progressive deterioration of homeostasis with age. There was a high error of estimation of the slope of the relationship between additive variance and age, so that some moderate degree of positive relationship cannot be ruled out. Nevertheless, it is clear that the change with age in additive genetic variance is not as dramatic as the change in mean fecundity. Kosuda (1985) reported an increase in the variance of the line means of male mating success for lines of *D. melanogaster* carrying different second chromosomes. Unfortunately, he did not carry out a full partitioning of variance into additive genetic, non-additive genetic and environmental components, so that the interpretation of this experiment is not entirely clear.

There was little evidence for non-additive components of genetic variance in female fecundity in the experiment of Rose and Charlesworth, in agreement with the results of Mukai and his collaborators for egg-to-adult viability (Mukai, 1985). This suggests that heterozygote advantage is not important for the maintenance of variation in these characteristics, since this would be expected to cause non-additive genetic variance in populations near equilibrium (Charlesworth, 1987). The magnitude of the additive variances, expressed as ratios of the population mean values, are similar for fecundity and viability. Adult female longevity, however, showed significant dominance but not additive variance, in contrast with the results of Maynard Smith (1959) for *D. subobscura*. No estimates of additive variances for age-specific survival rates are available, however.

If genes with the antagonistically pleiotropic effects on fitness components postulated in Williams' theory of senescence are segregating in natural populations, then negative additive genetic correlations would be expected between traits measured at different ages (Rose and Charlesworth 1980, 1981). Genetic correlations can be estimated from the correlations between relatives in the values of the traits concerned, using standard breeding designs (Kempthorne, 1957; Becker,1984). Owing to the need for large sample sizes in order to obtain reliable estimates of genetic correlations, relatively few studies of genetic correlations between life history traits have been conducted, and the results have been somewhat controversial (Clark, 1987). For *D. melanogaster*, Rose and Charlesworth (1980, 1981) found strongly negative correlations between early female fecundity and late female fecundity, and between early female fecundity and female longevity, using the same material as for the variance estimates described above. They interpreted this as evidence for Williams' pleiotropy theory, particularly as the effect of early female fecundity on longevity is consistent with experiments by Maynard Smith on *D. subobscura* in which environmental and genetic manipulations that reduced the rate of egg laying were found to increase female longevity (Maynard Smith, 1958). However, Giesel and co-workers (Giesel, 1979; Giesel and Zettler, 1980; Giesel *et al.*, 1982; Giesel, 1986) have reported positive genetic correlations for these traits, at least under certain experimental conditions.

Rose (1984) pointed out that the experiments of Giesel (1979), Giesel and Zettler (1980) and Giesel *et al.* (1982) partly involved the use of inbred lines, as opposed to the random-bred stock representative of a wild population used by Rose and Charlesworth. He suggested that homozygosity for deleterious recessive mutations with major effects on a suite of characters might bias the estimates of genetic correlations obtained from inbred stocks. This explanation of Giesel's results appears to be confirmed by Rose's own observations of positive genetic correlations in inbred lines extracted from his laboratory population, which contrasts with the negative correlations found in random-bred flies from this stock (Rose, 1984). But a later study by Giesel (1986) on random-bred flies derived immediately from the wild has again shown positive correlations. Giesel interprets this as meaning that the pattern of genetic correlations has itself undergone rapid change in the population since it was placed under laboratory conditions, so that the observations of Rose and Charlesworth (1980, 1981) are unrepresentative of a natural population. This interpretation has been disputed by Service and Rose (1985), who suggest that a population that is challenged by a new environment will be more likely to display positive genetic correlations between fitness traits, if there is variation with respect to the overall level of adaptedness to the new environment. They present some experimental evidence for an increase in genetic correlations between fitness traits when their standard laboratory population was placed in a new environment.

When assessing the significance of observations on genetic variation for life history evolution, it is important to bear in mind the fact that populations of higher organisms are known to carry a wealth of low frequency genes with generally deleterious effects on fitness (Simmons and Crow, 1977; Charlesworth and Charlesworth, 1987). This means that differences in life history traits with a polygenic basis will be found between almost any pair of inbred stocks. The properties of these differences may have no relevance for the evolution of life-histories and aging, or to the normal mechanisms of the genetic control of aging (Rose, 1984). Future studies of the genetics of life-histories and aging should be designed with this in mind.

Results for species other than *D. melanogaster* have been reviewed by Reznick (1985) and Bell and Koufopanou (1985). Their interpretations are superficially at variance; Reznick stresses the fact that negative genetic correlations are usually found when careful studies have been done (although the number of studies is small), whereas Bell and Koufopanou stress the frequent finding of positive correlations at the phenotypic level and at the genetic level in inbred populations Both studies agree that genetic correlations in outbred populations provide the most satisfactory basis for inferences about the nature of the variability available for the action of selection, although regrettably few estimates are available for life history characteristics. Bell and Koufopanou (1985) and Partridge and Harvey (1988) also review examples of the experimental manipulation of resource allocation which provide evidence for trade-offs. For example, Nur (1988) has shown that artificially induced changes in clutch-size in the great tit *Parus major* reveal a negative correlation between clutch size and female survival, presumably due to the expenditure of effort on parental care.

## CONCLUSIONS

As should be obvious from the foregoing material, we have a well-established body of theory concerning the evolutionary processes that influence life-histories. The discovery that the sensitivity of Darwinian fitness to changes in survival or fecundity declines with age, at a rate that is determined by the demography and ecology of the population to which the individual belongs, has led to major increases in our understanding. From the point of view of evolutionary theory, aging is no mystery: it is an evolved consequence of the greater selective significance of early life-history traits compared with characteristics expressed late in life. There is an abundance of data on species comparisons that fits well with the general predictions of the theory.

It should be stressed, however, that many of the conclusions of comparative studies are consistent with a variety of specific models of life-history evolution, and do not depend strongly on the physiological or developmental bases of life-history patterns. Instead, they reflect the consequences of demographic factors for the strength of the age-dependence of the sensitivities of $r$ to survival and fecundity changes, which mold the outcome of any process that involves age-specificity of selection pressures. Agreement of species or population comparisons with the qualitative predictions of optimization models, for example, does not necessarily imply that the particular constraints assumed in these models are operating in the species concerned; similar patterns could be produced by mutation-accumulation. For this reason, we are presently far from being clear about the details of the mechanisms underlying many evolutionary patterns, although it does seem likely that trade-offs between different traits play an important role. Even the *Drosophila* work on the genetics of life history variation does not unambiguously exclude a role for mutation-accumulation, although it provides strong support for antagonistic pleiotropy.

## REFERENCES

BECKER, W. A. (1984) *Manual of Quantitative Genetics.* 4th ed. Pullman, WA: Academic Enterprises.

BELL, G. and KOUFOPANOU, V. (1985) The cost of reproduction. *Oxf. Surv. Ev. Bio.* **3**: 83-131

CALDER, W. A. (1985) The comparative biology of longevity and lifetime energetics. *Exp. Geront.* **20**: 161-170

CAUGHLEY, G. (1977) *Analysis of Vertebrate Populations.* New York, NY: Wiley Interscience.

CHARLESWORTH, B. (1980) *Evolution in Age-Structured Populations.* Cambridge, U.K.: Cambridge University Press.

CHARLESWORTH, B. (1984) The evolutionary genetics of life histories. **In:** *Evolutionary Ecology* (Ed. B. Shorrocks), pp. 117-133. Oxford, U.K.: Oxford University Press.

CHARLESWORTH, B. (1987) The heritability of fitness. **In:** *Sexual Selection: Testing the Alternatives* (Ed. J. W. Bradbury and M. Andersson), pp. 21-40. Chichester, U.K.: John Wiley.

CHARLESWORTH, B. (1990) Optimization models, quantitative genetics and mutation. *Evolution* (in press).

CHARLESWORTH, B. and CHARLESWORTH, D. (1973) The measurement of fitness and mutation rate in human populations. *Ann. Hum. Genet.* **37**: 175-187

CHARLESWORTH, D. and CHARLESWORTH, B. (1987) Inbreeding depression and its evolutionary consequences. *Ann. Rev. Ecol. Syst.* **18**: 237-268

CLARK, A. G. (1987) Senescence and the genetic correlation hang-up. *Amer. Nat.* **129**: 932-940.

COLE, L. C. (1954) The population consequences of life history phenomena. *Quart. Rev. Biol.* **29**: 103-137

COMFORT, A. (1979) *The Biology of Senescence.* 3rd. ed. London, UK.: Churchill Livingstone.

DICKERSON, G. E. (1955) Genetic slippage in response to selection for multiple objectives. *Cold Spring Harb. Symp. Quant. Biol.* **20**: 213-224

DINGLE, H. and HEGMANN, J. P. (1982) *Evolutionary Genetics of Life Histories.* New York, NY: Springer.

EDNEY, E. B. and GILL, R. W. (1968) Evolution of senescence and specific longevity. *Nature* **220**: 281-282.

FALCONER, D. S. (1977) Some results of the Edinburgh selection experiments with mice. In: *Proceedings of the International Conference on Quantitative Genetics* (Ed. E. Pollak, O. Kempthorne and T. B. Bailey), pp. 101-115. Ames, IA: Iowa State University Press.

FALCONER, D. S. (1981) *An Introduction to Quantitative Genetics.* 2nd. ed. London, U.K.: Longman.

FELSENSTEIN, J. (1985) Phylogenies and the comparative method. *Amer. Nat.* **125**: 1-15

FINCH, C. E. and SCHNEIDER, E. L. (1985) *Handbook of the Biology of Aging.* New York, NY: Van Nostrand Rheinhold.

FISHER, R. A. (1930) *The Genetical Theory of Natural Selection.* Oxford, U.K.: Oxford University Press.

GIESEL, J. T. (1986) Genetic correlation structure of life history variables in outbred, wild *Drosophila melanogaster*: effects of photoperiod regimen. *Amer. Nat.* **128**: 593-603

GIESEL, J. T. (1979) Genetic co-variation of survivorship and other fitness indices in *Drosophila melanogaster*. *Exp. Geront.* **14**: 323-328

GIESEL, J. T. and ZETTLER, E. E. (1980) Genetic correlations of life historical parameters and certain fitness indices in *Drosophila melanogaster*: $r_m$, $r_s$, diet breadth. *Oecologia* **47**: 299-302

GIESEL, J. T., MURPHY, P. A. and MANLOVE, M. N. (1982) The influence of temperature on genetic interrelationships of life history traits in a population of *Drosophila melanogaster*: what a tangled data set we weave. *Amer. Nat.* **119**: 464-479

HALDANE, J. B. S. (1941) *New Paths in Genetics.* Allen and Unwin, London.

HAMILTON, W. D. (1966) The moulding of senescence by natural selection. *J. Theor. Biol.* **12**: 12-45

HARVEY, P. H. and READ, A. F. (1988) How and why do mammalian life histories vary? In: *Evolution of Life Histories of Mammals: Theory and Pattern* (Ed. M. P. Boyce), pp. 213-231. New Haven, CT: Yale University Press.

HARVEY, P. H. and ZAMMUTO, R. M. (1985) Patterns of mortality and age at first reproduction in natural populations of mammals. *Nature* **315**: 319-320

HILL, W. G. (1974) Prediction and evaluation of response to selection with overlapping generations. *Anim. Prod.* **18**: 117-139

HILL, W. G. (1977) Selection with overlapping generations. In: *Proceedings of the International Conference on Quantitative Genetics* (Ed. E. Pollak, O. Kempthorne and T.B. Bailey), pp. 367-378. Ames, IA: Iowa State University Press.

KEMPTHORNE, O. (1957) *An Introduction to Genetic Statistics.* New York, NY: John Wiley.

KOSUDA, K. (1985) The aging effect on male mating activity in *Drosophila melanogaster*. *Behav. Genet.* **15**: 297-303

LACK, D. L. (1954) *The Natural Regulation of Animal Numbers.* Oxford, U.K.: Oxford University Press.

LANDE, R. (1982) A quantitative genetic theory of life history evolution. *Ecology* **63**: 607-615

LAW, R. (1979) Ecological determinants in the evolution of life histories. In: *Population Dynamics* (Ed. R. M. Anderson, B. D. Turner and L. R. Taylor), pp. 81-103. Oxford: Blackwell.

MAYNARD SMITH, J. (1958) The effects of temperature and of egg-laying on longevity in *Drosophila subobscura*. *J. Exp. Biol.* **35**: 832-842

MAYNARD SMITH, J. (1959) Sex-limited inheritance of longevity in Drosophila subobscura. *J. Genet.* **56**: 1-9

MEDAWAR, P. B. (1946) Old age and natural death. *Modern Quarterly* **1**: 30-56

MEDAWAR, P. B. (1952) *An Unsolved Problem of Biology.* London, U.K.: H. K. Lewis.

MUELLER, L. D. (1987) Evolution of accelerated senescence in laboratory populations of *Drosophila*. *Proc. Nat. Acad. Sci. USA* **84**: 1974-1977

MUKAI, T. (1985) Experimental verification of the neutral theory. In: *Population Genetics and Molecular Evolution* (Ed. T. Ohta and K. Aoki), pp. 125-145. Berlin, W. Germany: Springer.

NUR, N. (1988) The consequences of brood size for breeding blue tits. III. Measuring the cost of reproduction: survival, future fecundity and differential dispersal. *Evolution* 42: 351- 362

PARTRIDGE, L. and HARVEY, P. H. (1988) The ecological context of life history evolution. *Science* 214: 1449-1455

REZNICK, D. (1985) Costs of reproduction: an evaluation of the empirical evidence. *Oikos* 44: 257-267

REZNICK, D. and ENDLER, J. A. (1982) The impact of predation on life history evolution in Trinidadian guppies (*Poecilia reticulata*). *Evolution* 36: 160-177

ROBERTSON, A. (1955) Selection in animals: synthesis. *Cold Spring Harb. Symp. Quant. Biol.* 20: 225-229

ROSE, M. R. (1982) Antagonistic pleiotropy, dominance and genetic variation. *Heredity* 48: 63-78.

ROSE, M. R. (1983) Theories of life history evolution. *Am. Zool.* 23: 15-23

ROSE, M. R. (1984) Genetic covariation in *Drosophila* life history: untangling the data. *Amer. Nat.* 123: 565-569

ROSE, M. R. (1985) Life history evolution with antagonistic pleiotropy and overlapping generations. *Theor. Pop. Biol.* 28: 342-358

ROSE, M. R. and CHARLESWORTH, B. (1980) A test of evolutionary theories of senescence. *Nature* 287: 141-142

ROSE, M. R. and CHARLESWORTH, B. (1981) Genetics of life history in *Drosophila melanogaster*. I. Sib analysis of adult females. *Genetics* 97: 173-186

SACHER, G. A. (1959) Relationship of lifespan to brain weight and weight in animals. In: *The Life-Span of Animals. CIBA Foundation Colloqia on Ageing* (Ed. G. E. Wolstenholme and M. O'Connor), pp. 115-133. London, U.K.: Churchill.

SACHER, G. A. (1959) Evolution of longevity and survival characteristics. In: *The Genetics of Aging* (Ed. E. L. Schneider), pp. 151-168. New York, NY: Plenum Press.

SAETHER, B. E. (1988) Pattern of covariation between life history traits of European birds. *Nature* 331: 616-617

SCHNEIDER, E. L. (1978) *The Genetics of Aging*. New York, NY: Plenum Press.

SERVICE, P. M. and ROSE, M. R. (1985) Genetic covariation among life history components: the effect of novel environments. *Evolution* 39: 943-945

SIBLY, R. M. and CALOW, P. (1986) *Physiological Ecology of Animals: An Evolutionary Approach*. Oxford, U.K.: Blackwell.

SIMMONS, M. J. and CROW, J. F. (1977) Mutations affecting fitness in *Drosophila* populations. *Ann. Rev. Genet.* 11: 49-78

STEARNS, S. C. (1976) Life history tactics: a review of the ideas. *Quart. Rev. Biol.* 51: 3-47

STEARNS, S. C. (1977) The evolution of life history traits: a critique of the theory and a review of the data. *Ann. Rev. Ecol. Syst.* 8: 145-171

TEMPLETON. A. R. (1980) The evolution of life histories under pleiotropic constraints and r-selection. *Theor. Pop. Biol.* 18: 279-289

WILLIAMS, G. C. (1957) Pleiotropy, natural selection and the evolution of senescence. *Evolution* 11: 398-411

WILLIAMS, G. C. (1966) Natural selection, the costs of reproduction and a refinement of Lack's principle. *Amer. Nat.* 100: 687-690

ZENG, Z.-B. (1988) Long-term correlated response, inter-population covariation, and inter-specific allometry. *Evolution* 42: 363-374

## DISCUSSION

1. In fact, many alleles that beneficially affect fitness early will also beneficially affect it later in life. The same will be true for harmful effects. How frequent are the types of genes that would be dealt with by his theories, that would be beneficial early, but harmful late? Charlesworth answered that there was no information on this.

2. There are several quantitative predictions: The extent of the premium on early gene action would be related to the species' chances of living to later ages. Also, if the population is growing rapidly, early reproduction would be more important, with more selective pressure for early beneficial gene action. Thus the ecology of the species should affect the evolution of life history patterns. For example plants with high mortality have early reproduction, although this may result in increased mortality. If a species in nature has low mortality, it will tend to have deferred reproduction and if it has high mortality it will tend to have early reproduction.

3. Body weights, clutch sizes, and ages at maturity are all important. In placental mammals, body size and age at maturity are related, so that the effects of one predict the other; oddly, maximum longevities are not as related to body sizes and age at maturity as fecundity. Nevertheless, despite poor data on maximum longevities, they still correlate well with fecundity.

4. Cutler points out that human beings live much longer than they should by such allometric considerations, mainly due to benefits of retained learning. This suggests that processes governing aging rates may be quickly and easily affected, and therefore may be much less complex than the processes causing the declines in function that come with age.

5. Will the fact that real populations are not in selective equilibrium affect this theory? Charlesworth answered that it would not affect the general, main conclusions.

6. Will self-fertilizing species have different strategies, since they may reproduce clonally with no selectively maintained variation? Charlesworth pointed out that this didn't affect answers relevant to man. Even insects and mammals should have fundamental similarities in general types of genes; it seems unlikely that different species would have widely different proportions of genes that are beneficial early in life, but harmful late.

# 4

# EVOLUTIONARY GENETICS OF AGING IN *DROSOPHILA*

Michael R. Rose

## INTRODUCTION

The experimental study of the evolutionary genetics of aging is reaching a point where it offers the prospect of new approaches to other types of gerontological research. This opportunity has arisen for two reasons. First, evolutionary genetic research on *Drosophila* spp. has revealed some of the essential features of the evolution of aging, thereby clarifying some of the basic issues in aging research. Second, this same line of research has produced stocks exhibiting postponed aging, stocks which provide suitable material for molecular and cellular analysis. This combination of theoretical clarification and new types of stocks for experimental work might accelerate the progress of gerontology as a whole. The present article will be concerned with conveying these findings in more detail. It cannot, of course, demonstrate that gerontology will necessarily derive much benefit from the evolutionary findings; the development of a field can't really be predicted, especially as such development depends on mobilization along lines of research whose success is necessarily uncertain. For this reason, valuable lines of research may be neglected for reasons of intellectual fashion alone. However, gerontological research that takes evolutionary genetics into account seems to me to offer particular promise at the present time.

Evolutionary biology has developed a general theory of aging based on the decline in the intensity of natural selection with respect to adult age (Medawar, 1952; Williams, 1957). This theory has been made mathematically explicit in the sense of showing that the evolution of aging follows deductively from the assumptions of age-specific genetic variation and separation of soma from germ line (*e.g.* Hamilton, 1966; Charlesworth, 1980). The basic requirement of age-specific genetic variation is known to be met in a reasonable number of species (Rose and Service, 1985; Hutchinson and Rose, 1987; Johnson and Foltz, 1987; other articles in this volume). At the level of comparative biology, the theory predicts that aging should be strictly associated with species in which there is a separate soma, as is the case in all insects and vertebrates, as opposed to those species with no such distinction, such as prokaryotes and most protozoa (Williams, 1957). This particular prediction has been experimentally corroborated in only one instance (Bell, 1984). While there are no extensive comparative studies of the presence and absence of senescence in taxa which exhibit both, the broad comparative patterns, alluded to above, clearly fit the predictions of the theory, and there are no reliable refutations. On these grounds alone, the evolutionary theory of senescence should command the interest of all those working on aging.

But it is the experimental research with *Drosophila* spp., particularly *Drosophila melanogaster*, which has provided the most striking evidence in favor of the evolutionary theory of aging. Furthermore, it is this work that has helped add empirical content to the evolutionary theory, particularly with respect to distinguishing among population genetic mechanisms for the evolution of aging. The reasons for this are not specific to the problem of aging. T.H. Morgan developed *D. melanogaster* as a laboratory system because he saw its numerous advantages for biological research: ease of laboratory culture, small size, rapid generation time, and so on. Add to this list only that *Drosophila* spp. are not too long-lived, and one sees clearly that *Drosophila* spp. have as many advantages for research on aging as they did for genetics. Furthermore, the fact that *Drosophila* spp. usually outbreed and can't self-fertilize make them more appropriate models for application to mouse breeding programs or the human population genetics of aging than is *Caenorhabditis elegans*, the other organism with a good claim to attention in fundamental aging research (cf. Johnson and Foltz, 1987).

It could be objected that *Drosophila* biology has a number of features which are unique, particularly features which make it unsuitable as a physiological model for mammalian aging. An example of such a feature is the absence of cell division in most somatic cells, evidently different from the vertebrate case. Leaving aside the obvious point that many post-maturational somatic cells, such as neurons, do *not* divide in mammals, many invertebrate taxa, from rotifers to insects, lack adult somatic cell division. As a general animal model, *Drosophila* is no worse than *Mus*. However, this entire line of criticism is spurious. Any gerontological research program grounded in evolutionary biology would have to concede that the physiological basis of aging in an insect would provide no specific guide to the physiology of aging in any other major taxon, including the rather minor, divergent, taxon of the Class Mammalia. In any case, *Drosophila* has proven itself to be a powerful workhorse for aging research in general (*vid.* Lints and Soliman, 1988), and here I will show how it has particularly led the way in developing our understanding of the evolution of aging.

Before turning to a detailed review of the *Drosophila* research, I wish to begin by outlining the four major issues that have been the focus for past research. The first, and most fundamental of these, is whether or not the pattern of aging can respond to selection. The evolutionary theory presumes that genetic variation in life-history patterns will give rise to evolutionary responses in aging patterns. This is a natural expectation, because the basic phenotype of aging, declining survival probability, is equivalent to marked changes in components of fitness. Indeed, if patterns of aging did not evolve in response to natural selection, then evolutionary biology as a whole would be under severe challenge. Evolutionary biology has as its foundation the evolution of fitness characters. A critical part of the theory pertaining to the evolution of these characters is that developed by Charlesworth (*e.g.*, 1980), the same theory that provides the fundamental evolutionary analysis of aging. Thus the experiments which test that theory are critical for both evolutionary biology and gerontology, including experiments in which selection is applied to late-age fitness components. It has in fact been suggested that aging does not evolve as other characters do (Lints, 1978; Lints and Hoste, 1974, 1977), so that this issue can not be taken as a matter of little controversy.

The second issue which has shaped research on the evolution of aging is the nature of the population genetic mechanisms that underlie this evolution. There are two cogent theoretical alternatives, both originally due to Medawar (1946, 1952), elaborated on by Williams (1957) and Edney and Gill (1968), and formally delineated by Charlesworth (1980) and others (*e.g.* Rose, 1985; Clark, 1988). The first population genetic mechanism is *antagonistic pleiotropy*. In this theory, it is hypothesized that alleles can have opposed effects at early and late ages. Those alleles with beneficial effects early and deleterious effects later, after the onset of reproduction, are selected upon primarily according to their effects at early ages, when natural selection is more intense. Thus alleles which enhance early fitness components, but depress later fitness components, will often be favored by natural selection, and therefore increase in frequency. This will enhance early net reproduction, but depress later viability and fertility, giving rise to aging.

The alternative mechanism is *mutation-accumulation*, or *age-specific adaptation*. In this theory, each life cycle epoch evolves independently of any other. It is also assumed that there is an unremitting pressure of new deleterious mutations affecting each age specifically. Since the intensity of natural selection falls with adult age in species with somata, the relative balance between selection and deleterious mutations in the determination of gene frequencies will shift in favor of deleterious mutations. Alleles with deleterious effects confined to later ages will accumulate in the population (note that this is not an accumulation of somatic mutations), giving rise to aging. Finally, it should be pointed out that these mechanisms are not incompatible with each other; both could act in the evolution of aging in a single species.

The third issue, or theme, of the evolutionary research has been the physiological mechanisms which give rise to particular population genetic mechanisms for the evolution of aging. Antagonistic pleiotropy and age-specific adaptation are hypotheses concerning allele action, which in turn implies hypotheses about the ways in which different functional components of the organism are genetically interdependent. Most genetic interdependence in turn requires some type of physiological interdependence, immediately raising the prospect of bridging the gap between population genetic and organismal or molecular research on aging.

Fourthly, a major issue in the evolutionary research has been the number of loci involved in the evolution of aging. If that number is small, then the prospects for unravelling the causation of aging using Mendelian genetic methods become great. If that number is large, then any such prospects are appreciably dimmed. While some have supposed that the former must be correct, and others have assumed that aging has to be polygenic, in *Drosophila* this is essentially an experimental question (*vid.* Luckinbill *et al.*, 1987).

While these four issues are perhaps the main ones which have shaped research over the last decade, they are not the only conceivable ones to be addressed. At the end of the present article, I shall discuss ideas for future research.

## RESPONSE TO SELECTION

Edney and Gill (1968) proposed that changes in the reproductive schedule of an experimental population should give rise to changes in the pattern of aging, after enough generations have passed for evolution to act. In particular, they proposed that populations reproduced at earlier ages, compared with those at which controls are reproduced, should age more rapidly, while populations reproduced at later ages should age more slowly. Sokal (1970) and Mertz (1975) provided some evidence from *Tribolium* which partially corroborated the predictions of Edney and Gill (1968), but there was some degree of inconsistency between replicates.

I should be clear at the outset about what is required to perform the proposed experiments correctly. First, there must be control populations that are handled as much like the selected populations as possible, except for the change in the timing of reproduction. *Drosophila* life-history characters are subject to too much variation from recondite sources to be effectively monitored without experimental controls.

Second, the selected and control populations should be given normal opportunities to reproduce. Keeping adults as virgins for long periods and then allowing them to reproduce, which does postpone reproduction, also gives rise to selection for a novel type of culture, confounding the selection mechanism of interest. For this reason, the *Drosophila* experiments of Glass (1960), in which mating was delayed within each generation, are not relevant.

Third, the experimental populations should not be inbred, initially. Evolution does not occur in the absence of genetic variation.

Fourth, there is a problem of a bias toward false positive results if the selected line is reproduced at a much earlier age than normal. If this reproduction is close to some physiological limit, then there may be fewer individuals reproducing in the selected line(s). If inbreeding depression then occurs, longevity will be relatively depressed in the selected line(s), because *Drosophila* is subject to inbreeding depression for longevity (Clarke and Maynard Smith, 1955; Rose, 1984a). Thus there will be a false positive result.

Fifth, enough generations should be allowed for evolution to act. In outbred *Drosophila* populations, 20 to 30 generations should normally be enough to get a response from relatively inefficient "culture" selection methods, given the success of artificial selection with this species (*vid.* Falconer, 1981). On the other hand, it is difficult to determine what a lower limit would be. If the negative result is of more interest, then selecting for at least 20 generations would seem imperative. As will be discussed, positive results can be obtained in fewer generations.

The first person to perform experiments of appropriate design was Wattiaux (1968a,b). In his first set of experiments, he established a line of *D. subobscura* which was subject to a 6 to 8 week postponement of reproduction (Wattiaux, 1968a). That is, new discrete generations were initiated only from females which had attained at least 6 weeks of age from pupal emergence. Control lines were maintained using females 3 to 9 days old at the time of reproduction. After 14 generations of the early-reproduced stock, there was a significantly greater mean longevity in the late-reproduced stock, in conformity with theoretical expectations. However, a freshly wild-caught sample had greater male longevity and greater early female fecundity than either selected or control lines, suggesting inbreeding depression. The founding of the laboratory populations from just 9 males and 62 females fits such an interpretation. The study of Wattiaux (1968b) which used *D. pseudoobscura* was similar in design except that the late-reproduced cultures used a turnover age of about 4 weeks. In six different pairings of control with selected lines, each pair having a different chromosomal morphology, 4 evolved increased longevity in the late-reproduced line. In all, Wattiaux (1968a,b) provided some corroborative evidence for the evolutionary theory of senescence, but none of it was unequivocal. It should also be said that Wattiaux (e.g. 1968a) seems to have favored some type of neo-Lamarckian interpretation of his results; he did not offer them as support for the views of Medawar (1952) or Hamilton (1966).

Lints and Hoste (1974, 1977) established cultures of *D. melanogaster* reproduced at 4 days after eclosion and 26 days after eclosion, the latter being changed later to the latest age at which 80-90 % of females still laid at least 20 eggs per day. The late-reproduced lines did not evolve increased mean longevity (Lints and Hoste, 1974), although they did evolve a shift in egg-laying toward later ages (Lints and Hoste, 1977). Luckinbill and Clare (1985) subjected this experiment to a penetrating analysis, which will be discussed below.

Until 1980, the published literature had only provided ambiguous corroborations, with some seeming refutations, of the predictions of Edney and Gill (1968). Rose and Charlesworth (1980, 1981b) provided a fairly clear corroboration. An outbred *D. melanogaster* stock, known to be genetically polymorphic (Rose and Charlesworth, 1981a) and normally reproduced at early ages, was used to found a selection line that was bred using females that had achieved at least 21 days from pupal eclosion. After 12 generations, the mean longevity of the selected line had increased by about 10 %, relative to that of the control, which was statistically significant. Late fecundity was also increased (Rose and Charlesworth, 1981b).

Rose (1984b) then repeated this experiment with a three-fold replication of both controls and selected lines. The females used to reproduce the selected lines were of progressively greater age, finally attaining 70 days of age from the egg. The results were essentially the same as those of Rose and Charlesworth (1981a), *i.e.* mean longevity and later fecundity were increased. The stocks studied by Rose (1984b) also had five-fold replication, with consistent differentiation between early-reproduced and late-reproduced flies (Hutchinson and Rose, this volume).

Luckinbill *et al.* (1984) performed an essentially similar experiment with *D. melanogaster* stocks founded from a base population entirely independent from that of Rose (1984b). Their study had two-fold replication of selected and control lines, with the four lines being measured every few generations. They found a clear trend toward increased longevity in the stocks reproduced at later ages.

Luckinbill and Clare (1985) and Clare and Luckinbill (1985) were particularly concerned with the basis for the discrepancy between the results of Rose (*e.g.* Rose, 1984b) or Luckinbill *et al.* (1984), which corroborated the evolutionary theory, and those of Lints and Hoste (1974, 1977), which did not. They noted that the experimental procedures used by Lints and Hoste entailed rearing of the *Drosophila* larvae at a density of 10 larvae per vial. They reasoned that this might have given rise to a genotype- environment interaction that suppressed expression of genetic variation affecting lifespan which *would* be expressed at higher rearing densities. In the experiments of Clare and Luckinbill (1985), they manipulated rearing densities and directly demonstrated the existence of such a genotype environment interaction. In Luckinbill and Clare (1985), they contrasted selection experiments with low rearing densities and high rearing densities, finding that the low-density rearing design prevented the predicted evolutionary response which was detected with high-density rearing. The corroborative results of Luckinbill *et al.* (1984) were also obtained with high rearing densities.

In conclusion, it is now well-established that lifespan and other aging characters can evolve in outbred populations kept in environments in which genetic variation can be expressed. This finding is of great importance for two issues. Firstly, the fact that populations that have the intensity of selection sustained at later ages evolve postponed aging is dramatic evidence in favor of the evolutionary theory of aging. Secondly, natural selection in the laboratory can be used to produce genetically-postponed aging in outbred organisms; such postponed aging then provides an avenue of attack for the study of the physiological mechanisms of aging, which will be discussed below.

## POPULATION GENETIC MECHANISMS OF AGING

Explicit attempts to test for alternative population genetic mechanisms of aging begin with Rose and Charlesworth (1980, 1981a,b). Their first experiment was a test for the exclusive action of mutation-accumulation in maintaining age-specific genetic variability for female fecundity. The additive genetic variance for age-specific female fecundity was measured over a range of adult ages, the expectation being that, if mutation-accumulation were occurring at later ages, then there should be greater additive genetic variance for age-specific fecundity at those ages. The results were negative: there was no tendency for genetic variance to increase with age, contrary to the hypothesis (Rose and Charlesworth, 1981a).

Other findings from these studies had significance for the antagonistic pleiotropy hypothesis. Negative genetic correlations were found between early fecundity and later life-history attributes, such as longevity (Rose and Charles- worth, 1981b). Antagonistic responses to selection were found, such that as longevity increased, early fecundity fell (Rose and Charlesworth, 1981a). These two findings are complementary, both indicating antagonistic pleiotropy between early reproduction and later reproduction, the latter including survival to later ages as well as later fertility.

Rose (1984b) found similar results with selection for postponed senescence. As longevity and later fecundity increased, early fecundity fell. This again fit antagonistic pleiotropy. Luckinbill *et al.* (1984) and Luckinbill and Clare (1985) also found that successful selection for increased longevity and later fertility resulted in decreased early fecundity.

In a number of studies (e.g. Giesel, 1979; Giesel and Zettler, 1980; Giesel *et al.*, 1982; Murphy *et al.*, 1983), the laboratory of Giesel has found generally positive genetic correlations between components of life-history. This is ostensibly contradictory to *both* mutation-accumulation and antagonistic pleiotropy theories, which require that genetic correlations between some of these characters be zero or negative. (Indeed, it is difficult to explain the evolution of aging if all genetic correlations between life-history characters are positive.) These results, however, can be explained in terms of two demonstrable artifacts: inbreeding depression (Rose, 1984a) and genotype-environment interaction (Service and Rose, 1985). These artifacts give rise to a bias toward positive genetic correlations between life-history characters and other fitness characters. One or the other of these arises in the experiments of the Giesel laboratory, as well as those of many other laboratories (reviewed in Rose and Service, 1985). All such experiments are of no certain scientific significance, from the standpoint of testing pleiotropy hypotheses, because of these artifacts.

More recently, evidence has been published indicating the action of mutation-accumulation in the evolution of senescence. Kosuda (1985) has found that the genetic variability for male mating success increases with age in *Drosophila*. Mueller (1987) has demonstrated a deterioration in the later fecundity of female *D. melanogaster* selected for reproduction only at early ages, although inbreeding and genetic drift may have played some role in these results. Service *et al.* (1988) showed an absence of antagonistic selection responses between early reproduction and some of the physiological characters involved in the evolution of postponed senescence in the lines of Rose (1984b). (See below for more on the physiological characters involved in postponed aging.)

In conclusion, it appears that *both* antagonistic pleiotropy and age-specific adaptation, or mutation accumulation, are involved in the evolution of aging in *Drosophila*.

## PHYSIOLOGICAL MECHANISMS FOR THE EVOLUTION OF AGING

Given that one has lines which exhibit evolutionarily postponed aging, it is obviously tempting to try to determine the mechanisms which underlie this postponement. This can be achieved by comparing replicated lines of postponed and control senescence patterns. Unreplicated selection lines are not adequate, because linkage disequilibrium and genetic drift may have given rise to spurious associations between postponed aging and a particular physiological character which does not play any role in postponing aging.

This line of research was begun by Rose *et al.* (1984). They studied the gross morphological differences between the long-lived and short-lived lines of Rose (1984b). They found that the only large detectable change at the morphological level was an increase in the early ovary weight of short-lived females, relative to females from the long-lived stocks. This increase in ovary weight corresponds to the period when these females are also more fecund than long-lived females. This is a direct manifestation of the antagonistic pleiotropy idea: longer-lived females have smaller ovaries when they are younger, sacrificing early reproduction for later survival. This finding did not, however, indicate what the benefit from this sacrifice was.

The study of Service *et al.* (1985) carried this line of work much farther. They found an enhancement of stress resistance in the longer-lived stocks of Rose (1984b), specifically resistance to starvation, desiccation, and ambient 15% ethanol solution. There was no enhancement in resistance to heat or more concentrated ambient ethanol solutions. This study began to get at the mechanistic roots of the enhanced survival of flies from the longer-lived stocks.

Service (1987) showed that the findings of Service *et al.* (1985) with respect to starvation resistance could be explained in terms of increased levels of lipids in longer-lived flies. However, he found that other patterns of increased stress resistance could not be explained in this manner. Nor could any other organismal attribute, such as metabolic rate, locomotory behavior, or water content explain the other results. Service also showed that some of these other variables also exhibited differentiation between longer-lived and short-lived stocks.

It should also be noted that Service and Rose (1985) found a large negative genetic correlation between early fecundity and starvation resistance. This suggests that there is a trade-off of lipid and other substances between fat body and ovary, this trade-off generating the evolutionary antagonism between survival and early fecundity, at least in part.

Luckinbill *et al.* (1988a) performed additional studies of the physiological basis of aging in their independently-derived long-lived stocks. Contrary to some of the suggestions of Partridge and Andrews (1985), they found that preventing flies from mating does not eliminate the postponement of aging found in their stocks, suggesting that this postponement is not a "reduced mating" effect upon short- term mortality risks. Service (1989) has replicated this finding with the stocks of Rose (1984b) and Service *et al.* (1985). Luckinbill *et al.* (1988a) also found that overall body weight was not affected by the evolution of postponed aging, corroborating the findings of Rose *et al.* (1984). Finally, Luckinbill *et al.* (1988a) found that one of their longer-lived stocks had a much greater flight endurance capacity than one of their short-lived stocks. Graves *et al.* (1988) replicated this finding with the same stocks, and showed that the flight endurance change was not due to decreased wing-beat frequency. Graves and Rose (this vol.) have found that the longer-lived stocks of Rose (1984b) also have increased flight endurance, relative to short-lived stocks.

Overall, a body of interesting information is accumulating about the physiological bases of postponed aging in two different sets of *Drosophila* stocks exhibiting postponed aging. One exciting feature of these results is simply that such differences in some, though not all, organismal functions are readily detectable. Another is that these differences appear to be consistent over replicated stocks derived by selection from common ancestral populations as well as consistent over stocks derived from different ancestral populations in different laboratories, often using different procedures. These findings, therefore, suggest that there are fundamental consistencies to be found in the physiological means by which evolution postpones aging, within a single species.

## LOCI INVOLVED IN THE EVOLUTION OF *DROSOPHILA* AGING

A fundamental question for studies of the evolution and genetics of aging in *Drosophila* is whether or not specific "senescence loci" can be identified (*cf.* Hutchinson and Rose, 1987). In this context, loci with mutant alleles that shorten lifespan are not necessarily appropriate material. They could be shortening life by introducing novel pathological processes. Rather, the loci of interest should modulate the processes which limit lifespan in normal flies.

The postponed senescence lines of Rose (1984b) or Luckinbill *et al.* (1984) provide material in which there is genetic differentiation affecting the processes which must normally limit lifespan. As such, they are attractive targets for genetic analysis aimed at identifying the loci involved in senescence. An initial step in this direction was taken by Luckinbill *et al.* (1987), who found that biometrical estimates of the number of loci involved in postponed aging in their stocks were quite low. Hutchinson and Rose (this volume) performed similar biometrical studies to those of Luckinbill *et al.* (1987). While they replicated the Luckinbill *et al.* findings, in terms of the average estimates of number of loci, they found that these estimates were statistically indistinguishable from a null hypothesis of arbitrarily many loci involved in aging. (This result was obtained with a considerably larger body of data than that of Luckinbill *et al.*). This raises doubt about the interpretations offered by Luckinbill *et al.*, as well as suggesting that the prospects for Mendelian analysis of aging are quite limited, in that the number of loci involved appears to be too large, relative to the amount of environmental variance.

Chromosome substitution analysis due to Luckinbill *et al.* (1988b) has in fact underscored this conclusion. They found that all three of the major chromosomes of *D. melanogaster* make a significant contribution to the postponement of aging in one of their longer-lived stocks. This means that a minimum of three loci must be involved in the postponement of aging in that stock. Moreover, since the *D. melanogaster* chromosomes studied include more than a thousand loci each, the likelihood is that there are many loci over the entire genome contributing to the postponed-aging phenotype in the stocks of the Luckinbill and Rose laboratories.

## FUTURE DIRECTIONS FOR RESEARCH

It would not be true to say that the research discussed above has reached its natural conclusion. Rather, it is only a beginning, the first steps of a research program which offers the promise of answering many of the most profound questions of biological gerontology, if this program is fully implemented.

The next question of obvious importance is that of the number of ways in which evolution can postpone senescence within a given species. Experimentally, this comes down to measurements of heterogeneity between evolutionarily distinct lines with postponed senescence, within a given species. The *Drosophila* stocks with postponed aging that have been created in the laboratories of Rose and Luckinbill are obvious material for addressing this question. It can be posed in two different ways. Firstly, are the replicate lines that were derived from a common ancestral population essentially homogeneous in patterns of postponed aging? Secondly, are the lines created in different laboratories from different ancestral populations essentially similar with respect to the genetic and physiological bases of postponed aging? Both of these subsidiary questions are now being answered using the available quantitative genetic techniques.

The other major question which the extant findings raise is the molecular genetic basis of postponed senescence in laboratory *Drosophila* stocks. Are there known electrophoretic loci which have played a major role in the postponement of aging? Are there loci involved which can be identified by some other molecular genetic technique, such as 2-D gel protein electrophoresis? These questions await the development of useful collaborations between those evolutionary geneticists and molecular geneticists who are interested in the problem of aging.

## ACKNOWLEDGEMENTS

I am grateful to L. S. Luckinbill for his comments on an earlier draft of this paper. I am also grateful to J. L. Graves and E. W. Hutchinson for numerous discussions of the points raised in the paper. Some of the research from my laboratory which is discussed here has been supported by the Natural Sciences and Engineering Research Council of Canada and is currently supported by the National Institute on Aging of the United States, Grant AG06346.

## REFERENCES

BELL G. (1984) Evolutionary and nonevolutionary theories of senescence. *Am. Nat.* **124**: 600-603

CHARLESWORTH B. (1980) *Evolution in Age-Structured Populations.* London: Cambridge University Press.

CLARE, M.J. and LUCKINBILL, L.S. (1985) The effects of gene-environment on the expression of longevity. *Heredity* **55**: 19-29

CLARK, A. G. (1988) Genetic correlations: The quantitative genetics of evolutionary constraints. In: *Genetic Constraints on Adaptive Evolution.* V. Loeschcke (Ed.). Berlin: Springer-Verlag.

CLARKE, J. M. and MAYNARD SMITH, J. (1955) The genetics and cytology of *Drosophila subobscura.* XI. Hybrid vigour and longevity. *J. Genet.* **53**: 172-180

EDNEY, E. B. and GILL, R. W. (1968) Evolution of senescence and specific longevity. *Nature* **220**: 281-282

FALCONER, D. S. (1981) *Introduction to Quantitative Genetics.* (2nd ed). London: Longman.

GIESEL, J. T. (1979) Genetic co-variation of survivorship and other fitness indices in *Drosophila melanogaster. Exp. Gerontol.* **14**: 323-328

GIESEL, J. T., MURPHY, P. A. and MANLOVE, M. N. (1982a) The influence of temperature on genetic interrelationships of life history traits in a population of *Drosophila melanogaster*: What tangled data sets we weave. *Am. Nat.* **119**: 464-479

GIESEL, J. T. and ZETTLER, E. E. (1980) Genetic correlations of life historical parameters and certain fitness indices in *Drosophila melanogaster*: $r_m$, $r_s$, diet breadth. *Oecologia* **47**: 299-302

GLASS, B. (1960) The influence of immediate versus delayed mating on the lifespan of *Drosophila*. In: *The Biology of Aging*. B. L. Strehler (Ed.).Washington, DC: American Institute of Biological Science.

GOWEN, J. W. and JOHNSON, L. E. (1946) On the mechanism of heterosis. I. Metabolic capacity of different races of *Drosophila melanogaster* for egg production. *Am. Nat.* **80**: 149-179

GRAVES, J. L., LUCKINBILL, L. S. and NICHOLS, A. (1988) Flight duration and wing beat frequency in long- and short-lived *Drosophila melanogaster*. *J. Insect Physiol.* **34**: 1021-1026.

HALDANE, J. B. S (1941) *New Paths in Genetics*. London: Allen and Unwin.

HAMILTON, W. D. (1966) The moulding of senescence by natural selection. *J. Theor. Biol.* **12**: 12-45

HUTCHINSON, E. W. and ROSE, M. R. (1987) Genetics of aging in insects. *Rev. Biol. Res. Aging.* **3**: 63-70

JOHNSON, T. E. and FOLTZ, N. L. (1987) Aging in *Caenorhabditis elegans*: Update 1986. *Rev. Biol. Res. Aging.* **3**: 51-61

KOSUDA K. (1985) The aging effect on male mating activity in *Drosophila melanogaster*. *Behav. Genet.* **15**: 297-303

LAW R. (1979) The cost of reproduction in annual meadow grass. Am. Nat. **113**: 3-16

LAW R., BRADSHAW, A. D.and PUTWAIN, P. D. (1977) Life-history variation in *Poa annua*. *Evolution* **31**: 233-246

Lerner, I. M. (1954) *Genetic Homeostasis*. Edinburgh: Oliver & Boyd.

LINTS, F. A. and HOSTE, C. (1974) The Lansing effect revisited. I. Lifespan. *Exp. Gerontol.* **9**: 51-69

LINTS, F. A. and HOSTE, C. (1977) The Lansing effect revisited. II. Cumulative and spontaneously reversible parental age effects on fecundity in *Drosophila melanogaster*. *Evolution* **31**: 387-404

LINTS, F. A., STOLL J., GRUWEZ G. and LINTS, C. V. (1979): An attempt to select for increased longevity in *Drosophila melanogaster*. *Gerontology* **25**: 192-204

LUCKINBILL, L. S., ARKING, R., CLARE, M. J., CIROCCO, W. C. and BUCK, S. A. (1984) Selection for delayed senescence in *Drosophila melanogaster*. *Evolution* **38**: 996-1003

LUCKINBILL, L. S. and CLARE, M. J. (1985) Selection for life span in *Drosophila melanogaster*. *Heredity* **55**: 9-18

LUCKINBILL, L. S., CLARE, M. J., KRELL, W. L., CIROCCO, W. C. and RICHARDS, P. A. (1987) Estimating the number of genetic elements that defer senescence in *Drosophila*. *Evol. Ecol.* **1**: 37-46

LUCKINBILL, L. S., GRAVES, J. L., TOMKIW, A. and SOWIRKA, O. (1988a) A qualitative analysis of life history characters in *Drosophila melanogaster*. *Evol. Ecol.* **2**: 85-94

LUCKINBILL, L. S., GRAVES, J. L., REED, A. H. and KOETSAWANG, S. (1988b) Localizing genes that defer senescence in *Drosophila melanogaster*. *Heredity* **60**: 367-374

MAYNARD SMITH, J. (1978) Optimization theory in evolution. *Ann. Rev. Ecol. Syst.* **9**: 31-56

MEDAWAR, P. B. (1946) Old age and natural death. *Mod. Quart.* **1**: 30-56.

MEDAWAR, P. B. (1952) *An Unsolved Problem of Biology*. London: H.K. Lewis.

MERTZ, D. B. (1975) Senescent decline in flour beetles selected for early adult fitness. *Physiol. Zool.* **48**: 1-23

MUELLER, L. D. (1987) Evolution of accelerated senescence in laboratory populations of *Drosophila*. *Proc. Natl. Acad. Sci. USA* **84**: 1974-1977

MURPHY, P. A., GIESEL, J. T. and MANLOVE, M. N. (1983) Temperature effects on life history variation in *Drosophila simulans*. *Evolution* **37**: 1181-1192

ROSE, M. R. (1982) Antagonistic pleiotropy, dominance, and genetic variation. *Heredity* **48**: 63-78

ROSE, M. R. (1984a) Genetic covariation in *Drosophila* life history: Untangling the data. *Am. Nat.* **123**: 565-569

ROSE, M. R. (1984b) Laboratory evolution of postponed senescence in *Drosophila melanogaster. Evolution* **38**: 1004-1010

ROSE, M. R. (1985) Life history evolution with antagonistic pleiotropy and overlapping generations. *Theor. Pop. Biol.* **28**: 342-358

ROSE, M. and CHARLESWORTH, B. (1980) A test of evolutionary theories of senescence. *Nature* **287**: 141-142

ROSE, M. R. and CHARLESWORTH, B. (1981a) Genetics of life-history in *Drosophila melanogaster.* I. Sib analysis of adult females. *Genetics* **97**: 173-186

ROSE, M. R. and CHARLESWORTH, B. (1981b) Genetics of life-history in *Drosophila melanogaster.* II. Exploratory selection experiments. *Genetics* **97**: 187-196

ROSE, M. R., DOREY, M. L., COYLE, A. M. and SERVICE, P. M. (1984) The morphology of postponed senescence in *Drosophila melanogaster. Can. J. Zool.* **62**: 1576-1580

ROSE, M. R. and HUTCHINSON, E. W. (1987) Evolution of aging. *Rev. Biol. Res. Aging.* **3**: 23-32

ROSE, M. R. and SERVICE, P. M. (1985) Evolution of aging. *Rev. Biol. Res. Aging.* **2**: 85-98

SERVICE, P. M. (1987) Physiological mechanisms of increased stress resistance in *Drosophila melanogaster* selected for postponed senescence. *Physiol. Zool.* **60**: 321-326

SERVICE, P. M. (1989) The effect of mating status on lifespan, egglaying, and starvation resistance in *Drosophila melanogaster* in relation to selection on longevity. *J. Insect Physiol.* **35**: 447-452.

SERVICE, P. M., HUTCHINSON, E. W., MACKINLEY, M. D. and ROSE, M. R. (1985) Resistance to environmental stress in *Drosophila melanogaster* selected for postponed senescence. *Physiol. Zool.* **58**: 380-389

SERVICE, P. M., HUTCHINSON, E. W. and ROSE, M. R. (1988) Multiple genetic mechanisms for the evolution of senescence in *Drosophila melanogaster. Evolution* **42**: 708-716

SERVICE, P. M. and ROSE, M. R. (1985) Genetic covariation among life-history components: the effect of novel environments. *Evolution* **39**: 943-945

SOKAL, R. R. (1970) Senescence and genetic load: Evidence from *Tribolium. Science* **167**: 1733-1734

WATTIAUX, J. M. (1968a) Cumulative parental age effects in *Drosophila subobscura. Evolution* **22**: 406-421

WATTIAUX, J. M. (1968b) Parental age effects in *Drosophila pseudoobscura. Exp. Gerontol.* **3**: 55-61

WILLIAMS, G. C. (1957) Pleiotropy, natural selection, and the evolution of senescence. *Evolution* **11**: 398-411

## DISCUSSION

1. Asked how much the maximum longevities of the selected lines are beyond maximum longevity for the *Drosophila* species, and what the record longevities are, Rose answered that the environments must be strictly defined to compare *Drosophila* longevities.

2. Examining the lines with intermediate longevities, as well as the shortest and longest-lived lines, are there changes in fecundity and other physiological parameters that correlate well with longevity? Rose answered that these are not consistent, but might be interesting. There is clear evidence

that amounts of lipid are directly proportional to longevity and inversely proportional to fecundity or ovarian contents; however there are many other factors involved.

3. Questions to be answered by further work include: Do long-lived lines have extended larval stages - retarded growth and development as well as aging? What do the flies die of - histological evidence?

# 5

# FLIGHT DURATION IN *DROSOPHILA MELANOGASTER* SELECTED FOR POSTPONED SENESCENCE

Joseph L. Graves, Jr. and Michael R. Rose

## ABSTRACT

This study tests for effects on tethered flight endurance arising from selection for increased lifespan. Flight durations were measured under ambient temperatures and humidities. Long-lived flies exhibited longer flight than short-lived, a pattern consistent with earlier studies of other, independently derived, long-lived stocks in the Luckinbill laboratory. Lifespan and flight duration were measured for 4 populations of B and O females simultaneously. A positive correlation between flight ability and lifespan was clearly demonstrated.

## INTRODUCTION

The success of selection in moulding life span and associated life history characters has been firmly established in several independent studies of laboratory populations. Rose and Charlesworth (1981), followed by Rose (1984), Luckinbill *et al.* (1984) and Luckinbill and Clare (1985) described extensive changes in patterns of longevity and fecundity resulting from selection for late-life fitness in *Drosophila melanogaster*. Subsequent investigations have compared the physiological responses to age-specific selection on those populations. These responses include improved resistance to starvation, desiccation and ethanol vapor in long-lived individuals (Service *et al.* 1985). Rose *et al.* (1984) and Service (1987) have also found differences in early ovary weight, lipid content, behavioural activity and metabolism. It was of particular importance that no overall difference in body size or weight could be found.

The analysis of stocks from the Rose and Luckinbill laboratories has thus far overlapped in assays of longevity, early and late fecundity, and body size. The results of these assays indicate that the responses to selection for late-life fitness in the Rose and Luckinbill stocks have generally corresponded, although slight differences in the nature of the selection regimes existed (Rose in this volume).

Luckinbill, Graves, Tomkiw, and Sowirka (1988) reported that large flight duration differences exist, favoring their long-lived line. Graves, Luckinbill, and Nichols (1988) corroborated that finding, also showing that the difference in flight duration observed in the stocks was not an artifact of any flight frequency difference. But a number of interesting comparisons between these stocks remain undone. For example, starvation, desiccation, and ethanol vapor resistances have been tested only in the Rose stocks, while flight duration has been tested only in the Luckinbill stocks. This study begins the much-needed comparison of these independently-derived stocks for the character of tethered flight duration.

## MATERIALS AND METHODS

The populations used in this study were originally described in Rose (1984) and Service *et al.* (1985). These populations have been subjected to strong selection for early-and late-life fitness. The $B_1$-$B_5$ populations were cultured in discrete generations of two weeks, while the $O_1$-$O_5$ populations were cultured on a ten-week generation schedule. These ten populations were derived simultaneously from a common ancestral population that had been maintained for the preceding five years under conditions favoring early-life fitness. The complete history and details of the selection procedures and culture conditions of the B and O stocks can be found in Rose (1984) and Service *et al.* (1985).

The techniques used for tethered flight measurement are the same as those used in Luckinbill *et al.* (1988) and Graves *et al.* (1988). Briefly, this involved lightly etherizing the fly and then tethering it to a light-test piece of fishing line by use of Duco Cement. The fly can then be stimulated to fly by utilizing the tarsal reflex or by lightly passing an air current along the head-tail axis. *Drosophila* stimulated in this way can be flown to exhaustion by an observer, providing the fly is immediately stimulated upon any momentary cessation of flight. Graves *et al.* (1988) demonstrated that the increase in tethered flight-duration capacity in the Luckinbill stocks did not seem to result from any difference in flight frequency during flight. Therefore, this study does not evaluate wing-beat frequencies.

Flight trials were performed on females 5-15 days of age from each population, with one population of each type paired. Males were not tested, because earlier studies have shown that they follow the same pattern as females, although they exhibit slightly lower flight duration (Graves *et al.* 1988; Luckinbill *et al.* 1988). The trials were performed on five successive days, under essentially uniform conditions. This of course does not rule out environmental variation that had unknown effects on the flies. Before the flight trial, the flies were allowed to eclose under standard culture conditions (60-100 larvae per shell vial), and then kept at adult densities of between 60-100 flies per shell vial until assayed. In an earlier study, it was shown that strong density-dependent effects alter both adult flight and longevity in *Drosophila melanogaster* (Graves 1989). Therefore, care was taken to maintain the vials at densities which allow the detection of flight differences.

Flight duration and longevity were correlated for four of the B and O populations. Longevity was measured as described in Rose (1984) and Luckinbill and Clare (1985). The procedure consists of pairing 30 male and female flies in standard shell vials. The flies are transferred without anesthesia, at two day intervals. When a fly died in a given vial it was replaced by a fly of the same sex, and the date of death recorded. This procedure was followed until all flies in the experiment were dead.

## RESULTS

Table 1 shows the mean flight durations together with the 95% confidence intervals, for females of the $B_1$-$B_5$ and $O_1$-$O_5$ populations and Table 2 gives the results of a nested analysis of variance which compares both the lines and the five populations in each. Table 2 shows that there was a highly significant difference in flight duration brought about by selection for late-life fitness in the B and O stocks. The variation within each population was also highly significant. Table 3 shows that if the mean flight duration is calculated for the 5 populations in both lines, the correlation between the amount of extension of life span and the relative increase in flight duration seems consistent with the earlier studies of Graves *et al.* (1988). In that study, Graves *et al.* found that an approximately 60% increase in longevity was associated with a four-fold increase in female flight duration at this age. That study also found that $F_1$ reciprocal crosses between the short-and long-lived lines, which exhibited intermediate longevity, also exhibited intermediate flight durations. This study reports that the 30% differential between the mean longevities of B and O stocks is associated with about a two-fold increase in female flight duration. This result is further evidence for the existence of a strong longevity/flight correlation.

The strongest evidence for a longevity/flight correlation is measuring the actual longevity of populations tested for flight duration. The earlier studies of Luckinbill et al (1988) and Graves et al (1988) could only infer the correlation. Table 4 presents the correlation for females of B and O popula-

**TABLE 1.** Mean Flight Duration And 95% Confidence Intervals For B And O Stocks, Aged 5-15 Days

| STOCK | N | MEAN | LOWER LIMIT | UPPER LIMIT |
|---|---|---|---|---|
| B1 | 28 | 27.8 | 14.4 | 41.2 |
| B2 | 31 | 77.5 | 64.4 | 90.2 |
| B3 | 22 | 27.6 | 12.4 | 42.7 |
| B4 | 28 | 31.0 | 17.5 | 44.4 |
| B5 | 26 | 41.7 | 27.7 | 55.6 |
| O1 | 27 | 67.6 | 52.7 | 82.5 |
| O2 | 29 | 117.0 | 102.6 | 131.3 |
| O3 | 28 | 87.5 | 72.9 | 102.1 |
| O4 | 28 | 70.3 | 55.7 | 85.0 |
| O5 | 28 | 74.2 | 59.6 | 88.9 |

**TABLE 2.** Nested Design Analysis Of Variance Of Flight Duration in B And O Stocks

| SOURCE | SUM OF SQUARES | DF | MEAN SQUARE | F RATIO | P |
|---|---|---|---|---|---|
| B1/O1 | 21783.7 | 1 | 21783.7 | 15.4 | 0.000 |
| B2/O2 | 23358.6 | 1 | 23358.6 | 16.5 | 0.000 |
| B3/O3 | 44256.0 | 1 | 44256.0 | 31.3 | 0.000 |
| B4/04 | 21685.7 | 1 | 21685.7 | 15.3 | 0.000 |
| B5/O5 | 14288.0 | 1 | 14288.0 | 10.1 | 0.002 |
| TREATMENT | 94336.4 | 4 | 23584.1 | 16.6 | 0.000 |

tions that were measured for flight duration and longevity simultaneously. The correlation was significant for the eight populations.

## DISCUSSION

This study shows that:

(1) Long-lived O populations exhibit an increase in tethered flight duration capacity similar to that of the Luckinbill stocks reported in Luckinbill *et al.* (1988) and Graves *et al.* (1988).

(2) The increase in flight duration was in proportion to the increase in longevity reported for these stocks in Rose (1984) and Service *et al.* (1985), further suggesting a consistent longevity/flight correlation.

(3) Longevity and flight duration shows a significant correlation in eight populations of B and O females that had both characters measured simultaneously.

In the studies of Service *et al.* (1985) and Service (1987), a prominent increase in lipid content was demonstrated in the O populations. Dipterans, unlike many insect groups, do not use lipid reserves during flight (Williams

| Table 3. T-test Comparison Of Average Mean Flight For B And O Lines | | | | | |
|---|---|---|---|---|---|
| POPULATION | MEAN | MEAN DIFFERENCE | df | t | SIG. |
| B | 41.1 | | | | |
| O | 83.3 | | | | |
| | | 42.2 | 8 | 9.12 | 0.001 |

Table 3 is the t-test comparison for average flight duration in females of 5 replicate B and O populations. The mean difference was 42.2 minutes and was highly significant.

| Table 4. Longevity-flight Correlation For Females 5-15 Days Old | | |
|---|---|---|
| | LONGEVITY (days) | FLIGHT (minutes) |
| B1 | 38.2 | 60.5 |
| B2 | 36.0 | 27.0 |
| B3 | 29.7 | 35.6 |
| B4 | 30.9 | 50.2 |
| | | |
| O1 | 43.2 | 76.6 |
| O2 | 44.5 | 78.3 |
| O3 | 59.5 | 74.4 |
| O4 | 47.5 | 87.1 |

Correlation  0.7271
R squared    0.5287
Prob r=0     0.041
D.F.         6

*et al.* 1943, Wigglesworth 1949). Wigglesworth (1949) demonstrated that *Drosophila* would continue flying until their glycogen reserves were exhausted. Therefore, it is highly likely that the increased flight duration capacity of the long-lived lines is due to a higher glycogen content available for flight, relative to that of the short-lived lines. It is also possible that selection for late-life fitness in these lines has caused some alteration of general energy metabolism, resulting in the long-lived line possessing both a higher lipid content and a higher glycogen content.

The recent study of Service *et al.* (1988) may be particularly important for understanding which physiological changes found in the long-lived line are most important in establishing increased longevity. That study demonstrated that, under reversed selection for early fecundity in the O stocks, starvation resistance retained its negative correlation with fecundity, while desiccation and ethanol resistance appeared to remain unchanged under the reversed selection regime. Service *et al.* (1985) had earlier hypothesized that the greater starvation resistance of the O lines was made possible by their greater lipid contents. If alteration of the overall energy utilization in the long-lived stocks has occurred, then a test of the flight duration capacity of the reverse selection lines should also exhibit a loss of increased flight capacity. [This experiment is currently underway in our laboratory.] The identification of physiological traits consistently and strongly associated with increased life span opens the way to genetical, molecular, and biochemical analysis of aging. For example, the enzymes responsible for variations in flight performance are known in *Drosophila*, and techniques are readily available for the measurement of their activity (Laurie-Ahlberg *et al.* 1985).

The analysis of physiological traits strongly associated with increased lifespan might also be applied to the analysis of longevity in mammals, since it is possible that selection may act in analogous ways to mould life span across widely different phylogenetic groups. This approach awaits, however, the creation of outbred laboratory mammals exposed to the type of selection regime used to create the Rose and Luckinbill *Drosophila* lines. Without these stocks, it is likely that comparisons such as the ones presented in this study will never be possible.

## ACKNOWLEDGEMENTS

We thank E.W. Hutchinson, Kelly Grimm, Suzanne Curtis, Christine Jeong, Janet Nelson, and Vinh Vu for assistance in the maintenance of the stocks and for participating in the flight trials reported in this study. This research was supported in part by a University of California President's Postdoctoral fellowship to JLG and in part by US-PHS Grant AG06346 to MRR.

## REFERENCES

GRAVES, J. L. (1989) Adult population effects on *Drosophila* melanogaster selected for postponed senescence. I. The longevity/flight correlation. Manuscript in preparation

GRAVES, J. L., LUCKINBILL, L. S., and NICHOLS, A. (1988) Flight duration and wing beat frequency in long-and short-lived *Drosophila melanogaster. J. Insect Physiol.* in press.

LAURIE-AHLBERG, C. C., BARNES, P. T., CURTSINGER, J. W., EMIGH, T. M., KARLIN, B., MORRIS, R., NORMAN, R. A., and WILTON, A. N. (1985) Genetic variability of flight metabolism in *Drosophila melanogaster*. II. Relationship between power output and enzyme activity levels. *Genetics* **111**: 845-868

LUCKINBILL, L. S., ARKING, R., CLARE, M. J., CIROCCO, W. C., and BUCK, S. A. (1984) Selection for delayed senescence in *Drosophila melanogaster. Evolution* **38**: 996-1003

LUCKINBILL, L. S. and CLARE, M. J. (1985) Selection for life span in *Drosophila melanogaster. Heredity* **55**: 9-18

LUCKINBILL, L. S., GRAVES, J. L., TOMKIW, A., and SOWIRKA, O. (1988) A qualitative analysis of some life history correlates of longevity in *Drosophila melanogaster. Evol. Ecol.* **2**: 85-94

ROSE, M. R. (1984) Laboratory evolution of postponed senescence in *Drosophila melanogaster. Evolution* **38**: 1004-1010

ROSE, M. R. and CHARLESWORTH, B. (1981) Genetics of life history in *Drosophila melanogaster*. II. Exploratory selection experiments. *Genetics* **97**: 187-196

ROSE. M. R., DOREY, M. L., COYLE, A. M. and SERVICE, P. M. (1984) The morphology of postponed senescence in *Drosophila melanogaster. Can. J. Zool.*. **62**: 1576-1580

SERVICE, P. M. (1987) Physiological mechanisms of increased stress resistance in *Drosophila melanogaster* selected for postponed senescence. *Physiol. Zool.* **60**: 321-326

SERVICE, P. M., HUTCHINSON, E. W., MACKINLEY, M. D., and ROSE, M. R. (1985) Resistance to environmental stress in *Drosophila melanogaster* selected for postponed senescence. *Physiol. Zool.* **58**: 380-389

WIGGLESWORTH, V. B. (1949) The utilization of reserve substances in *Drosophila* during flight. *J. Exp. Biol.* **26**: 150-163

WILLIAMS, C. M., BARNES, L. A., and SAWYER, W. H. (1943) The utilization of glycogen by flies during flight and some aspects of the physiological aging of *Drosophila. Biol. Bull. Woods Hole* **84**: 263-72

# 6

# QUANTITATIVE GENETIC ANALYSIS OF POSTPONED AGING IN *DROSOPHILA MELANOGASTER*

Edward W. Hutchinson and Michael R. Rose

## ABSTRACT

The quantitative genetics of postponed senescence in *Drosophila melanogaster* were investigated using postponed-senescence stocks created by selection and matched controls. There was little evidence of non-Mendelian inheritance, inbreeding depression, net directional dominance, or sex-linkage.

The apparently simple, additive inheritance of postponed senescence allowed the use of conventional quantitative genetic estimators for gene number. Assays of 24-hour fecundity, ovary weight, female starvation resistance, male starvation resistance, female longevity, and male longevity *did not* indicate a small number of loci involved in postponed aging.

Heritability estimates for early starvation resistance, a character closely related to longevity, revealed abundant genetic variability in selected and control lines, indicating that neither were near fixation. Selection experiments designed to push each of the two sets of lines towards fixation were performed, although a second series of heritability estimates, conducted after cessation of selection response, revealed that fixation had not occurred.

A genetic analysis was then performed on the newly selected lines. Again, there was little evidence of non-Mendelian inheritance, inbreeding depression, net directional dominance, or sex-linkage. The results for this second set of gene number experiments also did not indicate that the action of a single locus postponed senescence.

## INTRODUCTION

*Drosophila melanogaster* is one of only two species for which stocks having genetically-postponed aging are available (Rose, 1984a; Luckinbill *et al.*, 1984), the other being *Caenorhabditis elegans* (Johnson and Wood, 1982; Freidman and Johnson, 1988). These *D. melanogaster* stocks were not created by mutagenesis, but by selection on quantitative genetic variability. The use of selection is feasible for two reasons. Firstly, there is abundant quantitative genetic variability for life-history characters in outbred stocks of *Drosophila melanogaster* (Rose and Charlesworth, 1981a,b). Secondly, an indirect selection procedure can be used, in which natural selection is directed to act at later stages by the use of eggs laid by older females. When applied repeatedly over a number of generations, this type of selective screen leads to the evolution of postponed aging (Wattiaux, 1968a,b; Rose and Charlesworth, 1981b; Rose, 1984a; Luckinbill *et al.*, 1984), in which mean or maximum lifespan are increased. This procedure also allows population sizes large enough that inbreeding does not limit the gains made by selection.

The *D. melanogaster* populations that have been created using these methods have been analyzed in two different ways. Firstly, these populations have been compared with control populations, of identical origin but lacking postponed aging, with regard to morphology (Rose *et al.*, 1984; Luckinbill *et al.*, 1988a) and physiology (Service *et al.*, 1985; Service, 1987; Luckinbill et al., 1988a; Graves *et al.*, 1988). This research has endeavored to find mechanisms that could causally account for the postponed aging of the selected lines. Secondly, these populations have been examined genetically by means of biometrical analysis (Clare and Luckinbill, 1985; Luckinbill *et al.*, 1987) and chromosomal substitution (Luckinbill *et al.*, 1988b).

Table 1 provides a summary of the characteristics of short-lived (control) and long-lived stocks. For those characters which have to do with reproduction, early fecundity and early ovary weight, the short-lived stocks have higher values. For total body weight there is no difference between the stocks. For the rest of the characters (longevities, stress resistances, flight durations, and lipid contents), the long-lived stocks show higher values than the short-lived stocks. Since these findings were consistent over strains exhibiting increased lifespan, and outbred populations were used in selection, these characters are almost certainly involved in the biological changes which underlie postponed aging. There seems to have been a shift in the investment of energy from reproduction to survival capabilities.

The present article combines both the physiological and the biometrical avenues of research in an attempt to unravel the quantitative genetic basis of postponed aging in *D. melanogaster*. The basic techniques used involve crosses of populations, both within and between types of stocks. We report experiments in which: (i) the genetic variability present in postponed aging stocks was assayed by means of a sib analysis; (ii) artificial selection was applied to both control and postponed-aging stocks to make them diverge farther; (iii) sib analysis was used to assess the degree to which selection reduced genetic variability; (iv) diallel analysis and other types of population

| Table 1. Characteristics of short-lived and long-lived stocks. | | |
|---|---|---|
| Character | Short-lived "B" | Long-lived "O" |
| Generation Time | 2 weeks | 10 weeks |
| Early Fecundity [1,2,3,4,5,6,7] | + | - |
| Early Ovary Weight [6,8] | + | - |
| Female Total Body Weight [8,9] | 0 | 0 |
| Male Total Body Weight [8,9] | 0 | 0 |
| Female Longevity [1,2,3,4,5,6,9] | - | + |
| Male Longevity [9,6,10] | - | + |
| Female Starvation Resistance [6,7,11,12] | - | + |
| Male Starvation Resistance [6,11,12] | - | + |
| Female Desiccation Resistance [7,11,12] | - | + |
| Male Desiccation Resistance [11,12] | - | + |
| Female Ethanol Resistance [7,11,12] | - | + |
| Male Ethanol Resistance [11,12] | - | + |
| Female Lipid Content [12] | - | + |
| Male Lipid Content [12] | - | + |
| Female Flight Duration [9,13,14] | - | + |
| Male Flight Duration [9,13,14] | - | + |

The "+" indicates that the population type has a greater value for the character, the "-" that it has a lesser value, and the "0" that there is no statistical differentiation between the population types for that character.

[1] Rose (1984a)
[2] Rose (1984b)
[3] Luckinbill *et al.* (1984)
[4] Luckinbill and Clare (1985)
[5] Clare and Luckinbill (1985)
[6] Hutchinson and Rose (in prep.)
[7] Service *et al.* (1988)
[8] Rose et al. (1984)
[9] Luckinbill *et al.* (1988a)
[10] Service (in press)
[11] Service et al. (1985)
[12] Service (1987)
[13] Graves *et al.* (1988)
[14] Graves and Rose (this volume)

crosses were performed on the short-lived and long-lived crosses as well as on the selected lines derived from them; and (v) effective factor estimates were performed. Taken together, these results indicate additive inheritance and an absence of differentiation between lines within a given type. The number of loci involved in postponed aging in these stocks is not significantly different from infinity.

## STOCKS

### Long-lived and Short-lived Stocks

The postponed-aging stocks, called "O"s, were derived by culture selection from the Ives population studied by Rose and Charlesworth (1980, 1981a,b). The culture selection involved stock maintenance using discrete generations and females of progressively greater age. Eventually the females used were 10 weeks of age from the egg. For more details, consult Rose

(1984a) and Service *et al.* (1985). The control stocks, called "B"s, were maintained using the same media and procedures as the O stocks, except that females of 2 weeks of age were used to start the next generation. These two types of stocks exhibit those characteristics outlined in Table 1. There are 5 independent lines of each stock-type.

## Selected Stocks

The analyses of the short-lived and long-lived stocks may have been compromised since their genetic make-up is only indirectly known. Luckinbill *et al.* (1988a), using chromosome replacement, investigated the chromosomal location of the alleles contributing to postponed aging in *D. melanogaster*. They found that all three major chromosomes affected the character, but that some chromosomes from the stocks exhibiting postponed aging actually decreased longevity. This suggests the possibility of inconsistent differentiation between stock-types, a vitiating problem for effective factor estimation (Lande, 1981). Further selection would therefore be useful in providing selected stocks that are more differentiated from their controls, with reduced genetic polymorphism.

Three O stocks ($O_1$, $O_2$, and $O_3$) and three B stocks ($B_1$, $B_2$, and $B_3$) were therefore subject to selection for two different characters, early starvation resistance and early fecundity, respectively. The rationale for this is that O stocks have enhanced early starvation resistance relative to B stocks (Service *et al.*, 1985), while B stocks have enhanced early fecundity relative to O stocks (Rose, 1984a). More extreme differentiation is thereby obtainable by selecting further in those directions. In addition, since there is a negative additive genetic correlation between these characters of large magnitude (Service and Rose, 1985), selecting up on early fecundity should depress early starvation resistance and conversely.

In both cases, selection proceeded with three control lines matched to each of the three selection lines for the first 12 generations. Subsequently, the controls were dropped and a reduced level of selection was maintained for an additional 12 generations. Truncation selection was used, with the top 20 % of the mid-parent values being used to create the next generation, for the first 12 generations, with 50 % selection thereafter. In the case of selection on early starvation resistance, which is tested destructively, the progeny of each couple were obtained before selection. Details of the selection procedure are given in Hutchinson *et al.* (in prep.). The lines produced by selection for early fecundity are designated "F" lines and the lines produced by selection for early starvation resistance are designated "S" lines. Figure 1 illustrates the relationships between the various stocks created. In terms of notation, the $F_i$ popula-

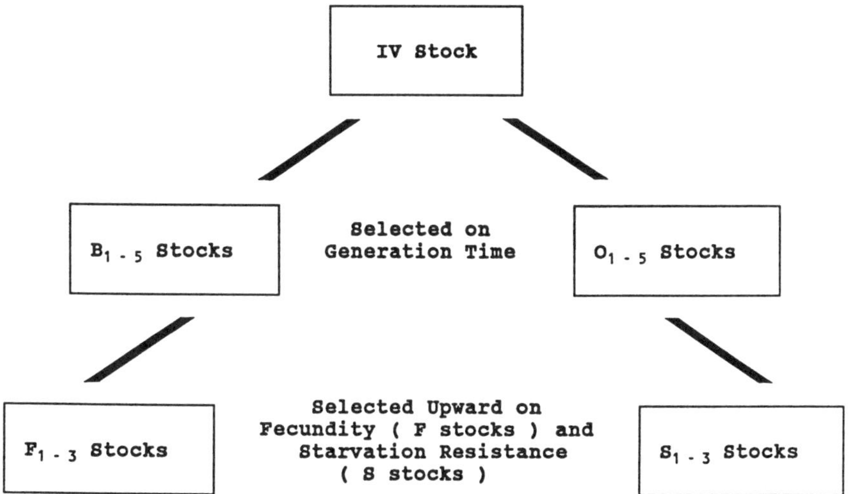


**Figure 1**. Creation of Short-Lived (B) and Long-Lived (O), and their derived Selected Stocks (F and S, respectively).

tion underwent derivation from the $B_i$ population, specifically, and similarly for the $S_i$ relative to the $O_i$.

Artificial selection produced significant direct responses to selection, as shown in Figures 2 and 3, which plot the generations for which the controls were retained. While there is always some variation in population averages from assay to assay, the O's have mean early starvation resistance levels from 30-40 hours, while the S's have early starvation resistances of 50-60 hours, almost a doubling. The F fecundities were increased by about 10 eggs per day over the mean fecundities of the B populations.

The realized heritability (*vid.* Falconer, 1981) for selection on early fecundity was $0.058 \pm 0.001$ (mean $\pm$ standard error). The realized heritability for selection on early starvation resistance was $0.203 \pm 0.004$. These findings indicate that the B and O populations were indeed polymorphic for the alleles involved.

## 24 HOUR FECUNDITY

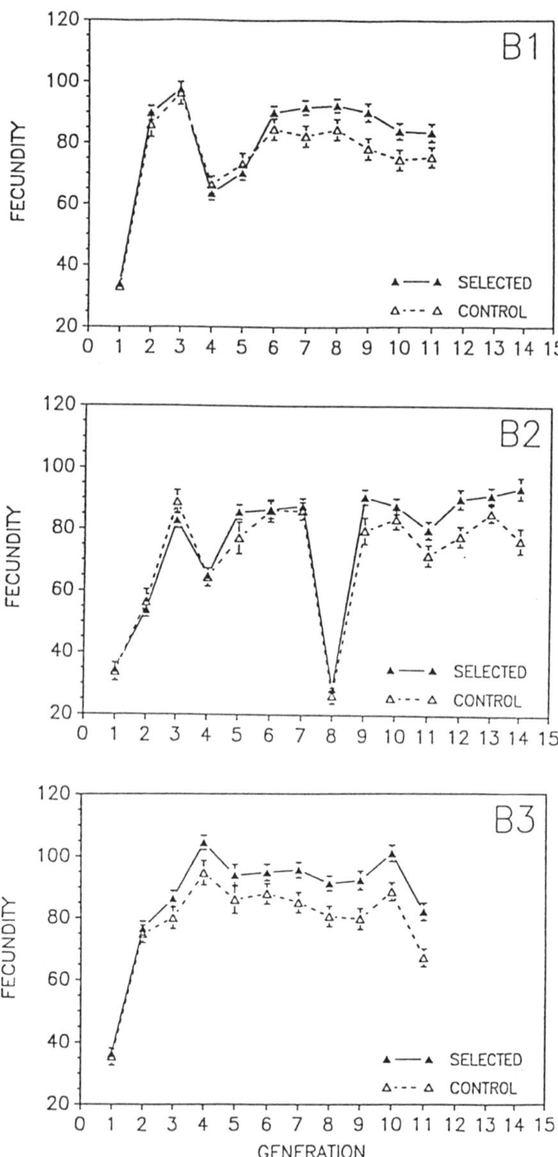


**Figure 2.** Direct response of the three B populations to selection for increased early fecundity. The selected group is represented by solid triangles connected by a solid line and the control group is represented by empty triangles connected by a dashed line. The 95% confidence intervals are shown around the means.

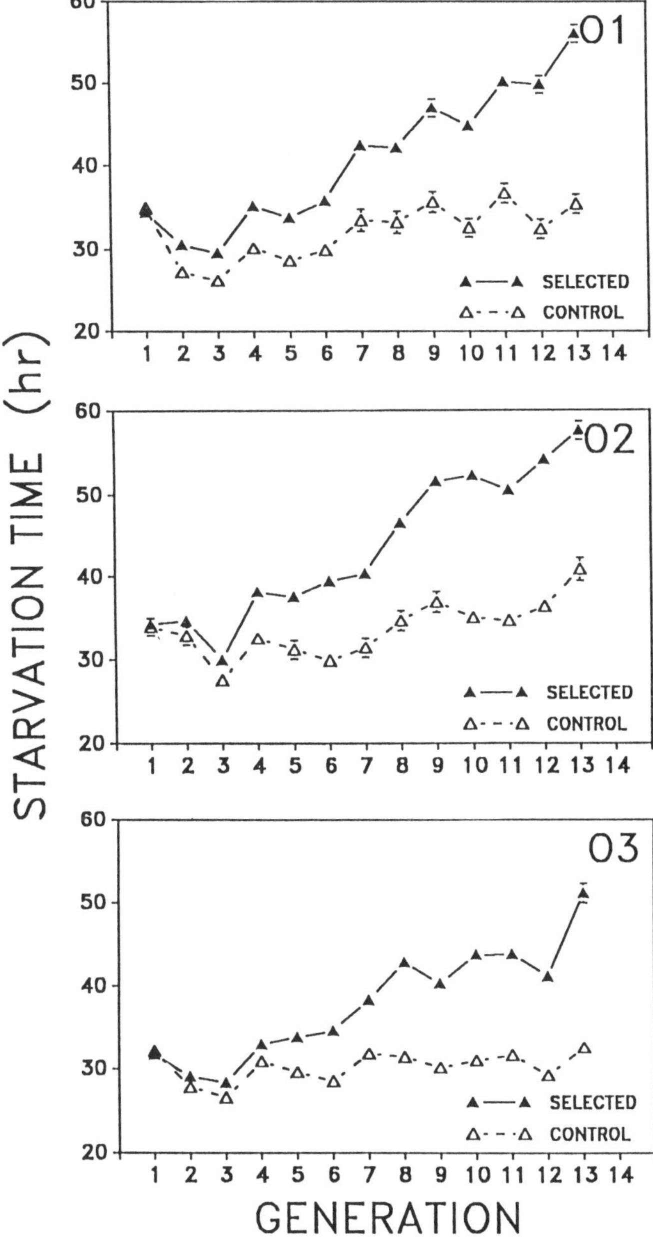



**Figure 3.** Direct response of the three O populations to selection for increased early starvation resistance. Symbols and lines are as in figure 5. Some of the 95% confidence interval bars are too small to show on the graph.

The total number of observations made in the course of the selection experiments exceeded 70,000.

## ASSAYS

All assayed flies were reared at a controlled density of either 30 or 90 larvae per 25 × 95 mm shell vial. The density was constant in any one experiment. Longevity, in both male and females, was measured in groups of flies transferred every 3 or 4 days. Fecundity was measured as the total number of eggs laid in 24 hours by one female, aged 3-5 days from pupal eclosion. Ovaries were dissected from females also aged 3-4 days, dried for 24 hours, and then weighed separately using a Cahn electronic microbalance, as in Rose *et al.* (1984). Starvation resistance was measured in both male and female flies aged 3-5 days. Flies were kept in vials without medium but with a source of constant humidity, as in Service *et al.* (1985). The time was recorded when the flies were dead, as determined by lack of movement, upon provocation.

## SIB ANALYSIS

Sib analysis was performed on the stocks before and after selection twice, making a total of twelve sib analyses. In each of these analyses, 50 sires were mated to 12 dams each, and a single progeny was obtained from each dam for assay. For details of the sib analysis, see Hutchinson *et al.* (in prep.). Components of variance were calculated using the standard quantitative genetics half-sib design (Falconer, 1981), from which heritabilities are readily determined.

### Sib Analysis Before Selection

The mean heritabilities ± standard error in the B stocks are 0.747 ± 0.325 for female early starvation resistance and 0.177 ± 0.118 for male starvation resistance. In the O lines, the mean heritabilities are 0.842 ± 0.273 and 0.592 ± 0.279 for female and male starvation resistance, respectively. These heritability estimates suggest that there has not been fixation of alleles involved in postponed aging. These findings motivated our artificial selection study.

### Sib Analysis After Selection

The mean heritabilities ± standard error in the F stocks are 0.425 ± 0.020 for female early starvation resistance and 0.370 ± 0.058 for male starvation resistance. In the S stocks the mean heritabilities are 0.516 ± 0.205 and 0.463 ± 0.057 for female and male starvation resistance, respectively. Therefore, in spite of the considerable increases in early starvation resistance among the Ss and increases in early fecundity among the Fs, there has been no statistical reduction in heritabilities among these populations. (This was tested using both pooled-group and paired-difference t-tests.) The reason for the reduction in the standard errors of the heritabilities is unclear. In any case, artificial selection failed to eliminate genetic variability within the F and S lines. However, these lines are considerably farther apart after selection, offering some hope of clearer results from population crosses. This lack of fixation in the presence of such a strong response to selection can be interpreted as evidence for the presence of many genes, since selection limits are less readily attainable the greater the number of loci involved (Falconer, 1981).

## DIALLEL ANALYSIS

A series of diallel analyses (*cf.* Mather and Jinks, 1982) were performed to test for heterogeneity among lines of a given type. In a diallel design, all possible crosses are performed between a set of populations, including the distinct reciprocal crosses.

There are two separate questions which are addressed in the diallel analysis. Firstly, is there any evidence for heterosis, or conversely inbreeding depression, in crosses between lines within stock-types? Secondly, to what extent are the lines within a stock-type differentiated from each other?

### Diallel Analysis of B and O Stocks

The results (Hutchinson and Rose, in prep.) consistently indicate an absence of heterosis. Table 2, giving line and crossed-line means for female early starvation resistance among the O populations, illustrates the kind of data obtained. These data were analyzed using analysis of variance designs with nesting as well as t-tests. In the present example, there was no significant heterosis effect nor was there a significant effect of the line of origin of father or mother (p > 0.05). In no case, over all crosses, was there any evidence of heteorsis. In a few cases there were significant line-of-origin effects, but in general, there is an absence of reproducible line effects, suggesting that there is no significant differentiation between lines within stock-types.

### Diallel Analysis of F and S Stocks

The results of the diallel analysis of F and S stocks (Hutchinson *et al.*, in prep.) are essentially the same as for the B and O stocks. In one case out of 16, female early starvation resistance exhibited significant heterosis. This was the only significant heterosis out of a total of 25 tests, with p < 0.05, which is about what would be expected by chance alone. Again, there were some cases

| Male Parent | Female Parent | | | | | Mean |
|---|---|---|---|---|---|---|
| | B1 | B2 | B3 | B4 | B5 | |
| B1 | 40.0 ± 1.5<br>52 | 37.9 ± 1.4<br>56 | 34.7 ± 1.2<br>56 | 34.1 ± 1.1<br>52 | 37.8 ± 2.0<br>56 | 36.9 ± 1.1<br>5 |
| B2 | 37.0 ± 1.5<br>56 | 45.0 ± 1.4<br>56 | 41.4 ± 1.3<br>52 | 39.7 ± 1.4<br>56 | 46.0 ± 1.7<br>56 | 41.8 ± 1.7<br>5 |
| B3 | 35.8 ± 0.9<br>56 | 39.6 ± 1.1<br>5 | 33.9 ± 1.2<br>56 | 38.2 ± 1.4<br>56 | 41.1 ± 2.2<br>56 | 37.7 ± 1.3<br>5 |
| B4 | 36.0 ± 1.2<br>56 | 38.6 ± 1.16<br>48 | 34.9 ± 1.4<br>52 | 37.8 ± 1.3<br>56 | 34.7 ± 1.5<br>52 | 36.4 ± 0.8<br>5 |
| B5 | 36.9 ± 1.5<br>56 | 39.8 ± 1.2<br>52 | 35.3 ± 1.9<br>56 | 43.1 ± 1.8<br>56 | 32.9 ± 0.9<br>56 | 37.6 ± 1.8<br>5 |
| Mean[*] | 37.2 ± 0.8<br>5 | 40.2 ± 1.2<br>5 | 36.1 ± 1.4<br>5 | 38.6 ± 1.5<br>5 | 39.9 ± 2.4<br>5 | 38.1 ± 0.3<br>1368 |

**Table 2.** Diallel Analysis.

Mean female starvation time (hours), standard errors, and number of individuals in the $B_i \times B_j$ diallel cross. The parental crosses are along the diagonal and the reciprocal hybrid crosses are above and below the diagonal.

of line-of-origin effects being significant, but these did not hold up over the experimental tests. This could be a reflection of the fact that choice of parent is confounded with line-of-origin in our analysis. As before, simple additive inheritance seems to arise.

## TRANSMISSION PATTERN EXPERIMENTS

In the transmission pattern experiments, B and O stocks (or F and S stocks) were crossed between lines, $B_1$ with $O_1$, $B_2$ with $O_2$, etc. The parental populations as well as both the reciprocal cross populations of the $F_1$ hybrids were then assayed for all six characters (male longevity, female longevity, female early starvation resistance, male early starvation resistance, early fecundity, and early ovary weight). Three features of the transmission data are of importance: (i) preservation of the B-O differences that had been detected before and documentation of the F-S differences; (ii) average dominance, as measured by the deviation of the crosses from the mid-parent value; and (iii) maternal effects, as measured by differences between two reciprocal cross means.

### Transmission Patterns of B and O Stocks

The results of a transmission pattern experiment on female longevity are shown in Table 3. The results indicate that the character differences have been preserved (p < 0.001). There is no evidence of significant dominance devia-

| Table 3. Transmission patterns. | | | | |
|---|---|---|---|---|
| Replicate | BB | BO | OB | OO |
| 1 | 60.7 ± 1.7 | 66.6 ± 1.9 | 56.4 ± 2.4 | 71.3 ± 2.0 |
|   | 60 | 60 | 60 | 60 |
| 2 | 46.7 ± 1.4 | 53.4 ± 1.9 | 50.0 ± 1.7 | 55.1 ± 1.7 |
|   | 60 | 60 | 60 | 60 |
| 3 | 49.5 ± 1.7 | 54.6 ± 1.7 | 51.9 ± 1.9 | 64.4 ± 2.3 |
|   | 60 | 60 | 60 | 60 |
| 4 | 47.2 ± 1.9 | 59.5 ± 2.1 | 58.0 ± 2.8 | 59.6 ± 2.8 |
|   | 60 | 60 | 30 | 30 |
| 5 | 46.3 ± 1.8 | 54.5 ± 2.0 | 63.3 ± 2.4 | 62.2 ± 2.3 |
|   | 60 | 60 | 60 | 60 |
| Mean | 50.1 ± 2.4 | 57.7 ± 2.2 | 55.9 ± 2.1 | 62.5 ± 2.4 |
|   | 5 | 5 | 5 | 5 |

tion or maternal effects. Figure 4 plots these results, showing the pattern of survivorship for the parental populations and their reciprocal crossed populations. The two parental populations, B and O, are well separated with the reciprocal crossed populations falling in between. These results clearly indicate the absence of inbreeding depression in the experimental populations, in that no hybrid means exceed the greatest parental mean. In general, the transmission data indicate additive inheritance without reproducible maternal effects or heterosis.

## Transmission Patterns of F and S Stocks

With the more differentiated F and S lines, there is the prospect of greater clarity in the transmission pattern results. Most of the tests for significant differentiation of F and S populations yield statistical significance (Hutchinson *et al.* in prep.). All the tests for maternal effects give non-significant results, excepting only male starvation resistance, in which the result was not consistent over experiments. There was only one case of significant dominance effects, for female starvation resistance, and this result was not reproduced in four other experiments.

## EFFECTIVE FACTOR ESTIMATION

Experiments were performed to estimate the number of "effective factors" (Lande, 1981) involved in postponed aging. Effective factors are loci of "equivalent effect" that are responsible for the differentiation of a quantitative character between two populations. These experiments have the same design as the transmission pattern experiments, except that $F_2$'s were obtained from the $F_1$'s of the B and O stocks and from the $F_1$'s of the F and S stocks. Two

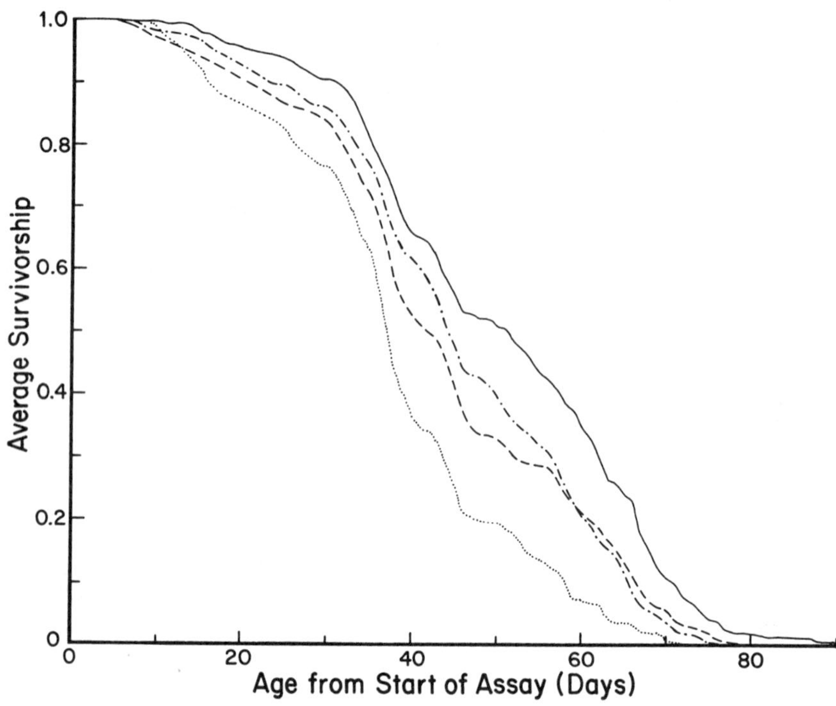



**Figure 4.** Survivorship curves for the O populations (solid line), the two reciprocal cross B x O populations (dashed and dashed-dot lines), and the B populations (dotted line), according to adult age from the start of assay.

separate sets of estimates were calculated. One for the differentiation between the B and O lines and one for the differentiation of the F and S lines. Effective factor estimates were calculated from the formula (Lande 1981)

$$n_e = (m_1 - m_2)^2 / 8V_s$$

where $m_i$ gives the mean of one of the parental populations and $V_s$ gives the segregation variance, where

$$V_s = Var(F_2) - Var(F_1)$$

This method of factor estimation is based on the relationship between parental and hybrid crosses with respect to their means and variances (Figure 5). It should be noted that the method hinges on the basic Mendelian phenomenon of $F_2$ segregation giving rise to increased variance relative to

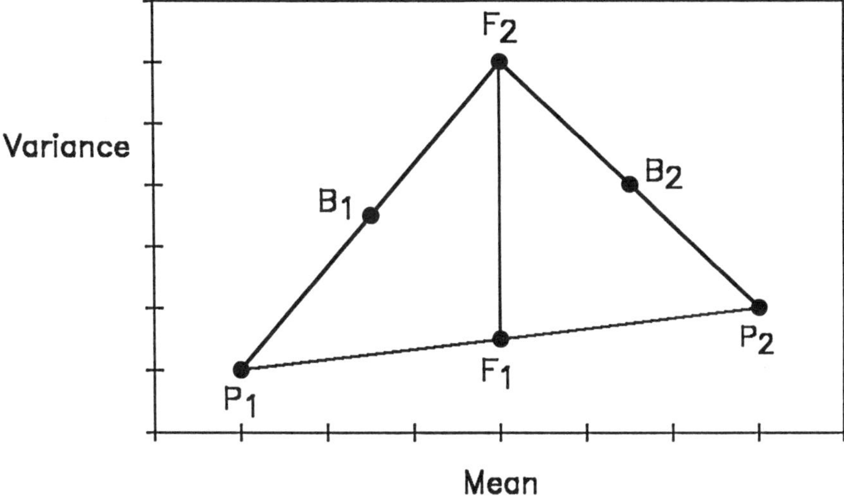


**Figure 5**. Relationship between parental lines (P1 and P2), hybrid crosses ($F_1$ and $F_2$), and backcrosses ($B_1$ and $B_2$) with respect to the means and variances of a quantitative character.

that of the $F_1$. In particular, with an infinite number of loci, we expect to have the $F_1$ and $F_2$ variances equal to each other.

As well as the $n_e$ estimates, we calculated the inverse estimates

$$1/n_e = 8V_s / (m_1 - m_2)^2$$

The reason for this is that there is a mathematical singularity in $n_e$ when $V_s = 0$. When $V_s$ is just above zero, $n_e$ diverges to positive infinity. When $V_s$ is just below zero, $n_e$ diverges to negative infinity. Figure 6 illustrates this situation. There is also the problem of interpreting negative values of $n_e$ when the data are replicated (*cf.* Luckinbill *et al.*, 1987). When $1/n_e$ is used as a test statistic, none of these problems arise, providing only that there is in fact differentiation between the parental lines under consideration. [And this proviso is almost always taken care in this type of experiment.] Figure 7 illustrates the function of $1/n_e$ against Vars. In addition, when $1/n_e = 0$, we must have $n_e$ approaching infinity. This is an appropriate null hypothesis, because $n_e$ is biased toward small values (Lande, 1981). Effectively, it constitutes a lower bound on the actual number of loci involved in population

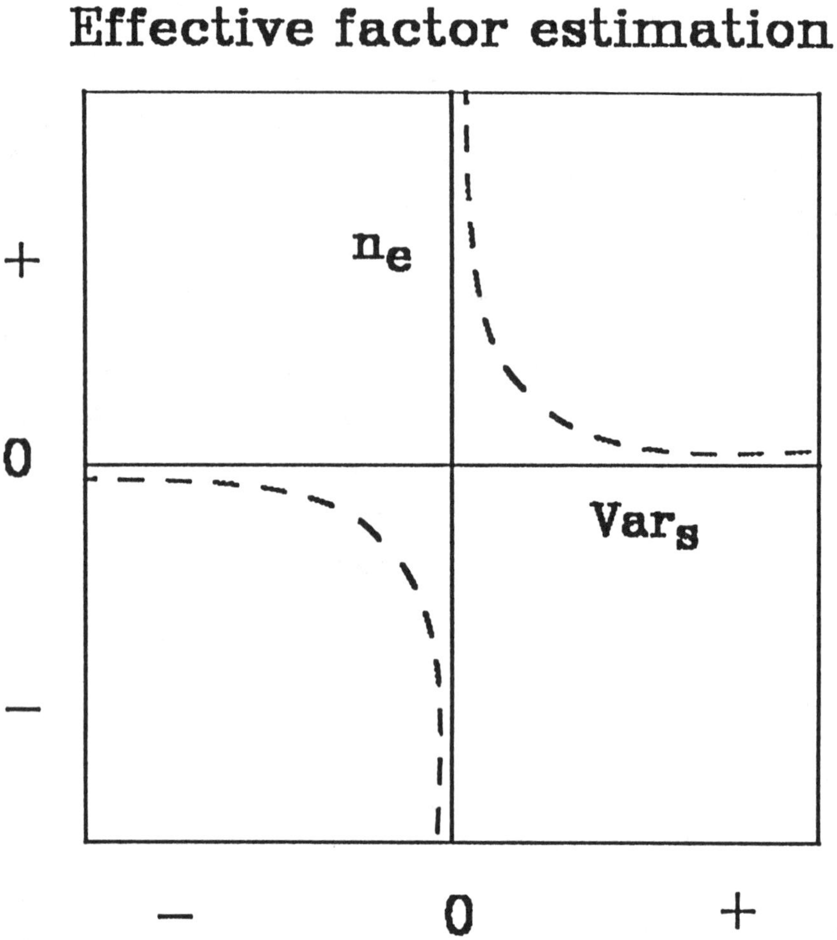

# Effective factor estimation

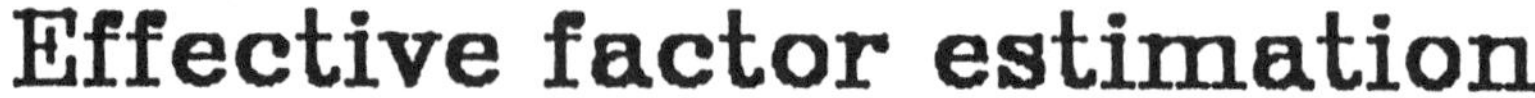


**Figure 6.** Effective Factor Estimation. Illustration of the general form of the function relating the number of effective factors, $n_e$, to the segregation variance, $V_{ars}$.

differentiation. Testing $1/n_e$ for significant deviation above zero tests whether or not there is any statistical reason to conclude that there are fewer than an arbitrarily large number of loci involved in population differentiation.

The factor effective number estimates for the B-O experiments are summarized in Table 4. They suggest that there are a small number of loci involved. The mean $n_e$ values over replicates tend to be below 1. It is only

# Inverse effective factor estimation

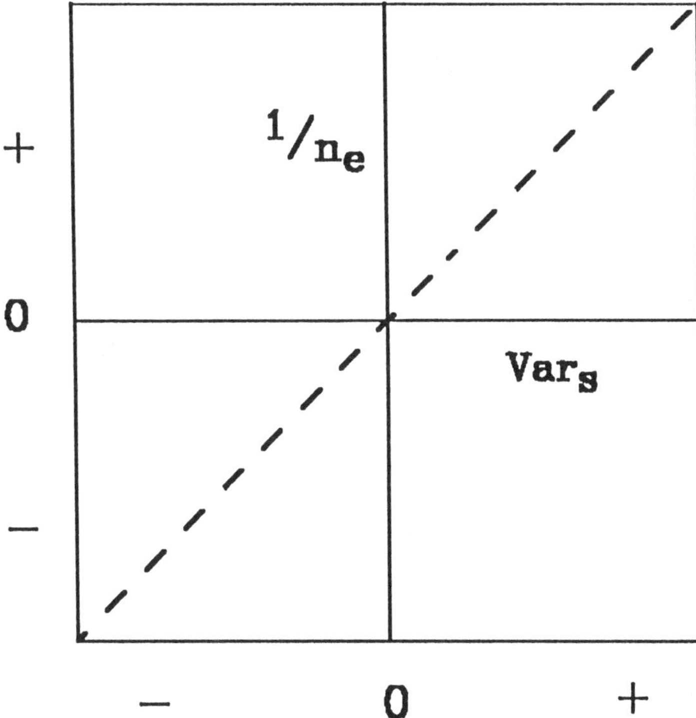


**Figure 7.** Inverse Effective Factor Estimation. Illustration of the general form of the function relating the inverse of the number of effective factors, $1/n_e$, to the segregation variance, $V_{ars}$.

once the inverse $n_e$ values are considered statistically that the results can be seen to be misleading. The $1/n_e$ estimates are not significantly different from zero in almost all cases. This different behavior probably arises from the role of the negative estimates in the two cases. Negative $n_e$ data decrease the average $n_e$ value, biasing the results toward underestimates, even though the negative data in fact indicate a large number of segregating factors. In the inverse effective factor data, negative estimates pull the mean toward zero, indicating more effective factors, which is the appropriate effect. Taken together, the results indicate the involvement of many loci in the postponed aging of the O stocks, relative to the B stocks.

**Table 4.** Effective factor estimates and inverse effective factor estimates for the B and O population cross experiments.

| Character  Experiment | Effective Factors<br>Mean ± SEM | Inverse Effective Factors<br>Mean± SEM |
|---|---|---|
| Ovary Weight | | |
| GN1 | 0.22 ± 0.19 | -3.67 ± 5.73 |
| Fecundity | | |
| GN2 | 0.02 ± 0.02 | 105 ± 105 |
| GN3 | 0.20 ± 0.36 | 10.46 ± 11.52 |
| Female Starvation | | |
| GN1 | 0.07 ± 0.03 | -1023 ± 1039 |
| GN2 | 0.19 ± 0.07 | 7.07 ± 2.55 |
| GN3 | 0.02 ± 0.58 | 1.50 ± 1.78 |
| Male Starvation | | |
| GN1 | 0.36 ± 0.24 | 1.46 ± 1.11 |
| GN2 | 0.72 ± 1.23 | 0.48 ± 0.76 |
| GN3 | -3.07 ± 3.86 | 0.88 ± 0.52 |
| Female Longevity | | |
| GN2 | 0.43 ± 0.25 | -5.19 ± 5.84 |
| GN3 | -0.19 ± 0.29 | -0.55 ± 1.55 |
| Male Longevity | | |
| GN2 | 0.61 ± 2.93 | 0.14 ± 0.17 |
| GN3 | -0.59 ± 3.78 | 0.18 ± 0.15 |

The factor effective number estimates for the F-S experiments are summarized in Table 5. Many of the effective factor number estimates obtained from crosses of F and S lines are negative or take on positive values greater than one, unlike the data from the B and O populations. There are only two cases, fecundity in experiment GN1 and female starvation in experiment GN2, having statistical evidence for fewer than an arbitrarily large number of loci involved in the differentiation of F and S stocks. In both cases the effective factor estimates indicate at least two loci. [It should be borne in mind that this is a systematic underestimate (*cf.* Lande, 1981).] Whatever is made of these two cases having a significantly small number of contributing loci, in general the F-S results indicate a large number of loci contributing to the differentiation of the suite of postponed aging characters.

| Table 5. Effective factor estimates and inverse effective factor estimates for the F and S population cross experiments. | | |
|---|---|---|
| Character Experiment | Effective Factors<br>Mean ± SEM | Inverse Effective Factors<br>Mean ± SEM |
| Fecundity | | |
| GN1 | 2.11 ± 0.73 | 0.64 ± 0.25 |
| GN2 | -0.01 ± 0.36 | 1.96 ± 1.93 |
| GN3 | -0.12 ± 0.21 | -1.38 ± 2.68 |
| Female Starvation | | |
| GN1 | -4.38 ± 16.27 | 0.50 ± 0.49 |
| GN2 | 1.75 ± 0.65 | 0.73 ± 0.21 |
| GN3 | 2.25 ± 1.00 | 0.64 ± 0.24 |
| Male Starvation | | |
| GN1 | 2.01 ± 0.80 | 1.07 ± 0.71 |
| GN2 | -0.14 ± 1.43 | 0.47 ± 0.44 |
| GN3 | 75.17 ± 76.52 | 0.17 ± 0.30 |
| Female Longevity | | |
| GN1 | -1.15 ± 0.89 | 0.61 ± 1.31 |
| GN2 | -4.53 ± 4.48 | 0.31 ± 1.87 |
| GN3 | 0.84 ± 1.42 | -1.15 ± 0.77 |
| Male Longevity | | |
| GN1 | -1.89 ± 1.80 | 0.02 ± 0.34 |
| GN2 | 9.14 ± 12.04 | 0.49 ± 0.77 |
| GN3 | -0.77 ± 1.14 | -0.13 ± 0.40 |

## DISCUSSION

There is little evidence in these results that suggests anything other than polygenic additive inheritance in the laboratory evolution of postponed senescence in the *D. melanogaster* stocks studied. Maternal or line effects, when present, are inconsistent over lines and characters. On average, hybrids of postponed-aging and control stocks appear to be intermediate; there is no consistent heterosis, inbreeding depression, or directional dominance. There is no statistical evidence that the results indicate a small number of loci involved in postponed aging. In general the characters examined seem to be classic "quantitative characters" (Falconer, 1981).

These results may be compared with those found by Luckinbill and co-workers. Like Clare and Luckinbill (1985), who studied fewer characters, fewer lines, and far fewer individuals, we find essentially additive inheritance in population crosses. Like Luckinbill *et al.* (1987), we found small estimates of effective factor number. However, we disagree with the interpretation that they give to their findings. They discarded negative estimates of $n_e$, failing to treat them as evidence for a large number of effective factors. Our method of averaging inverse effective factor estimates gives us hypothesis tests which are not as biased toward the conclusion that only a few loci are involved in the differentiation of the populations crossed. Our actual results, then, are not particularly different from those of Luckinbill *et al.* (1987); only our analysis is. Our findings fit those of Luckinbill *et al.* (1988b), who found evidence in at least some of their experiments for a hereditary contribution of all three major *D. melanogaster* chromosomes to postponed aging. This conclusion is incompatible with that of Luckinbill *et al.* (1987), in that it suggests that there are *at least* three contributory loci for postponed aging, and probably many more.

These studies, taken together, are simple in their implications: aging in laboratory cultures of *D. melanogaster* cultured from older females only, for a number of generations, appears to be postponed as a result of allele frequency changes at at least a moderate number of loci, those alleles having additive effects on average. There is no reproducible evidence for any type of maternal, or other non-genetic, effect. These findings also do not support the possibility of large epistatic effects on aging, since such effects would normally preclude additive inheritance.

What is the significance of all of these *Drosophila* results for our understanding of the genetics of aging in general? Firstly, what of the many known alleles, from that which causes Huntington's chorea in man to those aberrant mutants in *Drosophila* with shortened lifespan? These alleles are often supposed to cause "accelerated aging", and taken as evidence for few controlling elements for the aging process. In both man (e.g. Martin, 1978) and *Drosophila* (Hutchinson and Rose, 1987), mutants of this kind are only doubtfully aging mutants. They may kill adults, and induce chronic pathologies, but that is not evidence that they affect aging itself. Close inspection of their pathophysiology reveals a number of disparities with "normal aging" (Martin, 1978). Therefore, those alleles do not clash with the present conclusions, because they are of no genuine relevance to the genetic dissection of aging.

Secondly, are there any known alleles which can postpone aging in any model system? Such alleles are known in both *D. subobscura* (Maynard Smith, 1958) and *Caenorhabditis elegans* (Friedman and Johnson, 1988). In both these cases, lifespan is increased by homozygosity of a single allele as much or more than it is in the *D. melanogaster* stocks of Rose (1984a) or

Luckinbill *et al.* (1984). Interestingly, in both these cases, reproduction is greatly decreased in the longer-lived mutant strain. The *D. subobscura* mutants are in fact completely sterile (Maynard Smith, 1958). In a physiological sense, these other studies corroborate the results of Rose and Charlesworth (1981a,1981b), Rose (1984a), and Luckinbill and Clare (1985) in finding a clear association between postponed aging and reduced early reproduction.

Thirdly, is there any likelihood that the *D. melanogaster* results will prove to be generally true of the genetics of aging? We would argue that the present finding of polygenic inheritance is indeed quite likely to hold. Many loci are likely to affect later survival and reproduction, because survival and reproduction are the ends which natural selection strives toward. Loci which do not have alleles that directly or indirectly foster survival or reproduction are not going to be preserved, because natural selection will not oppose the accumulation of silencing mutations at those loci. Maintenance of polymorphism at those loci affecting aging is likely, because both of the population genetic mechanisms of aging, antagonistic pleiotropy (Williams, 1957; Rose, 1985) and mutation-accumulation (Medawar, 1952; Edney and Gill, 1968; Charlesworth, 1980), act to maintain genetic polymorphism. Antagonistic pleiotropy does so by generating overdominance and its higher-order analogues for fitness (Rose, 1982; Rose, 1985), without necessarily requiring dominance for individual character other than fitness. Mutation-accumulation does so because it allows deleterious mutations affecting later survival and reproduction to drift to high frequencies, because of the weakness of natural selection at later ages (Charlesworth, 1980). Therefore, almost all outbred species are likely to have allelic variation affecting aging at a great many loci, allelic variation which could be selected so as to postpone aging.

A case in point would be mammalian systems; these could readily be analyzed using all the same methods presented here and in Rose (this volume) and Graves and Rose (this volume) for *Drosophila*. Rose (1988) has argued strongly for this line of research as the most promising way to advance our knowledge of mammalian aging. The critical questions in any such experimental program are not fundamental scientific ones, since those are much more readily addressed using *Drosophila*. Rather, the problems of selective breeding rodents primarily revolve around the feasibility of specific experimental designs and the ways in which the resultant stocks could be analyzed. These are questions to be addressed by those working with rodents. In principle, the *Drosophila* findings show that stocks with postponed senescence are readily produced, though the genetic differentiation of such stocks depends on a number of genetic loci acting via a variety of different physiological mechanisms (*cf.* Service *et al.*, 1988). The detection of such loci and the determination of their specific mechanisms of action is the next major fundamental scientific problem in this area.

## ACKNOWLEDGEMENTS

The authors are grateful to P. M. Service for help in the planning, execution, and interpretation of the present experiments. We thank D. Arab, H. Gillis, G. Glazov, K. Grimm, L. E. Johnston, S. Johnson, D. M. Lane, J. Judah, M. D. MacKinley, B. Musgrave, J. Nelson, S. O'Keefe, D. Pringle, A. J. Shaw, B. Singh, D. Stewart, and B. Tremblay for technical assistance. This research was supported by NSERC of Canada grant U0178 and PHS grant AG06346 to MRR.

## REFERENCES

CHARLESWORTH, B. (1980) *Evolution in age-structured populations*. Cambridge: Cambridge University Press.

CLARE, M. J. and LUCKINBILL, L. S. (1985) The effects of gene-environment interaction on the expression of longevity. *Heredity* **55**: 19-29

EDNEY, E. B. and GILL, R. W. (1968) Evolution of senescence and specific longevity. *Nature* **220**: 281-282

FALCONER, D. S. (1981) *Introduction to Quantitative Genetics*. Ed. 2. London and New York: Longman.

FRIEDMAN, D. B. and JOHNSON, T. E. (1988) A mutation in the age-1 gene in *Caenorhabditis elegans* lengthens life and reduces hermaphrodite fertility. *Genetics* **118**: 75-86

GRAVES, J. L., LUCKINBILL, L. S. and NICHOLS, A. (1988) Flight duration and wing beat frequency in long-and short-lived *Drosophila melanogaster. J. Ins. Physiol.* **34**: 1021-1026

HUTCHINSON, E. W. and ROSE, M. R. (1987) Genetics of aging in insects. *Review of Biological Research in Aging* **3**: 63-70

JOHNSON, T. E. and WOOD, W. B. (1982) Genetic analysis of life-span in *Caenorhabditis elegans. Proc. Natl. Acad. Sci. USA* **79**: 6603-6607

LANDE, R. (1981) The minimum number of genes contributing to quantitative variation between and within populations. *Genetics* **99**: 541-553

LUCKINBILL, L. S., ARKING, R., CLARE, M. J., CIROCCO, W. C. and BUCK, S. A. (1984) Selection for delayed senescence in *Drosophila melanogaster. Evolution* **8**: 996-1003

LUCKINBILL, L. S. and CLARE, M. J. (1985) The effects of gene environment interaction on the expression of longevity. *Heredity* **55**: 19-29

LUCKINBILL, L. S., CLARE, M. J., KRELL, W. L., CIROCCO, W. C. and RICHARDS, P. A. (1987) Estimating the number of genetic elements that defer senescence in *Drosophila. Evol. Ecol.* **1**: 37-46

LUCKINBILL, L. S., GRAVES, J. L., TOMKIW, A. and SOWIRKA, O. (1988a) A qualitative analysis of life history characters in *Drosophila melanogaster. Evol. Ecol.* **2**: 85-94

LUCKINBILL, L. S., GRAVES, J. L., REED, A. H. and KOETSAWANG, S. (1988b) Localizing genes that defer senescence in *Drosophila melanogaster. Heredity* **60**: 367-374

MARTIN, G. M. (1978) Genetic syndromes in man with potential relevance to the pathobiology of aging. *Nat. Found.* **14**: 5-39

MATHER, K. and JINKS, J. L. (1982) *Biometrical genetics*. Ed. 3. London: Chapman and Hall.

MAYNARD SMITH, J. (1958) The effects of temperature and of egg-laying on the longevity of *Drosophila subobscura. J. Exp. Biol.* **35**: 832-842

MEDAWAR, P. B. (1952) *An unsolved problem of biology.* London: H.K. Lewis.

ROSE, M. R. (1982) Antagonistic pleiotropy, dominance, and genetic variation. *Heredity* **48**: 63-78

ROSE, M. R. (1984a) Laboratory evolution of postponed senescence in *Drosophila melanogaster. Evolution* **38**: 1004-1010

ROSE, M. R. (1984b) Artificial selection on a fitness-component in *Drosophila melanogaster. Evolution* **38**: 516-526

ROSE, M. R. (1985) Life history evolution with antagonistic pleiotropy and overlapping generations. *Theor. Pop. Biol.* **28**: 342-358

ROSE, M. R. (1988) Response to "Thoughts on the selection of longer-lived rodents" - rejoinders. *Growth Devel. Aging* **52**: 209-211

ROSE, M. R. and CHARLESWORTH, B. (1980) A test of evolutionary theories of senescence. *Nature* **287**: 141-142

ROSE, M. R. and CHARLESWORTH, B. (1981a) Genetics of life history in *Drosophila melanogaster.* I. Sib analysis of adult females. *Genetics* **97**: 173-186

ROSE, M. R. and CHARLESWORTH, B. (1981b) Genetics of life history in *Drosophila melanogaster.* II. Exploratory selection experiments. *Genetics* **97**: 187-196

ROSE, M. R., DOREY, M. L., COYLE, A. M. and SERVICE, P. M. (1984) The morphology of postponed senescence in *Drosophila melanogaster. Can. J. Zool.* **62**: 1576-1580

SERVICE, P. M. (1987) Physiological mechanisms of increased stress resistance in *Drosophila melanogaster* selected for postponed senescence. *Physiol. Zool.* **58**: 380-389

SERVICE, P. M., HUTCHINSON, E. W., MACKINLEY, M. D. and ROSE, M. R. (1985) Resistance to environmental stress in *Drosophila melanogaster* selected for postponed senescence. *Physiol. Zool.* **58**: 380-389

SERVICE, P. M., HUTCHINSON, E. W. and ROSE, M. R. (1988) Multiple genetic mechanisms for the evolution of senescence in *Drosophila melanogaster. Evolution* **42**: 708-716

SERVICE, P. M. and ROSE, M. R. (1985) Genetic covariation among life-history components: the effect of novel environments. *Evolution* **39**: 943-945

WATTIAUX, J. M. (1968a) Parental age effects in *Drosophila pseudoobscura. Exp. Gerontol.* **3**: 55-61

WATTIAUX, J. M. (1968b) Cumulative parental age effects in *Drosophila subobscura. Evolution* **22**: 406-421

WILLIAMS, G. C. (1957) Pleiotropy, natural selection, and the evolution of senescence. *Evolution* **11**: 398-411

# 7

## COMMENTARY - SELECTION FOR LONGER-LIVED RODENTS[1]

David E. Harrison

Recently, GDA sponsored a Genetics Effects on Aging Conference, with the emphasis on future work in mammals, but including advanced genetic studies in *Drosophila* and other model systems. The successful selection experiments for increased longevity in *Drosophila* by Rose and Charlesworth, and by Luckinbill *et al.*, caused vigorous discussions as to whether such experiments were feasible in mammals, especially in mice. These discussions were dominated by researchers close to the *Drosophila* experiments, who urged mammalian researchers to undertake selection for late female fecundity, the procedure that had produced extended *Drosophila* longevities. In response Dr. Johnson urged caution, summarizing reasons why selection might not be practical in mice. Dr. Rose answered these points, and their presentations are given together, both to stimulate further debate, and to assure that selection in mice, if done, is done under optimal conditions.

Everyone agrees that mice with substantially increased longevities would be extremely valuable to analyze mechanisms by which mammalian longevities can be increased. Intraspecies comparisons might be much clearer than those between long- and short-lived species, since it is very difficult to determine which of the many differences between species are responsible for the differences in longevity.

Everyone also agrees that strong selective advantages eventually can find ways to increase longevity. The question is whether significant increases will occur rapidly enough so that they will be useful, given practical limitations on selective pressures and mouse populations. I wonder whether new techniques, from combining molecular biology and mammalian genetics will make such selection experiments obsolete before they are completed. For example, might we soon produce longer-lived mouse strains with specific new genes inserted to reduce free radical damage, retard immune collagen aging, and so forth?

---

1    From: *Growth, Development and Aging* **52**: 207-211 (1988), reproduced with permission.

This would have the advantage of testing specific theories of causal mechanisms of aging, and the specific new genes would be well-defined. On the other hand, such experiments might not succeed in retarding aging rates.

Dr. Johnson and Dr. Rose have seen each others' original presentations, and thus have concentrated on points of disagreement. Dr. Charlesworth was asked for general comments, and cautions that a large breeding population is critical.

# THOUGHTS ON THE SELECTION OF LONGER-LIVED RODENTS

## Thomas E. Johnson

During the recent meeting at the Jackson Laboratory on the genetics of aging several speakers presented data that related to the selection of long-lived lines of invertebrates. The obvious utility of such lines in the dissection of the processes of aging provoked continued discussion among the participants, focused around the theme of performing such selections in rodents. The following observations are based on those subsequent conversations and pertain to such initiatives for the selection of long-lived rodents as may be undertaken by the National Institute on Aging or other interested parties.

Many considerations concerning feasibility and cost effectiveness must be made to insure the success of such a project. Some of those considerations occurring to me are listed below. First, I provide a partial list of alternative approaches to obtaining long-lived lines of rodents or to identifying genes responsible for longer life in rodents; this list is constrained so as to include only those alternatives that have been successfully used in other areas of genetic research in rodents and thus are, at least minimally, feasible. Second are a series of considerations that must be taken into account in choosing one strategy over another. A careful inquiry into the cost effectiveness, the scientific validity, and the likelihood of success of each approach should be carried out by a small but inclusive panel of experts so as to insure the effectiveness of the program or even to decide if such a program should be undertaken.

## ALTERNATIVE APPROACHES TO IDENTIFYING GENES INVOLVED IN AGING RODENTS

1. Selective breeding in mice for longer life.
   a. direct selection on life span.
   b. indirect selection on time of fertility
   c. indirect selection on another "aging biomarker or an index of such markers (*e.g.*, tail tendon break etc.)
2. Mutant induction and screens for longer-lived mutants.
   a. direct screen for longevity mutants.
   b. indirect screen for lengthened reproduction.
   c. indirect screen for slowing or delay in other biomarkers.
3. Construction of transgenic mice.
   a. using genes from other species (*e.g.*, H-2 from *Peromyscus*)

b. using select genes from mouse (*e.g.*, SOD, etc.).

4. Identification of genes in mouse "similar" to genes known to specify life span in other species.

a. identify by molecular homology with cloned genes.

b. identify by analogy from information in other species.

## CONSIDERATIONS WITH REGARD TO COST EFFECTIVENESS OF ALTERNATIVE APPROACHES

1. Specific uses of selected lines.

a. as model systems for biochemical, physiological studies in aging.

b. as tests of evolutionary theory.

2. End points and assessments of effectiveness.

3. Length of study (rounds of selection, etc.),

4. Number of animals involved.

5. Cost of study (based on best estimates from 3 and 4).

a. per animal costs.

b. inflation costs.

6. Possibility of error.

a. leading to lack of ability to obtain longer-lived strains.

b. leading to loss of important information.

c. leading to selection of invalid lines.

d. leading to lines that would not be able to be used effectively

7. Origin of selected lines.

a. genetic background.

   i. amount of variation.

   ii. amount of inbreeding.

   iii. how representative of wild genotypes.

   iv. genetic adaptation of wild genotypes.

b. environmental concerns.

   i. amount of variation.

   ii. reproductive schedule.

   iii. housing conditions (group, mating pairs, individual)

   iv. SPF or not.

## PROBLEMS IMPLICIT IN THE SELECTIVE BREEDING APPROACH

Since selective breeding was the approach most ardently promoted in subsequent discussions, I will first specifically address several potential problems that need to be seriously considered before this approach is pursued.

First, the selected lines will not be inbred at all; in other words they will still be segregating multiple genetic loci. This genetic heterogeneity will result in two difficulties: (i) the assessment of line means will entail more scatter or larger variances in physiological and molecular studies and may thus require the use of more animals to see statistically significant changes (2) it will not be possible to immediately relate the changes observed in the selected lines to known genes.

Second, phenotypic display of underlying genotype may be very sensitive to the environmental conditions under which selection is performed. For example, in *Drosophila*, merely controlling the density at which larvae develop results in a major decrease in the differential in life span between selected and unselected lines. Luckinbill and Clare, who performed these studies state " the failure of some previous attempts at selection, therefore, appears to have resulted from the introduction . . . of strong artifactual environmental effects that limit the phenotypic expression of genes for life span and the effectiveness of selection." Unfortunately, genotype/environment aspects of life span and/or heritability of reproductive capability have not been widely explored in the mouse and there is little basis on which to choose an environment appropriate for such selections.

Third, effective selection strategies in *Drosophila* have been based on direct selection for late age of reproduction and an indirect selection for extended length of life; however, there is scant information relating genetic covariance of these two phenotypic characters in the mouse. Moreover, unlike *Drosophila*, which reproduces up to a few days before death, the female mouse ceases reproduction about half way through its life expectancy - a life-history strategy also shared by humans and *C. elegans*.

These considerations lead me to conclude that *any immediate strategy to begin selection for long-lived rodents is premature* A cost-effective approach is to (1) begin pilot tests of some of the alternatives listed above and/or (2) start accumulating information upon which an informed decision can be based.

The final and most significant shortcoming is based on the inherent inability of the selective breeding strategy to identify, alleles that are genetically fixed. It is these alleles that make a mouse a mouse or a human a human, and that are responsible for endowing the species with the longevity and other life history traits which it enjoys. Alleles with significant negative effects on fitness components of life history traits will be found only at very low frequencies, so that the genetic variation necessary for effective selection will be lacking. This is not to say that alleles with effect on life history will not be polymorphic; rather, those genes that are highly polymorphic may not be the major genes specifying life-history characteristics in the species but only more minor players modifying these species-specific characteristics. The mode of action of these genetically fixed, species-specific alleles or genes will be most informative in understanding the genetic specification of senescence because it is these alleles that determine the senescence schedule in that species. Such genes may be identified by mutational studies, as has been demonstrated both by my work in the nematode and by classical studies in *Drosophila* by Maynard-Smith; however, little data is available upon which to judge the efficacy of such an approach in the rodent. In response to the rejoinder from Dr. Rose, he seems to have missed the point that "the existence of many alleles which segregate but have effects on life-history and fitness characters", is precisely the reason that these loci are fundamentally less interesting to the biochemist or physiologist and less relevant to the processes responsible for limiting life in the rodent.

In summary:

(1) I am greatly in favor of obtaining long-lived genotypes of rodents; the derivation of these lines is of fundamental scientific import and such genetic stocks would be potentially very useful.

(2) These aforementioned *caveats* argue for an intense exploration of alternate approaches, some of which were listed above without any attempt at explication. I am not proposing immediate initiation of a project to search for mutations leading to longer life (alternative approach 2) even though such mutations have been identified in *Caenorhabditis elegans* and in *Drosophila*.

(3) Other approaches in addition to those listed above should also be considered, and the many shortcomings of all of these approaches should be explored in depth by an expert panel.

## RESPONSE TO "THOUGHTS ON THE SELECTION OF LONGER-LIVED RODENTS"

Michael R. Rose

(1) As Tom Johnson has himself pointed out (Johnson and Wood, 1982), excluding species like *C. elegans* which normally inbreed, inbreeding in outbred species is associated with depressed longevity and other aging-related aging-related characters. Therefore, the fact that rodents selected for increased longevity should not be inbred is not a criticism. Indeed, if such rodents are to be a model for human intervention, a lack of inbreeding seems entirely appropriate. Admittedly, homozygous stocks are better for genetic analysis, all other things being equal. But in the present case, all other things are *not* equal.

(2) There can certainly be problems of genotype-environment interaction in the course of selection on aging characters (vid. Luckinbill and Clare, 1985; Service *et al.*, 1988). However, the *Drosophila* work, in which labs using different media and different flies obtained qualitatively equivalent results under at least some conditions (Rose, 1984a; Luckinbill *et al.*, 1984), suggest that these problems are not grievous. In particular, we expect genotype-environment interactions to be less severe with the more canalized physiology of a mammal, compared with insects or nematodes (Falconer, 1981). This does not address the question of the "basis on which to assess the environment in which selections should be performed," except that it suggests that the environment for selection is not that critical in mammals. It might be pointed out as a practical matter that there has been a great deal of success in selecting agricultural animals for a host of fitness-related attributes, attributes much like aging characters (Wright, 1977; Falconer, 1981).

(3) The third comment seems to be a plea for quantitative genetic research on the patterns of genetic covariance/variance affecting lifespan and reproductive schedule in mice, as has been done in *Drosophila* (*e.g.*, Rose and Charlesworth, 1981). This information would certainly be valuable. However, correlations between relatives do not prove to be a good guide to even medium- term responses to selection on fitness-characters (Rose, 1984b). Therefore, there are good reasons to doubt that they will be of much value. In particular, the results of Rose and Charlesworth (1981) could have been used to argue that selection was unlikely to produce a response in longevity, when such a response was in fact obtained from indirect selection (Rose, 1984a).

(4) Almost no quantitative characters lack genetic variation affecting them, and almost all loci have some all allelic variants, in populations with genetic structure like that of man, mouse, or *Drosophila*. The exceptions are organisms like *C. elegans* in nature or some laboratory lines which have been systematically inbred in the laboratory. In generalizing from *C. elegans* in this way, Johnson is adopting the "classical" (Lewontin, 1974) theory with respect to the nature of population genetic variation. This view is generally discredited within population genetics; "genetically fixed, species-specific genes" are hard to find, unless one compares broad phylogenetic groups. In particular, all the recent *Drosophila* research suggests the existence of many alleles which segregate but have effects on life history and fitness characters. The two major population genetic mechanisms for the evolution of aging, antagonistic pleiotropy and mutation-accumulation, specifically maintain genetic variability for aging. They do not exhaust or fix it.

## An Alternative Perspective

As I see it, the single most important task for the future of aging research is the creation of rodent stocks with genetically postponed aging. This project is of little general *scientific* significance, since we already have *Drosophila* and *C. elegans* stocks of this kind, and they can be used to address fundamental theoretical questions more readily than any mammal. [Accepting that mammals are trivial parts of the spectrum of organic diversity, and therefore not particularly important special cases to investigate]. But from the standpoint of doing something about human beings, the evolutionary theory of aging suggests that little insight into the physiology of postponed aging in mammals will be gained from work on vertebrates. Therefore, it seems clear to me that only rodent stocks with postponed aging can de used to address physiological problems involving the postponement of human aging.

There are three basic methods that could be used to create these stocks, solely or in combination: (i) mutagenesis, including transfection; (ii) stock-crossing; and (iii) selection. The idea of the first method is to look for mutant alleles or alleles in other organisms that dramatically enhance longevity, presumably when homozygous. Waiting for naturally-occurring mutations would take forever. Therefore, one needs artificial mutagenesis or transfection. In decades of research on a diversity of invertebrates, only two such alleles were found: *age-1* in *C. elegans* and *grandchildless* in *D. subobscura* (Maynard-Smith, 1959). Like other large-effect mutations, these alleles have dramatic deleterious effects. However, these deleterious effects are confined to the reproductive system, giving rise to sterility, in the case of *grandchildless*, or a considerable reduction in fertility, in the case of *age-1*. As a patent consequence of reduced reproductive capacity, the durability of the soma is enhanced. This conforms well with the antagonistic pleiotropy observed for segregating quantitative genetic variation in *Drosophila* and some other species (Rose and Hutchinson, 1987). However, the question becomes, can enhanced longevity achieved by genetic changes of this kind be used as an appropriate model for postponing human aging? It seems reasonable to conclude, form both Mendelian genetic and quantitative genetic evidence, that drastically reducing the physiological investment in early reproduction will enhance later survival in most species. [Note that male castrates in our species need not represent the extreme of what can be achieved in this direction.] But can this be proposed as a program of medical intervention? Mutagenesis is likely to provide only alleles with drastically deleterious effects, though alleles which greatly reduce reproduction may have antagonistically beneficial effects on later survival.

The second genetic technique is likely to be even more unpromising. It is easy in laboratory stocks of normally outbreeding diploids to create longer-lived stocks by crosses of inbred stocks. This has been known in *Drosophila* for 60 years, form the work of Pearl and colleagues. Such heterosis effects are well-known in corn, hogs, chickens and so on, for a variety of characters (Falconer, 1981). This heterosis effect arises at least in part from recessive deleterious alleles kept in the population by mutation-selection balance. It may also arise form overdominance, in which heterozygotes have an intrinsic advantage, but that is controversial. In any case, the technique requires the creation of inbred stocks and their subsequent crossing. The inbred stocks are of course available for both mice and rats. There are two overwhelming problems with experimental strategy. The first is that one cannot truly create a hybrid with sustained vigor, at least in mammals, because recombination in the $F_2$ and subsequent generations will lead to hybrid breakdown. The second problem is that there is little evidence that even the first-generation hybrid has postponed aging relative to many members of the outbred stock. Therefore, this entire line of work seems to bring about little more than what one finds with in an outbred stock, in terms of postponed senescence. And in terms of application to the human case, we are *already* outbred, so that no particular insights about inbred lines and hybrids would seem that germane to our case.

The third method is selection, which is known to work in both *Drosophila* and *C. elegans*. There is nothing surprising about this, in that selection has enhanced performance characters in a wide variety of animal and plant species, particularly agricultural breeds (wright, 1977). In the successful *Drosophila* experiments (*e.g.* Rose, 1984a), indirect selection is used, rather than direct artificial selection on longevity itself. This allows maintenance of large population sizes and the avoidance of interbreeding. Considerable progress has been made toward unravelling the physiological basis of postpones senescence in the longer-lived *Drosophila* lines (Rose *et al.*, 1984; Service *et al.*, 1985; Service, 1984; Luckinbill *et al.*, 1988a)

Once one has lines of these three types, the question becomes what use might be made of them. In terms of identifying particular loci, mutagenesis is the preferred method. However, handling and outbred mammalian line in this context is sure to result in inbreeding depression and some confusion in physiological analysis. In particular, dealing with an artificially inbred line raises the problem of selecting for alleles that directly or epistatically circumvent the recessive deleterious effects of alleles fixed by inbreeding. Therefore, I would argue that classical genetic analysis of such mutant stocks is not likely to help us understand how to postpone human aging.

Both hybridization and selection involve effects at many loci. But the hybridization method has some of the same problems as the mutagenesis design: hybridization may be circumventing specific pathologies associated with particular alleles in the inbred lines that are being crossed.

In normally outbred species, only selection is free of problems of inbreeding selection and idiosyncratic allelic effects. On the other hand, the response to selection has been found to be polygenic in both *Drosophila* (Luckinbill *et al.*, 1988b; Hutchinson and Rose, in preparation) and *C. elegans* (Johnson, 1986), making classical genetic analysis difficult. There are two avenues out of this ostensible impasse. The first is to compare the longer-lived and shorter-lived stocks at the molecular-genetic level, to look for specific loci (or marker loci linked to the actual loci) at which there is differentiation. This is already beginning in the *Drosophila* research, and the initial results indicate that a manageable number of molecular genetic differences can be identified. The second avenue out of the polygenic problem is to shift to a more physiological line of analysis. It turns out to be surprisingly difficult to find interpretable physiological differences associated with postpones senescence in fruit flies (*e.g.* Service, 1987). There are no obvious reasons why these same methods could not be applied to mouse or rat stocks selected indirectly for postponed senescence.

In conclusion, I have argued that, in principle, we can create selected rodent populations having postponed senescence, and that these lines can be profitably analyzed with a view to understanding the physiology of postpones mammalian senescence. The further work required from rodent to man I am not qualified to discuss; the evolutionary theory, however, suggests that it would be disastrous to go directly form invertebrate to man, since evolution is expected to be "local" in its shaping of organismal physiology.

# REFERENCES


FALCONER, D. S. (1981) *Introduction to Quantitative Genetics, 2nd. Edition*. London, Longman

JOHNSON, T. E. (1986) Molecular and genetic analyses of a multivariate system specifying behavior and life span. *Behav. Genet.* **16**: 221-235

JOHNSON, T. E. and WOOD, W.B. (1982) Genetic analysis of life-span in *Caenorhabditis elegans*. *Proc. natl. Acad. Sci. USA* **79** 6603-6607

LEWONTON, R. C. (1974) *The genetic basis of evolutionary change*. New York, Columbia University Press.

LUCKINBILL, L. S., ARKING, R., CLARE, M. J., CIROCCO, W. C. and BUCK, S. A. (1984) Selection for delayed senescence in *Drosophila melanogaster*. *Evolution* **38**: 996-1003

LUCKINBILL, L. S. and CLARE, M. J. (1985) Selection for life span in *Drosophila melanogaster. heredity* **55**: 9-18

LUCKINBILL, L. S. GRAVES, J. L., TOMKIW, A. and SOWIRKA, O. (1988a) A qualitative analysis of the life history characters in *Drosophila melanogaster*. *Evol. Ecol.* **2**: 85-94

LUCKINBILL, L. S. GRAVES, J. L., REED, A. H. and KOETSAWANG, S. (1988b) Localizing genes that defer senescence in *Drosophila melanogaster*. *Heredity* **60**: 367-374

MAYNARD-SMITH, J. (1958) The effects of temperature and of egg-laying on longevity of *Drosophila obscura*. *J. Exp. Biol.* **35**: 832-842

ROSE, M. R. (1984a) Laboratory evolution of postponed senescence in *Drosophila melanogaster*. *Evolution* **38**: 1004-1010

ROSE, M. R. (1984b) Artificial selection on a fitness-component in *Drosophila melanogaster*. *Evolution* **38**: 516-526

ROSE, M. R. and CHARLESWORTH, B. (1981) genetics of life-history in *Drosophila melanogaster*. I. Sib analysis of adult females. *Genetics* **97** 173-186

ROSE, M. R., DOREY, M. L., COYLE, A. M. and SERVICE, P. M. (1984) The morphology of postponed senescence in *Drosophila melanogaster*. *Can. J. Zool.* **62**: 1576-1580

ROSE, M. R. and HITCHINSON, E. W. (1987) Evolution of aging. *Rev. Biol. Res. Aging* **3**: 23-32

SERVICE, P. M. (1987) Physiological mechanisms of increased stress resistance in *Drosophila melanogaster* selected for postponed senescence. *Physiol. Zool.* **60**: 321-326

SERVICE, P. M., HUTCHINSON, E. W., MACKINLEY, M. D. and ROSE, M. R. (1985) resistance to environmental stress in *Drosophila melanogaster* selected for postponed senescence. *Physiol. Zool.* **58**: 380-389

SERVICE, P. M., HUTCHINSON, E. W., and ROSE, M. R. (1988) Multiple genetic mechanisms for the evolution of senescence in *Drosophila melanogaster*. *Evolution* **42**: 708-716

WRIGHT, S. (1977) *Evolution and the genetics of populations. volume 3. Experimental results and evolutionary deductions*. Chicago. University of Chicago Press.

## SELECTION FOR LONGER-LIVED RODENTS

## Brian Charlesworth

The question of whether or not it would be worth attempting to create longer-lived strains of rodents by means of selective breeding from surviving older individuals, as has been successfully achieved in *Drosophila*, is not an easy one to answer. Johnson has clearly pointed out the problems in such an approach, most notably the difficulty of carrying out a rigorous genetic analysis of a stock that is not homozygous for the loci of interest, and the small likelihood that a detailed molecular characterization of the genes responsible for any increase in longevity could be carried out. On the other hand, as Rose makes plain, alternatives such as screening for induced mutations that increase longevity face great practical difficulties in rodents.

From the *Drosophila* experience, it seems likely that a selection experiment to increase longevity would be likely to work in mice or rats, if carried out on an inbred stock maintained at a fairly large population size. It also seems likely that estimates of genetic parameters on the base population will not necessarily provide a useful guide to the outcome of selection, due to genetic correlations between traits; Rose and Charlesworth (1981a) found a low level of additive variance for longevity and late female fecundity (at the expense of a decline in early fecundity) by breeding from older individuals (Rose and Charlesworth, 1981b). There thus seems little alternative to actually practicing selection for several generations, if the creation of a longer-lived stock is regarded as a desirable goal.

The decision thus rests on an evaluation of the potential cost of such a project, in relation to the use that could be made of a longer-lived stock as a model for studying the basis of mammalian aging. This is not an issue which I feel competent to judge, but it seems clear that the main utility of such a stock would be for the study of physiological correlates of longer life, as has been done in *Drosophila*. In this regard, the maintenance of a large (100 plus) population of breeding individuals during the experiment is crucial, since the correlated responses to selection can be induced by small population effects (Rose and Charlesworth, 1981b). Such correlated responses would produce seriously misleading inferences concerning cause and effect, and should be avoided at all costs.

## REFERENCES

ROSE, M. R. and CHARLESWORTH, B. (1981a) Genetics of life-history in *Drosophila melanogaster*. I. Sib analysis of adult females. *Genetics* **97** 173-186

ROSE, M. R. and CHARLESWORTH, B. (1981b) Genetics of life-history in *Drosophila melanogaster*. II. Exploratory selection experiments. *genetics* **97**: 187-196

# Section 2

## AGING GENETICS IN NONMAMMALS

# 8

# GENETIC VARIANTS AND MUTATIONS OF *CAENORHABDITIS ELEGANS* PROVIDE TOOLS FOR DISSECTING THE AGING PROCESSES


Thomas E. Johnson, David B. Friedman, Norma Foltz, Paul A. Fitzpatrick, and Jo Ellen Shoemaker


## ABSTRACT


*Caenorhabditis elegans* is a short-lived species that has been widely used in the genetic dissection of development. This species is becoming important in the genetic analysis of aging because strains with mean life spans more than 70% longer than wild type have been identified both through the use of recombinant inbred lines and by the induction of single-gene mutants. Its unique hermaphroditic mode of reproduction leads to a lack of inbreeding depression and simplifies genetic analyses of quantitative traits such as length of life or behavior. Aging in this organism is composed of at least three independent processes: that specifying length of life, that specifying reproductive senescence, and that specifying senescence of the general motor system. These data suggest that aging is not a unitary process but that many different processes or independent components may be involved in various aspects of aging. Most importantly, an apparent single-gene mutation has been mapped to the middle of linkage group II; this mutation lengthens mean and maximum life span 60-110% and also decreases fertility about five-fold.


## INTRODUCTION AND BACKGROUND

*Caenorhabditis elegans* is a self-fertilizing hermaphroditic species of nematode that can be grown in petri plates on a simple diet of Escherichia coli. As such it has been widely used as a model experimental organism in many different areas of biology but especially in analyses of development, muscle physiology, and behavior. The almost invariant cell lineage of *C. elegans* has facilitated the complete cell lineage description of the 959 somatic cells of the hermaphrodite (Sulston and Horvitz, 1977; Kimble and Hirsh, 1979; Sulston

| **Table 1.** Advantages of *C. elegans* for the Genetic Analysis of Aging. |
| --- |
| -Small (1.2 mm) |
| - Rapid life cycle ( < 3 days) |
| - Short life span (20 days) |
| - Self-fertilizing hermaphrodite |
|   - easy isolation of recessive mutants |
|   - lack of inbreeding depression |
| - Spontaneous males (obligate outcrossers) |
| - Dauer larvae ( > 90 day survival) |
| - Cryogenic preservation of strains |
|   - no loss of mutants |
|   - no accumulation of modifiers or suppressors |
|   - all stocks in same genetic background |
| - Genetic transformation |
| - Transposon-mediated mutagenesis |
| - Physical map 98% complete in a series of cosmid arrays |
| - Many laboratories: many types of mutants (developmental, behavioral, Ts, amber suppressible, lethals, *etc.*) |

*et al.*, 1983). This analysis is aided by the small size of the animal (1.2 mm length), its 2-day period of development, and its optical transparency, which makes the analysis of cell lineage feasible.

## Genetics: Classical, Quantitative, and Molecular

Sophisticated tools that include simple techniques for classical and molecular genetic analysis have been developed. The recent beginnings of quantitative and population genetic analyses prove that unique applications are available in these areas as well.

The isolation of mutants is straightforward in *C. elegans*, and a large number of mutants have been identified after treatment with ethyl methanesulphonate or a wide variety of other mutagens (Brenner, 1974; Herman and Horvitz, 1980; Herman, 1988). Recently, molecular genetic analysis of this species has progressed rapidly. Many putative transposable elements have been identified in *C. elegans* (Emmons, 1988). Two of these have been shown to transpose at measurable frequencies in strains that have mobilized the Tc1 transposable element. Such "transposon-tagged" loci have facilitated the cloning of genes identified only by mutations (Herman, 1988). Efficient techniques for genetic transformation (Fire, 1986) and the availability of overlapping arrays of cosmids that cover as much as 95% of the genome (Coulson *et al.*, 1986, 1988), when combined with the long-lived genetic variants, offer possibilities for the analysis of aging unrivaled by any other species.

| **Table 2.** Comparisons of Genetic Approaches. | | | |
|---|---|---|---|
| | Induced Mutants | Selective Breeding | Molecular Approaches |
| Type of Phenotype | Qualitative | Quantitative | Molecular |
| Origin | Mutant Induction | Existing Variation | Molecular Construct /Transgenic Animals |
| Genes Involve | Usually Single Gene | Usually Polygenic | Single or Multiple Genes |
| Level at Which Understanding is Obtained | Organismic | Population | Molecular |
| Gene Localization Strategy | Classical Mapping | Interval Mapping | Physical Mapping |
| Method of Assessing Gene Number | Complementation | Numerical Estimates | DNA Sequence |

Several additional advantages in the use of *C. elegans* for genetic analyses of aging and senescence are listed in Table 1. The life style of *C. elegans* is such that during the fourth larval stages the worm produces sperm which are then stored in the spermatheca throughout the adult period when the worm produces only oocytes; both spermatocytes and oocytes result from regular meiotic divisions (Brenner, 1974). Two principal advantages, easy identification of recessive mutants and a lack of inbreeding depression, result from the fact that *C. elegans* is a self-fertilizing hermaphrodite. As a consequence, recessive mutations can be isolated with relative ease, and this has been quite important in the identification of long-lived mutants (Klass, 1983) and in their subsequent analysis (Friedman and Johnson; 1988a,b).

## Classical, Quantitative, and Molecular Approaches to Aging

Table 2 compares the mutational, selective breeding, and molecular genetic approaches in their ability to estimate genetic contributions, localize genetic effects to one region of the genome, and determine the physiological or molecular basis of phenotypes in any genetic system. Most of these approaches have already been applied to answering the question: What specifies length of life in *C. elegans*?

The approach of choice for the dissection of any biological process is the identification of single-gene mutations that alter the process of interest (Botstein and Mauer, 1982). Since there are relatively straightforward ways to clone a gene in *C. elegans* once mutants in that gene are available, the mutational approach leads directly to the molecular identification of the gene and the subsequent illumination of the molecular details of the process of interest. Moreover, the mutational approach has significant advantages over both selective breeding and molecular approaches. Unlike selective breeding (Rose, 1984; Luckinbill *et al.*, 1984), mutational analysis is not limited to allelic variants already present in the population, and unlike molecular approaches through transgenic stock construction there is no bias as to which genes are relevant for analysis nor limitations based on the availability of cloned genes. In studies on aging in metazoans, the mutational approach has proven effective only in *C. elegans*. [Two exceptionally long-lived (44 and 48 months) individual C57BL6/NIA mice were identified in colonies sponsored by the National Institute on Aging but post-mortem confirmation of age was not possible (Sprott, personal communication)]. Short-lived mutants have been identified in other species, but these mutants are likely to carry mutations in genes not specifically involved in aging. Problems of inbreeding depression that effectively prevent a simple assessment of underlying genotype based on the phenotype of one or a few related individuals may have prevented the identification of long-lived mutants in other genetic systems.

The selective breeding approach has been applied in Drosophila. Although the response usually results from the action of multiple genes and is limited to existing allelic variants, selective breeding has been effective in producing strains with increased maximum life span (Rose, 1984; Luckinbill *et al.*, 1984; see also Hutchinson and Rose, and Rose this volume). In contrast, mutations can be induced in any gene; the identification of these mutants is limited only by the time and ingenuity of the investigator.

A traditional, but non-essential, difference between these approaches has been the fact that quantitative phenotypes (characters that must be measured to assess genotype) have usually been studied using selective breeding, whereas qualitative traits (those that can be distinguished quickly by just looking at the wild type and mutant) are more amenable to mutant and molecular analyses. This distinction is, however, arbitrary in that any qualitative trait is potentially a quantitative trait if the distinction is small enough that measurements must be made or if a population must be monitored to assess genotype. Moreover, major effects of single-gene mutations that affect quantitative traits are well known. Thus, although the methodology and nomenclature are different (see Table 2), there is a surprisingly large amount of overlap between the information obtained by one technique and by an alternative approach.

## GENETIC CHARACTERIZATION OF LIFE SPAN

### Lack of Heterosis

Heterosis, or hybrid vigor, is defined as an improved performance of the $F_1$ hybrid in comparison with its two inbred parents. More precisely, heterosis is observed whenever the value of the $F_1$ hybrid is significantly different from that expected of the midparent as predicted by a model of simple additive genetic factors (Falconer, 1981). Although common in hybrid progeny resulting from crosses between inbred parents, the cause of heterosis is not completely understood and at least three major models have been proposed for the genetic basis of heterosis (Mitton and Grant, 1984).

There is little heterosis effect for life history traits in *C. elegans*. For example, the $F_1$ hybrid of two different wild-type strains (Bristol and Bergerac) that have significant genetic differences between them (Emmons, 1988) has a life expectancy not significantly different from either parent (Figure 1, Johnson and Wood, 1982). This result has been extended to other wild strains (Johnson, unpublished). This lack of heterosis is also seen in other life-history traits of the hermaphrodite, such as fecundity, rate of development, and fertility. Because *C. elegans* reproduces by self-fertilization in the wild, these populations are largely homozygous. Homozygotes cannot carry recessive alleles with significant deleterious effects; when a new deleterious allele enters a population by mutation, it is rapidly eliminated by selection against the recessive allele due to its expression in the homozygote. Thus, the unusual lack of heterosis effects and inbreeding depression may result from the self-fertilizing lifestyle of this organism.

For the genetic analysis of life history and other quantitative traits, the advantages of working with an organism that has little apparent over-dominance is extremely significant. This is seen especially in the genetic analysis of single-gene mutants where the ability to measure life history traits in homozygous populations has simplified the mapping of a major gene that affects length of life (Friedman and Johnson; 1988a; see also Figure 10 and below).

### Males, Dauers, and Cryogenic Preservation of Stocks

*C. elegans* spontaneously produces XO males by nondisjunction of the X-chromosome at frequencies of about 1 in 700 (Hodgkin *et al.*, 1979). These males are obligate outcrossers and thus can be used to construct new strains and to perform other crosses. Interestingly, males of the N2 wild-type strain

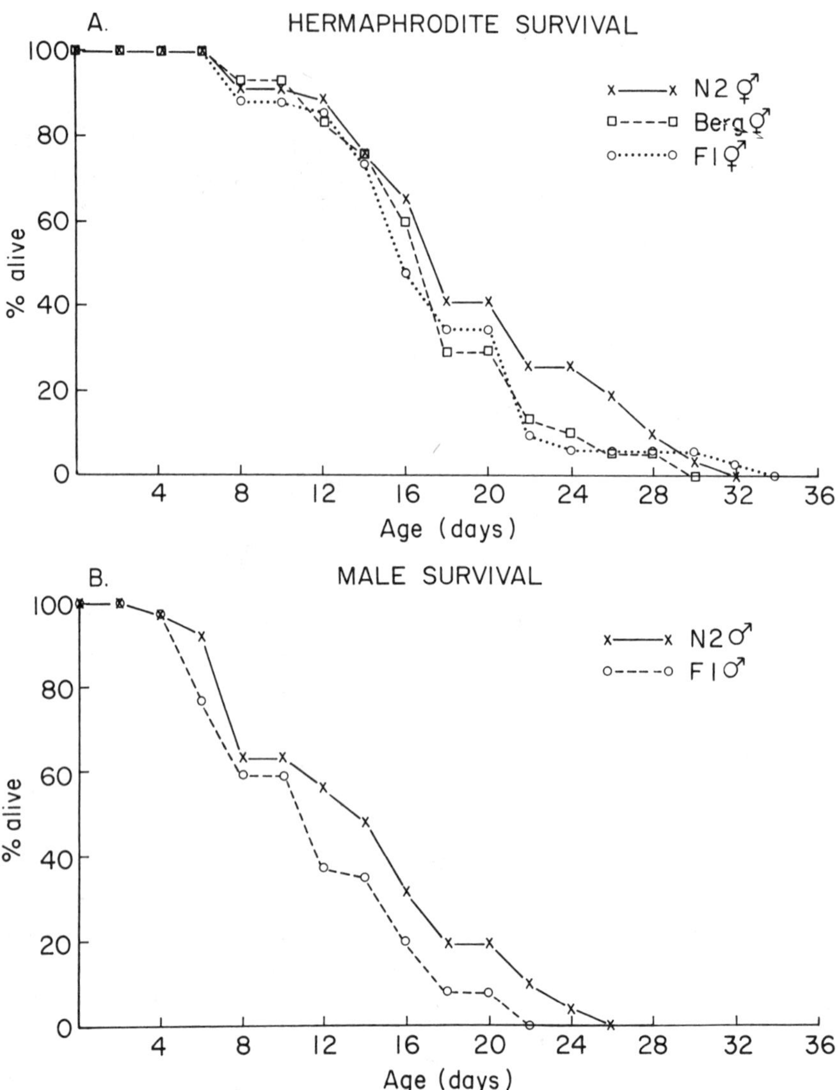



**Figure 1.** Survival curves for parental and $F_1$ hybrid populations. (A) Hermaphrodites. (B) Males. Mean ± SEM life spans for the Bristol, Bergerac, and $F_1$ hybrid hermaphrodites were 18.2 ± 1.1, 16.6 ± 0.8, and 16.6 ± 1.1 days, respectively. Mean life spans for the Bristol and $F_1$ hybrid males were 12.9 ± 0.8 and 10.7 ± 0.7 days, respectively. Comparisons of the hermaphrodite means by the Gehan and Log-rank tests indicated no significant differences in life span among the three populations ($P > 0.35$ in all pairwise tests). Similar comparisons of the male means also showed no significant differences ($P = 0.08$ and 0.10 from the Gehan and Log-rank tests, respectively). However, all pairwise comparisons between a male and a hermaphrodite population showed a significant differences ($P < 0.02$).

are shorter lived than the wild type (Johnson and Wood, 1982), although this is not true of all wild strains (Johnson, 1984).

Dauers are an alternative developmental stage to the normal third larva. They are resistant to desiccation and other environmental insults that would kill a normal worm (Riddle, 1988) and presumably evolved to survive harsh conditions. Dauers can be induced by starvation and survive up to 3 months with no apparent loss of remaining life span (Klass and Hirsh, 1976) while retaining normal or near normal levels of fertility. The dauer can be used in selection paradigms where genetically identical siblings of possibly long-lived mutants are kept in an immature stage until the long-lived cultures are identified, at which point the new mutations can be recovered by inducing the dauer to complete development (Klass, 1983).

A final, major advantage is that *C. elegans* strains can be preserved indefinitely by freezing in liquid $N_2$. This means that novel mutants are easy to maintain and even a small nematode lab can have several hundred mutants on hand. Most important for aging research is the fact that the strains do not accumulate new suppressor and modifier mutations as do Drosophila and mice, which must be maintained by continual passages. Such modifier muta-tions can significantly affect length of life and can lead to wide variation in quantitative aspects of supposedly identical strains (for examples of these types of problems in Drosophila, see Baker *et al.*, 1985). Thus, for example, almost all *C. elegans* laboratories work with the N2 wild type as a control, ensuring a common genetic background, identical with that of every other lab.


## Characterization of Length of Life

Interestingly, several different wild-type strains (Figure 2 and Johnson, 1984) have fairly similar life expectancies, maximum life spans, and survival curves, consistent with a functional significance for length of life or a tight relationship between length of life and some other life history traits. A number of different types of mutants have been identified in *C. elegans*. These include morphological variants such as short, squat "dumpies" (Dpy), longer than normal (Lon), etc.; behavioral variants such as uncoordinated (Unc), worms that roll instead of swimming smoothly (Rol), etc.; and more unusual mutants such as temperature-sensitive lethals which can affect almost any stage of life and transformer stocks that cause stocks of one sexual genotype to masquerade as the other sex. In a preliminary survey seeking strains that had normal life expectancy - and could therefore be used to map variants with longer life - we discovered that many strains (30%) have life expectancies not significantly different from wild type (Figure 3).

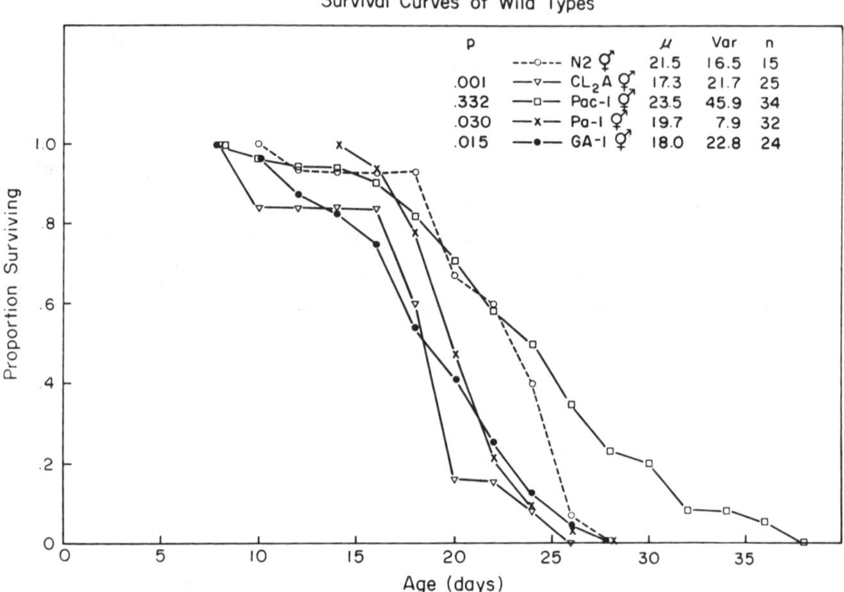


**Figure 2.** Survival curves of several wild-type strains of *C. elegans*.

We will describe two complementary genetic approaches used in our laboratory over the last seven years for the generation and analysis of long-lived lines of the nematode. The first approach, that of generating recombinant inbred lines (RIs) between two common laboratory strains of *C. elegans* (Johnson and Wood, 1982; Johnson, 1987), as well as the more recent analysis of mutants (Friedman and Johnson, 1988 a,b), have each resulted in strains with life expectancy more than 60% longer than that of the parental strains. The details of these studies will be reviewed herein.

## RECOMBINANT INBRED LINES

### Creation of Long-lived RIs

Two laboratory wild-type strains of *C. elegans*, the Bristol (N2) and the Bergerac BO, were crossed (Figure 4). F1 hermaphrodites were allowed to self-fertilize and the F2 hermaphroditic progeny were cloned and independently inbred through 19 subsequent rounds of self-fertilization. Within two months, recombinant inbred lines (Bailey, 1981), inbred to less than one part in $10^6$ (roughly equivalent to the rate of spontaneous mutation in *C. elegans*, Moerman *et al.*, 1986), were established.

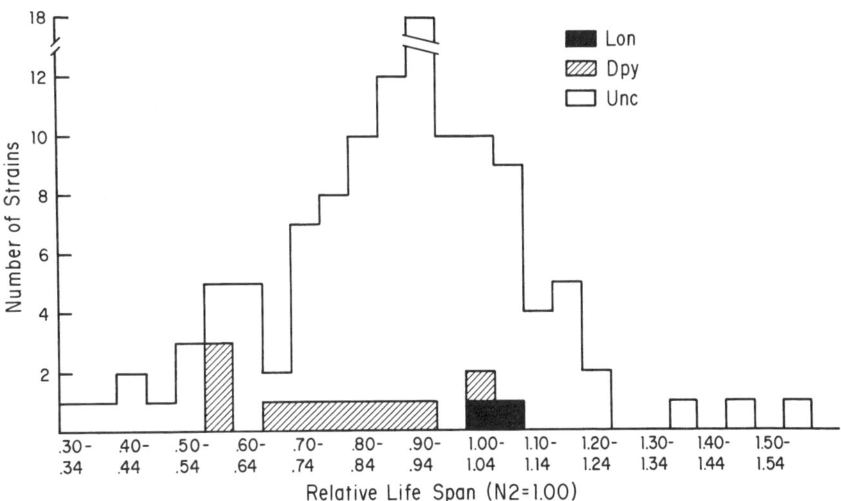


**Figure 3.** Distribution of life expectancies for 114 morphological and behavioral mutants: *Unc*, uncoordinated behavior; *Lon*, longer; *Dpy*, dumpy. For more information on strains see Brenner (1974).

These RI lines have been assayed several times for length of life. In typical experiments mean life spans of these lines vary three-fold, ranging from 13.8 days to 37.9 days (Figure 5A). More importantly, maximum life spans of the RI lines are also altered; maximum life spans both shorter (17 days) and up to 63% longer (63 days) than N2 (40 days) are observed among the RI lines. As expected, there are strong positive correlations between mean life span and the 90th percentile, the 95th percentile, or maximum life span (Figure 5B). These strong positive correlations are not trivial, because a higher mean life span can result either from decreased early life mortality or from increased maximum life span. In these lines, longer life results from an increase in life expectancy at all chronological ages.

The shape of the survival curve was examined in detail in three selected RI lines and in the two parental genotypes (Figure 6). The exact shape of the survival curves varies slightly between lines, but all are rectangular.

We undertook a more detailed analysis of the kinetics of mortality in the parent stocks and in five selected RI lines to see if mortality increases exponentially with chronological age as modeled by the Gompertz equation.

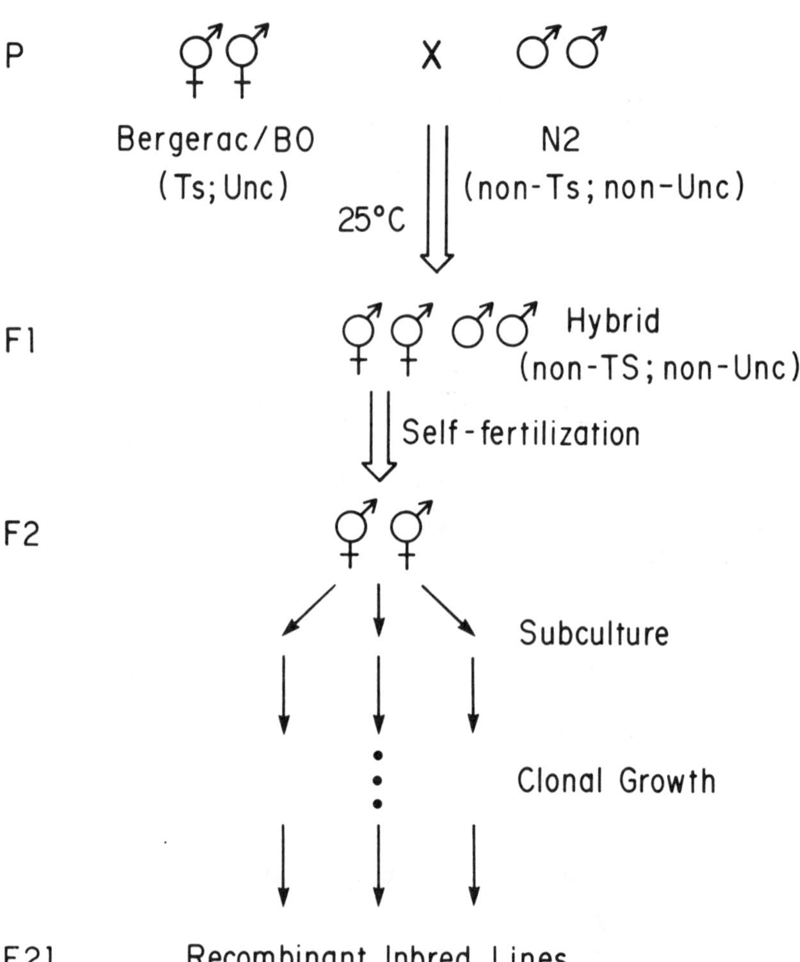


**Figure 4.** Scheme for constructing recombinant inbred lines in *C. elegans*. Two common laboratory wild types, N2 (Bristol) and Bergerac BO, were crossed. $F_1$ cross progeny were distinguished from self-progeny of the parental Bergerac hermaphrodites by the non-Ts, non-Unc phenotypes of the $F_1$'s. Individual fourth larval stage $F_1$ hermaphrodites were isolated to individual small petri plates. Subsequent generations were produced by self-fertilization. Fourth larval stage hermaphrodites were transferred to fresh NGM plates at each generation. This inbreeding procedure was continued for 21 generations (from Johnson *et al.*, 1988).

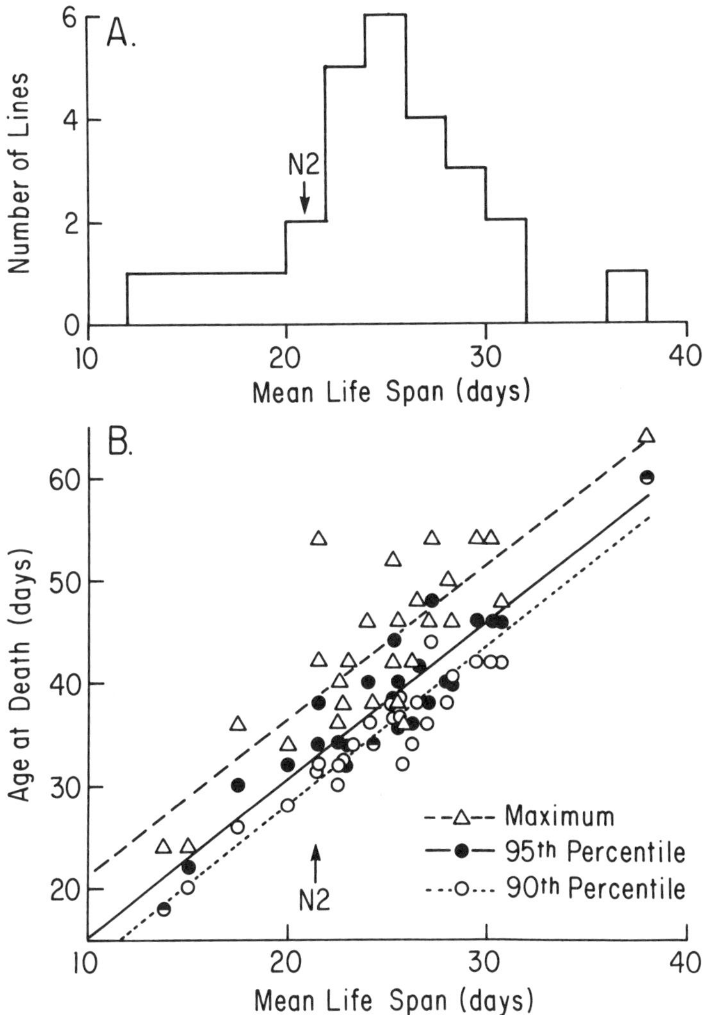



**Figure 5.** Life spans of hermaphrodites from RI lines. (A) Mean life spans of 27 RI lines. Data are the average of two survival experiments, each containing 50 nematodes. The entire experiment involved the assay of 2950 nematodes; 2206 died of natural causes. (B) Regression of mean life span (same nematodes described in Figure 4A) on either maximum life span, the 95th percentile of life span, or the 90th percentile of life span. Mean life span is highly correlated (P<.001) with maximum life span (r = 0.83), the 95th percentile of life span (r = 0.93), and the 90th percentile of life span (r = 0.96) (from Johnson, 1987).

In both wild type and RI strains, the age-dependent component increases exponentially with increasing chronological age. This is most clearly seen by plotting mortality rate against chronological age on a semilogarithmic scale (Figure 6 B, D). Because increased mean life span could result from lower basal mortality rate or from a slower rate of increase in mortality with chronological age, we asked how these components varied in the RI lines. The age-dependent component varies between lines and explains most of the variance in length of life (Johnson, 1987). No significant change in the age-independent component was observed.

## Coinheritance of Fertility and Life Span

Based on the findings with *age-1* and on theoretical models for the evolution of senescence we have also looked at the inheritance of fertility in these recombinant inbred lines (Foltz and Johnson, unpublished). A significant genetic component for life expectancy was observed in each of five trials, consistent with earlier observations (Johnson and Wood, 1982; Johnson, 1986). Hermaphrodite fertility also showed significant heritability in each of three trials. A significant positive phenotypic and genetic covariance for life span and fertility was also observed in two of three experiments (Table 3). Age-specific fertility was positively correlated with fertility on consecutive days but was negatively correlated with fertility on more distant days.

Three to five independently segregating genes are estimated to be specifying these traits within the RI lines; two of three single-gene markers used to generate strain distribution patterns for these lines were found to be associated with one or more loci which had a statistically significant effect on life span and/or fertility. There was also evidence for a significant environmental component affecting fertility and length of life, which leads us to be cautious about generalizing the observed positive covariances to the environment encountered in the wild.

## Dissecting the Aging Process

The length of developmental periods and the length of the reproductive period are unrelated to increased life span in these lines or in *age-1* mutants (Johnson, 1987; Friedman and Johnson; 1988a). Lengthened life is due entirely to an increase in post-reproductive life span. Development, reproduction, and life span are each under independent genetic control. General motor activity decays linearly with chronological age in all RI genotypes examined (Johnson, 1987). The decay in general motor activity is both correlated with and a predictor of mean and maximum life span, suggesting that both share at least one common rate-determining component. These observations can be

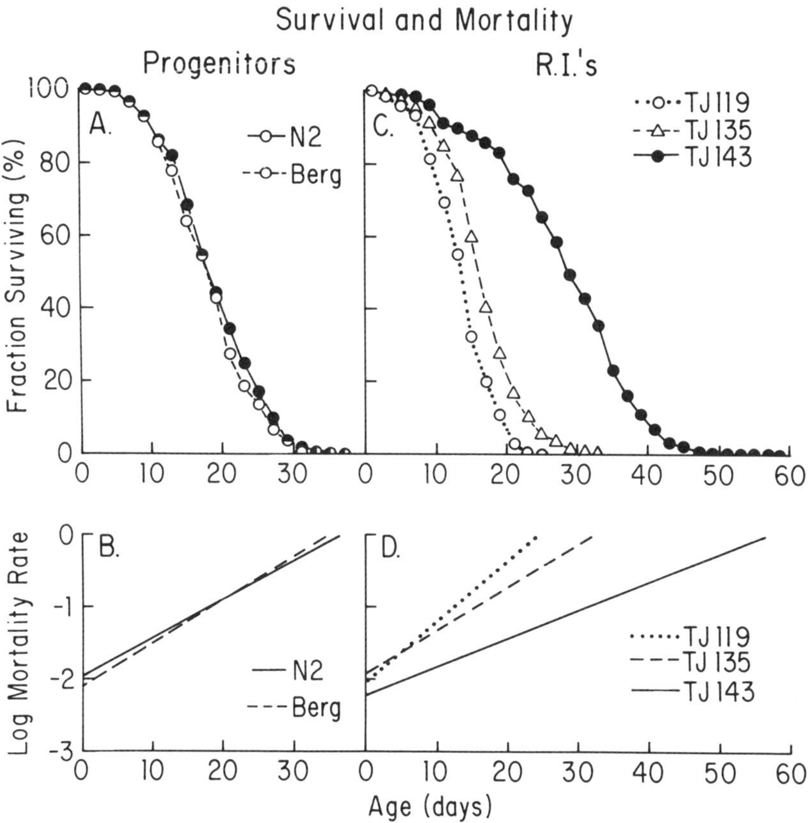



**Figure 6.** Survival data (A and C) and mortality rates (B and D) for the parental strains and three RI lines. Panels A and B show survival data obtained as described in Figure 5 except that each curve is the result of assays on 400 nematodes, 200 in each of two experiments, and that survival assays were performed every 12 hours. Subgroups of the same genotype were tested for consistency. One sample of 50 hermaphrodites (TJ143) showed significant differences in survival from the other three TJ143 subgroups and was excluded from this analysis; however, inclusion of that sample does not noticeably affect the results. Panels B and D are plots of age-specific mortality rates versus chronological age. Age-specific mortality rates were calculated for each 2-day period throughout life using SPSS subprogram, Survival. Lines are weighted regression estimates (SPSS). (A and B) Survival curves and mortality data for the parental stocks, N2 and Bergerac BO. (C and D) Survival curves and mortality data for TJ119, TJ135, and TJ143. TJ143 is one of the longest-lived stocks generated (from Johnson, 1987).

**Table 3.** Correlations[a] Among Age-Specific Self-Fertility, Total Self-Fertility, and Life Span

| Trial | Age: | 3 | 4 | 5 | 6 | 7 | >7[b] | Total Fertility | Life Span |
|---|---|---|---|---|---|---|---|---|---|
| | | | | | (days) | | | | |
| 1 | 3 | 1 | 0.55*** | 0.07 | 0.02 | 12 | 0.06 | 0.74*** | 0.11 |
| 2 | 3 | 1 | 0.60*** | 0.43** | -0.30** | -0.19** | -0.19* | 0.54*** | 0.15 |
| 3 | 3 | 1 | 0.57*** | 0.24** | -0.03 | -0.18** | -0.17* | 0.69*** | -0.13 |
| 1 | 4 | 0.54* | 1 | 0.48*** | 0.15 | 0.15 | -0.02 | 0.83*** | 0.40*** |
| 2 | 4 | 0.69** | 1 | 0.41*** | -0.50*** | -0.44*** | -0.29*** | 0.47*** | 0.08 |
| 3 | 4 | 0.64** | 1 | 0.65*** | 0.36*** | 0.07 | -0.07 | 0.88*** | 0.08 |
| 1 | 5 | 0.07 | 0.06 | 1 | 0.47*** | 0.32*** | 0.16* | 0.64*** | 0.24*** |
| 2 | 5 | 0.48* | 0.54* | 1 | 0.18* | 0.11 | 0.02 | 0.84*** | 0.11 |
| 3 | 5 | 0.38 | 0.79** | 1 | 0.68*** | 0.44*** | 0.21* | 0.84*** | 0.32*** |
| 1 | 6 | 0.02 | 0.13 | 0.45* | 1 | 0.54*** | 0.30*** | 47*** | 0.08 |
| 2 | 6 | 0.37 | -0.63** | 0.14 | 1 | 0.74*** | 0.42*** | 0.39*** | 0.06 |
| 3 | 6 | 0.20 | 0.61** | 0.85*** | 1 | 0.56*** | 0.32*** | 0.60*** | 0.28* |
| 1 | 7 | 0.11 | 0.13 | 0.31 | 0.53* | 1 | 0.41*** | 0.42*** | 0.10 |
| 2 | 7 | -0.23 | -0.62** | 0.13 | 0.96*** | 1 | 0.67*** | 0.38*** | 0.09 |
| 3 | 7 | -0.18 | 0.07 | 0.47* | 0.77*** | 1 | 0.67*** | 0.34*** | 0.14 |
| 1 | >7 | -0.06 | -0.04 | 0.16 | 0.29*** | 0.40*** | 1 | 0.14 | -0.02 |
| 2 | >7 | -0.28 | -0.63* | 0 | 0.92*** | 0.94*** | 1 | 0.24** | 0.03 |
| 3 | >7 | -0.29 | -0.19 | 0.21 | 0.57*** | 0.93*** | 1 | 0.17* | 0.01 |
| **Total Self-Fertility** | | | | | | | | | |
| 1 | | 0.73*** | 0.81*** | 0.62* | 0.47 | 0.42 | 0.13 | 1 | 0.30* |
| 2 | | 0.60** | 0.48* | 0.91* | 0.31 | 0.34 | 0.24 | 1 | 0.17 |
| 3 | | 0.69** | 0.91* | 0.90* | 0.80*** | 0.36 | 0.18 | 1 | 0.14* |
| **Life Span** | | | | | | | | | |
| 1 | | 0.08 | 0.37 | 0.20 | 0.06 | 0.08 | -0.03 | 0.25 | 1 |
| 2 | | 0.25 | 0.17 | 0.30 | 0.07 | 0.05 | 0.09 | 0.32 | 1 |
| 3 | | -0.16 | 0.27 | 0.60** | 0.43 | 0.32 | 0.21 | 0.34 | 1 |

a* Phenotypic correlations above diagonal; genetic, below diagonal; analysis of three trials.

b* Last progeny: Day 10 in trial 1; Day 13, trial 2; Day 14, trial 3. Significance: $P \leq 0.05$ (*); $P \leq 0.01$ (**); $P \leq 0.001$ (***); 2-tailed test.

combined with earlier studies suggesting a model in which development is completed before the onset of aging (Johnson *et al.*, 1984) to give a comprehensive summary of the independent processes involved in the specification of length of life (Figure 7).

## INDUCED MUTANTS

*age-1(hx546)* is a recessive mutant allele in *Caenorhabditis elegans* that results in an average 40% increase in life expectancy and an average 60% increase in maximal life span at 20° C (Figure 8; Table 4; and Friedman and

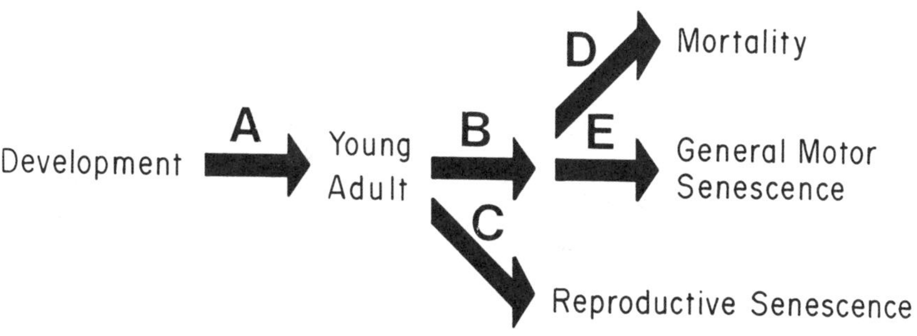


**Figure 7.** Diagram describing the order of dependency of events in senescence of *C. elegans*. Arrows indicate dependency relationships (from Johnson, 1987).

Johnson, 1988a,b); at 25°C, *age-1(hx546)* averages a 65% increase in mean life span (25.3 days *vs.* 15.0 days) and a 110% increase in maximum life span (46.2 days *vs.* 22.0 days for wild-type hermaphrodites; Friedman and Johnson, 1988a). Mutant males also show extended life spans. *age-1(hx546)* is associated with a 75% decrease in hermaphrodite self-fertility as compared to the *age-1*[+] allele at 20°.

## Physiological Characteristics of Long-lived Strains: Food Uptake

Klass (1983) reported that eight long-lived strains isolated in his screens had behavioral or developmental alterations that led to longer life and implied that the uncoordinated phenotype (Unc) might lead to the observed reduction in food uptake and thereby lead to longer life. In pilot studies on the segregation of life expectancy it became clear that the Unc character segregated independently of any locus or loci that specified long life (Johnson, 1986); the Unc mutation was subsequently shown to map to linkage group V and to be an allele of *unc-31* (Friedman and Johnson; 1988b). It was also clear that the long-lived mutant strains did not ingest less food than did wild type (Figure 8 C, E and Johnson, 1986). Pharyngeal pump rates were determined for age-synchronous cultures at the first larval stage (immediately after refeeding cultures starved at the time of hatching from the egg), second larval stage (20 hours after refeeding), and fourth larval stage (40 hours after refeeding), and on young adult (50 hours after refeeding) hermaphrodites of N2, DH26, MK7,

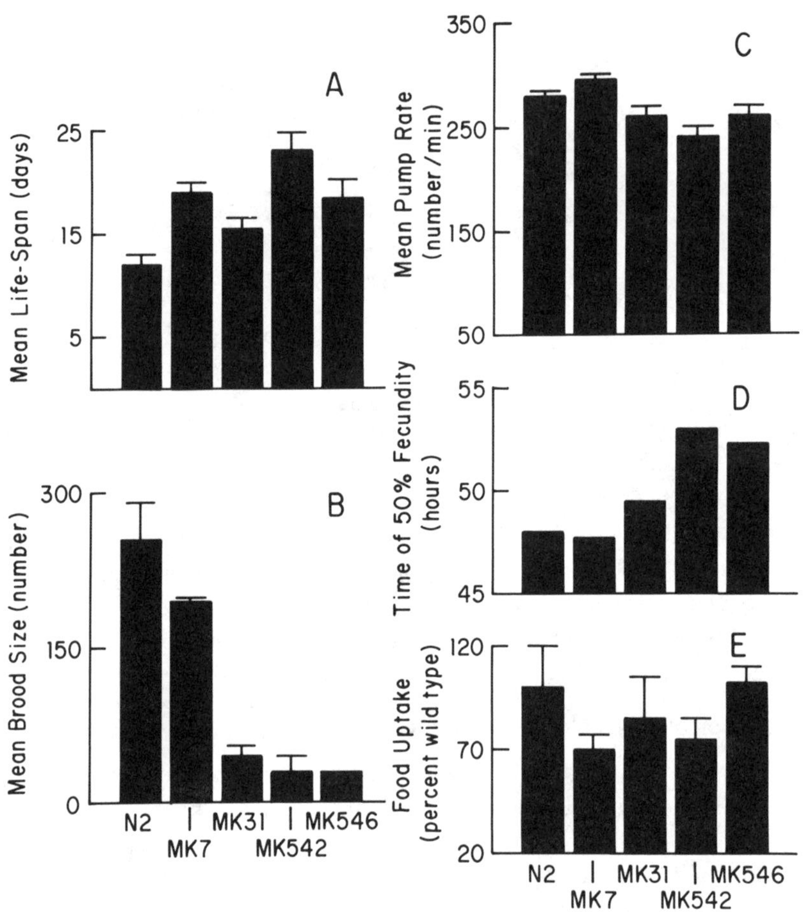



**Figure 8.** Physiological characteristics of four long-lived mutant strains and wild type, N2: (A) mean life spans; (B) average number of progeny; (C) pharyngeal pump rates; (D) length of time to 50% of population being fertile; (E) relative amount of radiolabelled *Escherichia coli* ingested. Procedural details can be found in Friedman and Johnson (1988a,b) and in Johnson and McCaffrey (1986).

MK31, MK542, and MK546. First stage larvae had lower pharyngeal pump rates than other larval stages. Pharyngeal pump rates (an indirect assessment of rate of food ingestion) and rates of radiolabelled food uptake of the long-lived stocks were comparable to the wild-type controls (Table 5).

| Table 4. Average Life of Age Mutants[a]. | | | |
|---|---|---|---|
| Strain | Number of Repeats | Average Life Expectancy ± SD | Average Maximum Life ± SD |
| N2 | 2 | 15.0 ± 1.3 | 22.0 ± 5.0 |
| DH26 | 3 | 15.7 ± 1.3 | 23.7 ± 2.9 |
| MK7 | 3 | 19.2 ± 1.6 | 29.3 ± 2.3 |
| MK31 | 4 | 18.4 ± 0.3 | 30.3 ± 1.1 |
| MK542 | 2 | 28.1 ± 6.3 | 46.5 ± 7.5 |
| MK546 | 5 | 25.3 ± 3.4 | 46.2 ± 3.4 |
| [a]. Data from Friedman and Johnson (1988b). | | | |

| Table 5. Pharyngeal Pump Rates and Food Uptake | | | | | | | |
|---|---|---|---|---|---|---|---|
| Strain | Geno-type | Mean Pump Rate ± SEM[a] (pumps/min) | | | | Mean Food Uptake[b] (cpm) | |
| | | First stage larvae | Second stage larvae | Fourth stage larvae | Young Adult | Experiment 1 (liquid) | Experiment 2 (agar) (liquid) |
| N2 | *age*[+] | 130 ± 12 | 225 ± 4 | 279 ± 4 | 281 ± 6 | 2648 ± 508 | — — |
| DH26 | *age*[+] | 107 ± 2 | 198 ±14 | 207 ± 25 | 295 ± 9 | — | 1799 ± 64 / 1372 ± 335 |
| MK7 | *age-?* | 110 ± 16 | 220 ± 20 | 259 ± 7 | 293 ± 6 | 1860 ± 187 | 1770 ± 163 / 660 ± 295 |
| MK31 | *age-1 (hx31)* | 163 ± 4 | 216 ± 10 | 256 ± 7 | 260 ± 9 | 2273 ± 636 | 7240 ± 90 / 1712 ± 45 |
| MK542 | *age-1 (hx542)* | 140 ± 3 | 174 ± 20 | 224 ±22 | 241 æ 13 | 1949 ± 333 | 2065 ± 10 / 2200 ± 628 |
| MK546 | *age-1 (hx546)* | 127 ± 16 | 232 ± 7 | 234 ±12 | 262 ± 13 | 2696 ± 257 | 3257 ± 238 / 1595 ± 8 |
| [a] Hatched larvae were fed and assayed at the following times: 0-1 hours for first stage larvae, 20- 21 hours for second stage larvae, 39-40 hours for fourth stage larvae, and 49- 50 hours for young adult worms. Data are from 20-second assays on 5 individuals. [b] 1000 worms were assayed except for experiment 2, liquid media, where 500 worms were used; assays are described in Johnson and McCaffrey (1986). | | | | | | | |

Further longitudinal studies of individual animals, as well as longitudinal studies on mass cultures (Johnson and Conley, unpublished), showed that the relationship between food uptake and chronological age is complex, with the mutants ingesting greater than normal amounts of food early in life and lesser amounts later. Thus, two apparently contradictory observations (Klass, 1983; Johnson, 1986), which had been obtained at different chronological ages, are not necessarily conflicting.

In an attempt to resolve this problem, we pursued another approach to answering the question of whether self-imposed food restriction leads to the longer life of *age-1*. Mean life spans of wild-type and long-lived mutants were determined in solutions of *E. coli* at concentrations ranging from $10^8$ to $10^{10}$ cells per ml. In these experiments we took advantage of observations by Nicholas *et al.* (1973), Schiemer *et al.* (1980), and Schiemer (1982) that food ingestion rates in other nematodes are proportional to bacterial concentration over concentrations from $2 \times 10^8$ to $5 \times 10^{10}$ cells per ml.

We reasoned that if the physiological processes affected by food restriction are independent of the process(es) affected in the long-lived mutants, then an additional component of life span might be added to the already longer life span of the mutants by food restriction. Alternatively, if the long life of the mutant strains is due entirely to food restriction, we would expect that no additional life extension due to food restriction would be observed in the mutants and that maximal life span would be observed at bacterial concentrations higher than those that maximize mean life span of DH26.

DH26 exhibited a bell-shaped response to varying bacterial concentrations, with a maximal mean life span at $10^9$ cells per ml (our standard survival conditions; Figure 9). With only one exception (MK7 at $3 \times 10^9$ bacteria per ml), each of the three mutant strains tested lived significantly longer than DH26 at comparable concentrations (P < 0.001). Maximal mean life span of MK546 was at $3 \times 10^8$ whereas MK31 and MK542 were maximal at $10^8$ bacteria per ml. This result suggests that whatever processes are acting to increase life span in the mutant strains, they function independently of, that is to say in addition to, the life-extension effects of food restriction.

## Mapping of the *age-1* Locus

Using two novel strategies for following the segregation of *age-1*, we obtained evidence that longer life results from a mutation in a single gene that increases the probability of survival at all chronological ages. The long-life and reduced-fertility phenotypes cosegregate in backcrosses to N2 (Figure 10). Surprisingly, both are tightly linked to *fer-15*, a locus on linkage group II; our current model suggests that *age-1* may be a further mutation in *fer-15* or tightly linked to it, and we are attempting to clone this region using overlapping deficiencies (Sigurdson *et al.*, 1984) and congenic strains (Link and Johnson, unpublished). *age-1(hx546)* does not affect the timing of larval molts, the length of embryogenesis, food uptake, movement, or behavior in any way tested.

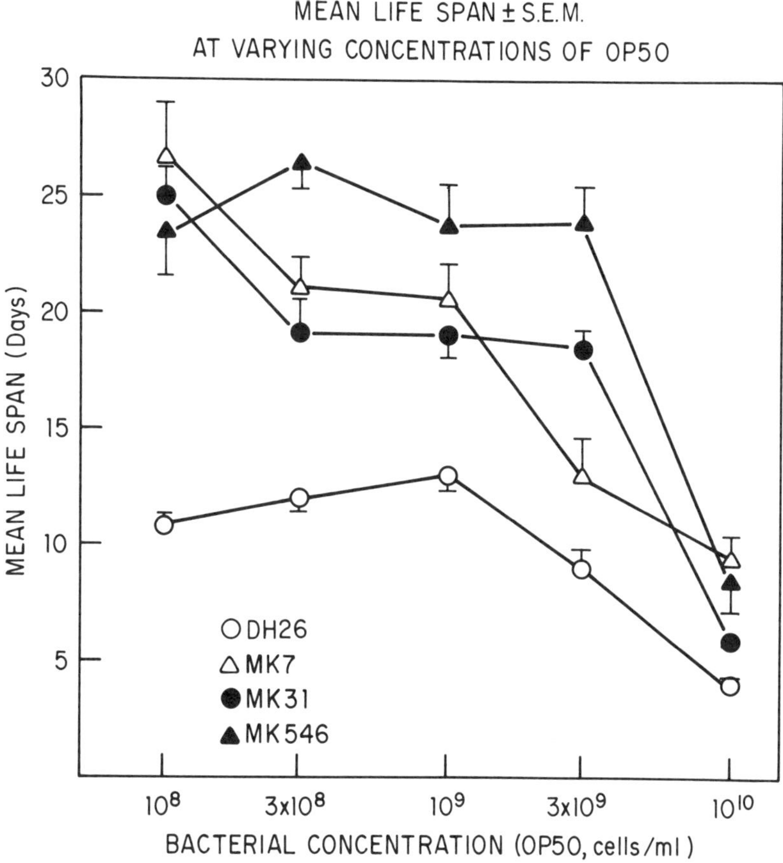



**Figure 9.** Survival populations of MK7, MK31, MK546, and DH26 at different concentrations of OP50. Mean life spans ± SEM were calculated from populations of 50 worms. Survivals of all mutants are significantly different from DH26 at the same concentration (P < 0.001) with the exception of MK31 at $3 \times 10^9$ bacteria per ml (P = 0.308).

In performing these mapping experiments we took advantage of the self-fertilizing nature of *C. elegans* and its lack of inbreeding depression in that we were able to establish homozygous populations for subsequent quantitative genetic analyses and that the lack of inbreeding depression simplifies the inference of genotype based on length of life of each resultant isolate. In contrast, sexually reproducing organisms face problems resulting from the segregation of alleles after crossing, as well as from inbreeding depression. These complexities are graphically illustrated by examining survival curves

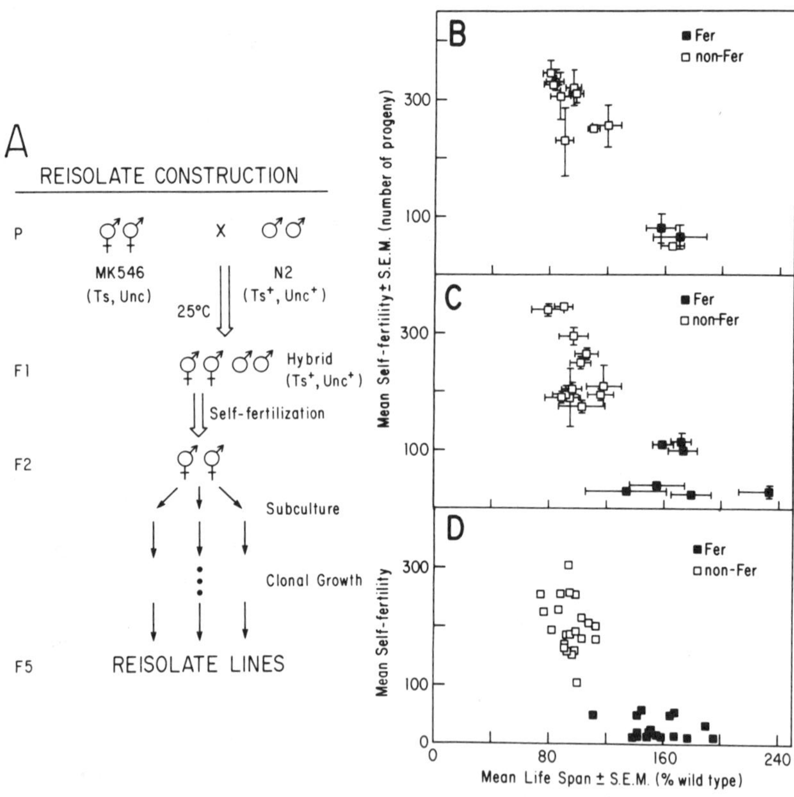



**Figure 10.** (A) Method for constructing homozygous populations from crosses between N2 and MK546. (B and C) Life expectancy at 20° of reisolates from the cross of MK546 [*age- 1(hx546) fer-15(b26ts)* II; *unc-31(z1)* IV] to N2 is plotted relative to hermaphrodite self-fertility; (B) $F_5$ reisolates from experiment 1, and (C) $F_{15}$ reisolates from experiment 2. (D) Life expectancy at 25° of $F_{10}$ reisolates from crosses of MK542 [*age-1(hx542) fer-15(b26ts)* II; *unc-31(z2)* IV] to N2. Fer (■) and non-Fer (□) stocks are indicated; because of the large number of points, standard errors are not shown in Figure 10D, but ranged from 5% to 15% of the mean life span, while self-fertility is the average of 3 to 5 hermaphrodites whose progeny were counted collectively rather than individually (from Friedman and Johnson, 1988a).

shown in Figure 11; the inference that a single gene specifies length of life would be quite difficult to make from these data alone.

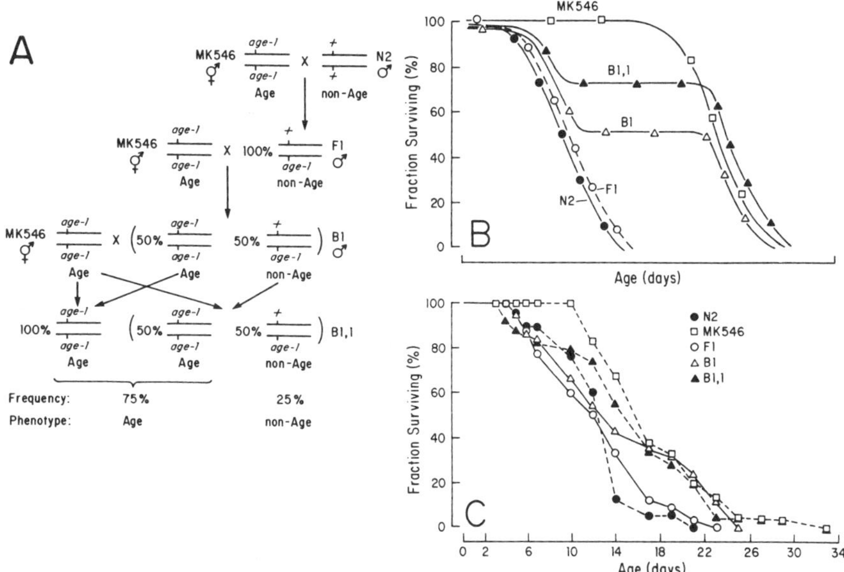



**Figure 11.** Scheme for following the segregation of a life-span determining gene in genetically heterogeneous populations. (A) MK546 hermaphrodites were backcrossed to N2 males to measure life span in the $F_1$. $F_1$ males were backcrossed to MK546 hermaphrodites to obtain a $B_1$ generation which were similarly backcrossed to obtain the $B_{1,1}$ generation. Also shown in this figure are the proportions of Age and non-Age progeny expected in each generation. (B) Idealized survival curves expected at each generation, assuming single gene segregation for *age-1*. (C) Actual survival curves obtained from the crossing scheme described in A (from Friedman and Johnson, 1988a).

## Fine Structure Mapping of *age-1*

Using both three-point crosses and deficiency analysis we have further localized *age-1* with respect to outside markers. In recombinants selected between *dpy-10* and *unc-4*, the lower fertility characteristic associated with *age-1* is shown to cosegregate with *fer-15* (Figure 12; Fitzpatrick and Johnson, unpublished). An alternate approach, deficiency mapping, uses a series of deficiencies covering much of the region between *dpy-10* and *unc-4* (Sigurdson *et al.*, 1984) and assigns *age-1* to a region between the nominal breakpoints of mnDf91 and mnDf92 which puts it into the region containing *fer-15* and *emb-27* (Figure 13; Shoemaker and Johnson, unpublished).

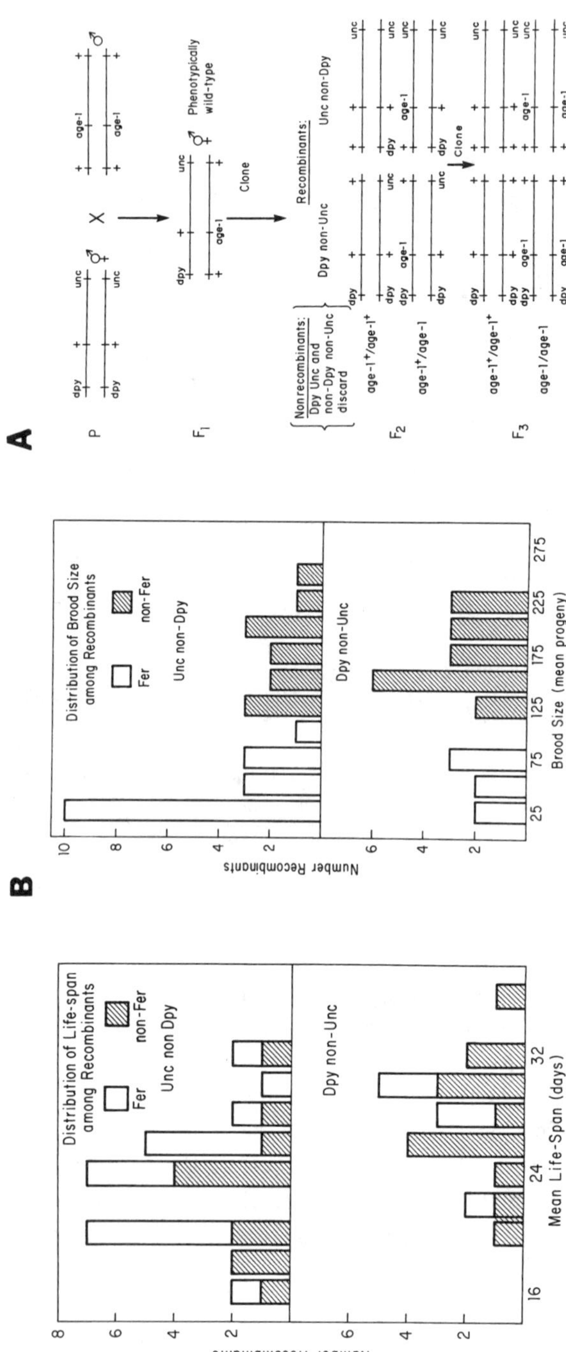


**Figure 12.** Scheme for performing three-point crosses (A) and results for fertility (B) and for life span (C).

**A**

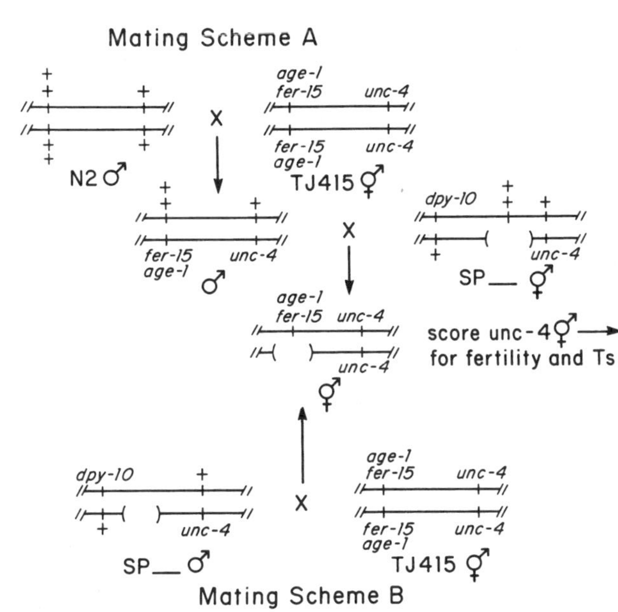


**B**

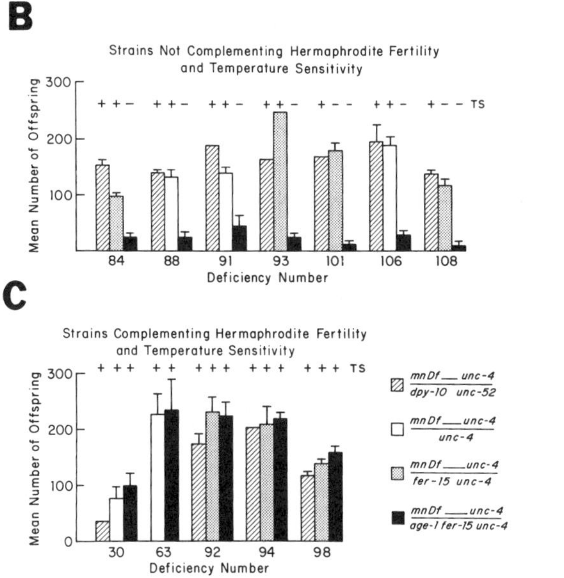


**Figure 13.** Scheme for performing deficiency analyses on fertility (A) and results (B).

## Effects on Other Physiological and Developmental Traits

Although *age-1(hx546)* lowers hermaphrodite self-fertility, it does not markedly affect the length of the reproductive period. All of the increase in life expectancy is due to an increase in the length of postreproductive life. Small changes in rate of movement at different chronological ages are seen when *age-1* and wild type are compared; similarly, changes in age-specific levels of lysosomal enzymes can be detected (Conley and Johnson, unpublished; Russell and Seppa, this volume). However, lipofuscin levels do not appear to be altered (Le Noir and Johnson, unpublished), suggesting that *age-1* changes one of the aspects of aging in *C. elegans* - that limiting length of life - without dramatically affecting other physiological systems.

## SUMMARY AND PERSPECTIVES

So far as we are aware, this mutation in *age-1* is the only instance of a well-characterized genetic locus in which the mutant form results in lengthened life. Consistent with the recessive nature of *age-1(hx546)* is the interpretation that longer life results from the elimination of normal gene function; deficiency analysis (Figure 13) suggests that *age-1(hx546)* is a null allele. Thus life span is shortened by the normal action of a gene whose function may be primarily involved in increasing reproduction. The *age-1* mutation dramatically displays a trade-off wherein reproductive effort is increased by the normal allele at a "cost" of loss of 1/2 of postreproductive life as is predicted by the Antagonistic Pleiotropy model for the evolution of senescence (Williams, 1957; Rose, 1985).

The molecular cloning and characterization of this locus is likely to provide significant insights into heretofore theoretical arguments concerning the evolutionary basis of senescence. Some of these arguments are described elsewhere in this volume (see Charlesworth, Rose, Kirkwood, Hutchinson, this volume; Partridge and Harvey, 1988) and may help to distinguish between rival theories. In light of such evolutionary arguments we favor a model in which the action of *age-1* in lengthening life results *not* from elimination of a programmed aging function but rather from the lack of the detrimental action of a gene whose primary function is involved in hermaphrodite reproduction. The existence of such genes offers an optimistic view about our ability to intervene in the aging processes to mimic the action of mutant alleles such as *age-1*.

## ACKNOWLEDGEMENTS

We thank N. L. Foltz, P. M. Cuccaro, W. L. Conley, and J. Le Noir for permission to cite unpublished data. Supported by grants from the National Institutes of Health (AG05720 and AG08322), from the National Science Foundation (8208652), and a Charles A. Dana Award from the American Federation for Aging Research. Some stocks were supplied by and are available through the Caenorhabditis Genetics Center, which is supported by contract NO1-AG-9-2113 between the NIH and the curators of the University of Missouri.

## REFERENCES

BAILEY, D. W. 1981. Strategic uses of recombinant inbred and congenic strains in behavior genetics research. **In**: *Genetic Research Strategies for Psychobiology and Psychiatry*, (Ed. E. S. Gershon, S. Matthysse, X. O. Breakefield, & R. D. Ciaranello), pp. 189-198. New York: The Boxwood Press.

BAKER, G. T. III, JACOBSON, M. & MOKRYNSHI, G. (1985) Aging in Drosophila. **In** *Handbook of Cell Biology of Aging* (Ed. V. J. Cristofalo), pp. 511-578. Boca Raton, FL: CRC Press.

BOTSTEIN, D. and MAUER, R. (1982) Genetic approaches to the analysis of microbial development. *Ann. Rev. Genet.* **16**: 61-83

BRENNER, S. (1974). The genetics of *Caenorhabditis elegans*. *Genetics* **77**: 71-94

COULSON, A., SULSTON, J., BRENNER, S., and KARN, J. (1986) Toward a physical map of the genome of the nematode *Caenorhabditis elegans*. *Proc. Natl. Acad. Sci. USA* **83**: 7821-7825

COULSON, A., WATERSTON, R., SULSTON, J., and KOHARA, Y. (1988) Genome linking with yeast artificial chromosomes. *Nature* **335**: 184-186

EMMONS, S. W. (1988) The genome. **In**: *The Nematode* Caenorhabditis elegans. (Ed. W. B. Wood), pp. 47-79. Cold Spring Harbor, NY: Cold Spring Harbor Laboratory.

FALCONER, D. S. (1981) *Introduction to Quantitative Genetics*. London: Longman.

FIRE, A. (1986) Integrative transformation of *Caenorhabditis elegans*. *EMBO J.* **5**: 2673-2680

FRIEDMAN, D. B. and JOHNSON, T. E. (1988a) A mutation in the *age-1* gene in *Caenorhabditis elegans* lengthens life and reduces hermaphrodite fertility. *Genetics* **118**: 75-86

FRIEDMAN, D. B. and JOHNSON, T. E. (1988b) Three mutants that extend both mean and maximum life span of the nematode, *Caenorhabditis elegans*, define the *age-1* gene. *J. Gerontol. Biol. Sci.* **43**: B102-109

HERMAN, R. K. and HORVITZ, H. R. (1980) Genetic analysis of *Caenorhabditis elegans*. **In**: *Nematodes as Biological Models*, **Vol. 1** Behavioral and Developmental Models (Ed. A. M. Zuckerman), pp. 227-262. New York: Academic Press

HERMAN, R. K. (1988) Genetics. **In**: *The Nematode* Caenorhabditis elegans. (Ed. W. B. Wood), pp. 17-45. Cold Spring Harbor, NY: Cold Spring Harbor Laboratory

HODGKIN, J. H., HORVITZ, H. R. and BRENNER, S. (1979) Nondisjunction mutants of the nematode *Caenorhabditis elegans*. *Genetics* **91**: 67-94

JOHNSON, T. E. (1984) Analysis of the biological basis of aging in the nematode, with special emphasis on *Caenorhabditis elegans*. **In**: *Invertebrate Models in Aging Research* (Ed. D. H. Mitchell and T. E. Johnson), pp. 59-93. Boca Raton, FL: CRC Press

JOHNSON, T. E. (1986) Molecular and genetic analyses of a multivariate system specifying behavior and life span. *Behav. Genet.* **16**: 221-235

JOHNSON, T. E. (1987) Aging can be genetically dissected into component processes using long-lived lines of *Caenorhabditis elegans. Proc. Natl. Acad. Sci. USA.* **84**: 3777-3781

JOHNSON, T. E., CONLEY, W. L. and KELLER, M. L. (1988) Long-lived lines of *Caenorhabditis elegans* can be used to establish predictive biomarkers of aging. *Exp. Gerontol.* **23**: 281-295

JOHNSON, T. E. and McCaffrey, G. (1985) Programmed aging or error catastrophe? An examination by two-dimensional polyacrylamide gel electrophoresis. *Mech. Ageing Devel.* **30**: 285-297

JOHNSON, T. E., MITCHELL, D. H., KLINE, S., KEMAL, R. and FOY, J. (1984) Arrest of development results in arrest of aging of the nematode *Caenorhabditis elegans. Mech. Ageing Devel.* **28**: 23-40

JOHNSON, T. E. and WOOD, W. B. (1982) Genetic analysis of life-span in *Caenorhabditis elegans. Proc. Natl. Acad. Sci. USA* **79**: 6603-6607

KIMBLE, J. and HIRSH, D. (1979) The postembryonic lineages of the hermaphrodite and male gonads in *Caenorhabditis elegans. Dev. Biol.* **70**: 396-417

KLASS, M. R. (1983) A method for the isolation of longevity mutants in the nematode *Caenorhabditis elegans* and initial results. *Mech. Ageing Dev.* **22**: 279-286

KLASS, M. R. and HIRSH, D. (1976) Nonaging developmental variant of *Caenorhabditis elegans. Nature* **260**: 523-525

LUCKINBILL, L. S., ARKING, R., CLARE, M. J., CIROCCO, W. C., and MUCK, S. A. (1984) Selection for delayed senescence in *Drosophila melanogaster. Evolution* **38**: 996-1003

MITTON, J. B. and GRANT, M. C. (1984) Associations among protein heterozygosity, growth rate, and developmental homeostasis. *Ann. Rev. Ecol. Syst.* **15**: 479-499

MOERMAN, D. G., BENIAN, G. M. and WATERSTON, R. H. (1986) Molecular cloning of the muscle gene *unc-22* in *Caenorhabditis elegans* by Tc1 transposon tagging. *Proc. Natl. Acad. Sci. USA* **83**: 2579-2583

NICHOLAS, W. L., GRASSIA, A. and VISWANATHAN, S. (1973) The efficiency with which *Caenorhabditis briggsae* (Rhabditidae) feeds on the bacteria *Escherichia coli. Nematologica* **19**: 411-420

PARTRIDGE, L., and HARVEY, P. H. (1988) The ecological context of life history evolution. *Science* **241**: 1449-1455

RIDDLE, D. L. (1988) The dauer larva. **In:** *The Nematode* Caenorhabditis elegans. (Ed. W. B. Wood), pp. 393-412. Cold Spring Harbor, NY: Cold Spring Harbor Laboratory

ROSE, M. R. (1984) Laboratory evolution of postponed senescence in *Drosophila melanogaster. Evolution* **38**: 1004-1010

ROSE, M. (1985) Life history evolution with antagonistic pleiotropy and overlapping generations. *Theor. Pop. Biol.* **28**: 342-358

SCHIEMER, F. (1982) Food dependence and energetics of free living nematodes. *Oecologia (Berl.)* **54**: 108-121

SCHIEMER, F., DUNCAN, A. and KLEKOWSKI, R.Z. (1980) A bioenergetic study of a benthic nematode, *Plectus palustris de Man 1880*, throughout its life cycle. *Oecologia (Berl.)* **44**: 205-212

SIGURDSON, D. C., SPANIER, G. J., and HERMAN, R. K. (1984) *Caenorhabditis elegans* deficiency mapping. *Genetics* **108**: 331-345

SULSTON, J. E. and HORVITZ H. R. (1977) Post-embryonic cell lineages of the nematode *Caenorhabditis elegans. Dev. Biol.* **56**: 110-156

SULSTON, J. E., SCHIERENBERG, E., WHITE, J. G., and THOMSON, J. N. (1983) The embryonic cell lineage of the nematode *Caenorhabditis elegans. Dev. Biol.* **100**: 64-119

WILLIAMS, G. C. (1957) Pleiotropy, natural selection, and the evolution of senescence. *Evolution* **11**: 389-411

## DISCUSSION

1. Asked where the variability comes from that makes the survival curve less than perfectly square Johnson pointed out that the environment affects a quantitative trait like aging, especially over time, so that all individuals do not die at the same time. This is also true in inbred mice.

2. An unanswered question was why do the worms die? Do they run out of something? This seems unlikely, as they are independent organisms. However, adults have no replicating cells except for reproductive cells. DNA repair should be no problem, as the worms can survive 100,000 R of irradiation.

3. Questioned whether *age-1* and *fer-15* may be alleles at the same locus, Johnson answered that he was testing this possibility with sequencing.

# 9

# EFFECTS OF SINGLE-GENE MUTATIONS ON AGING, AS MEASURED WITH BIOMARKERS

Richard L. Russell and Renée I. Seppa

## ABSTRACT

For the nematode *Caenorhabditis elegans* a set of 5 biomarkers of aging, including markers at levels from the populational (survival) to the biochemical (lysosomal enzyme levels), have been used to characterize perturbations of aging brought about by temperature reduction, nutritional restriction, and mutations in a few selected genes. The effects of temperature reduction and nutritional restriction are similar, but not identical, for all biomarkers; these two environmental perturbations appear to have broad general effects on aging. The effects of three mutations selected for extended longevity are less general; extended survival is accompanied by similar changes in some biomarkers, but not all, and there are significantly aberrant behaviors for at least one biomarker in each mutant strain studied. Thus, the affected genes do not have aging effects which are as broad or general as those of the environmental perturbations. Initial work on the complex gene *cha-1/unc-17*, which encodes the neurotransmitter biosynthetic enzyme choline acetyltransferase, shows that some mutant alleles reduce lifespan while others extend lifespan. There may be a correlation between these lifespan effects, the region of the complex gene affected, and the level of acetylcholine produced in these mutants.

## INTRODUCTION

As described in the preceding report (Johnson *et al.*, 1990), the genetic advantages of the small soil nematode *Caenorhabditis elegans* have been used in two general ways to approach the question of how lifespan may be genetically influenced in this organism. First, recombinant inbred strains between two separate wild isolates have been shown to have widely varying lifespans, and this has been used to estimate lifespan heritability, the number of major lifespan-affecting genes, and some relationships between lifespan and other characteristics (Johnson and Wood, 1982; Johnson, 1986). Second, mutants selected for extended lifespan have been used to ask how extensively lifespan can be affected by known single-gene mutations and to seek the nature of the genes exerting major lifespan effects (Klass, 1983; Johnson, 1986; Friedman and Johnson, 1988a, 1988b; Russell and Seppa, 1987).

One interesting result from the latter approach has been that simple mutations, apparently affecting only single genes, can produce a sizable extension of *C. elegans* lifespan. Because of the size of this lifespan effect, it was of interest to us to know whether comparable effects were exerted by the same mutations on other aspects of aging. Consequently we have examined in these mutant strains the progress of a series of 5 aging biomarkers, ranging in level from the populational to the biochemical. These biomarkers were chosen, based on our prior work to quantitate them in *C. elegans* (Bolanowski *et al.*, 1981; 1983), from a larger set which had been identified in earlier studies (for a review, see Rothstein, 1980; Zuckerman and Himmelhoch, 1980).

As a preamble to analysis of single-gene mutants, we used these 5 biomarkers to examine more closely the results of temperature reduction and nutritional restriction, two conditional alterations which can be used to extend lifespan in *C. elegans* as in other organisms (Klass, 1977; Johnson *et al.*, 1984; Russell and Seppa, 1987). Below we first review these results, which show that each of these alterations exerts broad aging effects; that is, all biomarkers are affected similarly by each. We then report how the same biomarkers have been used more recently to examine aging in single-gene mutants selected for extended lifespan. The results show that at least some aspects of aging are retarded in each, but the effects are certainly less broad and less consistent than with either temperature reduction or nutritional restriction. Lastly, we report the beginnings of similar biomarker-based studies of aging in single-gene mutants chosen not because of their known lifespan effects, but rather because the affected genes might conceivably be involved in controlling aging.

While these results are still fairly preliminary, they do suggest, surprisingly, that rather broad aging effects may be exerted by mutations in a gene governing synthesis of the neurotransmitter acetylcholine.

## STANDARD CONDITIONS AND BIOLOGICAL MARKERS OF AGING

We have chosen to conduct all our aging studies with *C. elegans* by maintaining animals (at a density of no more than 5 individuals per $cm^2$) on an agar surface seeded with a lawn of *E. coli* bacteria as food source. For convenience we have also chosen, after several preliminary tests, to use strain DH26 [*fer-15(b26ts)* II], grown at 25.5°C, as our standard, since this strain's sterility at 25.5°C permits us to maintain identified aging adults without continual removal of their progeny. (It should be noted that our strain choice

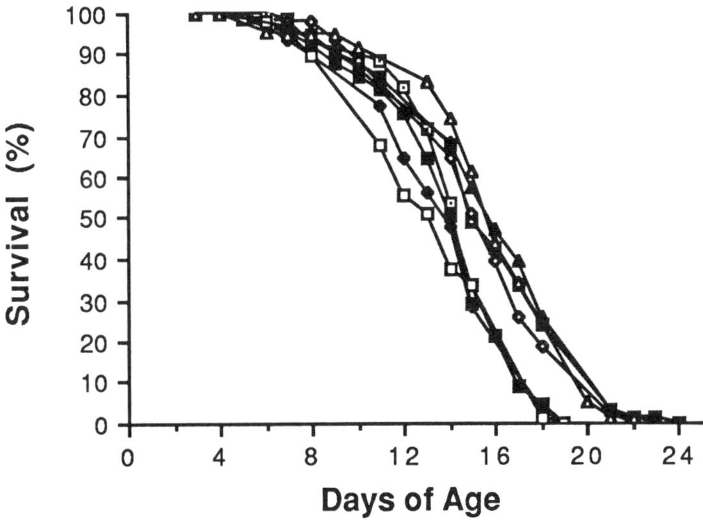

**Figure 1.** Reproducibility of Survival Curves under Standard Conditions. AU curves are for 96-animal cohorts of strain DH26 [*fer-15(b26ts)* II], maintained at 25.5°C, with lawns of *E. coli* strain OP50 as food source, on NGM agar (Brenner, 1974) in wells (2 ml of agar and 4 animals per well) of Linbro 24-well Tissue Culture Plates. Animals were transferred to these wells after 3 days of growth under the same conditions but on larger (95 mm diameter) Petri dishes containing 35 ml of NGM agar. Thereafter they were observed regularly (at 1- to 3-day intervals) without removing the plate cover. Death was determined by immobility, unresponsiveness to mechanical stimulation, lack of pharyngeal pumping, and degradation of internal anatomy. Results are for 8 experiments, conducted over a period of 24 months.

is the same as in the preceding report [Johnson *et al.*, 1988], but that our conditions are not. The liquid culture conditions used there undoubtedly differ from ours both in degree of exposure to the atmosphere and in nutritional richness, and differences in the details of results may derive from these conditional differences). The suitability of our choice of standard conditions is supported by the following evidence. First, as shown in Figure 1, survival curves under these conditions are quite reproducible. Second, as shown by example in Figure 2, survival curves for our standard strain, DH26, strongly resemble those for wild type *C. elegans* (N2), indicating that our strain choice has not had major unintentional effects on at least this one important aspect of aging.

Figure 3 shows, under our standard conditions, the age-dependent changes in the 4 additional biomarkers which we have chosen for our work. They are 1) movement rate, 2) lipofuscin level, 3) β-glucosidase activity, and 4) β-N-acetyl-glucosaminidase activity. (Elsewhere we have described in more detail

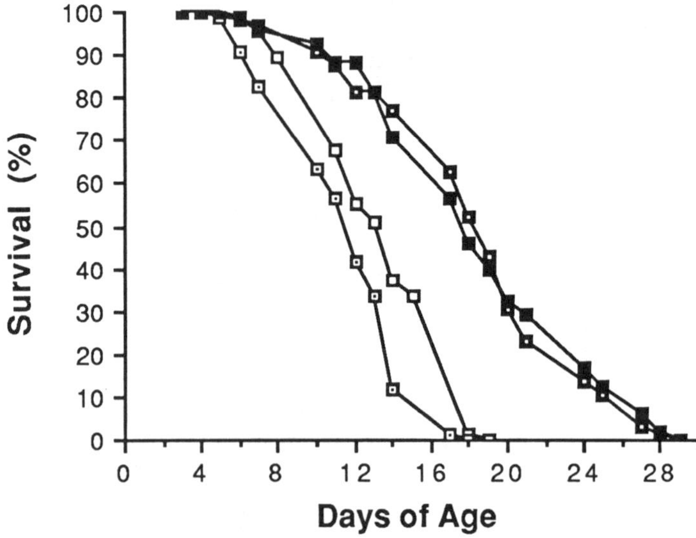


**Figure 2**. Survival curves for Strains DH26 and N2 [wild type] at 25.5°C and 16°C. Conditions as in Figure 1, except that regular removal from progeny, by transfer to fresh wells, was employed to maintain age synchrony. DH26, undotted symbols; N2, dotted symbols; 25.5°C, open symbols; 16°C, filled symbols. The lifespan extension achieved by temperature reduction from 25.5°C to 16°C is estimated at 38%, as judged by the fact that the best fit between survival curves could be obtained by rescaling the time axis for the 25.5°C curve by a factor of 1.38.

the measurement of these biomarkers and have documented the reproducibility of each [Russell and Seppa, 1987].) As the figure shows, each exhibits a large and relatively gradual change with age, and much of the change occurs post-reproductively, in what could be called the senescent phase of the life cycle. Figure 3 also provides further support for our choice of standard strain and conditions, since it shows that the age-dependent changes in these markers for our chosen strain (DH26) are essentially the same as for the wild type (N2).

## TEMPERATURE REDUCTION AND NUTRITIONAL RESTRICTION

Marked extensions of *C. elegans* lifespan by temperature reduction and nutritional restriction have already been reported (Klass, 1977; Johnson *et al.* 1984, Russell and Seppa, 1987). Figure 4 shows that for temperature reduction, the lifespan extension is accompanied by comparable changes in each of the other 4 biomarkers which we have chosen. In each case, the age-dependent change is markedly slower at 16°C than at 25.5° C, and in four of the five cases (lipofuscin being the exception) the general shape of the age-depend-

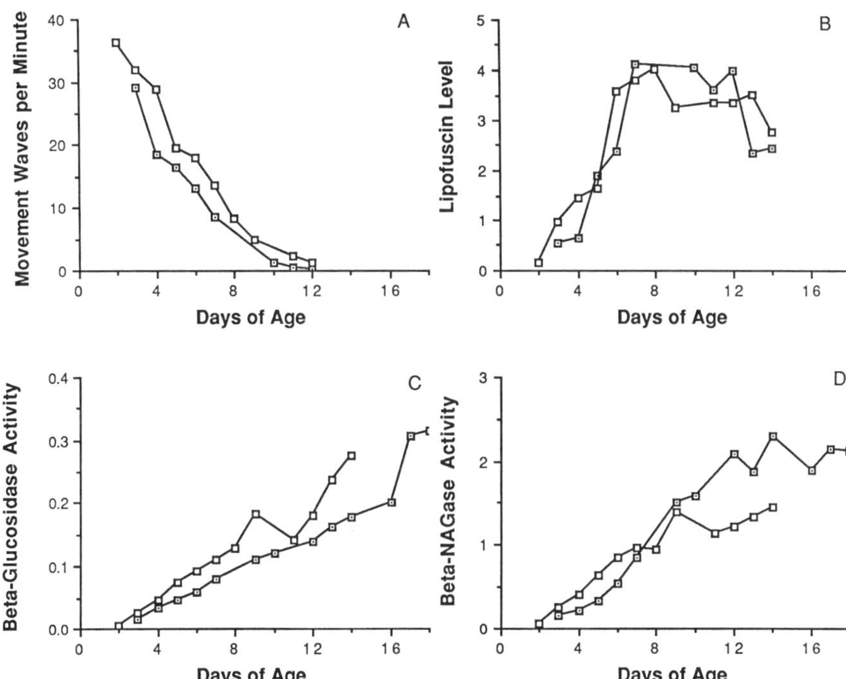



**Figure, 3.** Age-Dependent Changes in 4 Biomarkers for Strains DH26 and N2 at 25.5°C. Conditions as in Figure 2, except that populations were maintained throughout the lifespan on Petri dishes rather than Linbro Plate wells. Details of biomarker measurement are given in Russell and Seppa (1987). DH26, undotted squares; N2, dotted squares.

ence curve appears to be otherwise unaltered. Thus, temperature reduction has broad and comparable effects on each biomarker. It should be noted, however, that quantitatively the effects of temperature reduction are not equivalent; for example, survival is extended by a factor of 1.38, but the rates of change for the other biomarkers are slowed by factors ranging from 1.67 to 2.64.

For nutritional restriction, as shown in Figure 5, the lifespan extension is less marked (at least with the particular nutritional restriction regimen chosen), but again each of the other biomarkers is affected in at least a broadly similar way. Again, however, the effects are not equivalent; survival is extended by a factor of 1.18, but the rates of change for the other biomarkers are slowed by factors ranging from 1.25 to 2.01.

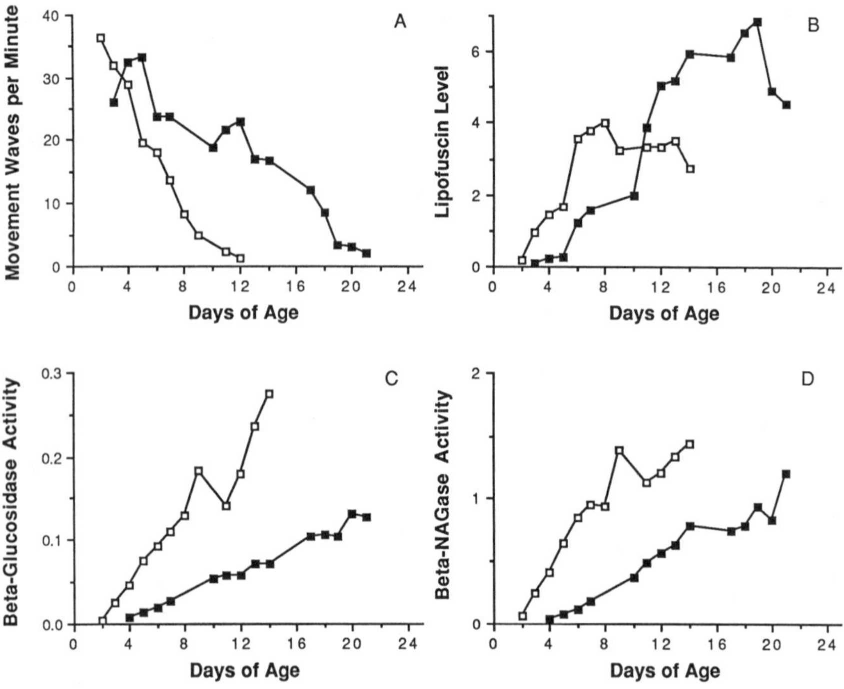

**Figure 4**. Effect of Temperature Reduction on Age-Dependent Changes in 4 Biomarkers. All results are for strain DH26. Conditions as in Figure 1, except that populations were maintained throughout the lifespan on Petri dishes rather than Linbro Plate wells. Optimal rescaling factors (as in Figure 2) are: Movement, 2.09; Lipofuscin, 1.67; β-Glucosidase, 2.64; β-N-acetylglucosaminidase, 2.61.


## MUTANTS SELECTED FOR LONGEVITY DIFFERENCES

To date, as far as we know, there are only two sources of *C. elegans* mutants which have been selected for their longevity differences from the wild type. The first source is a set of mutants originally isolated by Klass (1983) and subsequently backcrossed and studied more thoroughly by Johnson and his colleagues (Friedman and Johnson, 1988a,b). These mutants were selected by a "replica-plating" method based solely on lifespan differences. The second source consists of a single mutant isolated in our laboratory and briefly described elsewhere (Russell and Seppa, 1987). This mutant was selected for an extended period of reproduction, and was one of six so selected that also proved to have a lifespan extension. All of these mutants were

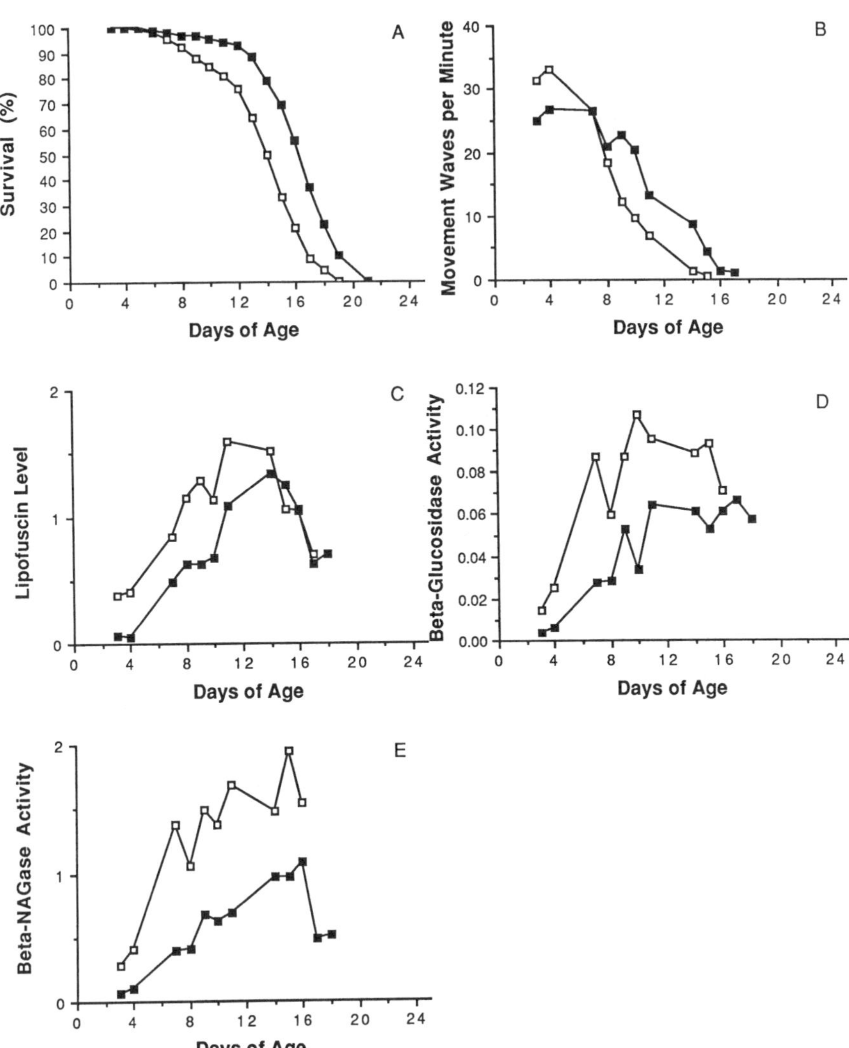

**Figure 5.** Effect of Nutritional Restriction on Age-Dependent Changes in 5 Biomarkers. All results are for strain DH26 at 25.5 °C, maintained throughout the lifespan on Petri dishes rather than Linbro Plate wells, and either fed normally (open squares) or nutritionally restricted by alternating 24 hr of normal feeding and 24 hr of starvation (filled squares). Two staggered populations were used so that markers could be measured daily, but always after feeding. Optimal rescaling factors (for time axis of normally fed curve to match restricted curve) are: Survival, 1.18; Movement, 1.25; Lipofuscin, 1.49; β-Glucosidase, 1.70; β-N-acetyl- glucosaminidase, 2.01.

isolated using DH26 as a starting strain, and thus all contain that strain's temperature-sensitive spermatogenesis mutation *fer-15* (*b26ts*), as well as one (or conceivably more) additional mutations.

For our work we chose 3 strains, our original mutant PR1400 (which has not been backcrossed and therefore may contain more than a single additional mutation) and backcrossed versions of two of the mutants isolated by Klass and studied by Johnson and his associates, TJ401 [*age-1(hx546)fer-15(b26ts)* II] and TJ412 [*age-1(hx542)fer-15(b26ts)* II]. Evidence has been presented elsewhere (Friedman and Johnson, 1988a,b) that the two *age-1* mutants harbor allelic mutations affecting lifespan and fecundity. However, the origin of these two mutants is somewhat clouded; 1) from his records, Klass cannot guarantee their independence of one another (M. R. Klass, personal communication), 2) neither mutation has yet been separated, despite energetic attempts, from the *fer-15 (b26ts)* allele which was included in the starting strain simply for technical reasons (Friedman and Johnson, 1988a), and 3) both mutant strains, when isolated, proved to harbor, in addition, mutant alleles of the unlinked, and apparently unrelated gene *unc-31*, from which the lifespan-affecting mutation has in each case been segregated by backcrossing (Friedman and Johnson, 1988a,1988b). These observations raise the possibility that these two mutants may not be independent in origin. However, we have treated them as separate during our work, in view of the uncertainty. Since our mutant has not been genetically characterized, it is unclear whether it also harbors an *age-1* mutation, as opposed to one or more mutations in other gene(s).

For each of the chosen "longevity" mutants, repeated survival curves are presented in Figure 6. Clearly, TJ412 reproducibly has a lifespan nearly twice that of the control, PR1400 has a much more modest, but nonetheless reproducible, lifespan extension, and TJ401, while falling somewhere between these two, is most accurately described as having a survival curve of rather different shape, beginning nearly coincident with that of the control but then diverging toward longer lifespan. For TJ412 and TJ401 both the magnitude of the lifespan effect and the nature of the survival curve are similar to those reported by Johnson and his colleagues (Friedman and Johnson, 1988a,1988b) for strains with the same mutant alleles under rather different culture conditions; this similarity supports the contention that these lifespan effects are not artifactual or somehow tied to nutritional peculiarities of either agar or liquid culture.

Figure 7 shows repeated measurements of the age-dependent decline of movement in the same strains. For TJ412, the rate of decline was considerably slower than for the control, in keeping with TJ412's much extended lifespan.

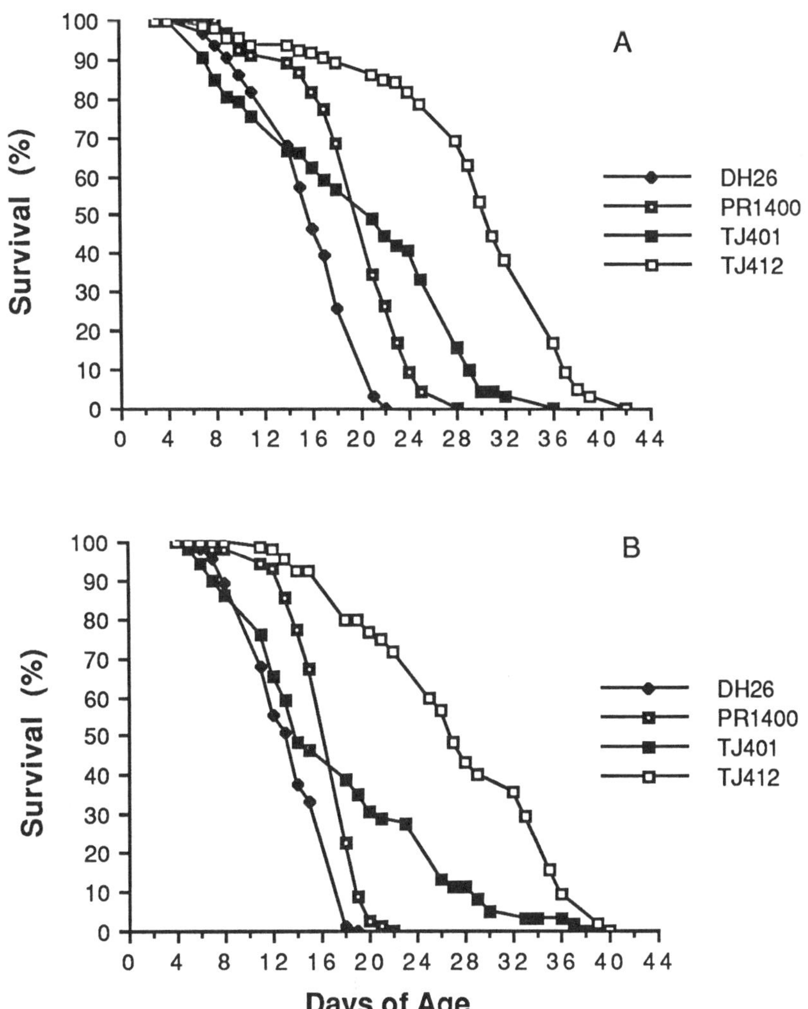


**Figure 6.** Survival Curves for DH26 and 3 "Longevity" Mutants. Conditions as in Figure 1. TJ401 and TJ412 harbor two apparently different mutant alleles of *age-1*. Panels A and B represent two experimental series, carried out over a period of 3 months.

Interestingly, TJ401, in this respect, was affected nearly as much as TJ412, despite the fact that its survival curve was decidedly different. Surprisingly, PR1400, despite having a small lifespan extension, nonetheless reproducibly exhibited the opposite sort of effect on movement, that is, a *more rapid* decline of movement rate than the control. This last result indicates that the

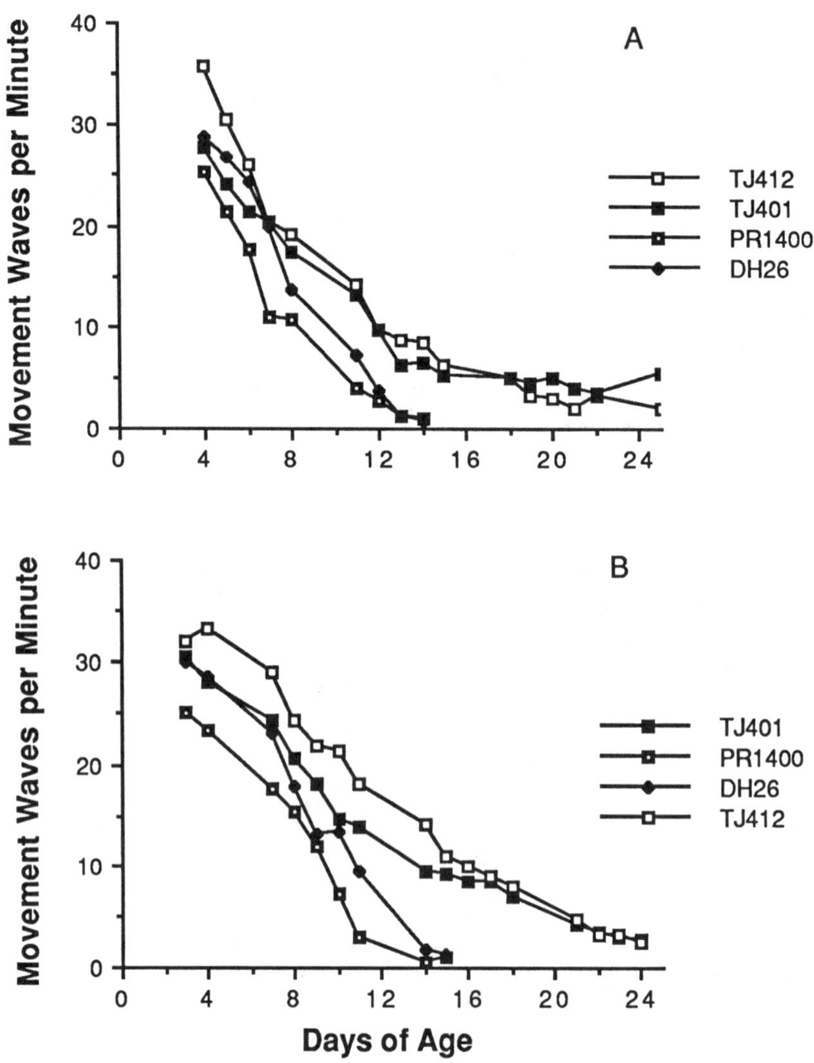


**Figure 7**. Age-Dependent Decline of Movement Rate for DH26 and 3 "Longevity" Mutants. Conditions as in Figure 4. Panels A and B represent the same two experimental series as in Figure 6.

rate of decline of movement can be genetically uncoupled from at least one other aspect of aging, namely an increased mortality rate.

Figure 8 shows, for the same strains, the age-dependent changes in the level of the fluorescent pigment lipofuscin. Despite extensive efforts at standardization, variability in these measurements is still a significant problem, as

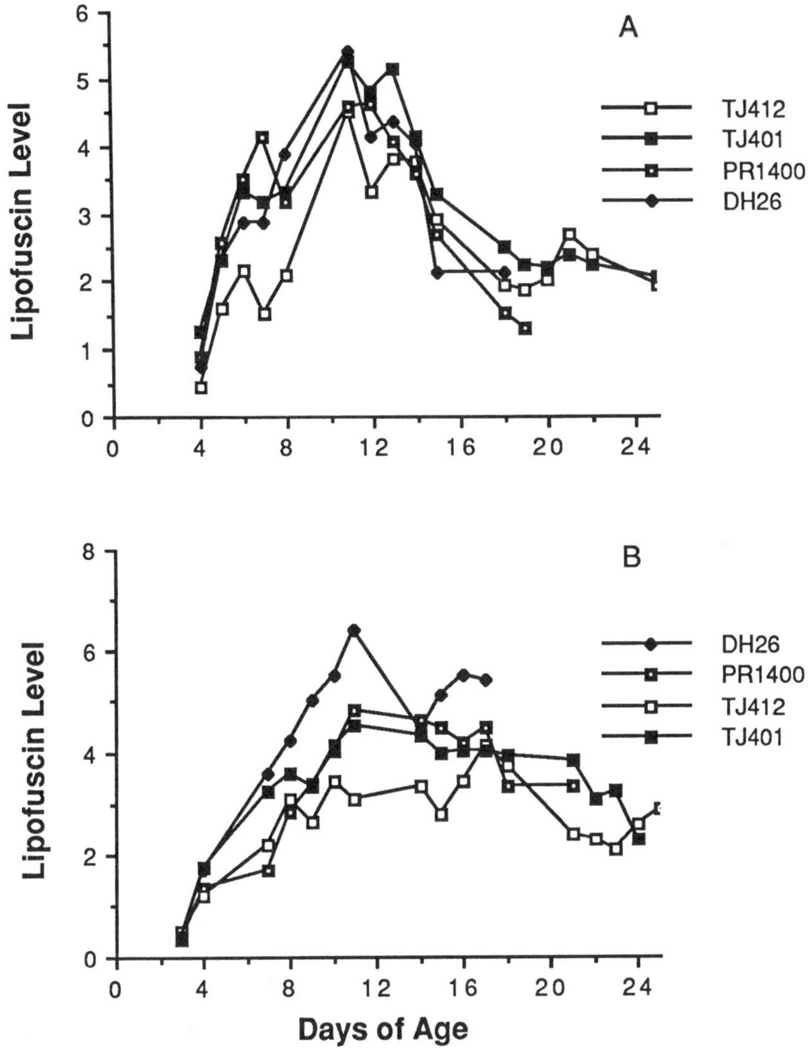

**Figure 8**. Age-Dependent Rise in Lipofuscin Level for DH26 and 3 "Longevity" Mutants. Conditions as in Figure 4. Panels A and B represent the same two experimental series as in Figures 6 and 7.

the presented repeat experiments demonstrate. However, it is clear that lipofuscin levels do rise markedly in all three mutant strains and, while the kinetics of the rise is not well characterized, there is a suggestion that the rate of rise may be diminished for TJ412. Whether there are comparable changes in PR1400 and TJ401 cannot be reliably judged, but if so the changes must be

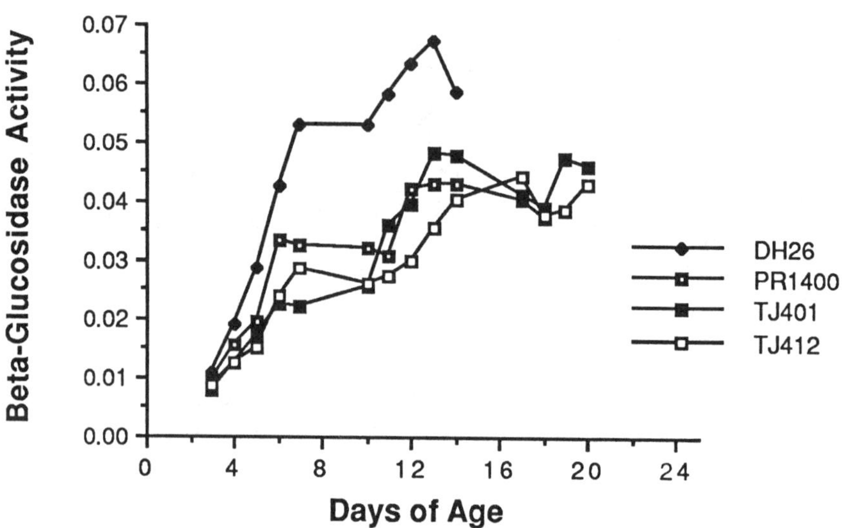


**Figure 9.** Age-Dependent Rise in β-Glucosidase Activity Level for DH26 and 3 "Longevity" Mutants. Conditions as in Figure 4. Separate experimental series from Figures 6, 7, 8, and 10.

small, and it is clear for all three strains that any effects on the rate of rise of lipofuscin are much less marked than those on lifespan.

Results with the two lysosomal enzyme biomarkers, β-glucosidase and β-N-acetyl-glucosaminidase, are presented in Figures 9 and 10. For β-glucosidase, all three mutant strains seem to have the same, significantly slower than normal, rate of rise with age, despite the clear differences among these mutants in survival and in decline of movement rate. And for β-N-acetyl-glucosaminidase, two of the mutant strains, PR1400 and TJ401, seem indistinguishable from the control, while the third, TJ412, has a perplexingly more rapid rate of rise and a higher final level than the control. From these results it is clear that the two lysosomal enzymes, while they change in quite parallel ways during normal aging, can be affected differentially by the mutations in these strains. It is also clear that TJ401 and TJ412 differ significantly from one another, suggesting that they contain different alleles of *age-1*.

## OTHER SINGLE-GENE MUTANTS

Recently we have begun to use a similar approach to test existing single-gene mutants for possible effects on aging. Among the many available *C. elegans* single gene mutants which might have been examined, we chose to

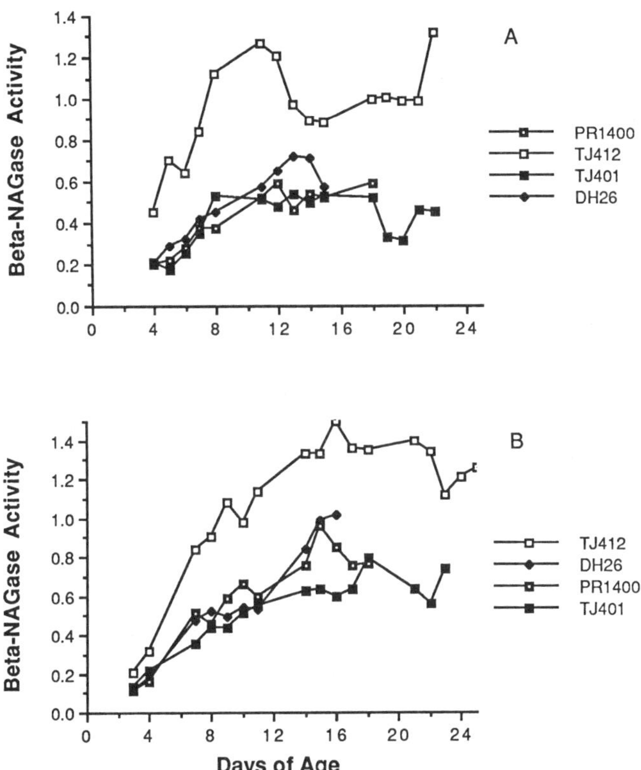


**Figure 10**. Age-Dependent Rise in β-N-acetylglucosaminidase Activity Level for DH26 and 3 "Longevity" Mutants. Conditions as in Figure 4. Panels A and B represent the same two experimental series as in Figures 6, 7, and 8.

concentrate initially on those concerned with metabolism of the neurotransmitter acetylcholine (ACh). In part this choice was based on our prior familiarity with and access to such mutants; our laboratory had previously identified and isolated multiple mutants in the genes encoding the degradative enzyme acetylcholinesterase, or ACHE, and the biosynthetic enzyme choline acetyltransferase, or CHAT (Johnson *et al.*, 1981; Culotti *et al.*, 1981; Rand and Russell, 1984; Kolson and Russell, 1985a, 1985b; Johnson *et al.*, 1988). But our choice was also based on somewhat more substantive grounds; we had previously used our mutants to show that marked genetic deficiencies for either ACHE or CHAT lead to significant growth impairments (Rand and Russell, 1984; Johnson *et al.*, 1988), the nature of which suggested that ACh itself might have a more profound role as a growth regulator than its activity as a simple neurotransmitter would suggest. In view of these impairments, we were anxious to see whether such deficiencies might also affect aging as well as growth.

Of the two enzyme activities, ACHE and CHAT, we focussed first on CHAT, because it is the easier to manipulate genetically. This is because CHAT is encoded-by a single (albeit internally complex) gene, *cha-1/unc-17*, on chromosome IV, whereas ACHE consists of three separate enzyme classes, A, B, and C, encoded by three separate genes, *ace-1*, *ace-2*, and *ace-3*, on chromosomes X, I, and II, respectively. Within the *cha-1/unc-17* gene encoding CHAT, fine structure mapping and characterization of many mutant alleles has revealed the presence of at least four distinct regions, as shown in Figure 11. Mutations mapping in each of these regions have overlapping but distinctive properties, and thus we chose to examine representatives of each type for possible aging effects.

For each of 15 mutant alleles of the *cha-1/unc-17* gene we constructed double mutants with the temperature-sensitive spermatogenesis-defective *fer-15* allele *b26ts*, and then carried out survival studies on these double mutants. A striking feature of the results, illustrated in Figure 12, is the wide range of lifespans exhibited by these strains, extending from considerably shorter than the control to considerably longer. For the most extreme cases we repeated the survival studies, and in these cases, at least, the differences were reproducible, as shown in Figure 13. Studies on these extreme cases are continuing and are not yet complete, but we have, in a single experiment so far, followed two more of the standard biological markers in these mutants, viz. $\beta$-glucosidase activity and $\beta$-N-acetylglucosaminidase activity. As shown in Figure 14, the two extreme mutant cases differ significantly from one another in both markers, and in each case the difference is consonant with the lifespan difference, that is, the shorter-lived mutant has a much more rapid rate of enzyme activity change with age than does the longer-lived one. Clearly, considerable work remains to be done with these and other mutant alleles, but so far, at least, these mutants appear to have unexpectedly broad effects on aging. A possible interpretation of the allelic differences is offered in the Discussion, below.

## DISCUSSION

In the work described above, we have used five selected biomarkers of aging to examine aging effects produced by two conditional alterations (temperature reduction and nutritional restriction) and a set of single gene mutations. The effects produced by the two conditional alterations have been rather broad, in that all biomarkers are affected similarly, albeit not identical-

## The ChAT Gene Complex of *C. elegans*

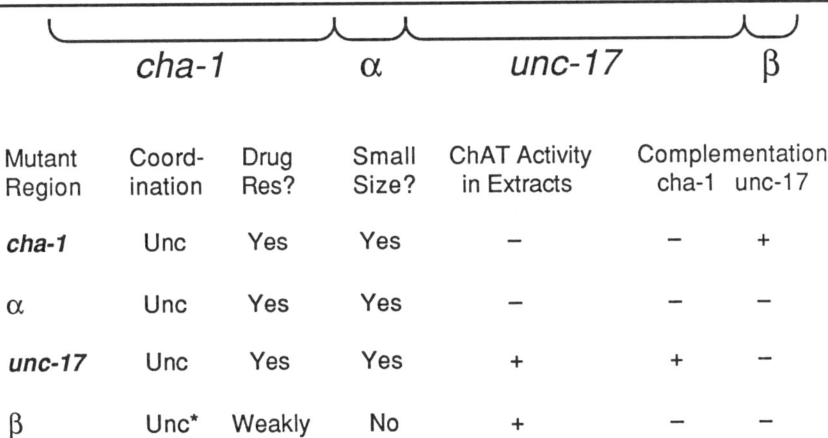



| Mutant Region | Coord-ination | Drug Res? | Small Size? | ChAT Activity in Extracts | Complementation cha-1 | Complementation unc-17 |
|---|---|---|---|---|---|---|
| *cha-1* | Unc | Yes | Yes | – | – | + |
| α | Unc | Yes | Yes | – | – | – |
| *unc-17* | Unc | Yes | Yes | + | + | – |
| β | Unc* | Weakly | No | + | – | – |

**Figure 11.** Structure of the *cha-1/unc-17* Complex Gene on Chromosome IV of *C. elegans*. Based on Rand and Russell (1984), Rand (1985), and personal communication from J. B. Rand. Of a total of 27 mutant alleles affecting this complex, 11 have been assigned a position on this fine structure map, serving to identify the 4 regions shown. *Unc* signifies coiling uncoordination typical of many of these mutants; *Unc* signifies a somewhat less severe curly uncoordination; *Drug Res* signifies resistance to a series of anti-cholinesterases of varying chemical classes, including carbamates and organophosphates; *SmaU* Size signifies a proportionately scaled-down adult size correlated with slowed growth during juvenile development; Complementation is scored by coordination in obligate double heterozygotes, + meaning coordination, - meaning uncoordination. As described elsewhere (Rand and Russell, 1984), the CHAT encoded by this complex gene is believed to be a functional homodimer, of which each monomer has a catalytic domain encoded by the *cha-1* region another essential domain encoded by the *unc-17* region, and a region important for dimerization, encoded by the 0 region; complementation between *cha-I* and *unc-17* mutants is thought to occur by formation of mixed dimers.

ly, by each. The effects produced by the single-gene mutations, however, have been more diverse, suggesting a variety of different ways in which single gene products can be involved in aging processes.

Of the aging effects examined, those produced by temperature reduction seem to be the most striking. All 5 of the examined biomarkers exhibited marked retardation at 16°C, relative to the standard temperature of 25.5°C. Furthermore, in 4 of the 5 cases, the age-dependence curve obtained at 16°C

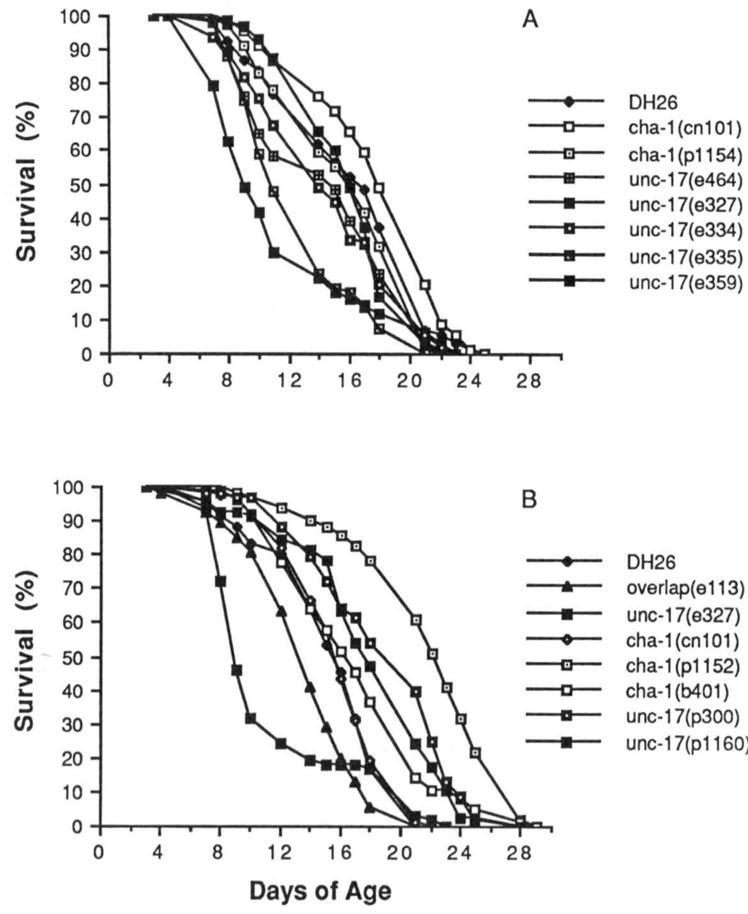


**Figure 12**. Survival Curves for DH26 and Several Strains with Mutations in the *cha-1/unc-17* Complex Gene. Conditions as in Figure 1. Each strain carried *fer-15(b26ts)* II in addition to the indicated allele of *cha-1/unc-17*. The "overlap" allele *e113* is one of two β -region alleles (see Figure 11).

could be fitted very closely to that obtained at 25.5°C by the simple transformation of rescaling the time axis; this indicates that the process of age-dependent change was apparently altered only in its rate, not in other aspects. Even in the 5th case, lipofuscin, where a higher level is reached at 16°C, the overall shape of the age-dependence curve at 16 °C still exhibits its characteristic and unusual property of rising to a peak and then dropping slightly. Overall, then, aging at 16°C, while slowed relative to 25.5°C, otherwise exhibits many similar properties.

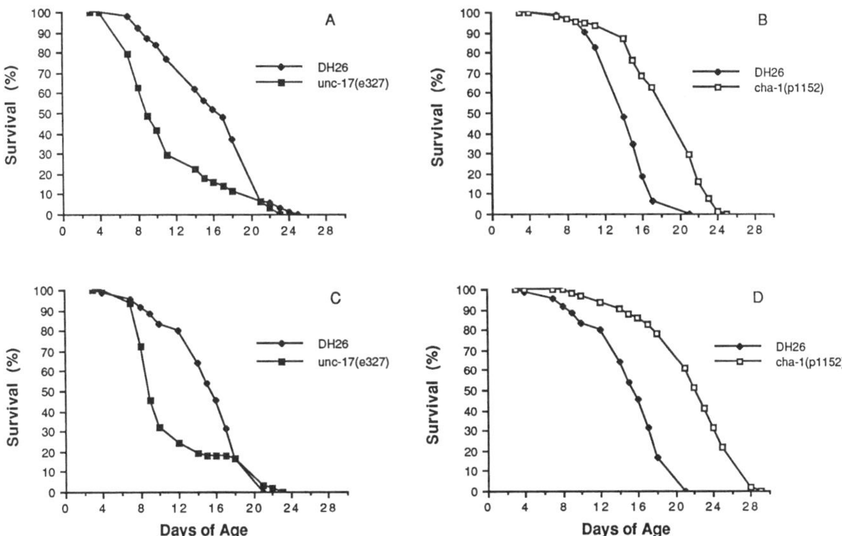



**Figure 13.** Reproducibility of Survival Curve Differences for Strains with Extreme Lifespan-Affecting Alleles of the *cha-1/unc-17* Complex Gene. Conditions as in Figure 1, strains as in Figure 12. Panel A is from one experimental series, panel B from a second, and panels C and D from a third. All were performed over a period of 4 months.

The general similarity of aging at these two temperatures is consistent with other work in which earlier aspects of the life cycle were examined at very nearly the same two temperatures (Byerly *et al.*, 1976). Growth curves for *C. elegans* at 16°C, including the four points of cuticular molting, can be fitted very closely to those obtained at 25°C, again by the simple transformation of scaling the time axis. The scaling factor which gives the best fit in this case is 1.94, within the range of 1.67 to 2.64 shown by the 4 non-survival biomarkers. Thus, whatever the reasons, temperature effects on both development and aging are quite similar for *C. elegans*.

The aging effects produced by nutritional restriction, or at least by the chosen regimen of alternate 24-hour periods of full bacterial feeding and starvation, are less marked than with temperature reduction, but otherwise appear about as broad. All of the biomarkers appear to have been affected in

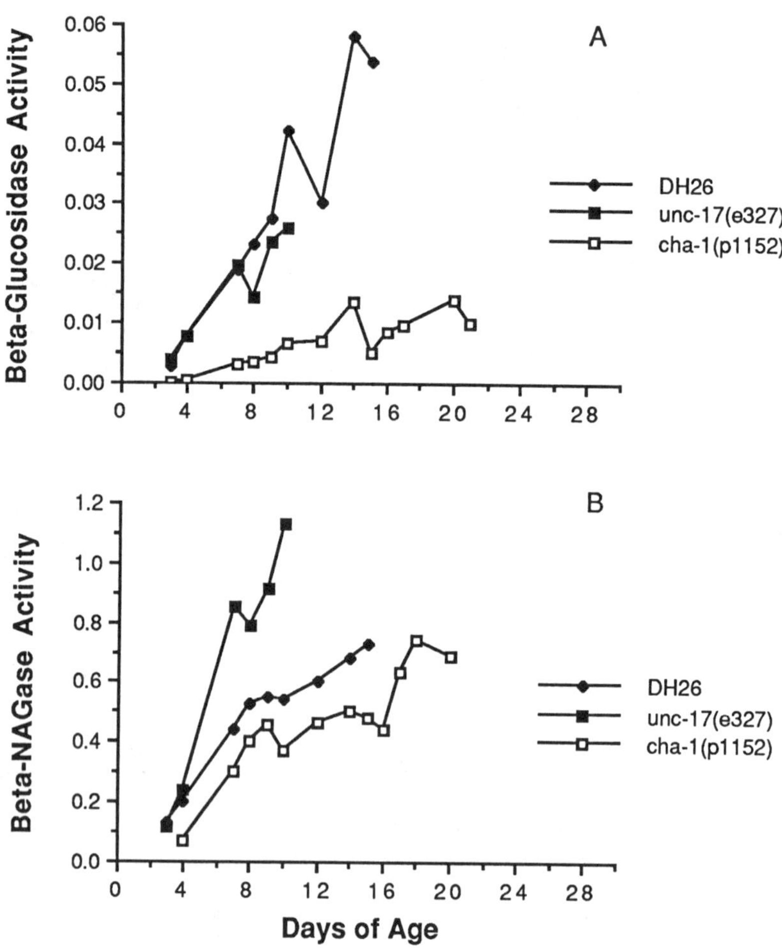

**Figure 14,** Age-Dependent Changes in Activity Levels of Two Lysosomal Biomarker Enzymes for DH26 and Extreme *cha-1/unc-17* Strains. Conditions as in Figure 4, strains as in Figure 12. Both panels are drawn from the same experimental series as panels C and D of Figure 13.

at least a broadly similar way, although the limited extent of the effects makes it difficult to make a more detailed comparison. Clearly, it would be desirable to explore the possibility that greater effects might be produced by more stringent nutritional limitations, and there is available evidence that such limitations can be tolerated, at least up to a point (Johnson *et al.*, 1984; Russell and Seppa, unpublished).

The available data on temperature reduction and nutritional restriction show that while the biomarkers are similarly affected by each, the effects on the individual biomarkers are not identical. In particular, both alterations apparently affect survival less markedly than the other 4 biomarkers. This is, of course, evidence against the extreme notion that each biomarker might somehow be temporally driven by tight coupling to a central clock, but at the same time it is consistent either with looser coupling to such a clock or with the complete absence of such a clock. The results may also indicate that survival is, in general, the least easily modified of the markers we have chosen, and if so, this would probably imply that future mutant searches should be focussed, as has the major past one, on screening directly for extended lifespan, rather than for slowed rate of change in some other biomarker.

For each of the 3 mutants selected for longevity differences, the pattern of change in biomarkers was more diverse than with either temperature reduction or nutritional restriction. In particular, although each mutant did show retardation of at least one other biomarker besides survival, none of the three mutants exhibited parallel changes in all biomarkers. One important corollary is that the chosen biomarkers can be *differentially* affected by mutations, and thus must have some degree of *independent* genetic control. But on the other hand, the fact that some biomarkers were *jointly* affected in some mutants indicates that they also have a degree of *common* genetic control. Thus it is feasible to envisage some sort of branched control pathway for these biomarkers (and similarly for other aging processes not measured), with specific gene products involved in particular branches. It seems too early to even attempt to sketch such a pathway from the current results, but it can reasonably be hoped that additional mutants, if analyzed adequately with respect to changes in several biomarkers, might be used to derive such a pathway.

The *age-1* gene, because it has received considerable attention, is of particular interest as regards these general issues of genetic control of aging. On the one hand, neither of the 2 *age-1* mutants examined exerts parallel effects on all 5 biomarkers. On the other hand, each of the 2 *age-1* mutants does affect more than one biomarker, in roughly parallel ways, suggesting that age-1 could produce a gene product involved specifically in some branch of a control pathway.

A distinctly puzzling aspect of *age-1*, however, is the significant difference in biomarker phenotype between the two *age-1* mutants examined. While both do show extended lifespan and a comparably retarded slowing of movement, their survival curves are reproducibly different in shape, and

TJ412 shows a paradoxically higher than normal level of β-N-acetyl-glucosaminidase, whereas TJ401 does not. Barring the trivial possibility of unintended differences arising from the backcrosses producing these strains, a first conclusion from these differences is that the contained *age-1* mutant alleles, *hx546* and *hx542*, probably are in fact different from one another, the uncertainties in their origins notwithstanding. At the same time, however, the differences make it impossible to judge what the biomarker phenotype for an *age-1* null allele might be, and thus it is difficult to specify more fully what the possibilities might be for a potentially controlling role for the *age-1* gene product. Clearly, if the function of *age-1* is to be better understood, a number of new mutant alleles are needed, and these should be extensively characterized with respect to changes in aging biomarkers.

The one additional "longevity" strain studied, PR1400, is currently of limited usefulness, primarily because its lifespan extension is quite modest. As a result it is hard to test whether PR1400 may have parallel alterations in other aging biomarkers, except that it clearly does not as regards loss of movement (where its rate of loss is accelerated rather than retarded). Fecundity has not yet been measured in this strain, but if it is as low as with the two *age-1* mutants (Friedman and Johnson, 1988a,b), the fecundity difference may permit backcrossing and complementation testing with those mutants; without such a difference, backcrossing and complementation testing based simply on lifespan seems technically unfeasible, and it may thus be impossible to decide whether PR1400 carries an *age-1* mutation. Even though PR1400 is currently of limited use, it is clear, in view of the very different origins of the few lifespan-extending mutants so far studied, that other such mutants, of independent origin, are badly needed to assess both the possible range of phenotypes and the number of genes which can yield such mutants.

Our results with mutations in the *cha-1/unc-17* gene are both intriguing and puzzling. Firstly, it seems surprising to find such extensive lifespan effects among mutant alleles of one of the first genes which we chose to examine. Perhaps the choice was simply fortunate, but we suspect that lifespan-extending effects may be more common than we would have expected, and that it may therefore be worth examining carefully a number of other already known genes for such effects. (If this approach is indeed adopted, it would seem wise to focus on genes for which multiple mutant alleles are available, and for which the finding of an effect would have clear and testable implications.) Secondly, it seems surprising to find such extensive interallelic differences among *cha-1/unc-17* mutant alleles; some produce marked shortening of lifespan, others marked extension. In one sense these results parallel those with *age-1*, in which the 2 tested mutant alleles also had significantly different effects on survival curves and on some biomarkers. But with *cha-1/unc-17* the differences are clearly more marked, and it becomes an interesting challenge to try to understand them.

One intriguing possibility, based on our current understanding of the structure and function of *cha-1/unc-17*, is that the opposite effects of some mutant alleles might arise because they fall in different regions of the gene, with putatively different roles in the final gene product, CHAT. As described in more detail elsewhere (Rand, 1985), the *cha-1* region of the gene is believed to encode a domain which possesses ChAT's active site for the synthesis of acetylcholine (from acetyl-CoA and choline), whereas the *unc-17* region is believed to encode a domain which is not catalytic but is nonetheless essential for the proper *in vivo* functioning of the full CHAT molecule (perhaps by ensuring proper regulation and/or localization of the catalytic domain). Part of the supporting evidence for these beliefs is that *unc-17* mutants, despite complementation patterns indicating that they belong to the same gene as *cha-1* mutants, do not reduce CHAT activity levels in extracts, nor do they have reduced levels of the CHAT product, acetylcholine. Indeed, at least some *unc-17* mutants actually have elevated levels of acetylcholine (Hosono, 1987; J. Rand, personal communication), which could be interpreted to signify that their CHAT activity is hyperactive because of altered regulation or inappropriate localization.

A quick glance at Figure 12 suggests how these ideas might be relevant to the lifespan differences among different *cha-1/unc-17* mutant alleles. While the pattern is not totally comprehensive, in general the strains with lifespan extensions carry *cha-1* mutant alleles, while those with lifespan reductions carry *unc-17* mutant alleles, and this is certainly true of the two extreme cases. In brief, then, there is a correlation among these mutants between the level of acetylcholine (measured in a few cases, expected in others) and the degree of lifespan shortening; mutants with probable higher than normal levels have shorter than normal lifespans, those with probable lower than normal levels have longer than normal lifespans. A possible implication, if this thinking is correct, is that acetylcholine level itself might play a major role in determining lifespan, perhaps in its role as a neurotransmitter, or perhaps because of some more general signalling function. (With regard to the latter possibility, it is noteworthy that *cha-1* and *unc-17* mutants are almost unique, among uncoordinated mutants, in being significantly smaller than normal as adults.)

While admittedly speculative, this notion does at least have the virtue of testability. One obvious testable prediction is that the level of acetylcholine, if measured for all *cha-1/unc-17* alleles, should show the expected correlation with lifespan shortening. Another prediction, although perhaps not as rigorous, is that an alternative manipulation of acetylcholine levels, by genetic alteration of the degradative acetylcholinesterase (ACHE) enzymes controlled by *ace-1*, *ace-2* and *ace-3* should also affect lifespans, and in predictable ways (appropriately lowered ACHE levels should raise acetylcholine levels and shorten lifespan). And if these predictions hold, it may even be possible to mimic genetic alterations of acetylcholine levels pharmacologically, with drugs targeted at CHAT and AChE; certainly, if it were to be true, the finding the *C. elegans* lifespan could be extended by judicious application of a CHAT inhibitor would be striking and potentially far-reaching.

In view of all the above speculation, it is probably best to end on a cautionary note. For all of the lifespan-extending effects shown above to be exerted by single genes there is a central and currently unavoidable caveat. Since nutritional restriction can lead to a marked lifespan extension in *C. elegans*, there exists the disturbing possibility that mutations which also extend lifespan may do so by an essentially secondary, nutritional mechanism. In particular, if a mutation leads to lowered food intake (as a result of a general behavioral impairment, say), then it may also extend lifespan secondarily, because the reduced food intake constitutes nutritional restriction. For such a mutation it would still be true that the affected gene has a role in determining lifespan, but the quest to understand that role would presumably result mostly in an understanding of how the gene affected food uptake, rather than how the affected food intake subsequently influenced lifespan. In this particular case, of course, direct tests of food intake rate would reveal the most important mutational effect, but it is well to realize that there is a host of additional downstream possibilities (*e.g.* defective intestinal absorption) where the essential lifespan-affecting mechanism would be similar, but where appropriate tests for the defect are currently non-existent and sometimes difficult to envisage.

While it is difficult to avoid the kind of trap represented by such mutants, it seems clear that measurement of several biomarkers can help to establish whether the pattern of changes brought about by a given mutation may differ from that produced by nutritional deprivation (in which case the mutation would seem unlikely to operate secondarily through nutrition). In addition, examining nutritional deprivation effects in a genetically long-lived mutant can, if carefully done, help to establish whether the nutritional effect is additive to that of the mutation (in which case, again, the mutation would seem unlikely to be operating secondarily through nutrition).

In general, as this caveat points out, the complexity of aging in any organism requires careful attention to detail, the entertainment and testing of alterative hypotheses, and sensitivity to possible artefacts. While *C. elegans* has some distinct advantages for the use of genetic tools in unravelling aging, and consequently offers some unusual hope, this general consideration should apply to it as much as to any organism and must not be forgotten. We believe that the evidence presented above illustrates that the use of several biomarkers to characterize perturbations of aging is an important part of the careful approach required.

## ACKNOWLEDGEMENTS

Our work reported above was supported by grant No. AG 01154 from the National Institutes of Health in the U. S. Dept. of Health and Human Services. We thank Lewis A. Jacobson for discussions and suggestions throughout, and Thomas E. Johnson for supplying strains TJ401 and TJ412. Some of the *C. elegans* strains used were obtained from the Caenorhabditis Genetics Center, whose help we gratefully acknowledge.

## REFERENCES

BOLANOWSKI, M. A., RUSSELL, R. L. and JACOBSON, L. A. (1981) Quantitative measures of aging in the nematode *Caenorhabditis elegans*. I. Populational and longitudinal studies of two behavioral parameters. *Mech. Ageing Dev.* **15**: 279-295.

BOLANOWSKI, M. A., JACOBSON, L. A. and RUSSELL, R. L. (1983) Quantitative measures of aging in the nematode *Caenorhabditis elegans*. II. Lysosomal hydrolases as markers of senescence. *Mech. Ageing Dev.* **21**: 295-319.

BRENNER, S. (1974) The genetics of *Caenorhabditis elegans*. *Genetics* **77**: 71-94.

BYERLY, W. L., CASSADA, R. C., and RUSSELL, R. L. (1976) The Life Cycle of the Nematode *Caenorhabditis elegans*. I Wild-Type Growth and Reproduction. *Dev. Biol.* **51**: 23-33.

CULOTTI, J. G., vonEHRENSTEIN, G., CULOTTI, M. R., and RUSSELL, R. L. (1981) A second class of acetylcholinesterase-deficient mutants of the nematode *Caenorhabditis elegans*. *Genetics* **97**: 281-305.

FRIEDMAN, D. B. and JOHNSON, T. E. (1988a) A mutation in the *age-1* gene in *Caenorhabditis elegans* lengthens life and reduces hermaphrodite fertility. *Genetics* **118**: 75-86.

FRIEDMAN, D. B. and JOHNSON, T. E. (1988b) Three mutants that extend both mean and maximum life span of the nematode, *Caenorhabditis elegans*, define the *age-1* gene. *J. Gerontol. Biol. Sci.* **43B**: 102-109.

HOSONO, R., SASSA, T., and KUNO, S. (1987) Mutations Affecting Acetylcholine Levels in the Nematode *Caenorhabditis elegans*. *J. Neurochem.* **49**: 1820-1823.

JOHNSON, C. D., DUCKETT, J. G., CULOTTI, J. G., HERMAN, R. K., MENEELY, P. M., and RUSSELL, R. L. (1981) An acetylcholinesterase-deficient mutant of the nematode *Caenorhabditis elegans*. *Genetics* **97**: 261-279.

JOHNSON, C. D., RAND, J. B., HERMAN, R. K., STERN, B. D., and RUSSELL, R. L. (1988) The Acetylcholinesterase Genes of *C. elegans*: Identification of a Third Gene (*ace-3*) and Mosaic Mapping of a Synthetic Lethal Phenotype. *Neuron* **1**: 165-173.

JOHNSON, T. E. (1986) Molecular and genetic analysis of a multivariate system specifying behavior and lifespan. *Behav. Genet.* **16**: 221-235.

JOHNSON, T. E., FRIEDMAN, D. B., FITZPATRICK, P. A. and CONLEY, W. L. (1987) Mutant genes that extend life span. **In**: *Evolution of Longevity in Animals* (Eds. A. D. Woodhead and K. H. Thompson), pp. 91-100.

JOHNSON, T. E., FRIEDMAN, D. B., FITZPATRICK, P. A. and SHOEMAKER, J. E. (1990) Genetic variants and mutations of *Caenorhabditis elegans* provide tools for dissecting the aging Processes. *Growth Dev. Aging* in press

JOHNSON, T. E., MITCHELL, D. H., KLINE, S., KEMAL, R. and FOY, J. (1984). Arrest of development results in arrest of aging of the nematode *Caenorhabditis elegans*. *Mech. Ageing Dev.* **28**: 23-40.

JOHNSON, T. E. and WOOD, W. B. (1982) Genetic analysis of life-span in *Caenorhabditis elegans*. *Proc. Natl. Acad. Sci. USA* **79**: 6603-6607.

KLASS, M. R. (1977) Aging in the nematode *Caenorhabditis elegans*: Major biological and environmental factors influencing life span. *Mech. Ageing Dev.* **6**: 413-429. @REFERENCES = KLASS, M. R. (1983) A method for the isolation of longevity mutants in the nematode *Caenorhabditis elegans* and initial results. *Mech. Ageing Dev.* **22**: 279-286.

KOLSON, D. L., and RUSSELL, R. L. (1985a) New aetylcholinesterase-deficient mutants of the nematode *Caenorhabditis elegans*. *J. Neurogenet.* **2**: 69-91.

KOLSON, D. L., and RUSSELL, R. L. (1985b) A novel class of acetylcholinesterase, revealed by mutations, in the nematode *Caenorhabditis elegans*. *J. Neurogenet.* **2**: 93-110.

RAND, J. B., and RUSSELL, R. L. (1984) Choline acetyltransferase-deficient mutants of the nematode *Caenorhabditis elegans*. *Genetics* **106**: 227-248.

RAND, J. B. (1985) Fine structure genetic analysis of the *cha-1* complex locus in *Caenorhabditis elegans*. *Genetics* **110**: s60.

ROTHSTEIN, M. (1980) Effects of Aging on Enzymes. In: *Nematodes as Biological Models* (Ed. B. M. Zuckerman), Academic Press, NY, pp.4-28.

RUSSELL, R. L. and SEPPA, R. I. (1987) Genetic and environmental manipulation of aging in *Caenorhabditis elegans*. In: *Evolution of longevity in Animals* (Eds. A. D. Woodhead and K. H. Thompson), Plenum Press, NY, pp. 35-48.

ZUCKERMAN, B. M., and HIMMELHOCH, S. (1980) Nematodes as Models to Study Aging. In: *Nematodes as Biological Models* (Ed. B. M. Zuckerman), Academic Press, NY, pp. 29-46.

# 10

# MUTATIONS IN *DROSOPHILA* THAT ACT IN THE LARVAL STAGE AND INFLUENCE LARVAL OR ADULT LONGEVITY

Thomas Grigliatti, Murray Richter, and Ian Whitehead

## INTRODUCTION

A number of theories exist regarding the etiology of aging. These theories can be generally classified into two groups. One group suggests that aging is genetically programmed, while the other group suggests that aging results from the natural deterioration of any biologically essential process. In their simplest form neither model is correct, nor do they need to be mutually exclusive.

Those that purport that longevity is genetically determined suggest that genes that limit lifespan are part of the normal developmental program. Hence there has been explicit interest in whether genes, or physiological events, that function or occur early in development influence longevity in the adult. This issue is very easy to address in *Drosophila*.

As a holometabolous organism, *Drosophila* goes through two distinct life forms, the larva and the adult. The larva is not only morphologically distinct from the adult, it also responds differently to its external environment. For example, the larva is positively geotactic and negatively phototactic while the adult responds oppositely. Hence they could be viewed as two separate organisms which share the same genome. This genome is quite small, with about 5,000 to 10,000 functioning genes. This low gene number obviously puts some constraints on the diversity of gene action that can occur between the two body forms. In fact, there are many physiological and regulatory similarities between the two forms. For example, there is virtually no cell division in either the larval body proper (excluding those cells that are set aside to give rise to the adult) or the adult soma. Hence it is quite possible that a large proportion of those genes that function to regulate cell physiology are shared between the two body plans. In contrast, the genes that act to differentiate the adult and larval external body plan may be limited in number and more exclusive in function.

We shall address three issues concerning genes that act in the larval stages. First, do genes that modify the lifespan of the larval form also influence the longevity of the adult? Second, does the duration or rate of larval development influence the longevity of the adult? Third, are there genes that function in the larva, but influence the longevity of the adult form only?

## MATERIALS AND METHODS

### Stocks and Mutant Strains

Descriptions of the standard genetic markers and strains used in these studies can be found in Lindsley and Grell (1968). Oregon-R, a standard laboratory wild-type strain of *Drosophila* melanogaster, was used as the paragon for longevity tests. A number of experiments in our lab suggest that this strain is certainly among the longest lived of the commonly used laboratory strains (Richter, 1986).

The temperature sensitive mutations described below are all heat sensitive. They display the mutant phenotype at the restrictive temperature (29°C), while they are functionally normal at the permissive temperature (22°C or lower). All of the special mutations described below were induced using ethyl methanesulfonate (EMS) as the mutagen. Since EMS has a propensity for inducing mutations that behave as point mutations, it has been used extensively for inducing temperature sensitive mutations.

The mutations that extend larval development (*eld*) are all X-linked, recessive, and temperature sensitive. They were induced in an Oregon-R strain; hence it serves as the control strain. The mutations were induced following a standard protocol for the isolation of sex-linked recessive mutations (Grigliatti, 1986). The developing cultures were placed at the restrictive temperature, 29°C, and pupae that formed at the natural time interval were removed from the culture bottles and discarded. Those individuals in which pupariation was delayed by 5 days or more were removed, shifted to 22°C, and allowed to survive to adulthood. Single males that eclosed from these pupae were used to establish individual lines and each line was tested for extended larval lifespan. Three temperature sensitive strains were recovered in which the larval lifespan at 29°C was extended by two to four-fold. These have been termed extended larval development (*eld*$^{ts}$).

The temperature sensitive mutagen sensitive mutations (*mus*) used in this study are located on the second chromosome. They were isolated following the protocol described by Henderson *et al.* (1987). The *mus* mutations were induced on an isogenic *b*, *pr*, *cn* strain (*b* = black body, *pr* = purple eyes, and *cn* = cinnabar eyes are recessive markers located on the second chromosome), that is, the second chromosome homologues were genetically identical. Hence the *b, pr, cn* strain serves as the proper control in these sets of experiments. Nevertheless, the adult lifespan of the *b, pr, cn* and Oregon-R strains do not differ (data not shown). Four temperature sensitive *mus* mutations were recovered. One of these is ts sterile at 29°C and was not used in the following sets of experiments. Genetic tests demonstrate that the three *mus*[ts] mutations used in this study represent lesions in three different genes.

A complete description of the genetic strains and special chromosomes used in these studies is given at the end of the manuscript (Table 3).

## Culture Conditions

The food that was used in all of these experiments is the standard cornmeal-agar medium with Tegosept added to inhibit mold growth and ampicillin and streptomycin added to reduce bacterial infection (Leffelaar and Grigliatti, 1984a). The cultures were either maintained at 17°C ± 1, 22 ± 1, or 29 ± 1/2°C continuously, or they were shifted once between two of these temperatures (see below). The relative humidity was maintained at 45 to 60%.

## Alteration of Duration of Development

Adult flies of a given genotype were separated into groups and placed at 17, 22, and 29°C and allowed to acclimatize for 5 days before eggs were collected. Synchronous cultures of developing flies were established by following the protocol outlined by Homyk and Grigliatti (1983). The culture density was 40 to 50 eggs per vial. At least one set of cultures (a minimum of 10 vials) was allowed to complete development at the temperature at which it was established. In addition, one set of cultures was shifted down from 29 to 22°C and another set was shifted up from 17 to 22°C at daily intervals throughout the course of development. Once shifted, these cultures were allowed to complete development at 22°C. The date of the shift, the developmental stage at the time the culture was shifted, and the total duration of development were recorded for each culture. For example, since the Oregon-R strain requires nearly 29 days to complete development at 17°C, thirty sets of cultures were established at 17°C. One culture was allowed to complete development at 17°C, and one set was shifted up to 22°C at day one post-ovaposition and each subsequent day until day 30.

## Longevity

The larval lifespan was determined by establishing synchronous populations of fertilized eggs on 5.5 cm. petri plates at 22 and 29°C. To obtain survival curves, the number of living larvae per petri plate was counted at daily intervals and the developmental stage of each larva was noted (determined by morphology of the anterior spiracles). A larva was considered dead when no voluntary movement was observed in response to prodding with a brush tip or when pupation occurred (the larva undergoes histolysis shortly after pupariation). A minimum of 200 larvae were used to determine longevity for a given population.

The longevity of adults was determined at both 22 and 29°C. Adults were collected within one day of eclosion, separated by sex, and placed in vials (10 flies/vial). The flies were transferred to vials with fresh medium every 3 days for populations maintained at 22°C and every two days for populations maintained at 29°C. The number of living flies was counted at each transfer, and the numbers were summed to obtain survival curves. Survival curves were based on a minimum of one hundred individuals of each sex.

## RESULTS

### Mutations that Alter Larval Lifespan

The tissues of both the larval and adult forms of *Drosophila* are essentially separated during embryogenesis. The cells that form the external body plan of the adult, and those that will be used to replace internal organs of the larva, are set aside as packets of cells called imaginal disc cells (imaginal since the adult body is the imago) and histoblasts, respectively. The developmental fates of the imaginal disc cells and histoblasts are determined during embryogenesis. These cells continue to undergo division and their developmental capacity becomes increasingly restricted during the larval and early pupal period. The adult precursor cells appear to lack function in the larval body plan. They can be removed, either by physical extirpation or by mutation,with no effect on the survival or function of the larva. Hence the larva can be viewed as an ambulatory embryo that functions solely to nurture and host the continued development of the adult precursors.

As part of this role of ambulatory host, the components of the larval body must be removed to allow complete morphogenesis and function of the adult. Hence the larva undergoes programmed cell death. Shortly after pupariation the larval cells undergo histolysis. Transplantation studies have shown that during development larval cells actually acquire the competence to undergo cell death and histolysis (Bodenstein, 1943). Hence genes for programmed cell death must exist in the genome. It is formally possible that these same genes could be used to limit the lifespan of the adult. To examine this possibility we isolated mutations that extend the lifespan of larva and asked whether these mutations also function in the adult to extend lifespan.

| Table 1. Duration of Development (days) | | | |
|---|---|---|---|
| Genetic Strain | Temperature | | |
| | 17°C | 22°C | 29°C |
| *Oregon-R* | 27 | 15 | 9 |
| *eld-1*[ts] | 30 | 17 | 34[a] |
| *eld-2*[ts] | 29 | 16 | 19[a] |
| [a] These cultures were shifted down from 29°C to 22°C less than one day after pupariation. | | | |

Two temperature sensitive mutations that increase larval lifespan have been isolated following the procedure outlined earlier in the Materials and Methods section. Each of these mutations is heat-sensitive, that is, they extend the lifespan of larvae maintained at 29°C (restrictive temperature) but have little or no effect on the lifespan of larvae maintained at temperatures of 22°C or lower (Table 1). To determine the effect of these mutations on longevity of the larvae, synchronous cultures were established on petri plates at both 22 and 29°C. The number of larvae surviving and the developmental stage were monitored daily. Since many of the larvae eventually pupate, we simply used the time of pupariation as the point of larval death (recall that the larva undergoes histolysis shortly after pupariation). The longevity curves for the wild-type strain (Oregon-R) and the most extreme mutant (*eld-1*[ts]) are shown in Figure 1. The mutation extends the lifespan of the larva about four to five-fold when larvae are maintained at the restrictive temperature (Figure 1A) and it has virtually no effect at the permissive temperature (Figure 1B). The *eld-1*[ts] mutation acts on all three larval stages. The duration of each stage is extended about two to five-fold compared to that expected at 29°C with the largest effect occurring in the third instar stage (Figure 2). Finally, this mutation has very little effect on the viability of the larvae at each developmental interval (Figure 1).

To determine whether *eld-1*[ts] acts in the adult, the flies were allowed to develop to adulthood at the permissive temperature (22°C). Adults were collected within 24 hours of eclosion, separated by sex and two groups were established. One population (males and females) were left at 22°C and the other cohort was immediately placed at 29°C. Survival curves for both populations were obtained by transferring the flies to fresh vials at two day intervals and recording the number of individuals surviving at each transfer. The lifespan of *eld-1*[ts] adults did not differ from the Oregon-R control strain in cultures maintained at either 22 or 29°C (Figure 3). Similar results were obtained for another mutation, *eld-2*[ts]. The lifespan of larvae bearing this mutation is extended two to three-fold when the larvae are maintained at

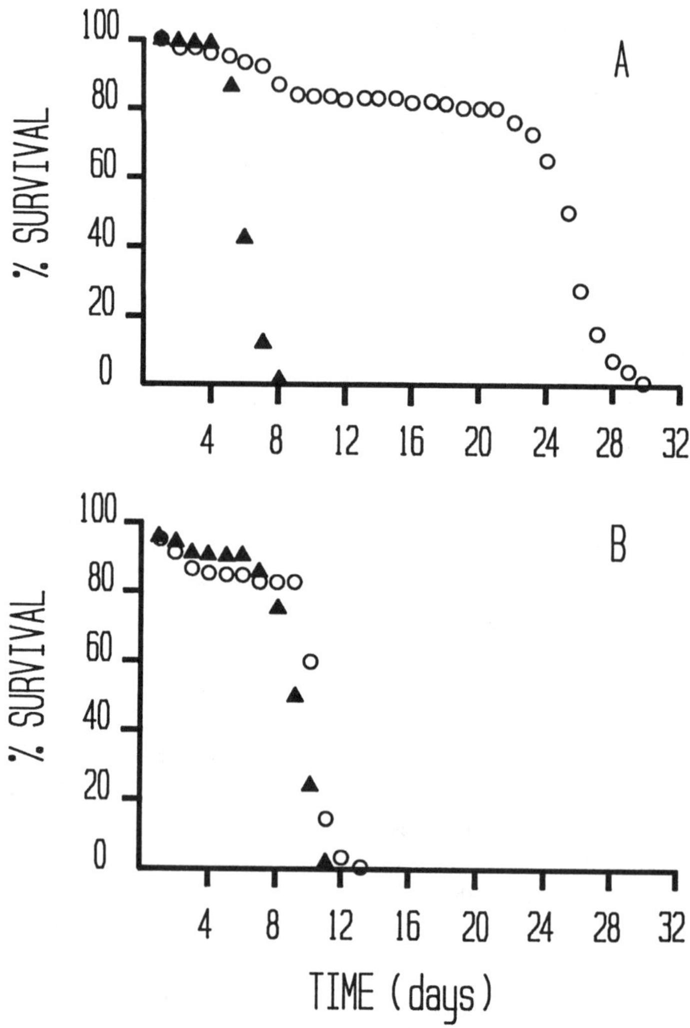

**Figure 1.** Survival curves for larvae. A) Populations established and maintained at 29°C. B) Populations established and maintained at 22°C. The filled triangle represent the wild-type strain Oregon-R; the open circles represent mutant strain *eld-1*[ts], no attempt was made to separate the sexes in either strain.

29°C. The mutation does not influence the longevity of adults maintained at 29°C (derived from cultures in which development occurred at 22°C).

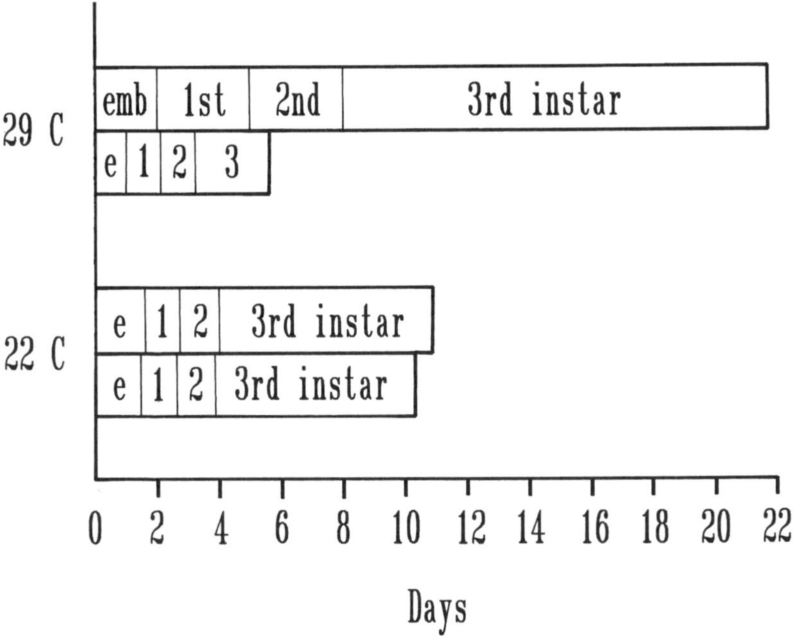


**Figure 2.** Duration of each of the larval stages at 22 and 29°C. At each temperature, the top bar graph refers to the mutant strain *eld-1*[ts] and the second bar graph refers to the wild-type strain Oregon-R. The vertical lines demarcate the first observation of transition from one stage to the next. The stages are embryo (e or emb), first instar (1 or 1st), second instar (2 or 2nd) and third instar (3 or 3rd).

While this represents a limited sample size, these data suggest that mutations that extend the lifespan of the larva do not necessarily influence the lifespan of the adult. This does not mean that the lifespan of the adult is not genetically programmed.

## THE INFLUENCE OF PRE-IMAGINAL DEVELOPMENT ON LONGEVITY OF THE ADULT

The lifespan of poikilotherms, cold blooded animals, is dependent on temperature. This is often used to support the rate of living theory of aging (Pearl, 1928). The $Q_{10}$, temperature coefficient, for longevity in *Drosophila melanogaster* is approximately 2 (Lamb, 1978; Leffelaar and Grigliatti, 1984b). That is, the lifespan decreases two-fold for every 10°C increase in temperature. However, the actual longevity curves for two populations of adults maintained at two different temperatures are identical when corrected for the difference in rate of living (Leffelaar and Grigliatti, 1984b ). Hence,

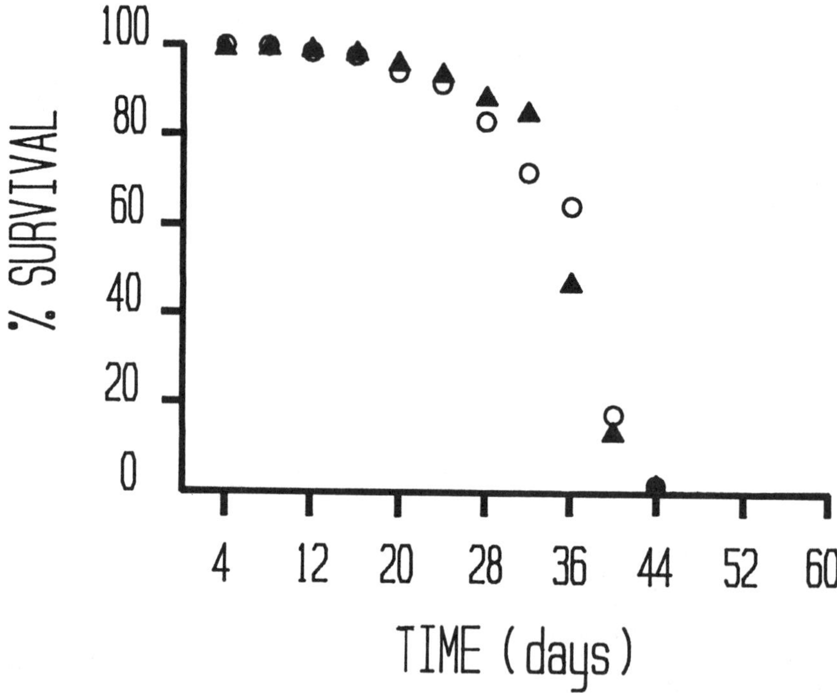

**Figure 3.** Survival curves for adult populations of wild-type and *eld-1*[ts] males maintained at 29°C post-eclosion. The filled triangles represent to the wild-type Oregon-R strain; the open circles represent the mutant *eld-1*[ts] strain.

alterations in body temperature result in temporal differences in lifespan but do not appear to cause any obvious physiological differences in aging and longevity.

In contrast, the duration of development has been observed to affect the longevity of adults. Alpatov and Pearl (1929) monitored the adult longevity of a wild-type strain of *Drosophila* that had been cultured at either 18 or 28°C during the pre-imaginal stages. They found that the flies that developed at the lower temperature lived longer regardless of the temperature at which the adults were maintained. Burcombe and Hollingsworth (1970) obtained similar results using first generation hybrid progeny derived from two wild-type strains. In contrast, Lints and Lints (1971) found a negative correlation between duration of development and adult lifespan. Both Burcombe and Hollingsworth (1970) and Lints and Lints (1971) argued that adult lifespan is somehow determined by the length of the developmental period. One might suggest that some physiological clock is set during development and that, once fixed, it influences the "rate of aging". If the adult lifespan is influenced by the rate of development then a series of temperature shifts during the pre-imaginal stages should delimit the interval during which the clock is set, that is, a temperature sensitive period for this phenotype should be identifiable.

Synchronously developing cultures of genetic siblings were established at 17, 22 and 29°C. Some cultures were allowed to complete development at the temperature at which they were established. In addition, each day a subset (5 vials) of the 29°C cohort were shifted down to 22°C and allowed to complete development at that temperature. Likewise, a subset of the cultures from the group established at 17°C were shifted up to 22°C and allowed to complete development. Two strains were used for these experiments: the wild-type strain (Oregon-R) and the temperature-sensitive strain *eld*$^{ts}$ which extends development in cultures maintained at 29°C (see above).

The duration of development in these strains varied depending on the temperature regime. The minimum and maximum duration of development for Oregon-R was 10 days (at 29°C) and 29 days (17°C) and for *eld-1*$^{ts}$ the minimum and maximum values were 17 (at 22°C) and 34 days (cultures shifted down from 29 to 22°C after pupariation), respectively. Shifting groups of developing cultures from 29 to 22°C, and from 17 to 22°C, produced adults in which the duration of development varied in daily intervals between these extremes. Shifting cultures from one temperature to another had a uniform affect on the rate of development (one stage was not affected more than another).

The lifespan of adults derived from these experiments was monitored at both 22 and 29°C. Adults were collected from each culture group within 24 hours of eclosion and separated into two populations, one of which remained at 22 while the other was placed immediately at 29°C. Hence, at each temperature (22 and 29°C), there were 42 populations of Oregon-R adults established (one from cultures that were allowed to develop at 17, 22, and 29 continuously, and one from each shift 29 to 22°C and 17 to 22°C). Likewise, 67 populations of *eld-1*$^{ts}$ were established at each temperature (22 and 29°C). The adults were transferred to fresh vials and monitored for viability at two or three day intervals. Examples of longevity curves for adults maintained at 29°C are shown in Figure 4. The duration of development for the Oregon-R males raised at 29, 22 and 17°C was 10, 15, and 29 days, respectively, and the longevity of these males at 29°C is shown in Figure 4A (survival curves for the females were also done and they are similar to those of the males). The duration of *eld-1*$^{ts}$ females raised at 29 (shifted down to 22°C on day 24), 22

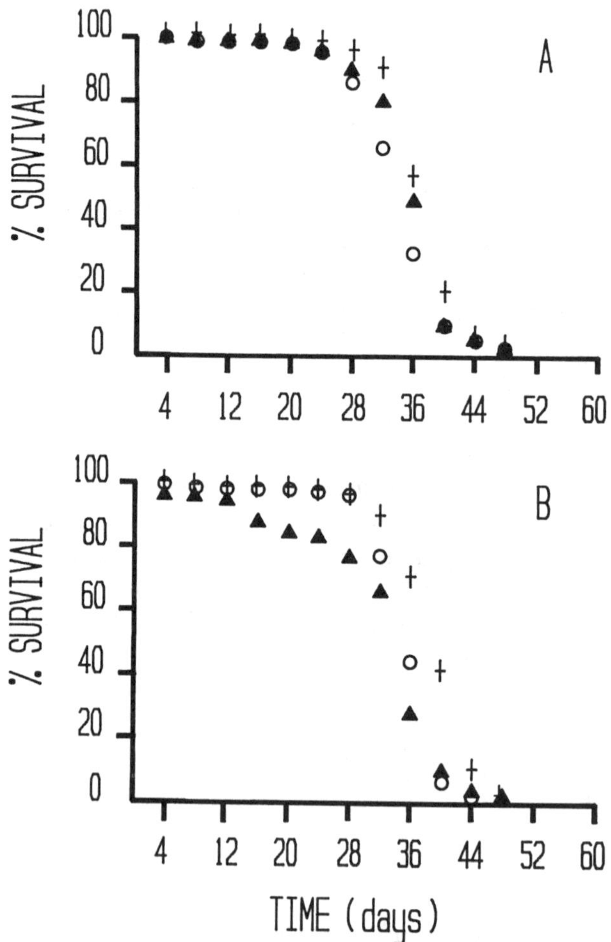

**Figure 4.** Survival curves for adult populations of wild-type and *eld-1*[ts] maintained at 29°C post-eclosion. A) Males of the wild-type strain Oregon-R. B) Females of the mutant strain *eld-1*[ts]. The adult populations were established from cultures in which pre-imaginal development occurred at 17, 22, or 29°C; the + symbol represents the 29°C group, the open circle represents the 22°C group and the filled triangle represents the 17°C group. In the case the *eld-1*[ts] (B) the + represent adult population derived from cultures that were maintained at 29°C for 24 days and then shifted down to 22°C for the remainder of development (recall that few *eld-1*[ts] survive if maintained at 29°C through pupation).

and 17°C was 36, 17 and 31 days, respectively and the longevity of these females at 29°C is shown in Figure 4B (survival curves for males were also done and they are similar to those of the females). Clearly, the duration, or rate, of development had no effect on the longevity of the adults.

## GENES THAT ACT IN THE LARVAL STAGE BUT INFLUENCE THE LONGEVITY OF THE ADULT

The results from the previous sections infer that mutations that influence the lifespan of larva do not necessarily influence the longevity of adults. In addition, no physiological clock appears to be set in response to variation in developmental rate. These results suggest that events which control the lifespan of larvae and those that control adult lifespan may operate independently. Indeed, in another set of experiments we were able to identify over a dozen mutations in separate loci that decrease the longevity of the adult (Leffelaar and Grigliatti, 1984a, and manuscript in preparation). Many of these genes appear to act only in the adult stage. However, even if the two processes are independent, it is quite possible that genes exist which function during the pre-imaginal stages, but only influence the lifespan of the adult. In this section, we attempt to identify such genes.

It has been postulated that aging in animals is a consequence of the accumulation of deleterious by-products of normal chemical events (i.e., free radicals) or damaged biochemical products (somatic mutation). This accumulation of damage, presumably reflects overload, decreased efficiency, or failure of one or more of the scavenging and/or repair systems in a tissue.

There has been much speculation, but little direct evidence, that DNA repair plays a major role in aging. Most of the support for the role of DNA repair in aging has come from studies using mammalian cells in tissue culture. For example, Price *et al.* (1971) found that DNA extracted from tissues of old mice had a higher template activity for DNA polymerase than DNA extracted from the same tissues of young mice. They concluded that the DNA from the older tissue had a greater number of single strand breaks. This interpretation was supported by Wheeler and Lett (1974) who found that the size of DNA extracted from tissues of old dogs was smaller than that from young dogs. Similar correlations between age and decline in repair capacity have been found in comparisons across species. For example, Hart and Setlow (1974) examined excision repair in primary fibroblast cultures derived from seven mammalian species and showed that there was a linear relationship between the maximum lifespan of the species and the amount of unscheduled DNA synthesis (DNA repair). Francis *et al.* (1981) found a positive correlation between mean lifespan and excision repair sites in DNA isolated from 21 mammalian species. These correlations between lifespan and DNA repair sites have been extended to include fibroblasts and primary lymphocytes cultured from primates (Hall *et al.*, 1984). Many researchers imply a causal relationship between loss of repair capacity (or increased unrepaired breaks) and aging. However, loss of repair capacity may be a consequence of aging. In fact, the evidence that aging is associated with increased DNA damage (or loss of repair capacity) is indefinite. For example, Woodland *et al.* (1980) and Kato *et al.* (1984) found no correlations between lifespan and DNA repair capacity in lower vertebrates and mammals, respectively. Hence, there is little evidence that suggests that a decline in DNA repair capacity actually leads to a decrease in longevity.

DNA repair has been extensively studied in *Drosophila*. Over 100 mutagen-sensitive (*mus*) mutations have been isolated (Boyd *et al.*, 1976; Smith *et al.*, 1980; Henderson *et al.*, 1987), and these identify at least 30 different genetic loci. Mutations that confer sensitivity to mutagens could reflect defects in metabolism rather than DNA repair. However, most of the *mus* mutations that have been characterized biochemically (18 of 19 to date) were found to be defective in one or more aspects of DNA repair. Indeed, *mus* mutations have been identified in all three major classes of repair: excision repair, post-replication repair and photo-repair (Boyd and Harris, 1985; Boyd and Shaw, 1982; Boyd *et al.*, 1982). The mutations we have isolated have not been analyzed biochemically; however, they are sensitive to several classes of mutagens including gamma radiation. We shall assume that these *mus* mutants are repair defective.

Several temperature-sensitive *mus* mutants have been identified (Henderson *et al.*, 1987) and these provide an ideal system for studying the role that DNA repair capacity may have on longevity. Three different recessive *mus*[ts] mutations, representing three different genes, were examined for their effect on longevity in the absence of any exogenous mutagens and then in the presence of very low (sub-lethal) doses of mutagen. The results for one of these will be presented here in some detail.

To demonstrate that the *mus A-1ts* is indeed temperature sensitive, matings were made between *mus/mus* and *mus/+* individuals and a single dose of mutagen was administered to their offspring at either 24, 48 or 72 hours after egg deposition. The ratio of *mus/mus* to *mus/+* survivors was scored. The data in Table 2 indicate that only the *mus* homozygotes that are kept at 29°C are sensitive to the mutagen. The *mus* homozygotes raised at 22°C are able to repair the mutations as well as the *b pr cn* (*mus*[+]) controls and the mus/+ heterozygotes are able to repair the damage at either temperature. This also demonstrates that the *mus* gene acts during the larval stages (first through early third instar).

To examine the effect of loss of DNA repair capacity on longevity in adults, synchronous cultures of the *mus* strains and their controls (*mus*[ts]/+ and *b pr cn/b pr cn*) were established at 22 and 29°C and allowed to complete

| Table 2. Viability After Exposure to MMS | | | |
|---|---|---|---|
| Dose % | Age at Exposure[a] (hours) | $mus^{+}/mus^{+b}$<br>22°C  29°C | $mus^{ts}/mus^{tsc}$<br>22°C  29°C |
| 0.0 | 48 | 1.01  1.05 | 1.01  0.96 |
| | 72 | 0.94  0.89 | 0.84  0.89 |
| | 96 | 0.96  1.02 | 0.83  0.86 |
| 0.01 | 48 | 0.92  0.89 | 0.86  0.89 |
| | 72 | 0.86  0.88 | 1.09  1.03 |
| | 96 | 0.93  1.06 | 0.84  0.91 |
| 0.04 | 48 | 0.89  0.79 | 0.86  0.05 |
| | 72 | 1.02  0.86 | 0.91  0.08 |
| | 96 | 0.96  0.92 | 0.91  0.09 |

[a] A single dose of methyl methanesulfonate (MMS) was administered at 48, 72, or 96 hours after egg deposition.

[b] The ratio of b pr cn (*mus⁺*) homozygotes to b pr cn/CyO homozygotes.

[c] The ratio of b pr cn *mus-A1^{ts}* homozygotes to b pr cn *mus-A1^{ts}*/CyO heterozygotes.

development at these temperatures. Adults were collected within 24 hours of eclosion and, for each genotype, two adult populations were established from each group: one at 22°C and the other at 29°C (see Figure 5). The survival of each population was monitored at two day intervals. The results of these experiments are shown in Figure 6. As one might predict, the *mus* mutation has no effect on the longevity of adults derived from cultures maintained at the permissive temperature (Figure 6A). Recall that at 22°C the *mus^{ts}* is able to repair mutations induced by moderate doses of mutagen (0.04% MMS). Therefore the gene product appears to function as well as that from the wild-type. In contrast, there is an obvious decrease in the lifespan of *mus/mus* individuals in cultures that were maintained at 29°C during development and adulthood (Figure 6B). This suggests that loss of DNA repair capacity during development reduces the lifespan of the adult. This notion is confirmed by the observation that *mus* homozygotes that were raised at the restrictive temperature (29°C) but maintained at the permissive temperature as adults also had a reduced lifespan (Figure 6C). Hence, loss of normal repair capacity appears to be associated with a decline in longevity. However, note that the reduction in lifespan was not as striking as that observed in the 29-29°C group. This suggests that perhaps some DNA repair function occurs in the adult. Indeed, *mus* homozygotes in the 22-29°C group show a slight reduction in lifespan relative to their controls (Figure 6D).

It could be argued that the reduction in lifespan observed in the *mus* strain is a consequence of a second lesion and hence does not result from loss of DNA repair capacity. If mutagen-sensitivity and reduced lifespan were inde-

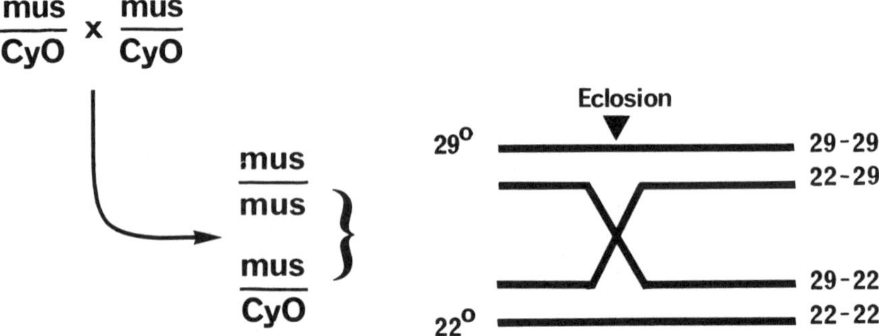


**Figure 5.** Protocol for establishing populations of *mus* flies and their controls for longevity studies. Synchronous cultures of fertilized embryos were established, and allowed to complete development, at 22 and 29°C. Adults from each group were collected within 24 hours of eclosion and divided into two groups one of which was placed at 22°C and the other at 29°C. Hence four groups were established for each genotype. 29-29 refers to the group in which the pre-imaginal stages occurred at 29°C and the adult longevity was then monitored at 29°C. 22-29 refers to the group in which development occurred at 22°C and the adult populations were maintained at 29°C post-eclosion, and so forth.

pendent, then one would predict that exposing the *mus* strain to very low doses of mutagen should not influence the longevity. The protocol described above was repeated, with a single dose of 0.01% MMS administered 24 hours after ovaposition. Recall that 0.01% MMS has no effect on survival of *mus/mus* larvae even in cultures maintained at the non-permissive temperature. The results are shown in Figure 7. There in no effect of the low doses of mutagen on *mus* strains maintained at 22-22°C (22°C through development and adulthood, Figure 7A) or at 22-29°C (22°C through development and 29°C as adults, Figure 7D). This suggests that the damage done by low doses of mutagen is effectively repaired at the permissive temperature. In contrast, exposure to low doses of mutagen under restrictive conditions (29°C during development) reduced the lifespan of adults maintained either at 22°C (Figure 7C) or 29°C (Figure 7B) post-eclosion. This suggests that failure to repair DNA damage in somatic tissues leads to a reduction in lifespan. More importantly, this result implies that the reduction in lifespan observed in the absence

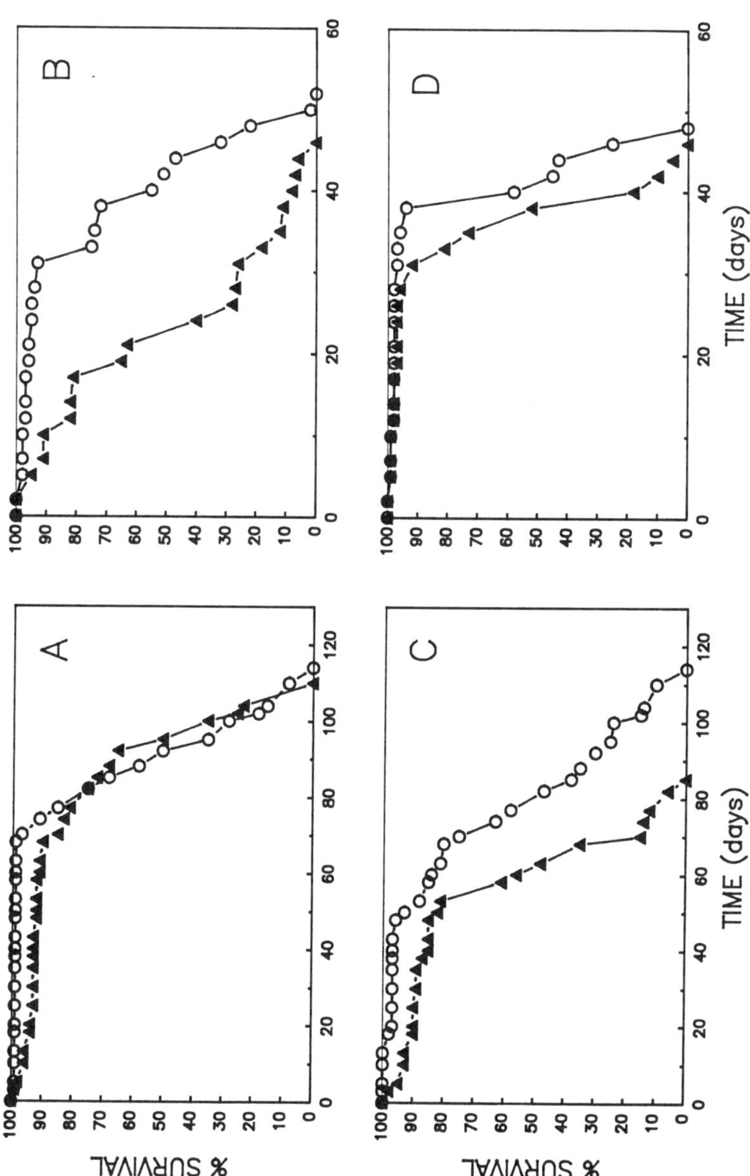


**Figure 6.** Male survival curves for adult populations of *mus-A1*[ts] and *mus*[+]. A) 22-22, development at 22 and adults maintained at 22°C. B) 29-29, development at 29 and adults maintained at 29°C. C) 29-22, development at 29 and adults maintained at 22°C. D) 22-29, development at 22 and adults maintained at 29°C. Open circles represent the isogenic *b pr cn* strain (*mus*[+]). Filled triangles represent the *b pr cn mus-A1*[ts] strain.

of any exogenous mutagen is associated with the dysfunction of the *mus* gene (*mus*$^{ts}$ maintained at 29°C during development).

## DISCUSSION

Some evidence had been advanced that the duration of development, or rate of growth, influenced the lifespan of the adult. By shifting synchronously developing cultures of a wild-type strain down from 29 to 22°C and up from 17 to 22°C adult populations were established whose duration of development was delayed, in daily increments, from 9 to 29 days. The longevity of each of these populations was monitored at both 22 and 29°C. The mean lifespan of males and females at 22°C was 73.4 and 84.7 respectively, and at 29°C it was 31.2 and 37.3, respectively. No correlation was observed between the duration of development and the mean lifespan of the adults.

The mutation *eld-1*$^{ts}$ delays all stages of larval development in 29°C cultures. By shifting synchronously developing cultures down from 29 to 22°C and up from 17 to 22°C, adult populations were established in which the duration of development varied, in daily increments, between 17 and 34 days. The longevity of each of these populations was also monitored at 22 and 29°C. The mean lifespan of the adult populations maintained at 29°C was 80.7 and 84.1 for males and females, respectively, and for the adults maintained at 29°C, it was 33.8 and 35.6 (males and females, respectively). Hence the mean lifespan of the *eld-1*$^{ts}$ adults was very similar to that of the wild-type strain. Again there was no correlation between duration of development and longevity of the adults.

We found no evidence of a link between the duration of the pre-imaginal interval (rate of development) and longevity of the adult. Furthermore, there was no stage of development that was sensitive to shifts from one temperature to another. The relationship between the total duration of development (egg deposition to eclosion of the adult) and the amount of time spent at 17 (shifts up to 22°C) or 29°C (shifts down to 22°C) was linear, with correlation coefficients ranging between 0.974 and 0.978, for both the wild-type and the *eld-1*$^{ts}$ strains. This suggests that there is no developmental interval during which a physiological clock is set to establish developmental rates for the rest of the pre-imaginal period. Hence we were not able to establish that the duration of any single developmental interval has an effect on either the rate at which subsequent development proceeds or the longevity of the adult (rate of aging).

In *Drosophila*, the larval tissues must be removed to allow proper metamorphosis and function of the adult tissues. Therefore, we assume that the larval tissue must be genetically programmed to undergo cell death and

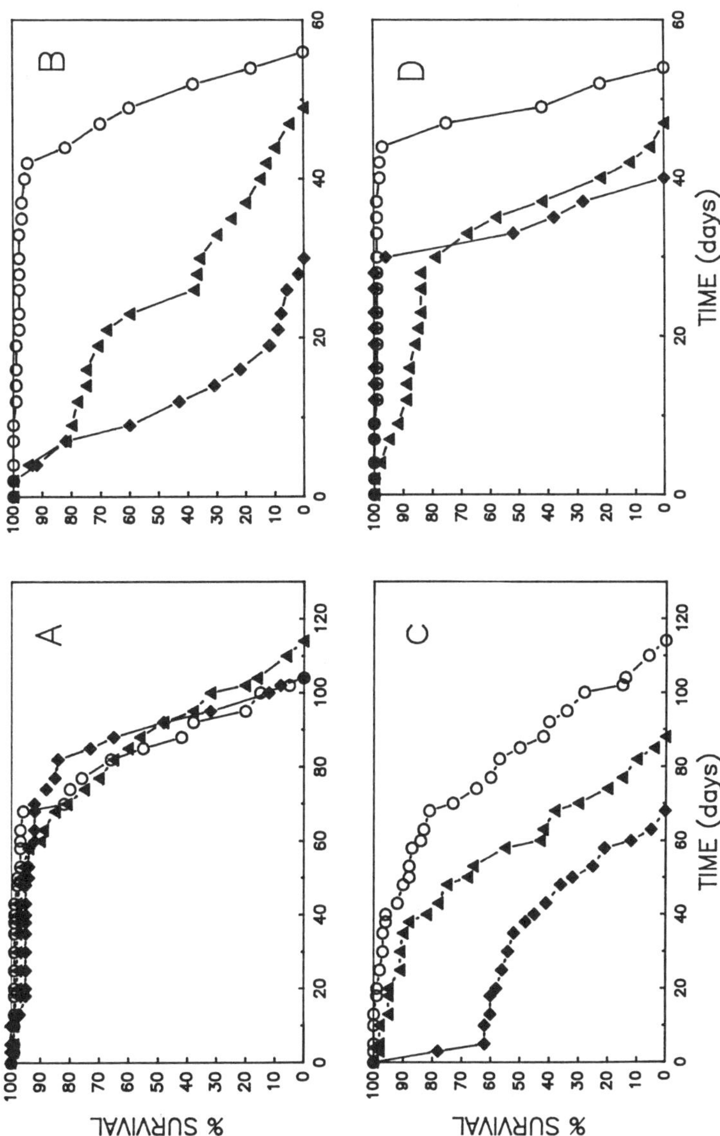

**Figure 7.** Female survival curves for adult populations of *mus-A1*[ts] and *mus*[+]. A) 22-22, development at 22 and adults maintained at 22°C. B) 29-29; development at 29 and adults maintained at 29°C. C) 29-22, development at 29 and adults maintained at 22°C. D) 22-29, development at 22 and adults maintained at 29°C. Open circles represent the isogenic *b pr cn* strain (*mus*[+]). Filled triangle represent the *b pr cn mus-A1*[ts] strain. Filled diamonds represent the *b pr cn mus A-1ts* strain exposed to a single sub-lethal dose of methyl methanesulfonate (MMS) 24 hours after egg deposition.

histolysis in response to some genetic trigger (i.e., large doses of ecdysone, or some other ecdysone-induced gene action). Indeed, transplantation studies have demonstrated that larval tissues acquire the competence to undergo cell death during development (Bodenstein, 1943). This suggests that the competence to respond to the appropriate inducer must be genetically programmed. Hence genes exist within the genome of *Drosophila* that are capable of causing cell death in response to some trigger. Since there is no evidence for loss of genetic information during development, it is logical to assume that these genes also exist in the adult. Are they used to limit the lifespan of the adult?

Mutations were isolated that extend the lifespan of the larva by delaying the onset of pupation. Two mutations that extend the lifespan of the larva by 2-fold and 4-fold were examined for their effect on the longevity of the adult. Neither influenced the longevity of the adult compared to wild-type strain in which the mutation was induced, suggesting that these particular genes do not function in the adult to cause cell death. Clearly, this does not eliminate the possibility that genes which cause programmed cell death function in the adult. It may mean that to identify such genes we should not select for mutations that extend the larval lifespan, but rather for mutations that interfere with histolysis of the larval tissues.

Nonetheless, when both of these data sets are taken together they suggest that larval and adult lifespans are regulated at least somewhat independently. Clearly those genes that cause cell death in the larva may perform the same function in the adult. However, at the very minimum they appear to respond to different genetic triggers.

The developmental fate of the adult precursor cells is actually determined during embryogensis. Once these cells have been specified they appear to be regulated differently from the larval cells. For example, the cells of the imaginal discs, which will eventually give rise to the external parts of the adult head and thorax, continue to undergo cell division and their developmental capacity becomes increasingly restricted. In contrast, the cells of the larva are post-mitotic. Since the two cell populations are physiologically insulated, it is possible that there are genes which act during the pre-imaginal stage to influence the lifespan of the adult, and that these genes have no effect on the lifespan of the larva.

It has been argued that the accumulation of somatic mutations might be a major force in the aging process. Others have argued that failure of repair systems in general might account for physiological aging and ultimately limit lifespan (for a discussion see Kirkwood, this volume). Like the larva, there is little or no cell division in the adult body. Loss of repair capacity, such as

DNA repair, in post-mitotic tissue should have a minimal effect on longevity unless the spontaneous mutation rate is exceedingly high. Hence, absence of DNA repair in the larva may not affect the longevity of the larva; likewise its loss in the adult may not influence longevity in the adult. However, loss of DNA repair during the larval stage may influence the longevity of the adult, since a mutation in a gene which is required in the adult may be amplified by cell division.

The temperature-sensitive *mus* mutations were induced on an isogenic second chromosome to minimize the variation resulting from differences in genetic background. The lifespan of the *b, pr, cn* and *b, pr, cn/CyO* strain did not differ from that of the Oregon-R control strain. Thus the results were not complicated by variations in genetic background. The lifespan of the *mus A-1ts* strain did not differ from controls when the cultures were raised at 22°C throughout development and maintained at 22°C as adults. Hence, at the permissive temperature, the A-1 mutation had no effect on longevity. In contrast, when raised at 29°C through development and maintained at 29°C as adults the lifespan of the A-1 strain was significantly reduced relative to the controls. In addition there was a significant reduction of lifespan in *mus A-1ts* adults derived from cultures grown at 29°C but maintained at 22°C as adults.

These results suggest that the loss of DNA repair capacity during development has a significant effect on longevity of the adult. Perhaps the simplest explanation is that, in the absence of DNA repair, spontaneous mutations accumulate in somatic tissue. Since the larval tissues are not undergoing cell division they will experience fewer mutations. The pre-imaginal cells, which are undergoing cell division, will accrue a fairly large quantity of mutations as a consequence of errors in DNA replication. Mutations that occur in housekeeping genes, that is, genes that are essential for the continued viability of the cell, would tend to be eliminated from the population by cell death. In contrast, mutations that occur in genes that are not expressed until the adult stage will have no apparent effect on the pre-imaginal tissue. Furthermore, the continued cell division will assure that these mutations become permanent, and that they will be passed on to many of the cells in a given tissue. Thus, the adults that eclose should vary in their somatic mutational load. The shape of the survival curves are certainly consistent with this notion. The control strains and the *mus*[ts] strain raised at the permissive temperature had normal shaped survival curves with a sigmoidal death phase, whereas the *mus*[ts] raised at the non-permissive temperature have survival curves that are more linear.

The *mus*[ts] mutation appears to reduce slightly the longevity of adults maintained at 29°C, derived from cultures that were allowed to develop at 22°C. The reduction in longevity is very slight in males and somewhat more

| Table 3. Description of *Drosophila* Strains and Mutations |
|---|
| **Strains** |
| *Oregon R*: |
| A wild-type strain which was isolated in 1925 and has been kept in the lab. This is one of the more commonly used wild-type strains. |
| *b pr cn*: |
| A strain in which the second chromosome is isogenic, that is the two homologous second chromosoms are genetically identical. This chromosome is marked with the recessive mutations b, pr, and cn (see below). When homozygous the flies have black bodies and orange eyes and are quite easily distriguished from wild-type. |
| *CyO*: |
| In(2LR)O, a second chromosome containing three different inversions that together encompass both the right and left arms of the chromosome and effectively nullify the effects of recombination on chromosome 2. Thus this chromosome acts to keep intact the allelic combinations on the homologous second chromosome. This inversion is marked with the dominant mutation Curly (*Cy*), which allows it to be distinguished from wild-type even as a heterozygote, and the recessive markers *pr* and *cn*, which allow identification of heterozygotes with the chromosome carrying the second chromosome *mus* mutations (see below) used in this study. This inversion chromosome is lethal when homozygous. |
| +: |
| The + symbol simply refers to a chromosome carrying the wild-type allele of a particular gene. |

noticeable in females. This suggests that there might be some DNA repair in wild-type adults. To the best of our knowledge, no one has actually attempted to estimate the amount of DNA repair that occurs in adult *Drosophila*. DNA repair capacity has been detected in very young embryos. This repair function appears to be maternally encoded (Graf *et al.*, 1979). Hence, DNA repair genes are expressed in the ovarian tissue of adult females. Therefore, it is reasonable to expect that DNA repair enzymes might function in somatic tissues in female adults. By analogy, a limited amount of DNA repair may also exist in adult males.

It should be emphasized that all three of the *mus*[ts] strains behaved similarly. When raised at the non-permissive temperature, even in the absence of any exogenous mutagen, the longevity of the adults was reduced. This phenotype, like the sensitivity to low doses of mutagen, is temperature sensitive. Since each mutation represents a lesion in a different gene, it is unlikely that this effect can be attributed to anything but loss of DNA repair. Therefore,

| **Table 3.** (Continued) Description of *Drosophila* Strains and Mutations |
| --- |

**Mutations**

*b* = *black*:
A second chromosome (autosomal) recessive mutation, located at map position 48.2, conferring black body instead of the wild-type tan body.

*cn* = *cinnabar*:
A second chromosome (autosomal) recessive mutation, located at map position 57.5, conferring a bright red eye instead of the wild-type deep red eye color; in combination with the mutation *pr* (see below) a light orange eye color is produced.

*Cy* = *Curly:*
A second chromosome dominant mutation located at map position 6.1. The wings curl upward making it very easy to distinguish heterozygotes for *Cy* from wild-type (straight wing); *Cy* is lethal when homozygous

*eld*$^{ts}$1 = extended larval development:
An X-linked recessive temperature sensitive mutation, at the restrictive temperature, 29°C, it delays embryonic and larval development. At the permissive temperature, 22°C or lower, the developmental rate is similar to wild-type. If maintained at 29°C throughout development few adults eclose, most of the individuals die during the pupal stage. If developing cultures are shifted down from the restrictive to the permissive temperature early in the pupal stage, adults will eclose.

*mus* = mutagen sensitive:
This designation refers to any of a number of recessive mutations, homozygotes for which are sensitive to one or more known mutagens. Approximately 30 different *mus* loci have been identified. They are found on all three major chromosomes (X, 2, and 3).

*mus-A1*$^{ts}$ = *mutagen sensitive A1*$^{ts}$:
A second chromosome temperature sensitive recessive *mus* mutation which was induced on the isogenic b, pr, cn second chromosome described above. At the restrictive temperature, 29°C, the mutation confers sensitivity to mono- and bifunctional alkylating agents as well as several other known mutagens. The permissive temperature is 22°C. .

*pr* = *purple*:
A second chromosome recessive mutation, located at map position 54.5, conferring a purplish red eye color instead of the wild-type dark red. The combination of cn and pr gives a light orange eye phenotype which is very distinct from the dark red eye color of wild-type flies.

In *Drosophila* mutations, are named according to their mutant phenotype (for example, *black* = black body). Dominant mutations are indicated by an upper case first letter; recessive mutations are indicated by a lower case first letter it appears that loss or reduction of DNA repair capacity can lead to a reduction in lifespan. It appears that this effect is seen only when the loss of repair occurs in tissues that are still undergoing cell division. It should be emphasized that we in no way imply, from this data, that decline in the efficiency of the DNA repair mechanisms determines longevity under normal circumstances. No one has attempted to measure DNA repair activity in adult *Drosophila*.

## ACKNOWLEDGEMENTS

We are very grateful for the assistance provided by Ms. Cathy Beynon, Kathy Kafer, and Susan Minaker, and Mr. Michael Tiu. We are indebted to the many members of the *Drosophila* laboratory for their very helpful discussions. This research was supported by N. I. A. grant AGO 3088-02, NSERC Strategic Grant G-1999, and NSERC Operating Grant 3005 to T. A. G.

## REFERENCES

ALPATOV, W. W. and PEARL, R. (1929) Experimental studies on the duration of life. XII. Influence of temperature during the larval period and adult life on the duration of the life of the imago of *Drosophila melanogaster*. *Amer. Naturalist* **63**: 37-67.

BODENSTEIN, D. (1943) Factors influencing growth and metamorphosis of the salivary gland in *Drosophila*. *Biol. Bull.* **84**: 13-

BOYD, J. B., GOLINO, M. D., NGUYEN, T. D., and GREEN, M. M. (1976) Isolation and characterization of X-linked mutants of *Drosophila melanogaster* which are sensitive to mutagens. *Genetics* **84**: 485-506.

BOYD, J. B., and HARRIS, P. V. (1985) Isolation and characterization of a photorepair-deficient mutant in *Drosophila melanogaster*. *Genetics* **110**: s85.

BOYD, J. B. and SHAW, K. E. (1982) Postreplication repair defects in mutants of *Drosophila melanogaster*. *Mol. Gen. Genet.* **186**: 289-294.

BOYD, J. B., SNYDER, R. D., HARRIS, P. V., PRESELEY, J. M., BOYD, S. F., and SMITH, P. D. (1982) Identification of a second locus in *Drosophila melanogaster* required for excision repair. *Genetics* **100**: 239-257.

BURCOMBE, J. V. and HOLLINGSWORTH, M. J. (1970) The relationship between developmental temperature and longevity in *Drosophila*. *Gerontologia* **16**: 172-181.

FRANCIS, A. A., LEE, W. H., and REGAN, J. D. (1981) The relationship of DNA excision repair of ultraviolet-induced lesions to the maximum lifespan of mammals. *Mech. Ageing Dev.* **16**: 181-189.

GRAF, U., GREEN, M. M., and WURGLER, F. E. (1979) Mutagen-sensitive mutants in *Drosophila*: Effects of premutational damage. *Mutation Res.* **63**: 101-112.

GRIGLIATTI, T. A. (1986) Mutagenesis. **In:** *Drosophila: a practical approach* (Ed. D. B. Roberts) pp. 39-58. Oxford: IRL Press.

HALL, K. Y., HART, R. W., BENIRSCHKE, A. K. and WALFORD, R. L. (1984) Correlation between ultraviolet-induced DNA repair in primate lymphocytes and fibroblasts and species maximum achievable lifespan. *Mech. Ageing Dev.* **24**: 163-173.

HART, R. W. and SETLOW, R. B. (1974) Correlation between deoxyribonucleic excision-repair and lifespan in a number of mammalian species. *Proc. Natl. Acad. Sci. USA* **71**: 2169-2173.

HENDERSON, D. S., BAILEY, D. A., SINCLAIR, D. R. and GRIGLIATTI, T. A. (1987) Isolation and characterization of second chromosome mutagen-sensitive mutations in *Drosophila melanogaster*. *Mutation Res.* **177**: 83-93.

HOMYK, T., and GRIGLIATTI, T. A. (1983) Behavioral mutants of *Drosophila melanogaster* IV. Analysis of developmentally temperature-sensitive mutations affecting flight. *Dev. Genet.* **4**: 77-97.

KATO, H., HARADA, M., TSUCHIYA, K., and MORIWAKI, K. (1980) Absence of correlation between DNA repair in ultraviolet irradiated mammalian cells and lifespan of the donor species. *Japan J. Genet.* **55**: 99-108.

LAMB, M. J. (1978) Ageing. **In:** *The Genetics and Biology of Drosophila.* **Vol 2c.** (Ed. M. Ashburner and T. R. F. Wright), pp. 43-104. London: Academic Press.

LEFFELAAR, D., and GRIGLIATTI, T. A. (1984a) A mutation in *Drosophila* that appears to accelerate aging. *Dev. Genet.* **4**: 199-210.

LEFFELAAR, D., and GRIGLIATTI, T. A. (1984b) Age-dependent behavior loss in adult *Drosophila melanogaster*. *Dev. Genet.* **4**: 211-227.

LINDSLEY, D. L., and GRELL, E. H. (1986) *Genetic Variations of Drosophila melanogaster.* Carnegie Institution of Washington Publication, No. 627.

LINTS, F. A., and LINTS, C. V. (1971) Influence of preimaginal environment on fecundity and ageing in *Drosophila melanogaster* hybrids - II. Developmental speed and life-span. *Exp. Geront.* **6**: 427-445.

PEARL, R. (1928) *The Rate of Living.* London: University of London Press.

PRICE, G. B., MODAK, S. P., and MAKINODAN, T. (1971) Age-associated changes in the DNA of mouse tissue. *Science* **171**: 917- 920.

RICHTER, M. D. (1986) *Environmental and Genetic Influences on the Life Span of Adult Drosophila melanogaster.* M. Sc. Thesis, University of British Columbia.

SMITH, P. D., SYNDER, R. D., and DUSENBERY, R. L. (1980) Isolation and characterization of repair-deficient mutants of *Drosophila melanogaster*. **In:** *DNA Repair and Mutagenesis in Eukaryotes* (Ed. W. M. Generoso, M. D. Shelby, F. J. de Serres), pp. 175-188. New York: Plenum Press.

WHEELER, K. T., and LETT, J. T. (1974) On the possibility that DNA repair is related to age in non-dividing cells. *Proc. Natl. Acad. Sci. USA.* **71**: 1862-1865.

WOODLAND, A. D., SETLOW, R. B., and GRIST, E. (1980) DNA repair and longevity in three species of cold-blooded vertebrates. *Exp. Geront.* **15**: 301-304.

## DISCUSSION

1. Asked where the genes are, Grigliatti noted that one is on the X chromosome. The genes are not allelic, but all complement each other. They are not on chromosome 3 and are not SOD (Superoxide Dismutase). The fecundity of the mutant strains has not yet been measured. As a result of Charlesworth's theories, any alteration in longevity would be expected to have the reciprocal effect on fecundity only if it acted through the genes naturally selected to control longevity and fecundity. Thus this question was often raised at the conference. It was pointed out that R. A. Fisher predicted that most mutations should reduce overall fitness. This would reduce fecundity as well as longevity, illustrating why both should be tested. Indeed, many mutations are known to reduce both fecundity and longevity.

2. Genes that increase longevity are the most interesting, although they may not truly extend normal lifespans in nature. There was disagreement as to whether there are any globally acting genes extending lifespan. Grigliatti noted that he had expected to find no effects of mutations on longevity and thus provide evidence against the hypothesis that aging occurs by accumulation of somatic mutations. If a "null" mutation increased longevity it would be most striking. We should be careful about saying that a mutation "accelerated aging". This requires a group of "landmarks" - obvious age changes in different biological systems at different stages of life - that would be compressed, occurring more rapidly.

3. An adult insect may be considered a parasite on its larva form, so it is not surprising if some mutations affect one and not the other. What would be more interesting would be an exception that increased both larval and adult lifespans.

# 11

# A FLY-BY VIEW OF AGING


Alan Garen


*He comes forth like a flower, and withers*
(Job 14: 1,2)

## ABSTRACT


Developmental events in *Drosophila* can generally be divided into three major phases: 1) determination of the primordial cells for a specified pathway of development; 2) proliferation of the determined cells to generate the population needed for each structure; 3) a switch from proliferation to differentiation of specialized cell functions. For the imaginal cells of *Drosophila*, which form most of the adult structures, proliferation and differentiation are clearly separated by the onset of pupation, when imaginal cells stop proliferating and begin to differentiate in response to a hormonal signal from the steroid ecdysone. In the absence of that signal, imaginal cells have a virtually unlimited capacity to continue proliferating without a significant loss of their potential for normal differentiation. Age-dependent degenerative phenomena in *Drosophila* are associated with imaginal cells which appear to have reached a terminal state of differentiation. The stability of the differentiated state is maintained during most of the adult lifespan, and the eventual loss of that stability could initiate the aging process. Aging might involve late stages of the genetic program for development or aberrant events, and therefore can be viewed either as a part of normal development or as a disease. Strategies for detecting age-dependent changes in gene function which might trigger the onset of aging are discussed.


Implicit in the theme of this symposium is a shared recognition of the importance of genetic effects on the aging process. However, identifying the significant genetic effects or even defining the aging process poses major difficulties, because aging involves a multitude of symptoms with disparate causes. There is general agreement that aging is a deleterious process, in the course of which desirable functions and features are steadily eroded. A widely accepted criterion of aging is the age-dependent probability of dying (Lamb, 1978), but that criterion has serious limitations. One is the exclusion of relevant age-dependent effects which may not alter lifespan. Another is the inclusion of age-dependent diseases such as cancer which contribute significantly to the probability of death in human populations but are induced by somatic mutation; a somatic mutation mechanism probably is not a major factor in aging, since it requires clonal proliferation of the mutant cells to exert a physiological impact. Rather than struggle with definitions of aging, the challenge for geneticists interested in the problem is to identify the relevant genes. Once identified, the molecular and biological properties of those genes and their roles in aging could be elucidated by the extensive armamentarium of molecular biology. A criterion of relevance to aging which avoids the problem of defining its effects is a change in gene expression in old individuals. In this chapter I will discuss the use of *Drosophila* as a model system for identifying and cloning genes which show a change in expression in old flies.

Shortly after the blastoderm stage, *Drosophila* development separates into two major pathways; one is the larval pathway for the differentiation of specialized larval structures, and the other is the imaginal pathway for the formation of the imaginal discs and histoblasts, which subsequently differentiate into specialized adult structures. The two pathways differ markedly during the larval stage: Most cells entering the larval pathway stop proliferating and develop polytene or polyploid chromosomes and differentiated characteristics, in contrast to cells entering the imaginal pathway which retain diploid chromosomes and relatively undifferentiated characteristics. The imaginal cells continue to proliferate at a constant exponential rate (Martin, 1982) until the end of the larval stage, when most of the imaginal cells also stop proliferating and enter the pupal stage of differentiation. The signal for the developmental switch from proliferation to differentiation of the imaginal cells is a sharp increase in the titer of the steroid hormone ecdysone, as indicated by two lines of evidence. One involves temperature-shift experiments with the temperature-sensitive mutant *ecd*-1, in which ecdysone synthesis is blocked after a shift from a permissive to a restrictive temperature (Garen *et al.*, 1977). When the shift is done a few hours before the end of the larval stage, no increase in ecdysone titer occurs and the larvae fail to pupate. The imaginal cells continue proliferating for several days after the shift, forming greatly enlarged discs which retain their capacity to differentiate when transplanted into wild-type larval hosts (Garen and Lepesant, 1980). The other evidence comes from the demonstration that permanent cultures of imaginal cells can be established *in vivo* by serial transfers of mature imaginal discs into the abdominal cavity of an adult female host (Hadorn, 1965), which has about the same ecdysone titer as third-instar larvae before the titer increases (Garen *et al.*, 1977; Richards, 1981). When long-term cultured imaginal cells are transplanted back into a late third-instar larval host, the cells stop proliferating and begin to differentiate synchronously with the imaginal discs of the host during its pupal stage (Hadorn, 1965). Differentiation of the cultured imaginal cells can also be elicited in an adult female host by injecting ecdysone (Postlethwait and Schneiderman, 1970). Thus, imaginal cells can either be maintained indefinitely as a proliferating population when the ecdysone titer is low, or can be induced to switch from proliferation to differentiation by an increase in ecdysone titer. The developmental switch in the larval pathway, which occurs early in embryogenesis, also appears to be induced by an ecdysone signal since there is a sharp increase in ecdysone titer at about the same time (Kraminsky *et al.*, 1980; Richards, 1981). *In vitro* cultures of *Drosophila* cells (whose lineage is uncertain) respond rapidly and irreversibly when the culture medium is supplemented with physiological concentrations of ecdysone: Cell proliferation stops and is usually followed by morphological changes (Cherbas *et al.*, 1980). In accord with the general function of steroid hormones, ecdysone probably serves as a cofactor for the regulatory proteins which induce or repress gene expression during all stages of *Drosophila* development (Ashburner, 1973; Garen *et al.*, 1977; Meyerowitz and Hogness, 1980; Lepesant *et al.*, 1978, 1982; Nakanishi and Garen, 1983). The genes involved in the ecdysone-induced developmental switch from proliferation to differentiation have not been identified.

There are two major conclusions from these findings that are especially relevant to the problem of aging in *Drosophila*. One conclusion is that proliferating populations of stably determined imaginal cells can be propagated indefinitely, unlike cultures of other normal cells which appear to have a sharply limited proliferative potential (Hayflick, 1965). That difference could reflect the developmental stage at which the cells are cultured, since there usually is a progressive loss of proliferative capacity as differentiation progresses. Recent studies of the *Drosophila* homeotic gene *deformed* suggest that the remarkable stability of the determined state of proliferating imaginal cells depends on an auto-regulatory interaction between homeotic genes and their encoded proteins (Kuziora and McGinnis, 1988). A second conclusion is that the degenerative phenomena associated with aging (Lamb, 1978) occur in differentiated imaginal cells which have stopped proliferating. These cells appear to have reached a terminal stage of differentiation in adults, since no further physiological or cytological changes are evident during most of the adult lifespan. Accordingly, adult vigor would depend on the stability of the fully differentiated state of imaginal cells, and the aging process could reflect a progressive loss of capacity to maintain that stability. An experimental approach to the problem of aging in *Drosophila*, which I favor, focuses on the components required to stabilize the fully differentiated state of imaginal cells and on the mechanisms which could interfere with their functions. Those components might include certain genes which continue to be expressed during the adult stage, or certain proteins or other molecules which are no longer being synthesized during the adult stage and therefore must retain their structural and functional integrity. Since different experimental approaches are involved in examining the possible role of gene expression or molecular stability in the aging process, I shall consider each in turn.

Differentiated imaginal cells continue to express a large number of genes, many of which are specific to one cell type or a few types. For example, the head region of *Drosophila* adults contains at least 500 species of messenger RNA which are not detected in young embryos (Palazzolo *et al.*, 1989). Such tissue-specific gene expression in fully differentiated cells might include regulatory genes controlling the stability of the differentiated state, analogous to the homeotic genes controlling the stability of the determined state. Aging might be triggered by a change in the auto-regulated expression of such genes. Ecdysone could be an important hormonal regulatory component for differentiated imaginal cells, since adults maintain a fixed concentration of ecdysone which is essential for fertility (Garen *et al.*, 1977) and probably also for various adult somatic functions. Therefore, aging in *Drosophila* could be affected by a reduced capacity of old adults to maintain the concentration of ecdysone or its receptors which is required for the expression of ecdysone-regulated genes.

A sensitive procedure for detecting differences in gene expression between two tissue samples is by subtractive-hybridization with cDNA libraries prepared from the two tissues. A recently improved procedure for subtractive-hybridization involves hybridizing an excess amount of biotinylated cDNA or cRNA from one of the libraries to non-biotinylated cDNA from the other library, and then removing the common species by binding the biotinylated component to a column containing an avidin matrix (Duguid *et al.*, 1988; Swaroop, personal communication); the cDNA remaining in solution will be enriched for species which are specific to the second library. The procedure is designed for direct cloning and amplification of the specific cDNA species, even when those cDNA species are as rare as one part in ten-thousand. One application of this procedure is to screen for differences in gene expression between the head tissues from young and old *Drosophila* adults, which might be relevant to the degenerative changes detected in the brain and nervous system of old adults (Herman and Miguel, 1971).

A full study of a complex developmental process such as aging requires the use of both genetic and molecular techniques, involving both mutants and DNA clones. For *Drosophila*, it should be feasible either to clone a gene once the mutant has been isolated, or conversely to isolate a mutant once the gene has been cloned. The first strategy has proved remarkably effective in studies of the control of early *Drosophila* development, principally because the relevant mutants were available for molecular analysis. However, the applicability of the same strategy to the study of aging is less clear, because the phenotype of a mutant affecting aging is not as evident as it was for the mutants affecting early development. A mutant with an extended adult lifespan would appear to be the most relevant to aging, but such a mutant has never been reported for *Drosophila*. Although significant hereditary differences in lifespans occur in *Drosophila* populations, those differences involve complex genetic polymorphisms which are difficult to resolve (Luckinbill *et al.*, 1988). If aging involves a loss of important gene functions, all of the relevant mutants might be deleterious and manifest a reduced rather than extended lifespan. The alternative strategy described above, using subtractive-hybridization to isolate cDNA clones for genes which might be relevant to aging, offers the advantage that no prior information about the function or phenotypic effect of the genes is required, and either a loss or gain of gene function could be detected.

The effectiveness of the subtractive-hybridization strategy depends on the assumption that aging results from age-dependent changes in the levels of specific messenger-RNA species. Since there is no evidence as yet to support that assumption, alternative mechanisms should also be considered, such as age-dependent changes in certain proteins or other cellular constituents which do not involve changes in messenger-RNA levels. For example, since there is no somatic cell division in *Drosophila* adults, some somatic cell constituents probably are no longer being synthesized, and a deleterious chemical modification of such a constituent might not be reparable or replaceable. Because the molecular composition of cells is so complex, and the variety of potential chemical modifications is so extensive, the technical problems involved in screening for such age-dependent effects are formidable. A full discussion of those problems is outside the scope of this symposium.

Since evolution tends to conserve basic mechanisms of development, as dramatically illustrated by the structural and functional conservation of homeotic genes (Manley and Levine, 1985), it seems reasonable to expect that significant homologies will emerge between age-dependent functions in *Drosophila* and mammals, and therefore that studies of aging in *Drosophila* could provide seminal clues to similar phenomena in humans.

## REFERENCES

ASHBURNER, M. (1973) Sequential gene activation by ecdysone in polytene chromosomes of *Drosophila melanogaster* I. Dependence upon ecdysone concentration. *Devel. Biol.* 34: 47

CHERBAS, P., CHERBAS, L., DEMETRI, G., MANTENFFEL-CYMBOROWSKA, C., SAVAKIS, C., YONGER, C. D., and WILLIAMS, C. M. (1980) Ecdysteroid hormone effects on a *Drosophila* cell line. **In**: *Gene Regulation by Steroid Hormones* (Eds. A. R. Roy and J. H. Clark) Springer-Verlag, New York, 278-308.

DUGUID, J. R., ROHWER, R. G., and SEED, B. (1988) Isolation of cDNAs of scrapie-modulated RNAs by subtractive hybridization of a cDNA library. *Proc. Natl. Acad. Sci. USA* 85: 5738-5742

GAREN, A. (1988) From cell proliferation to differentiation: the steroid connection. **In**: *Hormones, Cell Biology, and Cancer: Perspectives and Potentials* (Eds. W. David Hankin and T. David Puett), Alan R. Liss, Inc., New York, pp. 3-10.

GAREN, A., KAUVAR, L. and LEPESANT, J. A. (1977) Roles of ecdysone in *Drosophila* development. *Proc. Natl. Acad. Sci. USA* 74: 5099

GAREN, A. and LEPESANT, J. A. (1980) Hormonal Control of gene expression and development by ecdysone in *Drosophila*. **In**: *Gene Regulation by Steroid Hormones* (Eds. A. K. Roy and J. Clark) Springer-Verlag, New York, 255-262.

HADORN, E. (1965) Problems of determination and transdetermination. **In**: Genetic Control of Differentiation, *Brookhaven Symp. Biol.* 18: 148

HAYFLICK, L. (1965) The limited *in vitro* lifetime of human diploid cell strains. *Exper. Cell Res.* 37: 614-636

HERMAN, M. M. and MIQUEL, J. (1971) Electron microscopic studies of aging in D. Brain. *J. Neuropath. Exp. Neurol.* 30: 148-149

KLEIN, G. and KLEIN, E. (1985) Evolution of tumors and the impact of molecular oncology. *Nature* 315: 190

KRAMINSKY, G. P., CLARK, W. C., ESTELLE, M. A., GIETZ, R. D., SAGE, B. A., O'CONNOR, J. D., HODGETTS, R. B. (1980) Induction of translatable mRNA for dopa decarboxylase in *Drosophila*: An early response to ecdysterone. *Proc. Natl. Acad. Sci. USA* 77: 4175-4179

KUZIORA, M. and McGINNIS, W. (1988) Autoregulation of a *Drosophila* homeotic selector gene. *Cell* 55: 477-485

LAMB, M. J. (1978) Ageing. **In**: *The Genetics and Biology of Drosophila*, (Ed. M. Ashburner and T. R. F. Wright) Academic Press, New York, Vol. 2C, Chapter 20, 43-104.

LEPESANT, J. A., KEJZLAROVA-LEPESANT, J. and GAREN, A. (1978) Ecdysone-inducible functions of larval fat bodies of *Drosophila*. *Proc. Natl. Acad. Sci USA*. 75: 5570

LEPESANT, J. A., LEVINE, M., GAREN, A., KEJZLAROVA-LEPESANT, J., RAT, L., and SOMME-MARTIN, G. (1982) Developmentally regulated expression in *Drosophila* larval fat bodies. *J. Mol. Applied Genetics* 1: 371

LUCKINBILL, L. S., GRAVES, J. L., REED, A. H., and KOETSAWANG, S. (1988) Localizing genes that defer senescence in *Drosophila melanogaster*. *Heredity* 60: 367-374

MANLEY, J. L. and LEVINE, M. S. (1985) The homeo box and mammalian development. *Cell* 43: 1

MARTIN, P. F. (1982) Direct determination of the growth rate of *Drosophila* imaginal discs. *J. Expt. 2001.* 222: 97

MEYEROWITZ, E. and HOGNESS, D. S. (1980) Molecular organization of a *Drosophila* puff site that responds to ecdysone. *Cell* 28: 165

NAKANISHI, Y. and GAREN, A. (1983) Selective gene expression induced by ecdysterone in cultured fat bodies of *Drosophila*. *Proc. Natl. Acad. Sci. USA* 80: 2971

POSTLETHWAIT, J. H. and SCHNEIDERMAN, H. A. (1970) Induction of metamorphosis by ecdysone analogues: *Drosophila* imaginal disc cultured *in vivo*. *Biol. Bull.* **138**: 47
RICHARDS, G. (1981) The radioimmune assay of ecdysteroid titers in *Drosophila melanogaster*. *Mol. Cell Endocrinology* **21**: 181

# 12

# AVIAN LONGEVITY AND AGING

William A. Calder III

## ABSTRACT

Knowledge of longevity is important in ecology and physiology, which had to evolve together. Hence lifespan cannot be considered an isolated trait for understanding gerontological phenomena, rather one of a suite of traits which have been integrated through natural selection (see Charlesworth, this volume). Since maximum observed longevity, other life history traits, and metabolic intensity, show strong correlations with body size, I examine lifespan allometrically. From this, birds are seen to have exceeded the implied limitations on mammalian lifespan. Considering size and metabolic demands, hummingbirds have exceptional longevity. This has been explored in a study of the broad-tailed hummingbird.

## INTRODUCTION

We tend to focus on one aspect of biology at a time, necessarily limiting the scope of study to practical proportions. This initial simplification reveals how mechanisms work but may fail to provide insight into functional significance, such as when and under what circumstances they are utilized. Isolated disciplines may yield only fragmentary approximations.

Longevity and aging are important but often-overlooked phenomena in several disciplines. Ecologists need to know about not only annual natality, but also reproductive longevity as components of reproductive fitness. Natality can be measured in one season, though it may be atypical. The determination of vertebrate longevity requires several years of effort, which granting agencies have been reluctant to fund. Physiological values have been averaged from individual animals of usually unknown age and past history (except when studying simple, short-lived forms). Now we are urged to focus on within-population variability (Bennett 1987). This variability should include not only genetic but other factors such as health, experience, and age. Gerontological questions of when and why animals age and die must be answered in the context of reproductive replacement, a prerequisite for the species if it is to persist long enough to be studied. Hence I will argue that longevity can only be considered in the context of the animal's life history, a history lived out on a physiological time scale appropriate to that animal and its size. Hart and Turturro (1987) stated it well: " 'Why do we age?' may be the wrong question. The right question may be 'Why do we live as long as we do?' ". For the comparative biologist, this may be extended to ask "Why do animals live as long as they do?".

Aging is the alternative to early death; reproductive replacement is the alternative to the extinction of a genetic lineage. These parallels are connected by the fact that early death can also contribute to genetic extinction. Longevity is only one of several life history traits which are components of Darwinian fitness at any time, and subject to modification through natural selection over time (see chapter by Charlesworth in this volume). Reproductive fitness is the product of fecundity (offspring per year) and reproductive lifespan. The biological survival of the fittest must include the ability to perpetuate in kind at the replacement level or better before the potential parents expire. This is true whether longevity and aging are the manifestations of natural selection for the greatest possible longevity (preventative control *via* the existence of "longevity assurance (or determinant) genes"; Sacher, 1982; Cutler, 1983; Hayflick, 1985) or of selection for senescence genes that turn us off at a practical time (cessation control in accord with the "program theory of aging"; for review see Hayflick, 1985).

The comparative approach to biological mysteries can provide food for thought about life's limitations and constraints. We can study the extreme cases, the most vulnerable and the longest-lived, the smallest and the largest. We can also study the continuums between the extremes for general trends and relationships. For quantitative analysis, body-size-dependent characteristics are particularly helpful. As Sacher (1959) demonstrated, there is a significant interspecific correlation between size and record longevity, larger animals living longer than smaller ones. Other correlations may hint of underlying connections. For example, mass-specific metabolic rates (metabolic intensity) are inversely proportional to body size. The combination of this inverse (negative) correlation and the positive correlation of lifespan with size have suggested that the product of metabolic intensity and lifespan may approach a constant "lifetime metabolic potential". At any rate, size can either serve as an organizing handle, or it must be eliminated as a confounding variable (for additional references see Sacher 1978; Cutler 1976, 1978, 1983; Hart *et al.*, 1979; Lindstedt and Calder 1976, 1981; Calder 1982, 1984, 1985).

Cutler (1976) pointed out an exception to this well-known, approximately constant product of specific metabolic rate and maximum recorded lifespan, noting with reference to homeotherms that undergo daily torpor: "... the bat and hummingbird do not fit this relation when the waking specific metabolic rate is used. Life spans of the bat and hummingbird appear too long in relation to their size." Herreid (1964) observed an overall similarity in the longevity records for both tropical, non-torpor-utilizing bats and temperate species which do become torpid. Jurgens and Prothero (1987) found a slight difference in the allometries of lifespan for heterothermic *vs.* homeothermic bats, but size accounts for such a small percentage of the variation (2 and 23 percent, respectively) in the separate regressions, and the difference between them is not statistically significant. Thus it is not clear that longevity in bats is related to the proportion of life spent in suspended animation.

What about the hummingbirds? I would like first to look at comparative longevity in other vertebrate classes, among which we find that birds are masters of longevity. Then we can focus on hummingbirds, which among the birds are capable of amazing longevity, once size-effects have been factored out. The questions then, are: 1) "Why do birds live longer than mammals of equivalent size?" and, 2) "Why do hummingbirds live so much longer than the allometry says they should?"

## PHYSIOLOGICAL TIME

Physiological (or maximum recorded) lifespan is size-dependent, body size accounting for 60 per cent of the variability (r = 0.77; Sacher, 1959). Compared with the larger species, small mammals or birds are usually short-lived. This must generally be compensated by high annual fecundity (the shorter the period of opportunity, the more intense the effort must be to insure replacement). I will reexamine, on an interspecific and comparative intraclass basis, the scaling of maximum longevity. This can be related to metabolic or physiological time-scaling, reproduction, and, in a preliminary fashion, to aging. I will then proceed to examine specific natural histories in search for the functional connections between energetics, reproduction, and longevity.

Within a class or subclass of animals, metabolic rates do not increase in direct proportion to size ($\propto M^{1.0}$; where M= body mass in kg), but are scaled to a fractional power of body mass ($\propto M^b$) as in the well-known Kleiber relationship where b= 3/4. The metabolic turnover time, in which a fraction, say ten percent, of body mass consisting of stored energy such as fat is metabolized, is proportional to:

$$\frac{\text{amount} \propto 0.1m^{1.0}}{\text{rate} = \text{amount}/\text{time}, \propto M^{3/4}} = \text{time} \propto M^{1/4} \tag{1}$$

There is general consistency in the form of parallel scalings ($\propto M^{1/4}$) for the durations of a number of physiological cycles and life history stages, as well as the ecological times of populations of individuals (Figure 1 {from Figure 14.2, p. 370, Calder 1984}). Smaller animals do not live as long as do large animals, but their life cycles must include the same events and processes: development, growth, sexual maturation, and reproduction before death, with or without aging. Each step or stage of the life cycle of a small animal must therefore be completed in a smaller period of time (see Figure 12 in Cutler 1984).

## AVIAN AND MAMMALIAN LIFESPANS COMPARED

Lifespan can be expressed quantitatively in several ways. Hart and Turturro (1987) distinguished 3 measures of lifespan, to which we can add a fourth:

mean or median lifespan (ML): mean age at death or median age of survival. This is relatively rarely available because a survivorship curve or life table is required.

maximal achievable lifespan (MAL): maximum recorded under the best conditions, usually when protected from predation, starvation, and disease in zoological gardens and laboratory colonies.

maximum potential lifespan (MPL): generated from general allometric formulae not measuring but predicting lifespan from body or brain sizes, and is thus based on assumptions of trans-taxonomic similarity. "...requires the least amount of information...and is inordinately dependent upon one observation... [which] could be in error or could be very unrepresentative of normal maintenance conditions.

maximum wild lifespan (MWL): from banding and tagging studies in nature.

Longevity records indicate that maximal achievable (MALs) and maximum wild lifespans (MWLs) of birds and mammals scale to the 1/5 power of body mass (Lindstedt and Calder 1976,1981). Birds are of gerontological interest because they may live 2.4 times as long as mammals when compared on an equal-size basis (Figure 2) Natural (wild) longevity data are more abundant and systematically determined for birds than for any other vertebrates, due to the popularity of bird-banding (in Europe, bird-ringing) (Lindstedt 1985).

Turtles, crocodillians, and *Sphenodon* are remarkably long-lived (even after anecdotal and unverified records are excluded; Gibbons, 1987). Several of the record-holders were very large, but the relationship between maximum recorded lifespan and body size in the poikilothermic classes has received

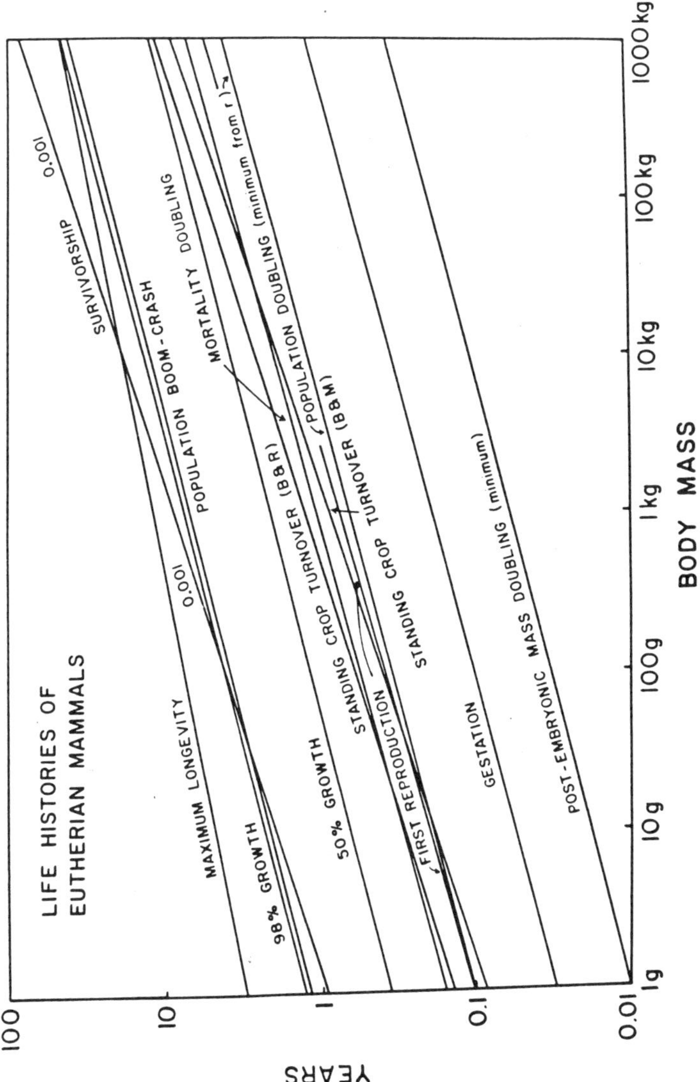


**Figure 1.** Each Life cycle must include embryonic development, growth, and time to insure reproduction if the species is to survive. The scaling of the physiological and developmental time scales extends with parallel size-dependency to the level of population dynamics. Whether the animal is small and short-lived, or larger and lives for a longer time, there is a proportional similarity for factors of longevity, mortality, population turnover, and the periodicity of population cycles (in those species like voles and varying hares, whose numbers fluctuate widely). (Reprinted with permission of Harvard University Press.)

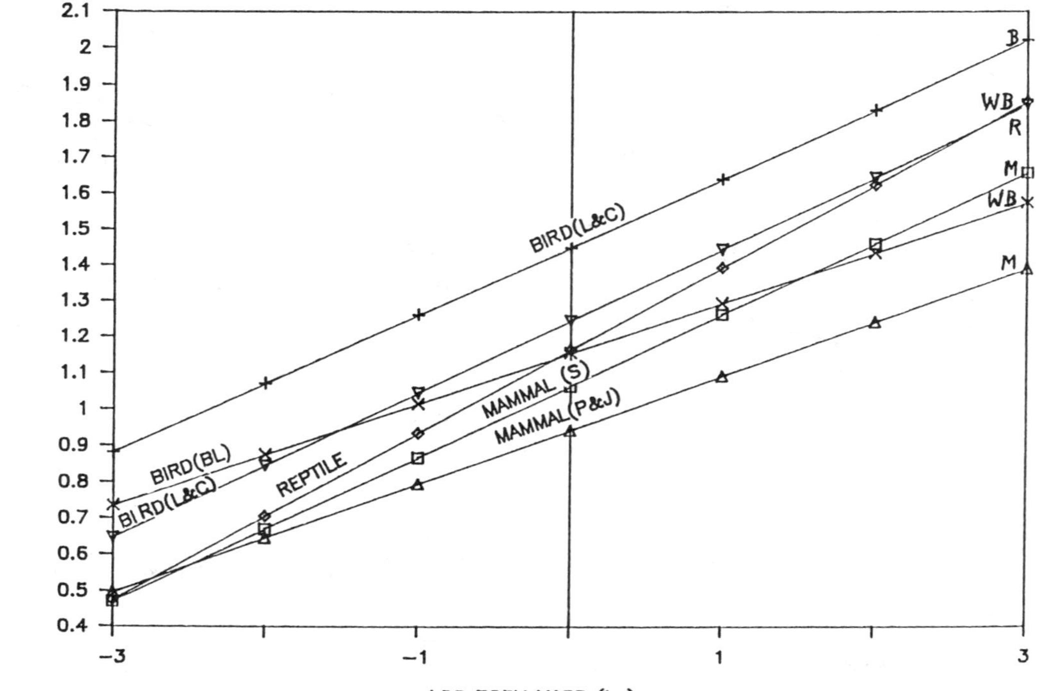


**Figure 2.** A comparison of maximum longevity of mammals (S = Sacher, 1959; P & J = Prothero & Jurgens, 1986; wild birds (L & C = Lindstedt & Calder, 1976; BL = banding records; see Figure 5)); captive birds (top line, from Lindstedt & Calder, 1976), and reptiles (Calder, 1984).

little (reptiles) or no (fish) attention, at least in part because body masses of the individuals of record longevity have not been published with the age, and given their indeterminate growth, "borrowed" species weights are relatively meaningless. The allometry is doubtless confounded further by variables of temperature (perhaps *via* metabolic rate) and nutrition (perhaps *via* growth rate). Longer life has been attributed to slow metabolic turnover and slow growth and development (Craig, 1985; Gibbons, 1987). Reptilian life span scaled to the 0.23 power of body mass in n = 8 spp. (Calder 1984). So far, on an equal-size basis, reptiles as a class do not appear to live longer than birds.

The size-dependence of longevity (MAL) has been noted to differ slightly from the component stages of a life history such as for gestation, growth, and maturation scaling (reviewed by Calder 1984). The consistently smaller body mass exponent of $\frac{1}{5}$ which characterizes MAL is thus a notable, though perhaps small exception to $M_{1/4}$ scaling of other physiological and life-history scalings (Sacher 1959, Lindstedt and Calder 1976, Calder 1985). Are these differences ($M^{0.2}$ for eutherian mammals, $M^{0.19}$ for marsupials, and $M^{0.19\text{.to}}$ $^{0.2.}$ for captive and wild birds respectively, *vs.* $M^{0.25}$ for metabolic turnover time) real, or do they reflect inadequacy or bias in the data from which the allometries have been derived? Lindstedt and Calder (1976) suggested that the avian MAL data could have been biased systematically by the fact that small birds with shorter lifespans had been more extensively sampled in the relatively short period of records from banding and recaptures.

A decade of additional bird recapture and recovery records and nearly three more decades of study and data gathering on mammals have made it possible to examine the scalings from more extensive data bases. For his pioneering examination of longevity scaling, Sacher (1959) included longevity records (MAL) for 63 spp. of mammals (in captivity). When this was expanded to a larger base (n = 239 spp) the regression was shifted downward in both coefficient ("intercept") and exponent ("slope") (Sacher 1975, cited by Prothero and Jurgens 1986). Prothero and Jurgens (1986) present a collection of regression equations derived from more extensive and critically selected data. For 578 species of mammals ("aggregated data base") they derived a scaling exponent of 0.187 for a regression that predicts lower MAL for all sizes compared to Sacher's (1959) equation. Most of the scaling exponents from their various reduced data sets are less than 0.187. Excluding 84 outliers, their regression predicts shorter MAL for all but the smallest mammals (< 10 g). From 236 data points from the very careful review of zoo longevity records by M.L. Jones (1979; his 1982 inventory was apparently overlooked) they obtained a mass exponent of 0.12. The regression predicts shorter MAL for all mammals 12 kg and under, compared with predictions from Sacher (1959). Restricting the regression to the maximum MAL from each of 76 mammal families, the mass exponent was 0.16 ± 0.17, predicting shorter MAL than Sacher's equations for mammals.

In none of these determinations do mammals, collectively, match birds for longevity records. Prothero and Jurgens (1986) claimed that bats outlived birds, but the correlation coefficient of their regression (0.234 for 28 spp.) is not significant at the p = 0.10 level. In a subsequent paper they reported only that bats outlive other mammals (compared on an equal-size basis; Jurgens and Prothero 1987). These authors found no significant sex difference in maximum longevity, and suggested that the scaling of mean longevity and maximum longevity were similar, and that wild mammals might possibly survive in the wild as long as they do sheltered in captivity.

Klimkiewicz (personal communication) has extracted the maximum longevity records for 498 species of wild banded birds from the computer files of the U. S. Fish and Wildlife Service Bird Banding Laboratory, through 1987. Some of these oldest records to date are based on limited sampling, so probably understate considerably ages actually attained for the species. Typically less than ten percent of banded birds are subsequently recaptured, collected, or found dead, except for colonial-nesting marine birds, and hunted species of fowl, waterfowl, and doves. Hence fairly intense banding/recapture efforts are necessary to obtain longevity records which actually reflect life's limits. Attempting to eliminate the understudied, I have used only the maximum longevity within each of the 215 genera represented. Combined with body weights from Dunning (1984), these yielded the least-squares regression shown in Figure 3:

$$\text{MAL, years} = 14.3 \ M^{0.14 \pm 0.016} \tag{2}$$

The correlation coefficient of 0.518 is significant at p < 0.001. Its square indicates that size accounts for 27% of the variance. The standard error of log 14.3 is 0.188. This regression predicts shorter MAL for all birds over 33g in body mass, compared to Lindstedt and Calder's (1976) equation for wild birds.

Is there a systematic bias towards smaller birds, more likely to be caught by back-yard banders, and more likely to be recorded as having attained the actual maximum by virtue of faster turnover relative to the history of the banding program. I have used the total numbers of bandings from which the records could have been sampled, as reported for 192 of these species by Clapp *et al.* (1982, 1983) and Klimkiewicz *et al.* (1983, 1987) regressing log number of bandings per species *vs.* log body mass. There is a suggestion of a

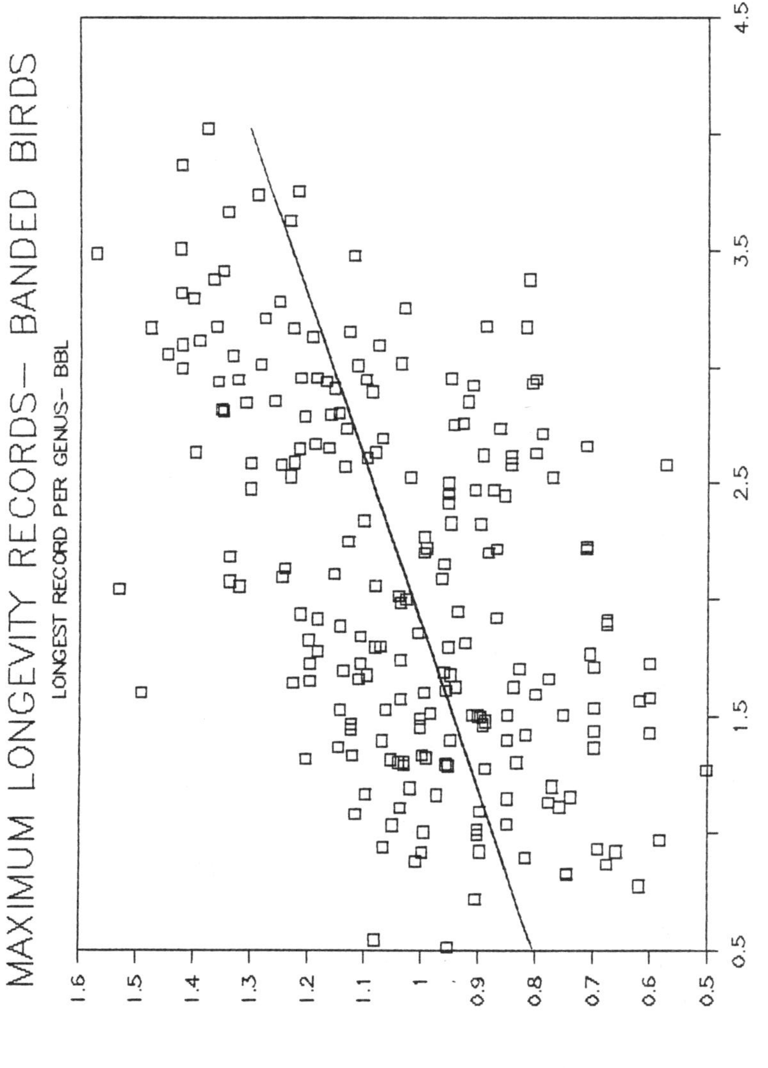


**Figure 3.** Maximum lifespans of birds from U.S. Fish and Wildlife Service Bird-Banding Laboratory records, using longest recorded lifespan per genus and typical body mass for the species exhibiting that maximum.

weak but statistically insignificant (r = 0.014) inverse relationship between banding frequency and bird size. The probability of recording a maximum longevity must increase with the extent of sampling (banding), but maximum lifespan did not correlate significantly with number of birds banded (r = 0.038).

Hence, there seems to be no ready explanation for why these scalings of MAL show exponents systematically less than the $M^{1/4}$ for physiological time. The addition of over two decades' worth of captive mammal and wild bird longevity records has not shown a significant increase in MAL, so perhaps we are approaching the point of diminishing returns in deriving generalizations about maximum longevity.

The maximum recorded longevity is an approximation to the maximum achievable lifespan. If this tends to be fairly characteristic of a species, chances are that it is genetically encoded, selected either to resist the ravages of time (longevity assurance) or in aging programmed to hasten disposal of bearers of transcription errors and metabolic malfunctions. Maximum longevity could thus be regarded as a genotype whose phenotypic expression is affected by environmental variables such as predation risks, diseases, capricious food supplies, etc. Mean lifespan or life expectancy is thus the mean phenotypic expression.

In birds and mammals, mean longevity scales more steeply than maximum longevity, the larger-bodied species being more likely to survive to senior citizen status, while smaller-bodied species are significantly less likely to survive to the genotypic maximum. This is expressed in scaling exponents of 0.46 for birds, compared to 0.24, 0.30, and 0.35 for mammals. This means that for small birds and mammals, the environment discourages full phenotypic realization of the genotypic potential (Damuth 1982, Calder 1983, Millar and Zammuto 1983, and Calder 1984). Prothero and Jurgen (1986) obtained smaller exponents from a much more extensive data set but these may not reflect any true mean longevity determined from life tables or survivorship, rather the averages of zoo records.

In captivity, mammalian survivorship is age-dependent, with an actuarial increase in annual mortality. Both the initial mortality rate and the aging increment scale with body-size (Calder 1982, 1983). According to Hayflick (1987): "Feral animals old enough to have decrements in physiological function comparable to that of a middle-aged human simply do not survive...If aging occurs at all in wild animals, its expression is quantitatively small and temporally brief."

Wild birds have generally failed to reveal evidence of senescent or age-dependent mortality. Either 1) the avian data have too much "noise" of age-independent death *via* accident, starvation, or predation, 2) the studies have not achieved the proportions and durations necessary to reveal age-dependence, or 3) birds do not age. The principal arguments that aging does occur in birds are theoretical ones (Botkin and Miller 1974, Calder 1983). One excellent empirical verification was obtained from long-term studies of the black-capped chickadee (*Parus atricapillus*) by Loery *et al.* 1987).

I suspect that the reason that age-dependent mortality is seldom recognized in birds is because of inadequate sampling. For many species of birds, one can only distinguish juveniles from adults, but not first year adults from second year, or older, adults. Without some morphological means of determining a bird's age, if I band one third of a local bird population one year, I do not know which birds in my Year 1 sample are really one year old, and how many are older. The next year, some of the unbanded birds I catch may have been present as adults, but not captured, so what I would be calling "Year class 1" for year 2 would be of mixed ages. Continuing this process, it would be hard to separate age-dependent from age-independent mortality, because ages were not clearly separated.

It is unknown whether the difference in maximum longevity of birds and mammals lies in their initial mortality (age-independent) or in the rate of aging, or in a combination of both. Loery *et al.* (1987) found that the chickadee's survival rate decreased with age at a rate of ~ 3.5% per year. A mammal of similar size (10.8 g, from Dunning (1984)) might be expected to show a survival rate decrease of only 2.4 % per year (eq. 11-52, Calder 1984).

## HUMMINGBIRDS

Hummingbirds have characteristics which make them excellent models for aging studies in the natural context: 1) they are not hunted by man, 2) predation does not seem to be significant in their mortality (Miller and Gass 1985), and 3) they have been selected for relatively generous longevity in nature. Hummingbirds, unlike several other species, can be attracted to artificial food sources, and if one can persist long enough, sooner or later, most members of a local breeding population can be caught, banded, and entered into one's data base. If capture tends to be random, or if one is sampling only a portion of a transient or migrant population, the age-dependency is swamped by imperfect knowledge of age itself. For example, Figure 4 shows the 242 returns (birds recaptured in years subsequent to banding) of 1641 ruby-throated hummingbirds banded by Baumgartner in Oklahoma (who now has a record lonegvity for that species of 9 years). After the typical, steeper disap-

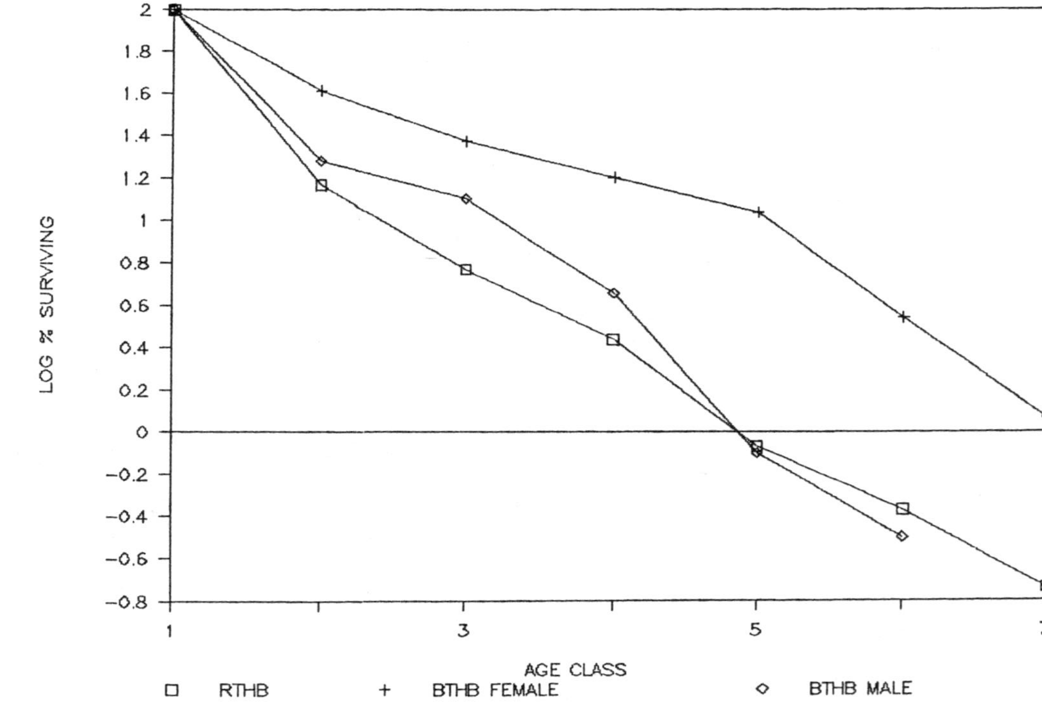



**Figure 4.** Apparent survivorship of the ruby-throated hummingbird (squares, lowest curve) shows no age-dependence after the first, presumably more transient, year (from which subsequent recapture would be less likely due to emigration). In contrast, a population of breeding broad-tailed hummingbirds, recaptured annually and almost competely, shows a progressively steeper rate of disappearance tentatively regarded as evidence of aging.

pearance rate from year 1 to year 2 which I would attribute to banding of some transients or migrants, there is no pattern of steepening that could be associated with aging.

The broad-tailed hummingbird (*Selasphorus platycercus*) breeds in Colorado, Wyoming, Nevada, Utah, Arizona, New Mexico, and through the Sierra Madres of Mexico to Guatemala. Birds breeding in the U.S. winter in the mountains of Mexico. In the only analysis of hummingbird population dynamics to date, this species shows that 46 percent of the nestings are successful and that 48 percent of the females and 73 percent of the males disappear from the population, from one year to the next. Disappearance does not necessarily mean mortality. In fact, we have recaptured some of our former breeding season residents at another location 6.7 km distant. However, the strong philopatry or site-fidelity of many birds suggests that failure to return may, in fact, represent death in most cases.

On 12 August 1987, a broad-tail with a minimum age of 12.1 years was recaptured at the Rocky Mountain Biological Laboratory. Two gray feathers on her crown were the only outward suggestion of aging. She had no "bags" under her eyes, like an aged garnet hummingbird (in excess of its 8 years in the New York Zoological Park; Conway 1961). In fact, the anodized numbers on her aluminum band (X-18025) were fading faster than she was. Although there is an aviary record of 14 y for the 5.9g planalto hermit (*Phaethornis pretrei*; see Skutch 1973, p.41), this was a new longevity record for wild hummingbirds. Allometrically, the maximum age expected for a bird of her size would be 6 years. Her twelve years is equivalent to 43 years for a large Canada Goose, but the record for that species is only 23 years. Within the birds, our maximum hummingbird lifespan was 2.1 times the predicted maximum wild avian lifespan (MWL) for its size. And since birds live 2.4 times as long as mammals, the product (2.1 times 2.4) says that this hummingbird lived 5 times the prediction for a hypothetical mammal of the same size, m = 3.5g.

Soon after our oldest female hummingbird set the 12.1 year record, Anna Eliza Williams of Swansea, Wales, the oldest living woman, died at an age of 114 years, four times what Sacher's (1959) mammalian equation would have predicted. Thus hummingbirds and humans have a quantitatively similar factor by which they outlive the typical longevity for similarly-sized mammals. Others of our species have reportedly lasted to 120 years, ten times the wild hummingbird maximum. Thus the female hummingbirds begin to show an increased mortality at the equivalent of 50 years for the human female.

Protected from natural hazards of predation, starvation, and migratory accidents, captive birds appear to be able to live 60% longer than wild birds. At 12.1 y, our oldest hummingbird exceeded the size-dependent predictions for captive birds by 25% and for wild birds by 100% Lindstedt and Calder 1976). Regardless of size, she was older than the records for 336 of 498 species in the Bird-Banding Laboratory computer files, and exceeded by 85% the allometric prediction from the genera represented (eq. 2 above).

This particular species and population is especially well-suited for field studies of longevity and aging because it has been pursued contemporaneously with other studies yielding considerable data relevant to survival and aging, such as body mass regulation, energetics, reproduction, and population biology. We have been banding and color-marking for individual recognition for 15 years, achieving capture rates that include virtually the entire adult population each year since 1979. "Data sets that are large, annually replicated and collected from animals that spend 100% of their lives living in an undisturbed condition are an ideal that most ecological studies cannot attain...estimates of rates of senescent mortality are notoriously hard to make for natural populations" (Dobson 1985).

Analysis of data on adult birds through 1985 showed overall annual return rates of 27% for males and 52% for females, a difference probably including migrant transients, and polygamy with male- territorial scarcity for the locals. If the initial adult year, in which transiency probably dilutes apparent survival, and the unreliable period of small sample sizes after year 7 are excluded, the tendency of the slopes to increase suggests that there is an age-dependent component to mortality, reasonable physiologically, but missing in most avian demographic studies.

Prior to 1979, we banded only incidentally at RMBL, but from that time forward have intensified the effort. Each year of banding most of the population improves the resolution of age-determinations. Figure 5 shows the survivorship curves through 1988, excluding the survivorship data of pre-1979 bandings. I have calculated two ways for each sex. The first is based on averaging the population-age class distributions for these years. The second treats longitudinal determinations of individual birds. The good agreement between the two methods is reassuring. From these curves, it appears mortality increases at age-class 5.

In comparison with the females, the male hummingbird survivorship curve begins to steepen downward at 4 years, equivalent to 40 years for man. Here we see another parallel between hummingbirds and men: as is well-established in humans (Holden, 1986), females outlive males. (Our oldest male hummingbird was at least 7.1 years old).

The lower limit for body and egg size is apparently related to physical constraints, although the explanatory details have not all been proven. The dimensions of the female hummingbird are such that she can incubate a clutch

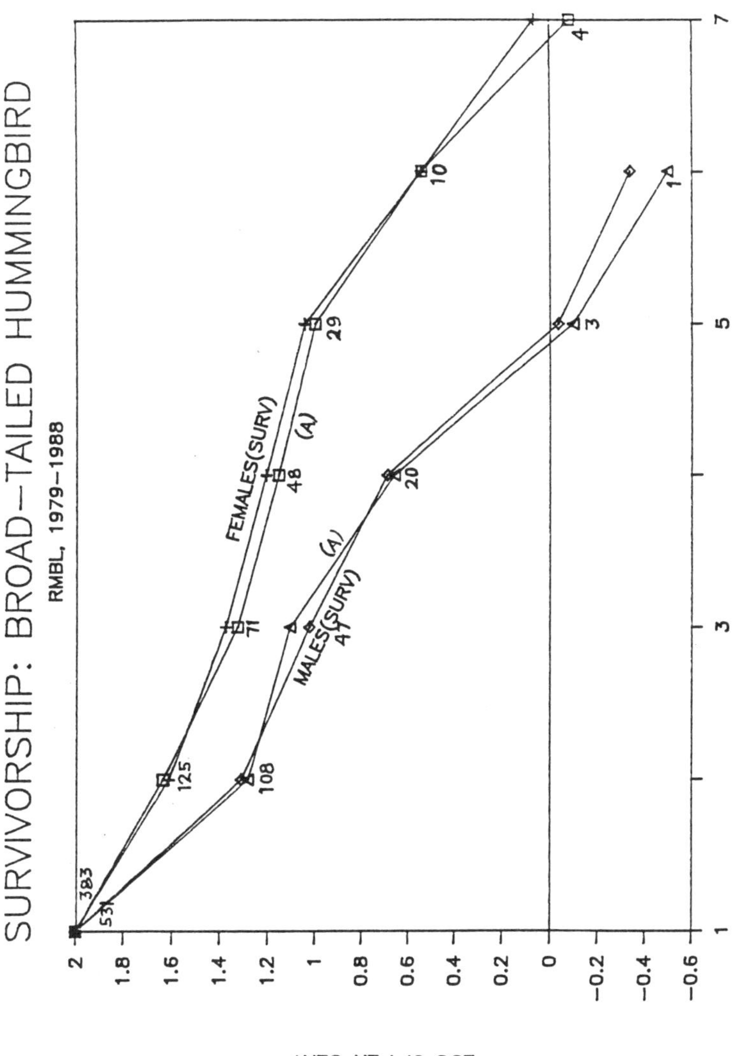



**Figure 5.** Survivorship curves of female (upper part) and male broad-tailed hummingbirds (lower part) determined by two methods, (SURV) by averaging eight years of longitudinal records on individual birds, and (A) by averaging annual population-age distributions in the captured population.

of only two eggs (most likely limited by brood patch size). Despite this limitation on reproduction, hummingbirds have managed to expand from the New World tropics to high altitudes and latitudes. At those extremes, the flowering season is so brief that only one clutch can be reared per year, posing a second limitation for reproduction. This low annual reproduction of one clutch per short montane summer, of only 2 eggs with 46% fledging success would necessitate a fair longevity just to achieve replacement (Calder *et al.*, 1983).

Given these limitations of success with a single small clutch per year, survival of northern temperate hummingbirds must be highly dependent upon (1) the quality of a female's nest site selection, care in construction, and attentiveness to eggs and chicks, and (2) extended lifespan, with relatively low vulnerability to predation and disease, perhaps surviving long enough for aging to be observed.

Thus one could conclude that the hummingbird might be a model for the study of physiological aging in birds. They are relatively long-lived for their size, practical for study in absolute time, and apparently fairly safe from non-age-dependent mortality.

## LONGEVITY AND TORPOR

Let us return to the suggestion that longevity and energetics may be connected. This has been set forth as the "rate-of-living" theory, that longevity is ultimately limited not so much by chronology as by cumulative metabolic turnover, a theory that suffers because it is not readily testable in nature. The best support to date for this idea is the strong positive correlation between age at death and proportion of life spent in hibernation by Turkish hamsters (*Mesocricetus brandti*; Lyman *et al.*, 1981).

Does "rate of living" apply to hummingbird longevity? The oxidative-energetic demands of hovering hummingbirds are well known. In the high montane environment, hypoxic and thermal stresses are added. However, after sustaining the metabolic intensity of daytime, hummingbirds can (and in my lab, the males do) enter hypothermic torpor at night (males do not participate in nesting). This could be a case of biological time extension through metabolic suppression (Hochachka and Guppy 1987), not strictly limited to emergency survival as hypothesized by Hainsworth *et al.* (1977). The view that torpor is used routinely has been strengthened by Kruger *et al.* (1982) who reported torpor in 18 species of hummingbirds, "independent of ambient temperature, feeding situation or the environment (biotope) of the species". If hummingbird males on territories and both sexes after the nesting season are normally going torpid for 8 hours or more each night, the daily metabolic turnover might be reduced by 25% (Calder 1974), possibly fitting the pattern found in hamsters by Lyman *et al.* (1981).

However, studies of free-living body mass changes now in progress indicate that even on the wintering grounds, these small dynamos are able to store an amount of energy that would normally support homeothermy all night. Hence "rate-of-living" may not explain the exceptional longevity of hummingbirds either. Whatever the secret of their potential longevity, it further enhances Darwinian fitness by allowing the animal to have additional breeding seasons. Considering the low annual fecundity of one to two off-spring in one or two litters or clutches per year characteristic of both bats and hummingbirds, enhanced longevity could be crucial to the persistence of species.

## HOMEOSTASIS AND LIFESPAN

One explanation for longevity is related to observations of tighter correlations between brain size and longevity than between body size and longevity, merely reflecting the smaller coefficients of variation for brain size than for body mass. This erroneous equation of correlation to causation is coupled with the argument that bigger brains can regulate more precisely than smaller brains, and longevity is favored by less variation in the *milieu interieur*. It should then follow that birds living longer would have more precise homeostatic regulation than mammals, but the opposite seems true. Birds have higher, and in smaller species, diurnally more variable, body temperatures, accompanied by higher protein turnover rates, and tolerate greater arterial acid-base and osmotic changes (2.8-fold alkalinity increase; Lindstedt and Calder 1981; Calder 1984). Prothero and Jurgens (1986) also rejected lifespan-organ size correlations as a real basis for longevity enhancement.

## CONCLUSIONS

Five points emerge from this interim analysis of avian longevity: 1. Birds may have considerable "safety margin" in their maximum longevities. A female hummingbird has survived in the wild to 12.1 y in a population with an average life expectancy of 2.8 y. Comparable ages for males are 7 y maximum and 2.05 y mean life expectancy. The apparent safety factors are 4.3 and 3.4 in these cases.

2. The rarity of outward evidence of aging in wild birds suggests that there is no need to program for aging to dispose of senior citizens. Predation, disease, accident, and starvation are probably adequate for termination of the non-productive.

3. By all comparisons, birds tend to last longer, so it is protoplasmically possible to live longer than mammals do.

4. Contrary to brain theories, which say that more brain allows closer homeostatic regulation and from it the preservation of life, birds live longer with less precise regulation - greater variation in plasma osmotic pressure, plasma pH, and body temperature.

5. This is an interim report of a continuing study. Three more years will provide an unbroken data set of consistent maximal effort to include the entire population for a period equal to maximum longevity, which will make these curves more precise and perhaps provide a unique record of aging in birds. It will provide a basis for analyzing the relative contributions of reducing initial vulnerability and slowing the actuarial aging rate relative to mammals.

## ACKNOWLEDGEMENTS

Research on hummingbird survival in nature has been funded in part by grants 2665-83, 2824-84, 3064-85, 3242-85, and 3513-87 from the National Geographic Society. I am grateful to Lorene Calder, Sara Hiebert, Denise Stevenson, Audrey Wagner, Dana Bradley, and Amy Seidl for field assistance, to Ken Williams (University of Arizona computer specialist) for setting up the database system, to Kathy Klimkiewicz (USF&WS Bird-Banding Laboratory), Nickolas Waser, David Inouye, and Natasha Kotliar of the Rocky Mountain Biological Laboratory for sharing unpublished data, to Grace J. Calder and James Linch for providing our trusty research vehicle, and to Perky-Pet Products for providing feeders to attract the birds for this study.

## REFERENCES

BAUMGARTNER, A. M. (1986). Longevity of selected species from a 50-year file. *N. Amer. Bird Bander* **11**: 6-9.

BENNETT, A. F. (1987). Interindividual variability: an underutilized resource. **In**: *New Directions in Ecological Physiology*. (Feder, M. E., Bennett, A. F., Burggren, W. W., and Huey, R. B.) Chap. 7, pp. 147-169 Cambridge University Press, New York.

BOTKIN, D. B. and MILLER, R. S. (1974). Mortality rates and survival of birds. *Amer. Nat.* **108**: 181-92.

CALDER, W. A. III. (1982). The relationship of the Gompertz constant and maximum potential lifetime to body mass. *Exper. Geront.* **17**: 383-85.

CALDER, W. A. III. (1984). *Size, Function, and Life History*. Harvard Univ. Press, Cambridge.

CALDER, W. A. III. (1985). The comparative biology of longevity and lifetime energetics. *Exper. Geront.* **20**: 161-70.

CHARLESWORTH, B. (1989). *Natural selection and life history patterns*. In this volume.

CLAPP, R. B., Klimkiewicz, M. K. and Kennard, J. H. (1982). Longevity records of North American Birds: Gaviidae through Alcidae. *J. Field Ornithol.* **53**: 81-124.

CLAPP, R. B., Klimkiewicz, M. K. and Futcher, A. G. (1983). Longevity records of North American birds: Columbidae through Paridae. *J. Field Ornithol.* **54**: 123-137.

CRAIG, J. F. (1985) Aging in fish. *Can.J. Zool.* **63**: 1-8.

CUTLER, R. G. (1976) Nature of aging and life maintenance processes. *Interdiscipl. Topics Geront.* **9**: 83-133.

CUTLER, R. G. (1978) Evolutionary biology of senescence. **In**: *The Biology of Aging* (Behnke, J. A., Finch, C. E., and Moment, G. B., Eds.) Ch. 20, pp.311- 60, Plenum, New York.

CUTLER, R. G. (1983) Species probes, longevity and aging. **In**: *Intervention in the Aging Process* (Regelson, W. and Sinex, F. M.) pp. 69-144, Liss, New York.

DOBSON, A. P. (1985) Age-dependent mortality rates of some British birds. **In**: *Statistics in Ornithology*, (North, P. and Morgan, B., Eds.) pp. 275-288. Berlin: Springer.

DUNNING, J. B. Jr. (1984). Body weights of 686 species of North American Birds. *Western Bird Banding Association Monogr.* **1**. 38 pp.

GIBBONS, J. W. (1987) Why do turtles live so long? *BioScience* **37**: 262- 269.

HAINSWORTH, F. R., Collins, B. G., and Wolf, L. L. (1977) The function of torpor in hummingbirds. *Physiol. Zool.* **50**: 215-222.

HART, R. W., SACHER, G. A., and HOSKINS, B. A. (1979) DNA repair in a short- and a long-lived rodent species. *J. Geront.* **34**: 806-17.

HART, R. W. and TURTURRO, A. (1987) Evolution of life span in placental mammals. **In**: *Modern Biological Theories of Aging* (Warner, H. R., Butler, R. N., Sprott, R. L., and Schneider, E. L. Eds.) pp.5-34, New York: Raven Press.

HAYFLICK, L. (1985) Theories of biological aging. *Exper. Geront.* **20**: 145-59.

HOCHACHKA P. W. and GUPPY M. (1987) *Metabolic Arrest and the Control of Biological Time*. Cambridge: Harvard U. Press.

HOLDEN C. (1983) Why do women live longer than men? *Science* **238**: 158-60.

JONES, M. L. (1982) Longevity of Captive Mammals. *Der Zool. Garten* **52**: 113-128.

JURGENS, K. D. and PROTHERO, J. (1987) Scaling of maximal lifespan in bats. *Comp. Biochem. Physiol.* **88A**: 361-7.

KLIMKIEWICZ, M. K., CLAPP, R. B., and FUTCHER, A. G. (1983) Longevity records of North American birds: Remizidae through Parulinae. *J. Field Ornithol.* **54**: 287-294.

KLIMKIEWICZ, M. K. and FUTCHER, A. G. (1987) Longevity records of North American Birds: Coerebinae through Estrildidae. *J. Field Ornithol.* **58**: 318-333.

KRUGER, K., PRINZINGER, R. and SCHUCHMANN, K.-L. (1982) Torpor and metabolism in hummingbirds. *Comp. Biochem. Physiol.* **73A**: 679-689.

LINDSTEDT, S. L. (1985) Birds. *Interdiscipl. Topics in Geront.* **21**: 1-21.

LINDSTEDT, S. L. and CALDER, W. A. (1976) Body size and longevity in birds. *Condor* **78**: 91-4.

LINDSTEDT, S. L. and CALDER, W. A. (1981) Body size, physiological time and longevity of homeotherms. *Q. Rev. Biol.* **56**: 1-16.

LOERY, G., POLLOCK, K. H., NICHOLS, J. D. and HINES, J. E. (1987) Age specificity of black-capped chickadee survival rates: analysis of capture-recapture data. *Ecology* **68**: 1038-1044.

LYMAN, C. P., O'BRIEN, R. C., GREENE, G. C., and PAPAFRANGOS, E. D. 1981. Hibernation and longevity in the Turkish hamster *Mesocricetus brandti. Science* **212**: 668-670.

MASORO, E. J., YU, B. P., BERTRAND, H. A., and LYND, F. T. (1980) Nutritional probe of the aging process. *Fed. Proc.* **39**: 3178-3182.

MILDVAN, A. S. and STREHELER, B. L. (1960) A critique of theories of aging. **In**: *The Biology of Aging*. (Streheler, B. L., Ebert, J. D., Glass, H. B., Shock, N. W., Eds.) Washington: Amer. Inst. of Biol. Sci. pp 216-235.

PROTHERO, J. and JURGENS, K. D. (1986) Scaling of maximal lifespan in mammals. **In**: *Evolution of Longevity in Animals*. (Woodhead, A. D. and Thompson, K. H. Eds:), pp.49-73, Plenum, New York.

ROSEN, P., WOODHEAD, A. D. and THOMPSON, K. M. (1981) The relationship between the Gompertz constant and maximum potential lifespan : its relevance to theories of aging. *Exp. Geront.* **16**: 131-135.

SACHER, G. A. (1959) Relation of lifespan to brain weight and body weight in mammals. **In:** *The Lifespan of Animals.* (Wolstenholme, G. E. W. and Connor, M. O. Eds.) Vol. 5, Ciba Foundation Colloquia On Aging. pp. 115-141, Little, Brown, and Co., Boston.

SACHER, G. A. (1977) Life table modification and life prolongation. **In:** *Handbook of the Biology of Aging.* (Birren, J., Finch, C., and Hayflick, L., Eds.) New York: Van Nostrand.

SACHER, G. A. (1978) Evolution of longevity and survival characteristics in mammals. **In:** *The Genetics of Aging.* (Schneider, E. L., Ed.) pp. 151-68, Plenum, New York.

SACHER, G. A. (1982) Evolutionary theory in gerontology. *Perspect. Biol. Med.* **25**: 339-353.

SCHNEIDER, E. L. (1987) Theories of aging: a perspective. pp.1-34, **In:** *Modern Biological Theories of Aging.* (Warner, H. R., Butler, R. N., Sprott, R. L. and Schneider, E. L., Eds), New York: Raven Press.

TIMIRAS, P. S. (1978) Biological perspectives on aging. *Amer. Sci.* **66**: 605-613.

WARNER, H. R., BUTLER, R. N., SPROTT, R. L., and SCHNEIDER, E. L., Eds. *Modern Biological Theories of Aging.* Raven Press, New York.

## DISCUSSION

1. There are some problems with this approach: the correlation doesn't explain underlying processes, male - female differences may be due to secondary effects, as males may migrate further, and, most serious, it can't distinguish death from migration. Nevertheless, a capture - recapture study is the best that can be done to give actual lifespans in the wild. This is where evolution actually occurs, and thus should be relevant to evolutionary theories, perhaps more relevant that studies in the laboratory environment. This is one of the first such studies in the wild.

2. The possibility that hummingbirds and small mammals may greatly retard their metabolic rates and thus extend lifespans by torpor must be examined to test metabolic theories of aging, including the free radical hypotheses. Hibernation seems to extend lifespans in chipmunks and ground squirrels.

3. Allometric studies are only the beginning. They hint at mechanisms, but further work is needed to define these mechanisms. Note that body sizes may affect natural niches and selection, thus molding patterns of aging. Birds may live long because their ability to fly greatly reduces predation and other accidental death. Thus their reproductive fitness later in life is enhanced, and natural selection will evolve mechanisms so that birds live long. What are these mechanisms, and may they offer ideas to increase "Healthspans" in man?

4. Males may live less long than females because their initial breeding ability was more important than their ability to raise the young. New mutations may be more important in males with only one X chromosome.

# Section 3

## GENETICS OF AGING RETARDATION

# 13

# PERSPECTIVES ON GENETIC VARIABILITY IN BEHAVIORAL AGING OF MICE

Donald K. Ingram

## ABSTRACT

Data are reviewed and ideas are discussed concerning the use of inbred mouse strains for investigating genetic mechanisms involved in behavioral aging. Strain comparisons and test crosses using A/J and C57BL/6J inbred strains and B6AF$_1$ hybrids are used to identify possibly interesting analyses to explore with respect to psychomotor and learning performance. Questions are posed concerning the agreement between patterns of behavioral and actuarial aging in inbred strains. Manipulation of the aging rate through dietary restriction in these strains is considered with respect to whether behavioral tests reflect alterations in the aging rate. Behavioral aging in CBA/HT6J and C57BL/6J genotypes is also compared with respect to possible strain differences in the nigro-striatal dopamine system. Several models representing different hypotheses of genetic influence on behavioral aging are proposed.

## INTRODUCTION

Aging is viewed as a universal phenomenon among mammalian species, yet a cardinal feature of this phenomenon is the marked degree of variability in aging rate between species (Cutler, 1984) and possibly within species as measured by performance in clinical and functional tests (Rowe and Minaker, 1985; Shock *et al.*, 1984). While for many scientific disciplines variability in experimental measures of a phenomenon presents a problem of interpretation, the acknowledgment of variability in gerontological studies can lead to an examination of possible causal mechanisms of aging.

Figure 1 presents a hypothetical function that illustrates the principle of an age-related increase in variability. At any age there exist individual differences in performance, but the variability in the measure increases as a function of age. This cross-sectional perspective is considered to reflect different rates of aging among individuals on a longitudinal basis. This view of aging can be supported empirically to some degree (Welford, 1958) but still

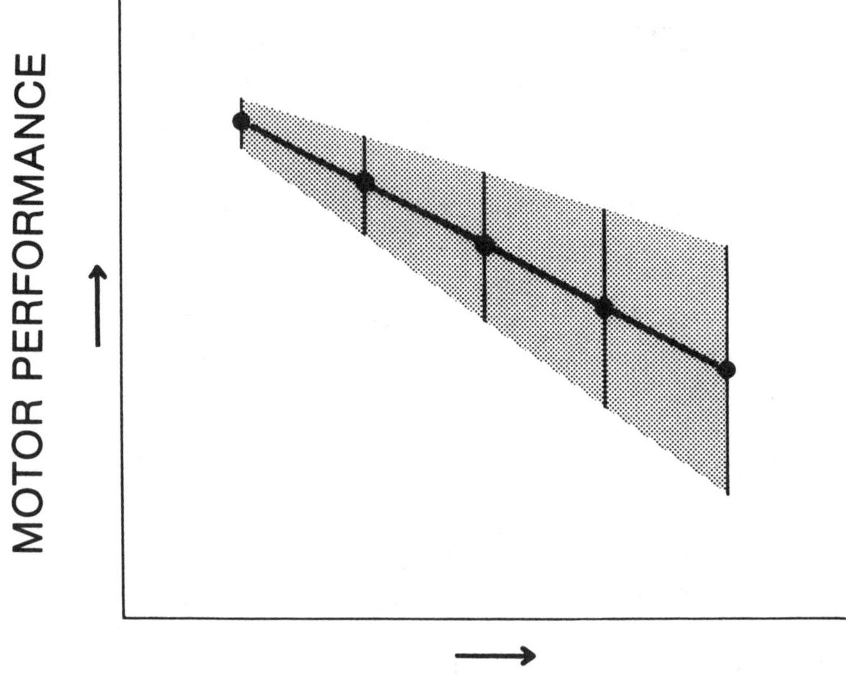



**Figure 1**. Hypothetical function depicting age-related increase in performance variability.

requires greater investigation to understand the nature and importance of age-related increases in variability (Sprott, 1988).

Among natural populations, the age-related increase in performance variability observed in the results of cross-sectional studies represents a complex mixture of possible genetic, environmental, and measurement error factors (Ingram, 1988b). From the genetic perspective, it can imply that different genotypes age at different rates. From the environmental perspective, it can imply that different environmental factors can modulate the genetic program for aging even for the same genotype. And then measurement errors must also be considered and how these might change with age. Finally, there is the conceptual confound of disease, the incidence of which increases with age and the prevalence of which can produce variability in results.

Teasing out the contribution of each of these factors is a particularly difficult task in human studies. Investigations utilizing registries of human twins have begun this arduous process but only on a small scale until recently (McClearn and Foch, 1985). However, it is obvious that the use of laboratory animals would yield more easily obtainable, and possibly more accurate, information concerning the contribution of specific genetic and environmental factors to intra-individual variability during aging (Elias *et al.*, 1977).

## INBRED MOUSE STRAINS

The objective of this paper is to focus attention on the possible uses of inbred mouse strains in elucidating genetic mechanisms of aging. This approach has been addressed several times previously in much more detailed fashion (Elias *et al.*, 1977; McClearn and Foch, 1985; Russell and Sprott, 1974; Sprott, 1976; Sprott 1980). The current intent is to provide additional data and ideas concerning the identification of possible fruitful investigations in the behavior genetics of aging.

The practical advantages of using inbred mouse lines are manifest. Their relatively short lifespans (<4 years), rapid development, small size, fecundity, adaptability to the laboratory, identified morbidity and pathology—all offer significant advantages compared to the problems confronted in studies of longer-lived species, especially humans. Most importantly with inbred strains, the investigator is able to specify, and to control to a certain extent thereby, the genetic and environmental conditions of the subjects. With the use of genetically homogeneous strains, comparisons can be made between genotypes reared in specified environments. Conversely, the influence of different environmental treatments can be compared within the same genotype. By controlling one source of variation, the other can be manipulated to assess the existence and magnitude of genotype-environment interactions (Sprott, 1980). Many other advantages are also offered by the use of inbred mouse lines. Further genetic analysis to identify the single gene or polygenic influence on a parameter of interest can be conducted using conventional Mendelian techniques of hybridization and backcrossing or with the use of more modern techniques such as recombinant inbred lines or bilineal congenic lines (Bailey 1971; Sprott, 1980). Although either approach can be used, the latter techniques significantly short-cut the process of identifying the number and location of genetic loci possibly involved in the phenomenon of interest. With success in this venture, techniques of modern molecular genetics offer the potential of dissecting out the genetic code and manipulating it with transgenic strategies. Of course, the use of inbred lines already offer natural experiments with the presence of single-gene mutations at identified locations (Elias *et al.*, 1977; Russell and Sprott, 1974).

## BEHAVIOR GENETICS OF AGING

As a highly ubiquitous phenomenon, aging is manifested at virtually all levels of biological organization in mammals. Behavior is the interaction of the organism with its environment. As such, it represents a complex product involving many different levels of biological organization.

The analysis of aging at a behavioral level is important for at least two reasons. First, because behavior represents such a high level of biological organization, an analysis of behavioral aging concerns the manifestation of many interacting systems and may thus represent aging of the whole organism (primary aging) more accurately than does analysis at lower levels. This sword cuts both ways, though, since this complexity makes the task of identifying specific genetic pathways more difficult. However, the fact that many complex behaviors influenced by single genes have been identified suggests that the task is not an impossible one (Elias *et al.*, 1977; Sprott, 1976; 1980). A second important rationale for an analysis of behavioral aging is that such assessments reflect what the organism is capable of doing in its environment. As such, behavioral analysis reflects "quality of life" performance which is important for assessing the status of health and vigor of the organism in relation to specific variables that exist or that are being manipulated.

A behavior genetics of aging has not formally emerged (McClearn and Foch, 1985) although its potential value has been emphasized for a long time (Elias *et al.*, 1977; Sprott, 1980; Russell and Sprott, 1974). Some progress has been achieved in invertebrate models in identifying loci possibly involved in age-related behavioral decline (Johnson, 1986; 1988). In mouse models, research has been directed primarily to identifying possibly interesting strain differences in behavioral aging. The current discussion will focus on the potential that such observations hold with respect to identifying possible mechanisms of behavioral aging under genetic control. These comparisons will be made between strains of male mice housed under similar environmental conditions in our laboratory.

## STRAIN DIFFERENCES IN BEHAVIORAL AGING

Several reports have documented differences in psychomotor performance among inbred mouse strains assessed across adult lifespans (Goodrick, 1975a; Ingram *et al.*, 1981; Sprott and Eleftheriou, 1974). Figure 2 provides a perspective on how differences between two strains can be manifested at a behavioral level of analysis in a cross-sectional aging study.

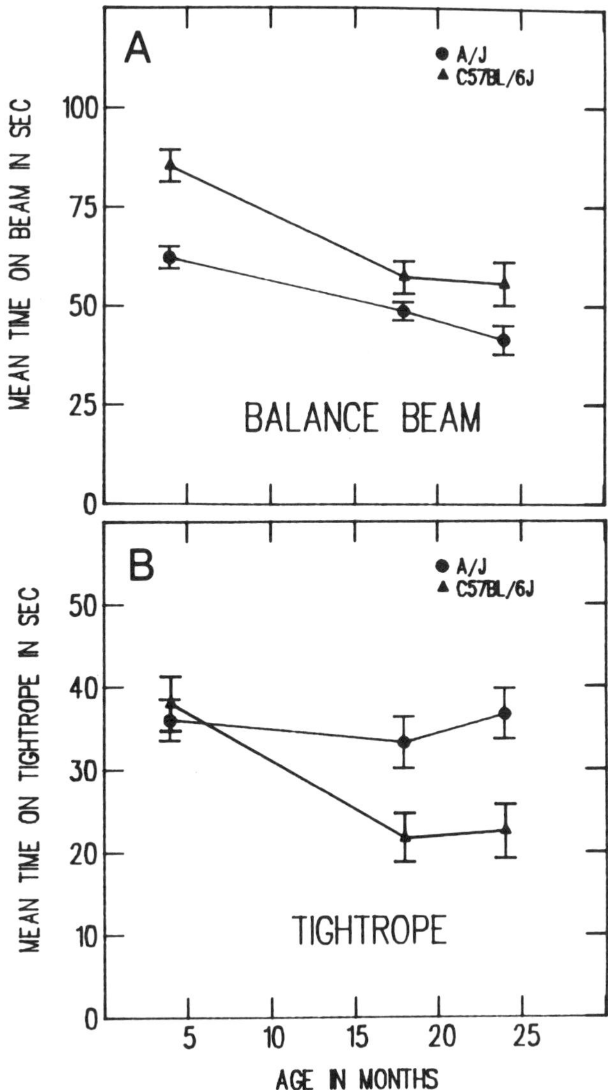



**Figure 2.** Age differences (mean +/- sem) in psychomotor performance of A/J and C57BL/6J strain in a balance beam task (A) and a tightrope task (B). Data from Ingram et al (1981); ns = 18-37.

From Figure 2A it is clear that C57BL/6J exhibit superior performance over their lifespan compared to A/J mice in a balance beam task, the procedural details of which have been described previously (Ingram *et al.*, 1981). In general, the amount of time that a mouse can remain on a narrow wooden dowel before falling is averaged over several trials. It would appear that C57BL/6J mice were genetically endowed to perform better in this task under the specified conditions. Both strains exhibit an age-related decline in performance as measured in this cross-sectional study; however, the slope of age-related decline appears similar. This perspective would indicate that whatever genetically mediated processes were acting on this behavior were similar in both strains across their lifespans.

This perspective on strain differences can be contrasted with that in Figure 2B, which represents the mouse's ability to remain suspended by its front paws from a taut string as averaged over several trials (Ingram *et al.*, 1981). At the youngest age, no strain difference was noted. This observation would indicate an equivalent genetic endowment for the abilities required in this task. However, genetic involvement in the rate of aging would appear different between the strains. Whereas the C57BL/6J strain demonstrates an age-related decline in performance, A/J mice exhibit stable performance across age in this task.

Differential effects of aging on performance in learning and memory tasks have also been reported (Sprott, 1978; Stavnes and Sprott, 1975). Sprott (1978) argued that the age differences he observed in a simple passive avoidance task were probably due to health factors and suggested that more complex tasks might be necessary to observe meaningful age differences. In our laboratory, we have applied a complex, 14-unit T-maze for the assessment of age differences in the learning abilities of rodents (Goodrick, 1968; Ingram, 1985; 1988a). This task has proven to be very robust with respect to reflecting age differences under a variety of procedures and in a variety of rodent strains (Ingram, 1985; 1988a). A comparison of error performance between A/J and C57BL/6J strains is presented in Figure 3. Cross-sectional age differences are apparent in both genotypes. However, the age-related increase in error performance is much greater in A/J mice even though both strains exhibit equivalent performance at the youngest age. This pattern of behavioral aging suggests genetic influence that appears opposite in direction to the pattern observed in the tightrope task in which the C57BL/6J strain exhibited an age-related decline while the A/J strain did not.

To what extent can the genetic factors underlying these strain differences be further assessed? To address this question in earnest would require much additional analysis to determine the pattern of inheritance for each strain

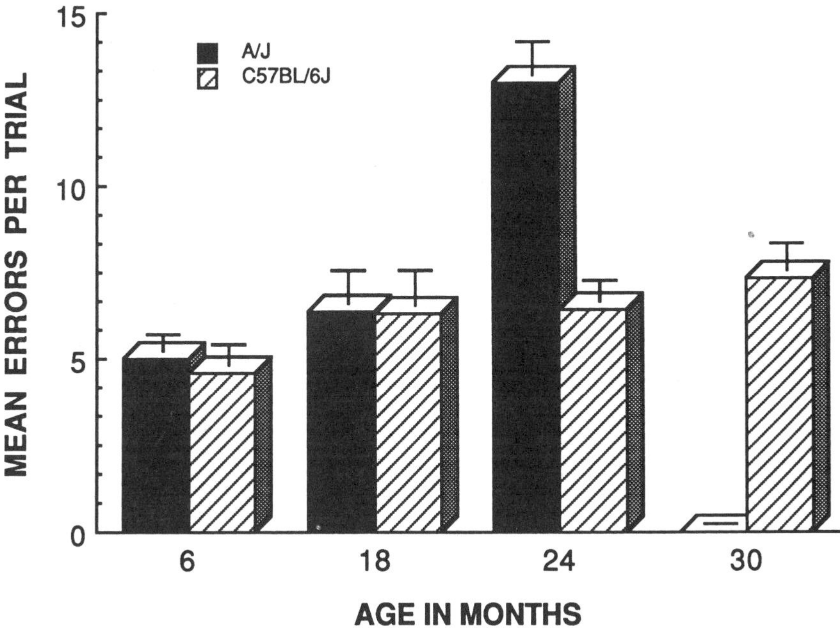


**Figure 3.** Age differences (mean +/- sem) in error performance of A/J and C57BL/6J strains in a 14-unit T-maze. Data from Ingram (1988a); ns = 6-10.

difference. A first step in this process would be to determine the pattern of behavioral aging in the hybrid of these two inbred strains.

Figure 4 presents data comparing C57BL/6J and A/J strains and their $F_1$ hybrid (B6AF$_1$) in an exploratory activity test described previously (Goodrick, 1973; Ingram *et al.*, 1981). Essentially, locomotor activity is assessed by counting the number of revolutions each mouse makes in an oval runway during a 15-min session. The test is conducted under bright illumination (white light: Figure 3A) and then under darkened (red light: Figure 3B) conditions. Again, as in the balance beam test, the basic strain difference is very evident over the lifespan in this cross-sectional study. C57BL/6J are generally much more active in this test compared to A/J mice. However, the comparison under different conditions offers an important observation with respect to analyzing genetic differences in behavioral aging. When performance under the white light was compared, an age-related decline in activity was noted in C57BL/6J mice but not in the A/J strain. Under darkened conditions, an age-related decline was noted in both strains. Comparing both conditions, it is clear that A/J mice had greatly increased activity under the

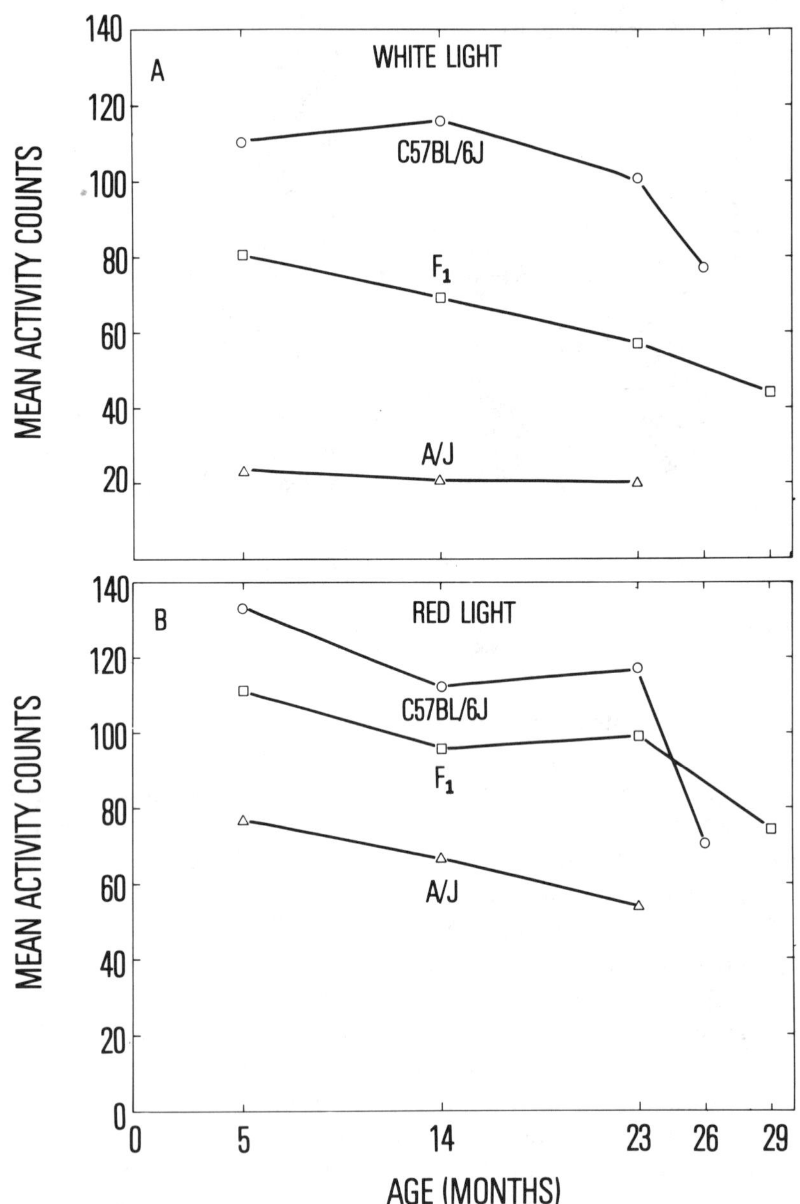


**Figure 4.** Age differences (means) in exploratory activity of A/J and C57BL/6J strains and their $F_1$ hybrid (B6AF$_1$) under two illumination conditions (ns = 16).

red light. This albino strain is photophobic and therefore was inhibited in its exploratory activity under bright illumination. Thus, rather than reflecting motor behavior, performance in this task may reflect motivational factors to a greater extent under this condition. These aspects of test construction and procedure should always be evaluated with respect to what aspect of behavior is being analyzed.

Regarding strain differences in the rate of aging in exploratory activity under darkened conditions, it would appear that A/J mice exhibited a greater age-related decline (29%) compared to C57BL/6J mice up to 23 months of age (12%). This pattern contrasts with that observed in Figure 2B. It should be noted that a marked performance decline in the C57BL/6J strain is observed after 23 months of age.

The performance of the $F_1$ mice indicated an intermediate mode of inheritance which has been observed in this type of behavior previously (Goodrick, 1973; McClearn, 1959). The $F_1$ pattern of aging in this behavior, however, appears to approximate that of the C57BL/6J parental strain. Thus, these data would indicate that factors of a polygenic nature endow these strains with differences in locomotor behavior but that aging in this parameter may be under different genetic controls.

Figure 5 provides another perspective on the inheritance of behavior and behavioral aging. This also reflects age and strain differences in locomotor behavior in a cross-sectional study. However, rather than in a novel environment, as in the exploratory activity test described above, this measure is obtained in the home cage of the animal. As described previously (Goodrick, 1975a; Ingram *et al.*, 1981), the dependent measure in this test reflects the mouse's activity in a runwheel cage over an extended period of time (1-week). The issue of photophobia is reduced in this context, but the test is still motivationally weighted to some extent, since the runwheel must be activated voluntarily. As in the exploratory activity test, C57BL/6J are much more active than are the A/J mice. Both strains show an age-related decline in performance, but the slopes across age appear equivalent to 23 months, at which time C57BL/6J exhibits a steep decline in activity. The interesting aspect of these results is the indication of a dominant mode of inheritance, as evidenced by the near parallel performance of the age function observed in hybrid animals with that of the C57BL/6J parents. Using analysis of recombinant inbred strains, a major locus controlling differences in wheel-running behavior between C57BL/6By and BALB/cBy strains has been suggested previously (Eleftheriou *et al.*, 1976).

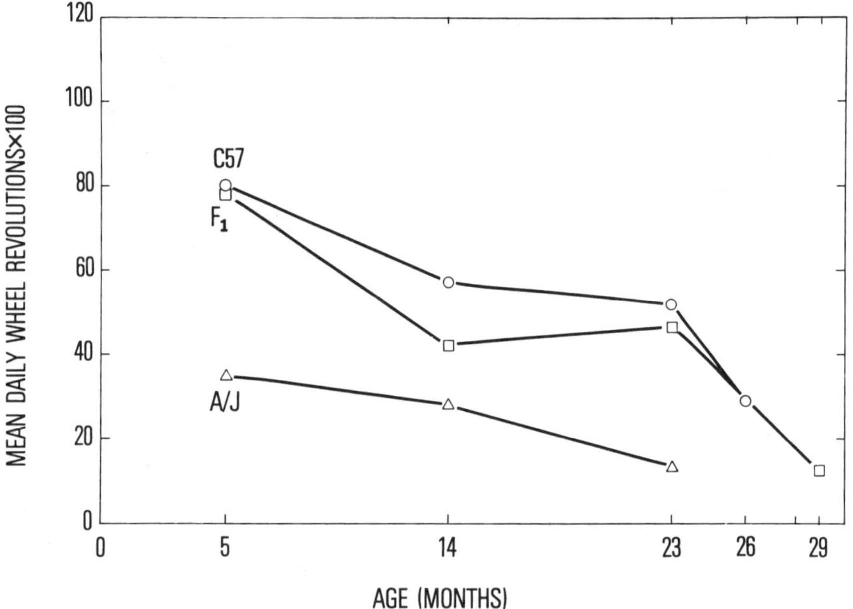



**Figure 5**. Age differences (means) in runwheel activity of A/J and C57BL/6J strains and their $F_1$ hybrid, B6AF$_1$ (ns = 16).

Another aspect of runwheel activity that can be assessed is the distribution of this behavior across circadian cycles. Wax (1977) noted that an age-related loss of circadian periodicity in runwheel activity appeared more frequently in the A/J genotype than in the C57BL/6J strain and the $F_1$ hybrids. Under both high and low levels of illumination, aged (23-mo) A/J mice exhibited a loss of 24-hr periods of activity cycling, whereas C57BL/6J and $F_1$ mice did not.

Thus, strain comparisons and the inclusion of $F_1$ hybrids provide clues to possibly interesting genetic analyses related to behavioral aging in inbred mice. No further sophisticated genetic analysis has been conducted in mice to determine the degree of heritability, the number of genetic loci involved, or the map location of candidate genes of these or any other similar behaviors as affected by aging. Goodrick's (1978) lifespan analysis of the inheritance of ethanol selection by inbred mice represents a model of further Mendelian analysis that can be conducted when given different patterns of behavioral aging among parental strains.

In summary, the importance of these types of simple analyses is in identifying possibly interesting behavioral parameters to explore further. From this perspective, patterns that show strain differences maintained throughout the lifespan which change at a similar rate appear less appealing than those that are manifested as differential rates of aging. Another perspective can also be gained by these simple strain comparisons. The differential pattern of results suggests that rather than global effects on aging, genetic influences on behavioral aging can be manifested along specific avenues that relate to specific performances.

## RELATIONSHIP BETWEEN BEHAVIORAL AND ACTUARIAL AGING

With respect to identifying behavioral parameters that reflect aging rate in general rather than in a particular performance, attention should be given to strain differences in actuarial aging and the manipulation thereof. Figure 6 presents a comparison of survival curves among A/J and C57BL/6J genotypes and their $F_1$ and $F_2$ hybrids. These data demonstrate that survival is greater in the C57BL/6J strain compared to A/J mice with clear differences in median and maximum lifespans. Survival in the $F_1$ hybrid demonstrates heterosis but not to a marked extent superior to the survival experience of C57BL/6J parents. The $F_2$s exhibit a possible pattern of segregation, with early deaths resembling those of the A/J genotype and late deaths resembling those of the C57BL/6J genotype. Based on analysis of variability in $F_2$ hybrids in this study, Goodrick (1975b) estimated the heritability of lifespan in these strains to be about 50 percent.

Whether these different survival profiles indicate differences in the rate of aging among different strains is controversial. Sacher (1977) indicated that differences in log slope of mortality between groups (Gompertz analysis) was evidence of differential rates of aging. Others have argued against exclusive reliance on this technique (Smith, 1966). Grahn (1972) reported that the log slopes of mortality for BALB/cJ and C57BL/6J were parallel although there were marked differences in mean lifespans. Storer (1978) reported similar results for a large number of female inbred genotypes and four male genotypes (A/J, DBA/2J, LP/J, and SM/J). In general, he concluded that the probability of dying was equivalent across age for all strains and that survival differences were probably due to differential vulnerabilities to specific pathologies. No comprehensive analysis of this question using a large number of male inbred mouse strains under more rigorously controlled (disease-free) conditions has yet been conducted. Thus, at present it cannot be concluded that differences

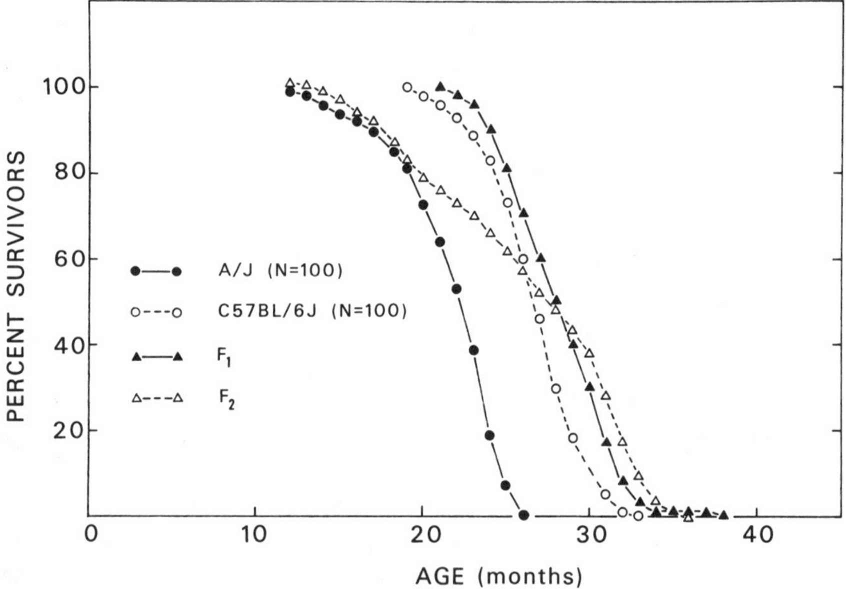



**Figure 6**. Survival distributions of A/J and C57BL/6J strains and their $F_1$ and $F_2$ hybrids. Data from Goodrick, 1975b; ns for hybrids 50.

in mean and maximum lifespan between inbred mouse strains indicate differences in the rate of aging. However, such differences in the slopes of mortality have been observed in recombinant inbred strains of nematodes (Johnson *et al.*, 1988).

If one assumes that actuarial differences in mortality between genotypes reflect differences in the rate of aging, then the question is whether strain differences in behavioral aging are representative of these differences and reflect underlying genetic influences. This question has been addressed in the nematode model with some success (Johnson *et al.*, 1988). In the mouse strain comparisons of behavioral performance made previously, some results reflect this possibility while others do not. For example, in the exploratory activity and maze learning tests, the rate of behavioral aging appeared to be greater in the short-lived A/J genotype than in C57BL/6J mice, observations which would be consistent with the actuarial perspective. In contrast were the tightrope test results which indicated that A/J mice did not exhibit an age-related decline in this performance. The assumption to be made here is that further genetic analysis of exploratory activity and maze learning performance as a function of age would yield greater insight into genetic control of aging processes than would analysis of tightrope performance. This is an intriguing assumption in view of the predictability that individual differences in tightrope performance had in the C57BL/6J genotype. Specifically, Ingram and Reynolds (1986) noted that performance of aged C57BL/65 mice in this test was predictive of lifespan. Of course, this within-strain variability was reflective of environmental influences.

The concept of a generalized aging rate and whether it can be altered is brought to bear most pointedly in studies manipulating the caloric content of diets in rodents. Again applying the results of a Gompertz analysis as evidence, Sacher (1977) argued that aging rate is altered by reducing the caloric content of the diet from *ad libitum* levels in laboratory rodents. With a regimen of intermittent feeding, the actuarial rate of aging is altered in rats and mice in our laboratory (Goodrick *et al.*, 1983; Goodrick *et al.*, submitted).

Results of numerous studies have also documented that age-related decline in many (but not all) biologic parameters are retarded in calorically restricted rodents compared to controls fed *ad libitum*, or close to this level of intake (Weindruch and Walford, 1988). Ingram *et al.* (1987) reported that aspects of behavioral aging were also probably retarded in mice undergoing a chronic regimen of caloric restriction compared to controls.

Regarding the current subject of genetic regulation of behavioral aging, the question is whether strain differences in behavioral performance react to this presumed environmental manipulation of aging rate in a manner indicative of genetic influence. Figure 7 provides a comparison of survival distributions for A/J and C57BL/6J genotypes and their hybrid, B6AF$_1$, undergoing ad libitum or intermittent (every-other-day) feeding beginning at different ages (Goodrick *et al.*, submitted). When the intermittent feeding regimen is begun at weaning, all genotypes express an increase in survival. However, it is clear that the increment in survival in A/J mice is smaller compared to the similar effect observed in the C57BL/6J strain and the F$_1$ hybrid. The similarity in survival between the latter two genotypes is also manifested when the intermittent feeding regimen is initiated at 6 mo of age, as is their difference compared to A/J mice in which no significant effect of diet on lifespan is observed. When the diet treatment was begun at 10 months of age, again C57BL/6J mice and the hybrid responded similarly with no diet effect on mean survival in either genotype (maximum lifespan was affected). In contrast, the intermittent feeding regimen had a significant negative impact on

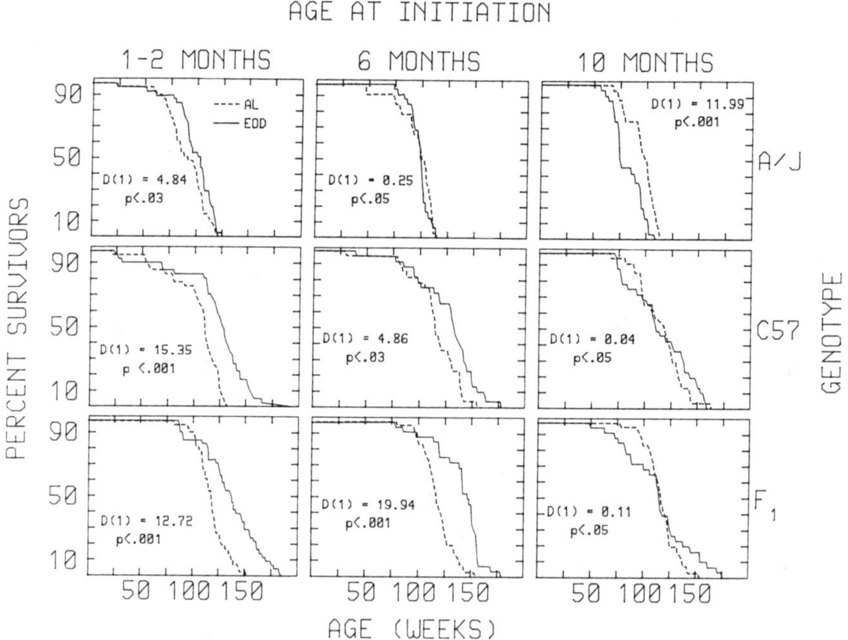


**Figure 7.** Survival distributions of A/J and C57BL/6J strains and their $F_1$ hybrid (B6AF$_1$) fed ad libitum (AL) or every other day (EOD) beginning at different ages (ns = 30-40). Data from Goodrick *et al.*, submitted (ns = 30-40). D statistic refers to results of Lee-Desu survival analysis.

the survival of A/J mice when begun at 10 months of age. Thus, similar to the data on aging in runwheel performance, this survival "behavior", as influenced by caloric restriction of $F_1$ mice, tends to match that of the C57BL/6J parents.

As presented in Figure 8, a similar correspondence of behavioral performance between C57BL/6J and $F_1$ mice was observed in the results of a psychomotor test battery administered at 26-28 months of age in groups undergoing either ad libitum or intermittent feeding initiated at 6 mo of age. As observed in Figure 7, this regimen significantly increased survival in both genotypes and reduced body weight (Figure 8E). Unfortunately, data were not

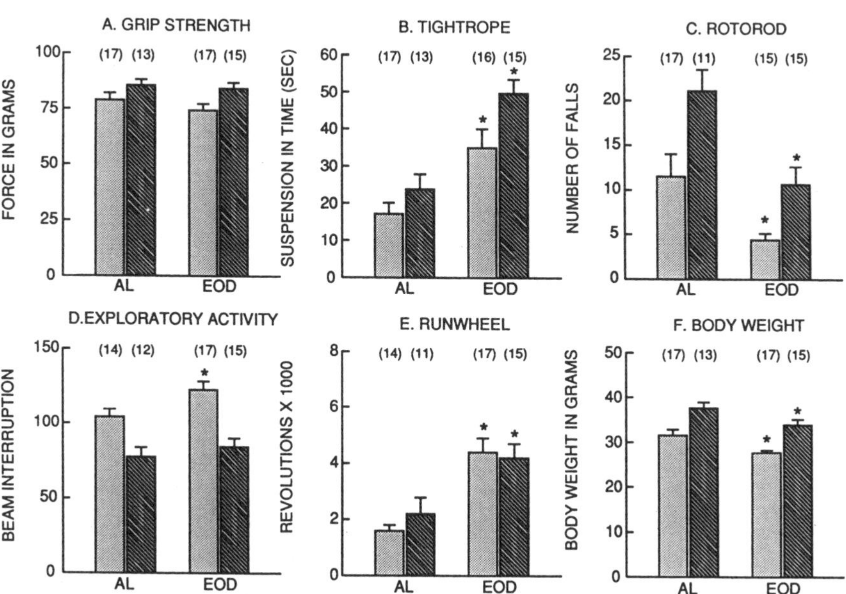



**Figure 8.** Comparison (mean +/- sem) of psychomotor performance of 26-28 mo old C57BL/6J and B6AF₁ mice fed ad libitum (AL) or every other day (EOD) beginning at 6 mo of age (ns = 8-14). *p < 0.05 compared by t-test to control group of same genotype.

available for the A/J strain because not enough of these mice survived for testing at this age. All procedures have been described previously (Ingram *et al.*, 1981; Ingram, 1983; Ingram *et al.*, 1987). The grip strength test (Figure 8A) was a measure of the ability to pull on a strain gauge averaged over three trials. C57BL/6J and F₁ mice did not differ in this performance, and there was no significant diet effect. The tightrope test (Figure 8B) has been mentioned previously. Similar to aged A/J mice, aged F₁ mice appeared to be better performers compared to C57BL/6J mice, and the diet treatment affected these genotypes in a similar fashion. The rotorod test (Figure 8C) assesses the ability of the mouse to remain on a rod rotating at 3 rpm. Similar to the performance of A/J mice on the stationary rod mentioned earlier, $F_1$ mice exhibited inferior performance (more falls) compared to C57BL/6J mice in this task, but they manifested a similar diet effect. The exploratory activity test (Figure 8D) has already been described (under red-light), and the results confirm the lower level of activity observed in $F_1$ mice compared to their C57BL/6J parents. The dietary treatment significantly increased activity among the C57BL/6J mice but not among hybrids. Again matching the results described earlier for runwheel behavior, C57BL/6J mice and their $F_1$ hybrid were similar in activity levels (Figure 8E), and were similarly affected by the diet manipulation. Thus, even though data for A/J mice were unavailable for comparison, it would appear that the $F_1$ hybrids closely resembled their C57BL/6J parents in response to this dietary manipulation that affected the actuarial rate of aging.

These results must be contrasted with those of Harrison and Archer (1987). Using a calorically restricted regimen, these investigators noted that the psychomotor performance (tightrope and open field tests) of C57BL/6J mice and their $F_1$ hybrid from a different parent (CBA/HT6J) responded similarly at an advanced age. Both were superior in performance to that of ad libitum fed controls. However, in the case of actuarial aging, the caloric restriction regimen applied in their study impacted negatively upon survival of C57BL/6J mice. Although these investigators suggested that a nutrient deficiency in their diet might explain this negative influence of survival, it is premature to conclude that strain differences in behavioral performances that parallel manipulations of actuarial aging are likely under genetic control. These observations, however, do suggest some reasonable candidates for further genetic analysis.

## NEUROBIOLOGY OF STRAIN DIFFERENCES IN BEHAVIORAL AGING

The analysis of the genetic modulation of behavioral aging can focus on any of several levels of biological organization, individually or collectively. Focussing on a neurobiological level of organization involves a search for possible links between behavioral performance and specified parameters of neuronal function. Attention to differences among inbred mouse strains in various parameters related to neurotransmitter systems may yield valuable information about genetic influence on aging along neural lines of expression (Finch, 1988).

Concerning the effects of aging on psychomotor performance, Reis (1983) noted the potential value of the CBA/J mouse strain in the genetic analysis of neurobiological mechanisms involved in aging of the nigro-striatal dopamine

(DA) system. Compared to young mice of the BALB/cJ genotype, CBA/J mice had significantly lower concentrations of DA containing cells in the midbrain and less tyrosine hydroxylase (the synthetic enzyme for catecholamines) activity in the substantia nigra (SN) and striatum, which is the terminal for DA-containing axons from the SN (Ross *et al.*, 1976). These neurobiological differences were reflected in the strain differences in locomotor activity in an open field test and in response to DA agonist and antagonist drugs. BALB/cJ mice were much more active in the open field and exhibited a greater response to DA-sensitive drugs (Reis, 1983). Thus, the CBA/J mouse was considered an excellent candidate for assessing a possible predisposition of psychomotor aging due to its deficient endowment of DA-containing cells. Such deficiencies have been suggested as a possible model of differential vulnerability to various age-related pathologies, with particular reference to Parkinson's and Huntington's diseases (Finch, 1988).

To assess this possibility, lifespan representative groups of male CBA/HT6J mice (n = 39), a close variant of the CBA/J strain, were obtained and compared to male C57BL/6J mice (n = 40) in psychomotor performance in our laboratory. These results are presented in Figures 9 and 10. Linear regression of age on each psychomotor variable is computed for each genotype, and the elevations and slopes are compared statistically (t-tests; statistical significance accepted as p 0.05).

The open field test differed from the exploratory activity test described previously (Goodrick, 1973) in that this was a square open field (42.2 cm on each side) which was dimly illuminated, and activity was automatically scored by a matrix of infrared sensors interfaced to a computer (Optovarimex: Columbus Instruments, Ohio). The actual distance traveled during a 10-min test could be computed. As noted in Figure 9A, C57BL/6J mice again exhibited a relatively high level of locomotor activity compared to the other strain. However, the slopes of the age functions were parallel between strains.

Locomotor activity was also assessed in the runwheel cages described previously (Goodrick, 1975a; Ingram *et al.*, 1981). Measurement over a 72-hr period revealed a generally higher level of activity among the CBA/HT6J mice compared to C57BL/6J mice (Figure 9B), a finding which contrasted to that observed in the open field. However, although the slopes appear slightly different, the statistical analysis indicated they were equivalent, a pattern which was similar to that observed in open field activity.

In the tightrope test previously described (Ingram, 1983), CBA/HT6J mice were generally superior to C57BL/6J, primarily at the older ages as had been observed in A/J mice (Figure 9C). Again, however, the analysis of slopes indicated statistical equivalence in aging between the genotypes.

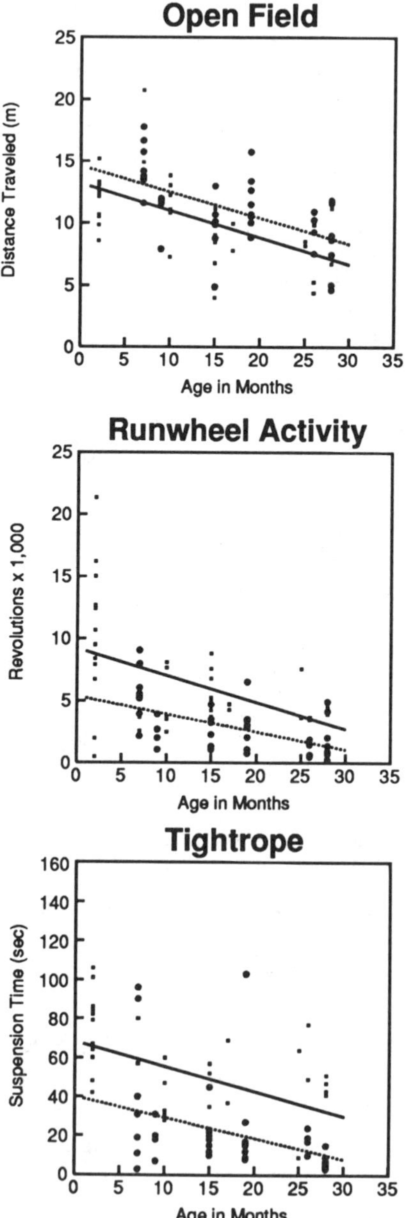

**Figure 9.** Comparison of psychomotor performance of CBA/HT6J mice (closed squares and solid line) and C57BL/6J (closed circles and dotted line) mice in open-field activity, runwheel activity, and tightrope test (ns = 39-40).

## Rotorod

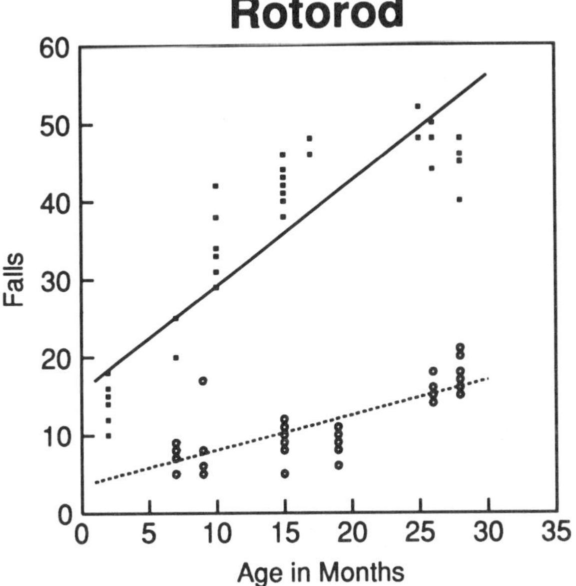


## Maximum Running Speed

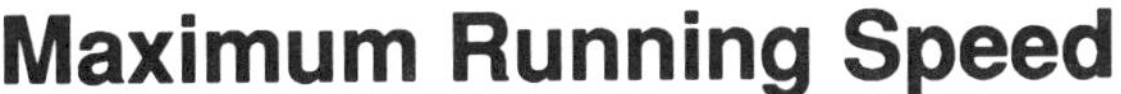

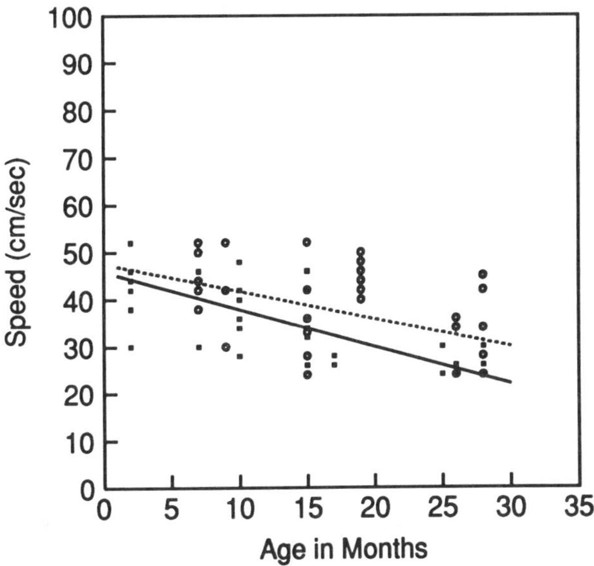


**Figure 10.** Comparison of psychomotor performance of CBA/HT6J mice (closed squares and solid line) and C57BL/6J mice (open circles and dotted line) in rotorod and maximum running speed tests (ns = 39-40).

In the rotorod test also previously described (Ingram, 1983), a divergence of aging rates was observed (Figure 10A). CBA/HT6J mice were clearly poorer performers (more falls) in this task compared to C57BL/6J, and this difference was magnified as a function of age.

The last test was a variation of the rotorod test in which a drum was accelerated over several trials to the point that the mouse could no longer stay on it. The details of this maximum running speed task have been described previously (Ingram, 1988b). In this test, as in the rotorod task, C57BL/6J were superior performers, and the slopes diverged significantly as a function of age (Figure 10B).

Thus, in three of the five tests, behavioral aging rate was similar between the two strains even though they differed in performance level. In the rotorod and running speed tests, there was divergence of aging rate with the CBA/HT6J strain exhibiting the worst performance and the greatest age-related decline. How do these strain comparisons in psychomotor performance relate to neurobiological differences in these strains and to differences in actuarial aging rates?

Regarding strain differences in DA parameters, Severson *et al.* (1981) compared the concentration of striatal DA receptors among young (3 month) BALB/cJ, C57BL/6J, and CBA/J mice. As indicated by the results of Reis and associates, BALB/cJ mice can be characterized as a high DA strain, and CBA/J mice as a low DA strain. As measured by two receptor ligands (spiroperidol and [$^3$H]ADTN), the BALB/cJ genotype had a higher concentration of striatal DA receptors compared to C57BL/6J and CBA/J strains. With respect to differences between the latter two genotypes, DA receptor concentration in C57BL/6J mice was significantly higher compared to CBA/J mice only for [$^3$H]ADTN binding. For spiroperidol binding, these strains were equivalent. The significance of this finding is that spiroperidol binding is specific to a D2 receptor subtype; whereas, the [$^3$H]ADTN ligand has more general binding capacity to D1 and D2 receptor subtypes. In terms of behavioral responses related to DA receptor pharmacology, CBA/J and C57BL/6J mice responded similarly to the DA agonist, apomorphine, with increased stereotyped behavioral responses compared to lower levels observed among CBA/J mice. In response to the DA antagonist, haloperidol, CBA/J mice were much more sensitive, as demonstrated by their higher catalepsy scores compared to CBA/J and C57BL/6J genotypes, and this response among CBA/J mice would be consistent with their lower concentration of striatal DA receptors. In addition to these behavioral differences, the DA receptors of CBA/J mice compared to the other two strains were also less sensitive to up-regulation following a chronic regimen of haloperidol.

The behavioral assays associated with DA receptor pharmacology in the study of Severson *et al.* were not duplicated in the present study. The open field measure was similar to that used in the studies by Reis and colleagues and appears to be a sensitive measure of nigro-striatal DA involvement. In the present study C57BL/6J mice exhibited a slightly higher level of open field activity compared to CBA/T6J mice, but the age-related performance decline was parallel for both strains. Thus, the strain difference in genetic endowment of striatal DA receptors would not appear to matter with respect to the rate of age-related decline in open field performance. Since striatal DA receptors were not assayed across the lifespan in the present study, it is not clear how age-related declines in this neurobiological parameter influenced the current behavioral results. Age-related loss in striatal D2 receptor concentration has been established in C57BL/6J mice (Severson and Finch, 1980).

Both the runwheel and tightrope tests also yielded parallel age slopes for both strains. Performance in the latter test has been shown to be influenced by striatal cholinergic mechanisms in C57BL/6J mice (Barclay *et al.*, 1981). No comparison of age-related loss in striatal cholinergic receptors has been made between these strains, although a decline in cholinergic muscarinic receptor concentration has been observed in the striata of C57BL/6J mice (Strong *et al.*, 1980). Performance in the runwheel task is probably not strongly related to DA systems, since the CBA/HT6J strain exhibited greater activity in this situation unlike their inhibited activity in the open field test.

The two tasks demonstrating divergence of behavioral aging rate between the C57BL/6J and CBA/HT6J strains were the rotorod and running speed test, neither of which has been well characterized with respect to which neurotransmitter systems are involved. The latter test has been developed only recently (Ingram, 1988). In C57BL/6J mice, an impairment in rotorod and balance beam performance has been correlated with a loss in total and terminal dendritic length of medium spiny neurons in the striatum of aged animals, and these neurons have been suggested as a target for DA fibers arising from the SN (McNeill *et al.*, 1988). This age-related alteration in dendritic arborization might underlie the age-related loss of DA receptors in this strain. However, poor rotorod performance in aged rats has also been correlated with loss of cerebellar Purkinje cells from the molecular layer, and this would likely involve norepinephrine systems (Rogers, 1988). Thus, it remains uncertain whether performance in this task involves the nigro-striatal DA system. To further ascertain the significance of the divergent aging rates in rotorod and running speed performance between these strains, additional investigation concerning specific neurotransmitter involvement in these tasks would be needed. These tasks would appear to offer the greatest potential for assessing genetic modulation of aging.

Finally, the correspondence of these patterns of behavioral aging to actuarial aging should be considered. Harrison and Archer (1983) reported that the survival distributions of C57BL/6J and CBA/HT6J mice were virtually identical with mean (SEM) lifespans of 815 (16) and 830 (14) days, respectively. Therefore, for those tests reflecting the primary rate of behavioral aging, this observation would dictate that the aging slopes should be parallel for these two strains. And this was the case for tightrope, open field, and runwheel performance. Those tests showing divergence in slopes, such as in the rotorod and running speed test, would appear to reflect aging in a specific neural system independent of those more generalized, primary aging processes reflected in actuarial aging.

## CONCLUSIONS

The value of comparing the behavioral performance of inbred mouse strains across the lifespan has been considered with respect to identifying candidates for assessment of possible genetic mechanisms of behavioral aging. As such, these comparisons are only a perusal of possibilities, a necessary first step to determine the value of further effort. Resulting patterns suggest a variety of perspectives concerning possible models to pursue as outlined in Table 1. The table indicates conclusions and directions that can be drawn about genetic influences on behavioral aging when making comparisons between inbred rodent strains.

Model A suggests that behavior may be related to primary processes of aging, although baseline differences in performance may be present over the lifespan. Equivalent slopes indicate that the age-related decline in performance is general among strains with similar rates of actuarial aging. Examples of Model A would be open-field and runwheel activity (Figure 9) and tightrope performance (Figure 10) in C57BL/6J and CBA/HT6J mice. Because of the parallel appearance of both behavioral and actuarial aging, there would be little interest in investigating differences in the genetic regulation of aging as reflected in such cases.

Model B is probably the least interesting of models to pursue. The subject genotypes would differ in actuarial rates of aging but the subject behavior would exhibit parallel change across the lifespans of these mice to indicate little difference in its genetic regulation. This model was best represented by the performance of A/J and C57BL/6J mice in the balance rod task (Figure 2A).

| Table 1. Possible Models of Study for the Behavior Genetics of Aging | | | | |
|---|---|---|---|---|
| Model | Behavioral Aging | | Actuarial Aging | |
| | Parallel Slopes | Divergent Slopes | Parallel Slopes | Divergent Slopes |
| A | * | | * | |
| B | * | | | * |
| C | | * | * | |
| D | | * | | * |
| * Indicates presence of condition in the model. | | | | |

Model C stimulates interest since the subject genotypes would display divergent change with age in the behavioral performance being examined. Because of the lack of differences between strains in actuarial rates of aging, however, the behavioral observations would indicate differences in genetic regulation related to a secondary aging process of possible neural origin. Performance of the C57BL/6J and CBA/HT6J strains in the rotorod and running speed tasks (Figure 10) fit this model.

Model D represents perhaps the greatest potential for additional assessment of the genetic regulation of behavioral aging. This model proposes divergent slopes in the behavioral parameter of interest, the performance of which matches the divergence in actuarial rates of aging, *i.e.*, the strain with the greatest increase in mortality also shows the greatest decline in performance as a function of age. Examples of this model were observed for A/J and C57BL/6J mice in exploratory activity (Figure 4) and maze learning (Figure 3). Tightrope performance (Figure 2B) did not fit this model since the shorter-lived A/J strain exhibited the least age-related decline in performance.

A caveat should be made to the suggestion that models A and B might have limited interest for pursuing genetic mechanisms of aging. All the models assume that a linear decline in performance with age reflects aging processes. However, the rate of this decline might be less relevant if one considers that thresholds to pathology may differ across strain and may be more functionally significant (Smith, 1966). In other words, even if the slopes of two genotypes are parallel, but the elevations differ, then it is possible that one genotype will reach a threshold to pathology at an earlier age than the other. This is the model proposed for genetic differences in the endowment of SN dopaminergic cells (Finch, 1988). However, in such cases, I would emphasize that interest in genetic involvement is directed more to mechanisms involving the initial endowment rather than to genetic modulation of performance decline with aging. The major complicating factor to this argument is if genotypes differ in threshold levels. If one assumes this reality, then analysis of rates of aging may be much less relevant.

Once marked and reliable differences are identified from whatever perspective, the investigator can pursue further analyses from any number of strategies. The difference can be analyzed at a relatively proximate level by attempting to link the differences in behavioral aging to a neurobiological parameter. Or the genetic mechanisms can be pursued in earnest with classic Mendelian techniques or with more modern short-cut tools of recombinant inbred strains or bilineal congenic strains. The number of genetic loci can be identified (if reasonable in number), linked, and mapped. Given the product of this extensive investment, the investigator would hope that modern techniques of molecular biology might permit the genetic material to be extracted, cloned, or otherwise manipulated for further experimental tests of its role in the behavioral aging phenomenon of interest. This would be the ultimate value of this strategy and its reliance on inbred mouse strains. At this juncture, though, the utility of a behavior genetics of aging in a mouse model remains only a possibility. Thus far, the field has been involved in searching for suitable phenomena to pursue.

## ACKNOWLEDGMENTS

This paper would not have been possible without the valuable contributions of; John Freeman and Edward Spangler in animal husbandry and testing; Richard Hiner, Maurice Zimmerman, Raymond Bannar, and Gunther Baartz in the construction of equipment; William Yee and Sharon Davison for data analysis and graphs; Paul Ciesla for computer-assisted graphs; David Harrison and John Archer for supply of CBA/HT6J mice; and Rita Wolferman for clerical assistance.

## REFERENCES

BAILEY, D. W. (1971) Recombinant inbred strains: An aid to finding identity, linkages, and function of histocompatibility and other genes. *Transplantation* 11: 325-331

BARCLAY, L. L., GIBSON, G. E. and BLASS, J. P. (1981) Impairment of behavior and acetylcholine metabolism in thiamine deficiency. *J. Pharmacol. Exp. Ther.* 217: 537-543

CUTLER, R. G. (1984) Evolutionary biology of aging and longevity. **In:** *Aging and Cell Structure*, Vol. 2, (ed. J. E. Johnson), pp. 1-147, New York: Plenum Press.

ELEFTHERIOU, B. E., ELIAS, M. F., CHERRY, C. and LUCAS, L. A. (1976) Relationship of wheel-running, plasma testosterone, and corticosterone levels: A behavior-genetic analysis. *Physiol. Behav.* 16: 431-438

ELIAS, M. F., ELIAS, P. K. and ELIAS, J. W. (1977) *Basic Processes in Adult Developmental Psychology*, St. Louis: C.V. Mosby.

FINCH, C. E. (1988) Neural and endocrine approaches to the resolution of time as a dependent variable in the aging processes of mammals. *The Gerontologist.* 28: 29-42

GOODRICK, C. L. (1968) Learning, retention, and extinction of complex maze habit for mature-young and senescent Wistar albino rats. *J. Gerontol.* **23**: 298-304

GOODRICK, C. L. (1973) Exploration activity and emotionality of albino and pigmented mice. *J. Comp. Physiol. Psychol.* **84**: 73-81

GOODRICK, C. L. (1975a) Behavioral differences in young and aged mice: Strain differences for activity measures, operant learning, sensory discrimination, and alcohol preference. *Exp. Aging Res.* **1**: 191-207

GOODRICK, C. L. (1975b). Life-span and the inheritance of longevity of inbred mice. *J. Gerontol.* **30**: 257-263

GOODRICK, C. L. INGRAM, D. K., REYNOLDS, M. A., FREEMAN, J. R. and CIDER, N. L. (1983) Differential effects of intermittent finding and voluntary exercise on body weight and lifespan in adult rats. *J. Gerontol.* **28**: 36-45

GOODRICK, C. L., INGRAM, D. K., REYNOLDS, M. A., FREEMAN, J. R. and CIDER, N. L. Effects of intermittent feeding upon body weight and lifespan in inbred mice: Interaction of genotype and age. *Mech. Aging Devel..*, submitted.

GRAHN, D. (1972) Data collection and genetic analysis in the selection and study of rodent systems in aging. In: *Development of the Rodent as a Model System of Aging* (Ed. D.C. Gibson), pp. 55-65. DHEW Pub. No. (NIH) 72-121. Washington: U.S. Government Printing Office.

HARRISON, D. E. and ARCHER, J. R. (1983) Physiological assays for biological age in mice: Relationship of collagen, renal function, and longevity. *Exp. Aging Res.* **4**: 245-251

HARRISON, D. E. and ARCHER, J. R. (1987) Genetic effects on responses to food restriction in aging mice. *J. Nutr.* **117**: 376-382

INGRAM, D. K. (1983) Toward the behavioral assessment of biological aging in the laboratory mouse. Concepts, terminology, and objectives. *Exp. Aging Res.* **9**: 225-238

INGRAM, D. K. (1985) Analysis of age-related impairments in learning and memory in rodent models. *Annals N.Y. Acad. Sci.* **444**: 312-331

INGRAM, D. K. (1988a) Complex maze learning in rodents as a model of age-related memory impairment. *Neurobiol. Aging* **9**: 475-485

INGRAM, D. K. (1988b) Motor performance variability during aging in rodents: Assessment of reliability and validity of individual differences. In: *Central Determinants of Age-Related Declines in Motor Function* (Ed. J.A. Joseph) *Annals New York Acad. Sci.*, 515, 70-96.

INGRAM, D. K., LONDON, E. D., REYNOLDS, M. A., WALLER, S. B. and GOODRICK, C. L. (1981) Differential effects of aging on motor performance in two mouse strains. *Neurobiol. Aging.* **2**: 221-227

INGRAM, D. K. and REYNOLDS., M. R. (1986) Assessing the predictive validity of psychomotor tests as measures of biological age in mice. *Exp. Aging Res.* **12**: 155-162

INGRAM, D. K., WEINDRUCH, R., SPANGLER, E. L., FREEMAN, J. R. and WALFORD, R. L. (1987) Dietary restriction benefits learning and motor performance of aged mice. *J. Gerontol.* **42**: 78-81

JOHNSON, T. E. (1986) Molecular and genetic analyses of a multivariate system specifying behavior and lifespan. *Behav. Genet.* **16**: 221-235

JOHNSON, T. E., CONLEY, W. L. and KELLER, M. L. (1988) Long-lived lines of *Caenorhabditis elegans* can be used to establish predictive biomarkers of aging. *Exp. Gerontol.* **23**: 281-295

McCLEARN, G. E. (1959) Strain differences in activity of mice: Influence of illumination. *J. Comp. Physiol. Psychol.* **53**: 142-143

McCLEARN, G. and FOCH T. T. (1985) Behavioral genetics. In *Handbook of the Psychology of Aging* (Ed. J. E. Birren and K. W. Schaie), pp 113-143. New York: Van Nostrand Reinhold.

McNEILL, T. H., KOEK, L. L., BROWN, S. A. and RAFOLS, J. A. (1988) Age-related changes in the nigrostriatal system. In: *Central Determinants of Age-Related Declines in Motor Function* (Ed. J. A. Joseph), *Annals New York Acad. Sci.* **515**: 239-248

REIS, D. J. (1983) Genetic differences in numbers of chemically specified neurons in brain: A possible biological substrate for variations in onset of symptoms of cerebral aging in man. **In:** *Aging of the Brain* (Eds. D. Samuel, S. Algeri, S. Gershon, V.E. Grimm, G. Toffano) pp. 257-269, New York: Raven Press.

ROGERS, J. (1988) The neurobiology of cerebellar senescence. **In:** *Central Determinants of Age-Related Declines in Motor Function* (Ed. J.A. Joseph), *Annals New York Acad. Sci.,* **515:** 251-268.

ROSS, R. A., JUDD, A. B., PICKEL, V. M., JOH, T. H. and REIS, D. J. (1976) Strain- dependent variations in number of dopaminergic neurones. *Nature.* **264:** 654-656

ROWE, J. W. and MINAKER, K. L. (1985) Geriatric medicine. **In:** *Handbook of the Biology of Aging,* 2nd edition (ed. C.E. Finch and E.L. Schneider), pp. 932-959. New York: Van Nostrand Reinhold.

RUSSELL, E. S. and SPROTT, R. L. (1974) Genetics and the aging nervous system. **In:** *Survey Report on the Aging Nervous System* (ed. G.J. Maletta), pp. 511-519. Washington: U.S. Government Printing Office.

SACHER, G. A. (1977) Life table modification and life prolongation. **In:** *Handbook of the Biology of Aging* (Eds. C.E. Finch and L. Hayflick), pp. 582-638. New York: Van Nostrand Reinhold.

SEVERSON, J. A. and FINCH C. E. (1980) Reduced dopaminergic binding during aging in the rodent striatum. *Brain Res.* **192:** 147-162

SHOCK, N. W., GREULICH, R. C., ANDRES, R., ARENBERG, D., COSTA, P. T., LAKATTA, E. G. and TOBIN, J. D. (1984) *Normal Human Aging*: The Baltimore Longitudinal Study of Aging. NIH Pub. No. 84-2450. Washington, D.C: U.S. Government Printing Office.

SMITH, J.M. 1966. Theories of aging. **In:** *Topics in the Biology of Aging* (ed. P.L. Krohn) pp. 1-35. New York: John Wiley.

SPROTT, R. L. (1978) The interaction of genotype and environment in the determination of avoidance behavior of aging inbred mice. **In** *Genetic Effects on Aging* (Ed. D. Bregsma and D.E. Harrison), pp 109-120. New York: A.R. Liss.

SPROTT, R. L. (1980) An appraisal of the utility of genetic techniques for the study of neurobiology and aging in mice. **In:** *Psychobiology of Aging: Problems and Perspectives* (ed. D. Stein), pp. 21-34. New York: Elsevier/North-Holland.

SPROTT, R. L. (1988) Age-related variability. **In:** *Central Determinants of Age-Related Declines in Motor Function* (Ed. J.A. Joseph) *Ann. New York Acad. Sci.* **515:** 121-122

SPROTT, R. L. and ELEFTHERIOU, B. E. (1974) Open-field behavior in aging inbred mice. *Gerontologia.* **20:** 155-162

STAVNES, K. L. and SPROTT, R. L. (1975) Effects of age and genotype on acquisition of an active avoidance task. *Devel. Psychobiol.* **8:** 437-445

STORER, J. B. (1978) Effect of aging and radiation in mice of different genotypes. **In:** *Genetic Effects on Aging* (Ed. D. Bregsma and D.E. Harrison), pp. 55-70. New York: A.R. Liss.

STRONG, R. HICKS, P., HSU, L., BARTUS, R. T. and ENNA, S. J. (1979) Age-related alterations in the rodent brain cholinergic system and behavior. *Neurobiol. Aging.* **1:** 59-64

WAX, T. M. (1977) Effects of age, strain, and illumination intensity on activity and self-selection of light-dark schedules in mice. *J. Comp. Physiol. Psychol.* **91:** 51-62

WEINDRUCH, R. and WALFORD, R. L. (1988) *The Retardation of Aging and Disease by Dietary Restriction.* Springfield, IL: Charles C. Thomas.

## DISCUSSION

1. In the $F_2$ survival curve, about a quarter of the animals paralleled the A/J inbred strain. Could differences in longevities be due to one gene? This was not known, although some people speculated that it might be H-2. Others

claimed that the use of inbred strains was confusing and that the study should have been done with outbred stocks having interpretable differences, such as those shown by the long and short lived *Drosophila* lines with a 500% difference in flying ability. Since no such lines are available for mammals, this emphasised the importance of the discussion in Chapter 7 of this volume.

2. $F_1$ hybrids should have less variance than inbred strains as they should have more effective homeostasis. Why wasn't this observed in the $B6AF_1$? This is not the only example where the variance in an $F_1$ exceeds that in the parent lines. Maybe the hybrids can tolerate larger differences, as younger animals sometimes can, so that the floor or ceiling is further from the mean in $F_1$ hybrids or younger individuals. Thus the variance is higher depending on the scale of measurement. In fact the slope giving the rate of decline in function for individuals is not the same for every genetically identical individual in creatures from worms to mice. This statement caused disagreement, with a claim that genetically identical *Drosophila* do show the same slope of age change.

# 14

# BIOMARKER CHARACTERISTICS AND RESEARCH ON THE GENETICS OF AGING

Gerald E. McClearn

## ABSTRACT

Behavioral measures of exploratory and motor activity, strength, coordination and autonomic reactivity were examined for age-relatedness and gerometric properties in three studies of mice. The first animals examined were C57BL/6NNia, DBA/2NNia and B6D2F1/NNia of about 5 and about 25 months of age in a two-cohort, cross-sectional study. The second was a cross-sequential study with three birth cohorts of these same genotypic groups measured on three occasions each so that adjacent cohorts were of the same chronological age on the third and first measurement occasions, respectively. The total age span of the study was from about 2 to about 21 months. The third study involved measurement of two cohorts of genetically heterogeneous (HS) mice, about 3 and about 22 months of age. The results showed age differences or changes for all of the measures, but showed that susceptibility to confounding effects of cohort, previous testing, residence time in colony or occasion of measurement differed greatly, and was dependent upon sex, genotype and age.

Substantial genetic effects were found for many of the variables, and age X genotype interactions for some measures reveal a genetic influence on aging rate.

## PROLOGUE

This is a preliminary report from a multi-disciplinary, collaborative program of research on the genetics of lifespan development of the laboratory mouse. The program is based on a set of assumptions:

1. Aging is a complex of subprocesses, probably hierarchically organized, at least in part, with varying degrees of interaction and covariation among subprocesses. This orientation does not deny the possible existence of one or a few major "pacemakers" of aging, but does aver that the observable consequences are, in any case, manifold and imperfectly correlated.

2. These subprocesses are influenced by a sufficiently large number of genetic loci that they cannot be effectively studied by Mendelian methods.

3. Throughout the lifespan there are both continuities and discontinuities in aging subprocesses. The continuities will be sufficiently great as to warrant a lifespan examination of predictability of late life states or changes from earlier states or changes. The discontinuities will be sufficiently great, at least at the manifest variable level, as to require multivariate approaches to the solution of measurement issues.

Following from assumption 1, it is necessary to measure a broad array of age-related phenotypes, because no single one can be expected to reveal more than a small part of the aging process(es).

Following from assumption 2, the methods of quantitative genetics will be required to estimate the contributions of additive and non-additive genetic sources and of various types of environmental sources to variance of the phenotypes and to the covariances among them.

The implication of assumption 3 is that the research should be longitudinal, and that the entire lifespan should be sampled. These assumptions set the general strategic outline for the program - that of a longitudinal multivariate study of resemblance of relatives that adequately samples animals, variables and occasions of measurement (ages) in relation to the research issues. Tactical decisions on the specific design and methods to be employed have required a series of preliminary studies which form the basis of this report.

Three major areas required investigation: the measures to be utilized, the subjects to be employed and the chronological ages to be examined. Issues in these areas may be expected to be highly interdependent, with answers to questions about measures depending upon subjects and ages, and so on. However, they may be separated temporarily for purposes of discussion.

## Measures

As old as the field of gerontology itself, and at its definitional core, is the question of "marker" variables, the measures to be utilized in the assessment of biological age and aging. Were they available, we should of course employ direct measures of the aging subprocesses. At the present state of knowledge, no such measures exist, and it is arguable from an operational point of view (see McClearn, 1988) that they never will. In any case we are presently constrained to theorize or hypothesize about the unobserved *latent* variables of aging, and to measure *manifest* variables (see Loehlin, 1987). These latter are often described as substitute, indicator, proxy, index or marker variables, and, at least in some usages, can be generically described as "biomarkers." Interest in biomarkers has recently grown dramatically, due in considerable measure to programmatic interest in the identification of dependent variables that will permit systematic evaluation of proposed interventions in aging processes. An examination of the issues involved in biomarker selection suggests that they do not differ necessarily or fundamentally from any other variable employed in the study of basic mechanisms of aging (McClearn, 1988). Thus, biomarkers may be regarded as consisting of all age-related variables, a particular subclass of which possesses attributes that may be useful for evaluation of interventions; on the other hand, the label may be applied to the latter subclass only. In either case, these latter, intervention-sensitive measures are not restricted to intervention research, but may be involved in any gerontological research, including the most basic. In this presentation, no distinction is drawn, and the terms "biomarker," "measure" and "phenotype" are used interchangeably.

Many considerations enter into the selection of biomarkers for any particular study - theoretical salience, weight of empirical evidence, interests of the investigator, laboratory capabilities, expense of measurement, etc. Whatever the basis for nomination, however, prospective measures should be evaluated with respect to their measurement properties, including reliability, validity, sensitivity, range and susceptibility to confounding effects. A complete evaluation of any measure in respect to all of these "gerometric" attributes would require very considerable effort; a thorough characterization of a whole prospective battery would be a formidable project in its own right. Nonetheless, some appreciation of a biomarker's properties is necessary for the proper interpretation of research results using the biomarker. Each may have its own pattern of strengths and weaknesses, making it relatively more or less useful for particular applications. Following is a brief discussion of some of the pertinent issues in gerometric evaluation.

*Reliability*

Accuracy is, of course, a fundamental requirement of a measurement. One way of assessing accuracy is to measure repeatedly in order to determine the degree to which different occasions of measurement give the same result. If measurements are taken on a number of individuals on two occasions, the correlation between the first and second occasions is often taken to be the *reliability* of the measure. It is, in fact, a combination of reliability and *stability*. A variable measured with great reliability may show low stability; some process between the first and second measurement occasions might alter the ordinal status of the (reliably) measured individuals so that the correlation between the occasions is attenuated. Similarly, ordinal status could be perfectly preserved across occasions, yielding a high inter-occasion correlation, but intervening processes could reduce or elevate all measures; thus, high reliability is compatible with substantial discrepancy between means of consecutive measurement occasions, which latter outcome might be viewed in certain contexts as inaccuracy.

Individual differences in aging clearly imply individual differences in rates of change in some biomarker of age between specified chronological ages. These rate differences will result in a change of ordinal status of the individuals and thus will affect the test-retest correlation. The resulting value, if low, is not necessarily a gerometric condemnation of the measure, but, regarded as *stability* rather than as *reliability* (Nesselroade *et al.*, 1986), is a descriptive statistic of intrinsic interest in its own right.

Among the processes that can initiate or mediate change between test and retest is the initial test itself. For many biomarkers, we may expect that the act of measurement alters subsequent values. This possibility may be particularly believable in respect to behavioral measures, where learning or memory clearly can alter second or later responses to a measurement situation. For example, assessment of exploratory behavior in a novel situation can, by definition, be done only once. However, the whole array of biological measures is potentially susceptible to this class of effect, which can yield an artifactual impression of aging.

*Validity*

There are various definitions of validity and various methods of assessing it (see Ghiselli *et al.*, 1981 for a general discussion; for gerontological applications, see Ingram, 1983; Ingram and Reynolds, 1986; McClearn, 1988), none of which is exhaustive. In the gerontological biomarker context, these definitions relate to the notion of age-relevance. Perhaps the conceptually simplest manifestation of age-relevance is a cross-sectional mean difference between or among groups of differing chronological age, or a longitudinal mean change within a group from one chronological age to another. More subtle age-relevance might be discerned in a difference or change in the relationships of a particular biomarker to other biomarkers as a function of chronological age. Such changes could take place without any alteration of mean or variance, yet be of profound gerontological importance, indicating differences in the basic "structure" of different biological ages.

It is also important to note a limitation of definitions of age-relevance that require changes or differences of population statistics. Changes taking place in an individual can be of vital importance to that individual's life course, yet not be detectable at the group level, depending upon the relative frequency of individuals undergoing the particular change, the sample size, the standard error, *etc.*

*Sensitivity*

Sensitivity may be thought of as the minimum chronological age interval over which a significant age-relevance is demonstrable. Although this demonstration could be of changing covariance structure, in practice it will usually be a significant change or difference in means. It is apparent that sensitivity assessment will be strongly influenced by sample sizes, and, in the case of longitudinal studies, by stability of the measure.

*Range*

Range may be defined as the portion of the lifespan in which age-relevance can be shown, *i.e.*, the sensitive portion of the life-course trajectory. Some measures may change continuously throughout the entire lifespan, others may only begin to change after puberty, others in mid-life, others only in the terminal phase of the lifespan. Obviously, sensitivity of a measure might differ in different ranges.

*Susceptibility to Confounding Effects*

The identification of classes of effects that can mimic age processes has led to an intense scrutiny of gerontological methodology (*e.g.*, Schaie, 1975), that has greatly influenced current experimental and study design. Perhaps usually seen as more pertinent to human researches, variants of these confounding influences may be of great importance even in the well-controlled environment of animal models. For example, if animals are imported to a laboratory for study, the "adaptation" time to the new laboratory must be an important matter in respect to recovery from travel stress and adaptation to new conditions of husbandry, including food, temperature, humidity, cage-changing schedule, handling styles of personnel, exposure to previously unencountered pathogens, etc. Seasonal effects on reproduction are well-known in mouse breeding laboratories in spite of stringent environmental control. Presumably, such effects might also influence the outcomes of biomarker measurement. Studies requiring concurrent comparisons of groups of different chronological ages necessarily involve animals which were born at different times with attendant possibilities of persisting cohort effects due to season, differing conditions of husbandry, or other conditions prevailing at the time of birth or early development.

If a biomarker is a part of a battery or panel it may well be influenced by the particular nature and order of the other measures preceding it. In addition to such effects of concurrent measurement, the effects of previous measurement discussed above will be of special significance for longitudinal research.

There appear, thus, to be numerous possibilities for confounding effects in animal aging research, and the susceptibility of nominated biomarkers to these effects is an important part of their qualifications.

## Subjects

In the selection of subjects for animal model research, the first choice naturally is that of the species. The mouse was selected for the present work as a useful combination of short life span, well-known husbandry requirements, extensive previous literature on age-related processes, and richness of pertinent genetic knowledge.

Of particular importance, there are available in the laboratory mouse many different genetically specifiable groups. These different groups constitute a richly equipped toolbox for the study of the genetics of a phenotype and of the mechanisms through which the genetic effects are mediated. Each of the tools has its particular strengths and weaknesses, and it is important that the most appropriate tool be used for the job at hand.

Inbred strains have been extensively employed in gerontological research. These inbred strains and defined groups derived from them are useful for certain types of genetic analysis utilizing comparisons of means and variances, and for explorations of possible mechanisms underlying any differences in longevity or age-related phenotypes. For research requiring correlational statistics, however, either in seeking mechanisms or in assessing heritabilities and genetic correlations, animals of a genetically heterogeneous stock are appropriate. Recombinant inbred strains, congenic and coisogenic strains, and selectively bred lines are other important approaches offered in particular abundance by the mouse (see McClearn, 1981, 1988).

## Chronological Ages

The lifespan perspective suggests a connectedness of different parts of the lifespan. If it is true that successive parts of the life course trajectory have some of their determinant mechanisms in common, then study of change during any part (at least any post-maturity part) of the trajectory should be informative about "aging." Even if the age-defining network of mid-life processes is only modestly related to end-stage processes, it would constitute part of the total system that moves us from conception to senescence and death, and would thus be part of aging. Insofar as this argument is correct, it has important time-saving implications for animal model research, in that it would not be necessary always to follow animals to the end of their lives to obtain relevant information. However, the argument is most persuasive when applied to a total network of determinants. In respect to any single biomarker, as implied above in the discussion of range, there may be an onset of measurable, age-related change at any point in the life course, and measurements prior to that time may be uninformative. For the purpose of initial evaluation of a candidate biomarker, then, it is useful to select chronological ages that are rather extreme, permitting a "bottom line" assessment of whether the marker shows differences or changes over a major part of the lifespan.

## THE STUDIES

In an attempt to address some of the issues raised in the preceding section, several pilot or preliminary studies were performed. Three of these will be described here.

Study I. The first study was cross-sectional using mice from the NIA contract colonies of Charles River. Mice of both sexes and three genotypes were employed: C57BL/6NNia, DBA/2NNia, B6D2F1/NNia. Animals were about 5 and 25 months old at time of testing, approximately 5 weeks after importation to our colony. Sample sizes varied somewhat from measure to measure, with approximately 6 to 10 per sex/genotype/age class.

Study II. The second study was cross-sequential with three birth cohorts each of the three genotypes used previously. After 21 days of adaptation to the laboratory following importation from Charles River Laboratories, first measurements were taken when the animals were about 2, 8, and 15 months old (these groups are described hereafter as cohorts 1, 2 and 3, respectively). At approximately 3 month intervals, second and third measurements were taken. Thus, the third occasion of cohorts 1 and 2 were about the same chronological age as the first occasion of cohorts 2 and 3, respectively. There were about 6 to 8 animals per sex/genotype/age class at the time of first testing, but severe losses occurred in the DBAs.

Study III. Study III was a longitudinal study utilizing two birth cohorts of HS mice, approximately 2 to 3 and 22 months of age at time of first testing. The older animals were imported from the Institute for Behavioral Genetics, Boulder, at about 10 months of age; the younger animals were imported from the same source at about 6 to 8 weeks of age. There were five measurement occasions, approximately 50 days apart, beginning when the younger and older had been in the laboratory about 4 and 48 weeks, respectively. There were 24 male and 29 female mice in the younger cohort; 33 male and 27 female in the older cohort at the time of first testing. Substantial attrition was experienced in the older cohort, so only the first 3 occasions of measurement will be reported here.

## Biomarkers

The biomarkers assessed in these studies were selected to represent major theoretical perspectives or empirical data domains in gerontology that are also pertinent to the interests of the collaborators in the program and for which their laboratories are suitable. The total battery included measures of behavior, immune system (natural killer) function, glucose tolerance, glutathione peroxidase activity, tail tendon break-time and hematocrit. This report will concern only the behavioral measures, which were assessed first in the battery sequence.

## Behavioral Measures

### File apparatus

The File apparatus (File and Wardill, 1975) was selected to provide multiple behavioral measures from a single measurement occasion. The apparatus, constructed of black, opaque plexiglass, consists of an arena (40cm × 40 cm × 15cm deep) set on top of 12 cm legs with a low level of overhead illumination. The floor is divided into four square quadrants with a 15 mm diameter hole in the center of the floor of each quadrant. Mice were tested individually. A trial began when the mouse was lowered into a clear cylinder (5 cm diameter × 5 cm tall) in the center of the field. After 10 sec, the cylinder was lifted to begin a 5 min scoring period. The observer was seated with the floor at eye level and a mirror overhead permitted observation of the full arena. FACTIV is the locomotor activity scored as the number of quadrant borders crossed by all four feet during the scoring period. FHDPK is the number of times the nose of the mouse protruded through the holes in the floor. FREARS is the number of times the animal stood on its hind legs with both forepaws off the floor. FBOLI is the count of the number of fecal pellets deposited during the scoring period, and FURINE is the amount of urine deposited, scored on a 3-point scale (0=none; 1=small amount; 2=more than a few drops).

### Rod

The rod apparatus was modified from the work of Dean *et al.* (1981). In our version, a wooden dowel rod 1.6 cm in diameter and 89 cm long was suspended horizontally 23 cm above a foam pad. The rod was marked into 5 sectors of 17.8 cm each. Each animal was tested separately. The animal was placed on the rod at the center and was timed until the first fall or until one minute had elapsed. The animal was then placed back in its home cage for one minute, and replaced on the rod. This procedure was repeated so that each animal was tested three times. On each occasion, fall time (RODROP), activity in terms of the number of sectors entered (RODACT), fecal pellets dropped (RODBOLI) and urination (RODURINE) were recorded.

## Cord

The cord apparatus was based upon the work of Miquel and Blasco (1978) and Ingram *et al.* (1982). In our version, a monofilament of 0.4 mm diameter was suspended 29 cm above a foam pad. The animal was held in the center of the cord until it had grasped it and was able to cling when released. The procedure followed was the same as for the rod described above, yielding a measure of fall time (CORDROP).

## RESULTS AND DISCUSSION

### Stability/reliability

The best evidence available from these studies on stability/reliability of the biomarkers is the set of correlations among occasions 1, 2 and 3 of Study III. With an inter-occasion interval of approximately 50 days, there was presumably sufficient time between occasions for individual differences in aging phenomena to rearrange ordinal positions. Table 1 shows the significant ($p < .05$) correlations.

Regarded as *reliabilities*, the values would be described as modest. For only RODROP 2 - 3 does the correlation exceed 0.8. However, as *stabilities*, the data indicate that there is some continuity of ordinal ranking of individuals over both successive 50 day intervals and over the combined 100 day interval. These data do not permit the unambiguous disentangling of reliability and stability, so no strong interpretation can be made of the magnitude of the coefficients. Some interesting comparisons can be made, however. Overall, the old cohort, relative to the young cohort, appears more stable with respect to Rod behavior, equally stable for the measures involving bodily activity (FACTIV and FREARS), but less stable for the measures of autonomic reactivity (FBOLI and FURINE). In general, evidence of stability is more plentiful for the File apparatus measures than for the Rod measures.

Stability from the first to second occasion does not appear to be markedly different from that from the second to third occasion. Furthermore, overall, the stability over the 100 day interval from first to third occasion does not appear to be particularly reduced from that of the two 50 day intervals for either cohort.

**Table 1.** Correlations among testing occasions in longitudinal study of genetically heterogeneous (HS) mice

| Measure | Young Cohort | | | Old Cohort | | |
|---|---|---|---|---|---|---|
| | 1 - 2 | 2 - 3 | 1 - 3 | 1 - 2 | 2 - 3 | 1 - 3 |
| FACTIV | 43 | 59 | — | 67 | 45 | 34 |
| FREARS | 53 | 68 | 35 | 62 | 48 | 51 |
| FHDPK | — | 37 | — | 39 | — | — |
| FBOLI | 49 | 51 | 58 | — | — | 34 |
| FURINE | 48 | 30 | 41 | — | — | — |
| RODROP | —[1] | 86 | —[1] | 69 | 87 | 61 |
| RODACT | — | — | — | — | 79 | 32 |
| RODBOLI | — | — | — | — | — | — |
| RODURINE | — | — | — | — | — | — |
| CORDROP | — | — | — | 39 | 57 | — |

[1] correlation not calculable due to absence of variance on occasion 1

## Validity

Using the simple criterion of detectable mean difference, age-relevance was established for all variables by analysis of variance of Studies I and III. Table 2 displays the results for main effects of age, sex (Studies I and III), genotype (Study I) and the interaction terms. Attention here is on the age main effect, which is significant for all measures in each study, with the exception of RODROP and CORDROP which are significant in Study III and not significant in Study I. Thus, for the uniform genotypes of C57BL/6, DBA/2 and $F_1$, at the ages of about 5 and about 25 months, and the genetically heterogeneous stock at about 2 and about 22 months, cross-sectional differences can be demonstrated.

## Sensitivity

From the evidence just cited, the sensitivity of these measures is at least 20 months, but that constitutes faint gerometric praise. A more refined assessment of sensitivity can be attempted by testing mean differences in successive occasions of Study III. Results of appropriate t-tests are given in Table 3.

In the young cohort, all File apparatus measures and no Rod or Cord measure display apparent 50 day or even 100 day (occasion 1 to occasion 3) sensitivity. However, the fact that no differences are obtained in the File apparatus between occasions 2 and 3 (an equal chronological interval to that from occasion 1 to 2) suggests that the difference between occasions 1 and 2 may be a matter of previous testing rather than genuine aging. In the old cohort, the File measures also display apparent sensitivity; the continuation of change between occasions 2 and 3 for FREARS and FHDPK in this older

| Table 2. Significance of Main Effects of Age, Genotype and Sex in Longitudinal and Cross-sectional Studies | | | | | | | | | | |
|---|---|---|---|---|---|---|---|---|---|---|
| | Study III | | | Study I | | | | | | |
| | A | S | A×S | A | G | S | A×G | A×S | G×S | A×G×S |
| FACTIV | * | *** | * | *** | *** | | | | *** | |
| FREARS | *** | *** | *** | *** | | | | *** | * | |
| FHDPK | *** | ** | ** | *** | ** | | | | | * |
| FBOLI | ** | * | ** | ** | | ** | | ** | * | |
| FURINE | *** | *** | | *** | | *** | | | | * |
| RODROP | *** | | | | | | | | | |
| RODACT | *** | | * | *** | * | | * | | | |
| RODBOLI | *** | | * | *** | | | | | *** | * |
| RODURINE | *** | * | | *** | ** | | | | | |
| CORDROP | * | | | | | | | | | |
| A - Age | | | | | | | | | | |
| S - Sex | | | | | | | | | | |
| G - Genotype | | | | | | | | | | |

group may represent real aging, or simply a continuation of previous testing effect. Unlike the younger cohort, the older animals show some inter-occasion differences for ROD and CORD measures.

## Susceptibility to Confounding Effects

Study II was explicitly designed to assess susceptibility to confounding effects, by comparing successive cohorts at the "seam," where the animals are of the same chronological age, but tested at different times with different numbers (zero or two) of previous testing occasions. In study II, there were two coincident age ranges: the third and first occasions, respectively, of the youngest and middle cohort (about 9 to 10 months) and the third and first occasions, respectively, of the middle and oldest cohort (about 14 to 15 months). Significant differences between cohorts at these chronological ages could be due to any combination of the potential confounding variables described earlier. Results from an overall evaluation of combined genotypes by t-tests are presented in Table 4.

All possible combinations of outcomes appear: one class of variable is "robust," in the sense that the compared means do not differ, at either testing age (FBOLI, RODBOLI, CORDROP); one is susceptible at each testing age (FREARS, FHDPK, FURINE); one susceptible at 9 - 10 mos., but not at 14 - 15 mos (RODROP, RODACT, RODURINE); and one susceptible at 14 - 15 mos., but not at 9 - 10 mos. (FACTIV). These results must be regarded as extremely tentative, given the relatively small sample sizes. The "robust"

**Table 3.** Results of t-tests for mean differences between occasions in longitudinal study of genetically heterogeneous (HS) mice

| Measure | Young Cohort | | | Old Cohort | | |
|---|---|---|---|---|---|---|
| | 1 - 2 | 2 - 3 | 1 - 3 | 1 - 2 | 2 - 3 | 1 - 3 |
| FACTIV | * | — | ** | *** | — | *** |
| FREARS | ** | — | *** | *** | * | *** |
| FHDPK | *** | — | *** | * | * | *** |
| FBOLI | ** | — | *** | — | — | — |
| FURINE | ** | — | *** | — | — | — |
| RODROP | — | — | — | * | — | * |
| RODACT | — | — | — | — | — | — |
| RODBOLI | — | — | — | — | ** | * |
| RODURINE | — | — | — | — | — | — |
| CORDROP | — | — | — | ** | — | ** |

*   p<.05

**  p<.01

*** p<.001

category must be particularly suspect, since membership only requires absence of significant evidence of mean differences. Such an outcome might arise simply from large standard errors. However, the results for CORDROP and RODBOLI are actually rather convincing, as illustrated for the latter by Figure 1, which shows the results for combined genotypes. The between cohort trends are matched closely by within cohort trends, and the differences at the overlapping chronological ages are not significant. A typical cross-sectional comparison involving what are here first occasion results or a longitudinal comparison within any one of the cohorts would suggest an aging effect, and that suggestion would probably be veridical.

On the other hand, Figure 2 shows extreme susceptibility to confounding by FHDPK for both sexes, but particularly in the case of females, where the dramatic within-cohort decline is not matched by appropriate across-cohort differences. Similar results are seen for FREARS. For these and similar biomarkers, cross-sectional results would reveal no evidence of aging, but longitudinal results could give misleading evidence of age changes.

The intermediate sensitivity of other biomarkers is well illustrated by female (and, again, somewhat less well by male) results for FACTIV (Figure 3). Scores from previously tested animals differ in the direction of inferred aging change from those with less previous testing. The amount of previous testing is thoroughly confounded with season, time in laboratory and cohort, of course. This class of measure offers genuine age validity, but it is accompanied by a susceptibility to confounding effects that imposes a need for great care in interpretation.

**Table 4.** Significant mean differences between cohorts at same chronological ages but different occasions of measurement.

| Measure | Measure  Cohort 1 vs. cohort 2 (9 - 10 mos) | Cohort 2 vs. cohort 3 (14 - 15 mos.) |
|---|---|---|
| FACTIV | — | *** |
| FREARS | *** | *** |
| FHDPK | *** | *** |
| FBOLI | — | — |
| FURINE | *** | ** |
| RODROP | * | — |
| RODACT | * | — |
| RODBOLI | — | — |
| RODURINE | ** | — |
| CORDROP | — | — |

* p<.05

** p<.01

*** p<.001

## Range

Whereas some of the biomarkers such as FACTIV and RODBOLI show a more-or-less steady decline beginning as early as 2 to 3 months, several give evidence of being late-stage markers. An example is provided by RODROP in Study II. Figure 4 shows that there is no evidence of change during the time span covered by the first cohort. However, the males of cohort 2 may show a decline beginning about 8 months, and the females of cohort 3 show a rather sharp drop beginning about 16 months.

## Sex Differences

Table 2 shows the variables for which a mean difference between sexes was demonstrable by analysis of variance. A larger number of such measures (all of the File measures plus RODURINE) was identified in Study III than Study I, due, perhaps to the greater power of Study III.

Of particular interest are those variables for which an Age X Sex interaction term was significant. In Study I these are confined to the File apparatus measures (FACTIV, FREARS, FBOLI); in Study III these are all confirmed, and FHDPK, RODACT and RODBOLI are added. The results for FBOLI, shown in Figure 5, are particularly pronounced, with significant age, sex, age X sex and genotype X sex interaction effects. The age effect reflects overall lower scores for the 25 month old than for the 5 month old animals; the sex effect is evident in the overall lower scores of females; the age X sex interaction arises from the fact that the older females have higher average scores whereas the males have lower scores; the genotype X sex interaction is due to

# RODBOLI
## GENOTYPES COMBINED

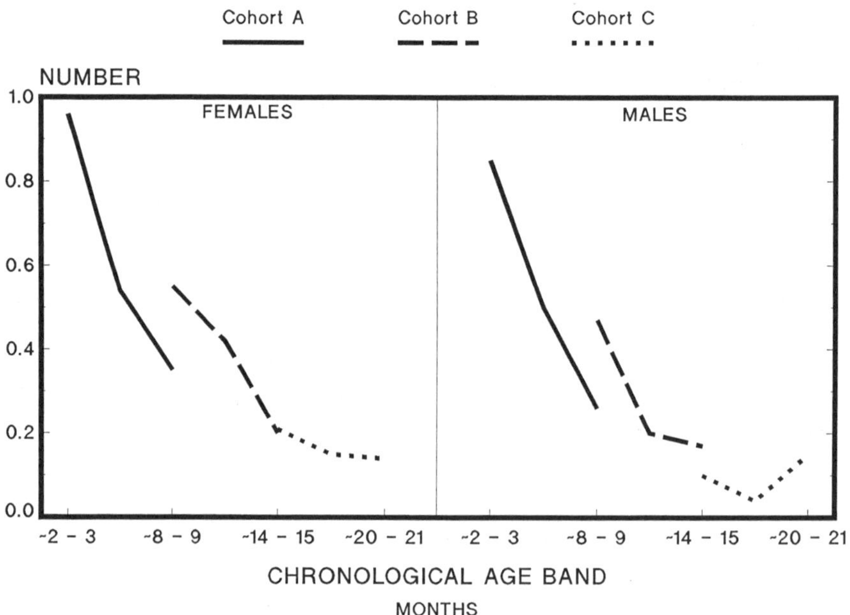


**Figure 1.** Mean RODBOLI scores for three age cohorts of mice, separately by sex, for C57BL/6, DBA/2 and $F_1$ groups combined.

the fact that the older female value is dependent largely on the very high scores of one group, the DBA/2.

These results suggest that differing age functions for males than for females may be characteristic of many biomarkers. Together with the evidence cited earlier of sex differences in susceptibility of a biomarker to confounding effects, these interaction data emphasize the need to characterize the sexes separately. From a positive point of view, these sex differences and interactions can be perceived as identifying a useful approach to the study of putative aging mechanisms through comparisons of the sexes.

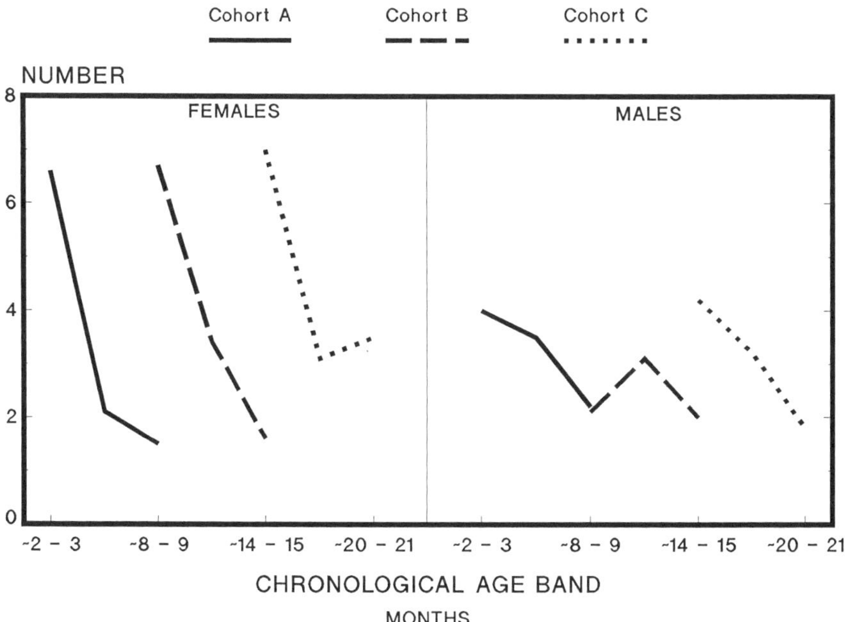


**Figure 2**. Mean FHDPK scores for three age cohorts of mice, separately by sex, for C57BL/6, DBA/2 and $F_1$ groups combined.

## Genotype

Study I offers evidence of genetic influence through mean differences among the inbred strains and their $F_1$. A useful first level of information, such comparisons are limited in that only the genetic loci for which allelic differences existed in the parent strains are being assessed. A positive outcome is thus strong in demonstrating that loci exist which can influence the phenotype; a negative outcome is weak in that an unknown number of loci remain unevaluated.

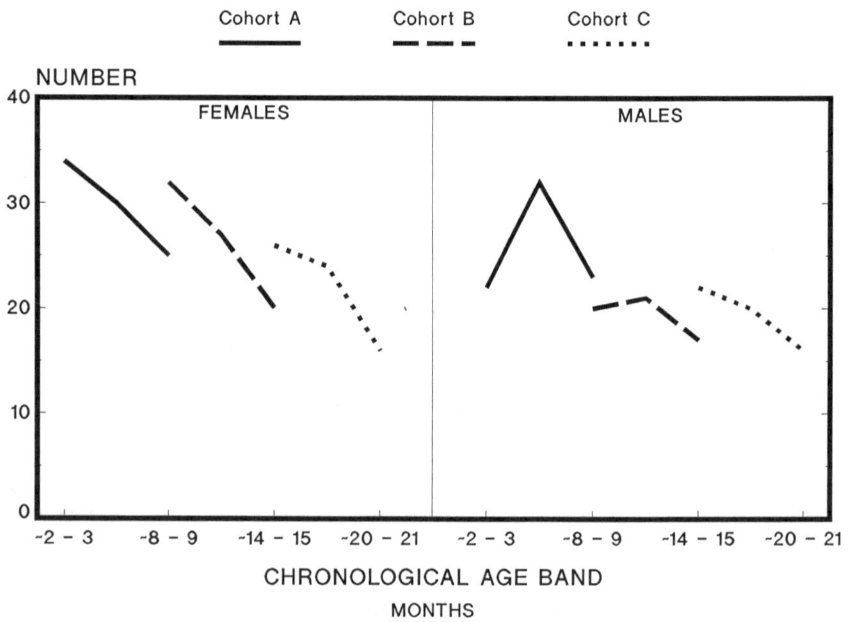



**Figure 3.** Mean FACTIV scores for three age cohorts of separately by sex, for C57BL/6, DBA/2 and F$_1$ groups combined.

In Table 2 significant main effects of genotype are shown for FACTIV, FHDPK, RODACT and RODURINE. Table 5 reports the mean values of the separate groups for these measures.

The direction of mean differences between the strains is of particular interest in relation to the generally reported shorter longevity of DBA/2 relative to C57BL/6 mice (Committee on Animal Models for Research on Aging, 1981). For the old cohort in the case of FACTIV, for both cohorts in the case of FHDPK and RODURINE and for the young cohort in the case of RODACT, the means of DBA animals are, relative to the C57BL, in the

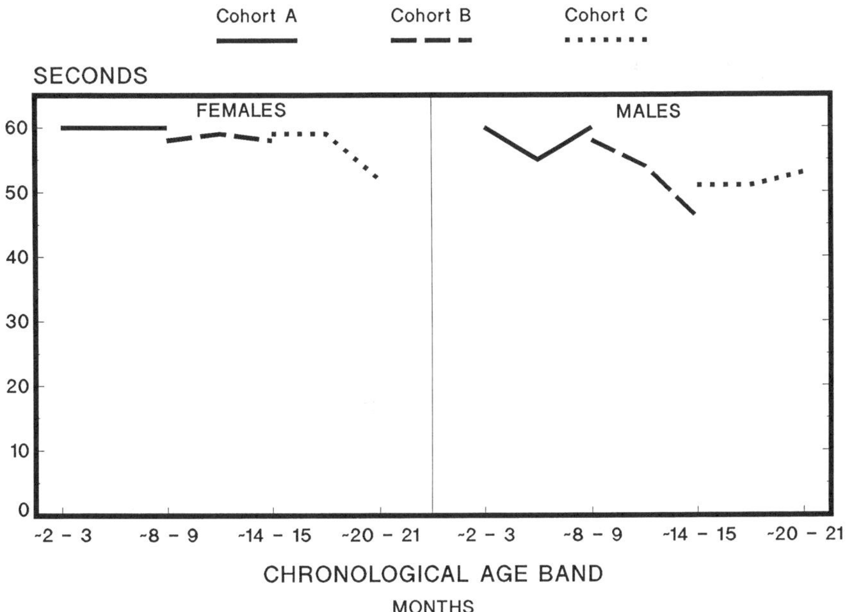



**Figure 4.** Mean RODROP scores for three age cohorts of mice, separately by sex, for C57BL/6, DBA/2 and $F_1$ groups combined.

direction of age differences. In the exceptional cases, (young/FACTIV and old/RODACT) the differences are very small. In general, then, the results would seem to suggest that these biomarkers are related to longevity. From the evidence on longevity of hybrid animals, however, we would expect the $F_1$ values for these measures to be near to or to exceed the value of the C57BL/6 parent strain, which is not the case.

Significant interaction terms involving genotype and age provide further evidence of genetic influence on age-related processes. Age X genotype interactions are shown for FREARS and RODACT; Age X genotype X sex

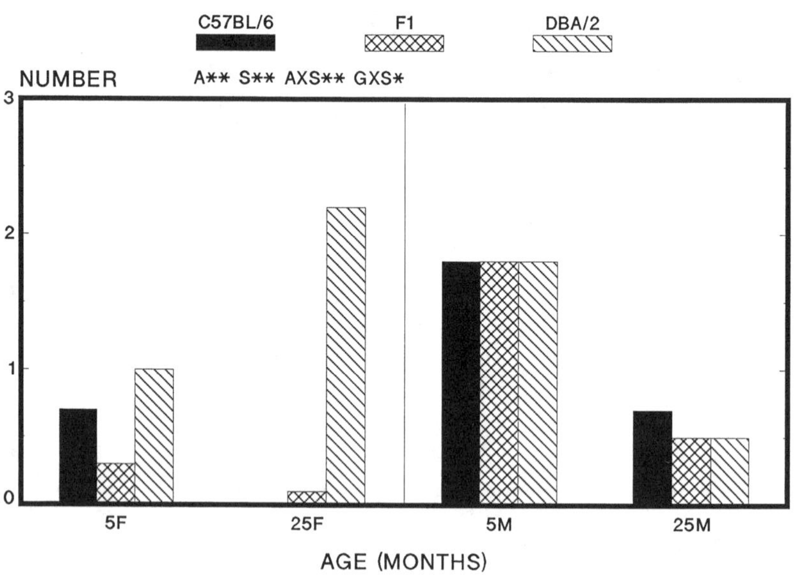



**Figure 5.** Mean FBOLI scores for two age cohorts of mice, separately by sex, age and genotypic group. Significant effects are indicated for age, sex, age X sex and genotype X sex.

interactions appear for FHDPK, FURINE and RODBOLI. These results are consistent with the position that variability in aging rates may be under genetic influence. For illustration, RODACT results are shown in Figure 6. The nature of the age X genotype interaction is clearly revealed. Substantial differences among the three genotypes at 5 months of age have disappeared at 25 months. This type of outcome could be interpreted as indicating a decline in genetic influence in the later part of the lifespan with respect to this variable, but interpretation is somewhat constrained by the difficulty of dis-

| Table 5. Means of biomarkers showing significant main effect of genotype in cross-sectional study | | | | |
|---|---|---|---|---|
| | FACTIV | FHDPK | RODACT | RODURINE |
| **Young** | | | | |
| C57BL/6 | 27.9 | 10.8 | 6.2 | 0.4 |
| F1* | 21.4 | 7.5 | 3.7 | 0.2 |
| DBA/2 | 30.4 | 6.2 | 1.9 | 0.1 |
| **Old** | | | | |
| C57BL/6 | 22.0 | 3.2 | 0.8 | 0.1 |
| F1* | 12.9 | 3.6 | 1.3 | 0.0 |
| DBA/2 | 15.1 | 2.0 | 0.9 | 0.0 |

entangling what may be a genuine biological effect from a scalar one imposed by the apparent "floor" effect.

These collective results indicate some genetic influence on age-related changes in FACTIV, FREARS, FHDPK, FURINE, RODACT, RODBOLI and RODURINE, but reveal little about the genetic system involved. Some useful further information, on the average dominance of the alleles at relevant loci for which the parent strains differ, is provided by the location of the $F_1$ means relative to the parent strain means. The presence of dominance was evaluated by t-tests of departure of the $F_1$ mean from the midparent value by sexes and by age cohort separately. Results can be summarized briefly as follows: for FACTIV, dominance was present for all groups, in the direction of the C57BL/6 parent for the young and in the direction of the DBA/2 parent for the old; for FBOLI, dominance in the direction of the C57BL/6 parent was present for females of both age cohorts, but not for the males of either age; old males alone showed dominance in the direction of the DBA/2 parent (and in the direction of age differences) for FURINE and for RODBOLI.

This information can further be interpreted in respect to natural fitness in that the direction of departure of the $F_1$ mean from midparent values indicates the "more fit" direction on the phenotypic scale. An obvious question is whether this Darwinian fitness, defined ultimately in terms of reproductive success, can be related to the concept of "vitality," defined in terms of likelihood of survival. It is presumed that older animals are in general possessed of less vitality than younger ones. If there is a mean difference between age groups on some variable, the value of the variable typical of the older animals might be assumed to be related in some way to lower vitality. Thus, in those cases where a significant difference is found between strains at the same chronological age, that strain which exhibits a mean in the direction of the older age groups might be regarded as less "vital." The mixed results

## RODACTMX

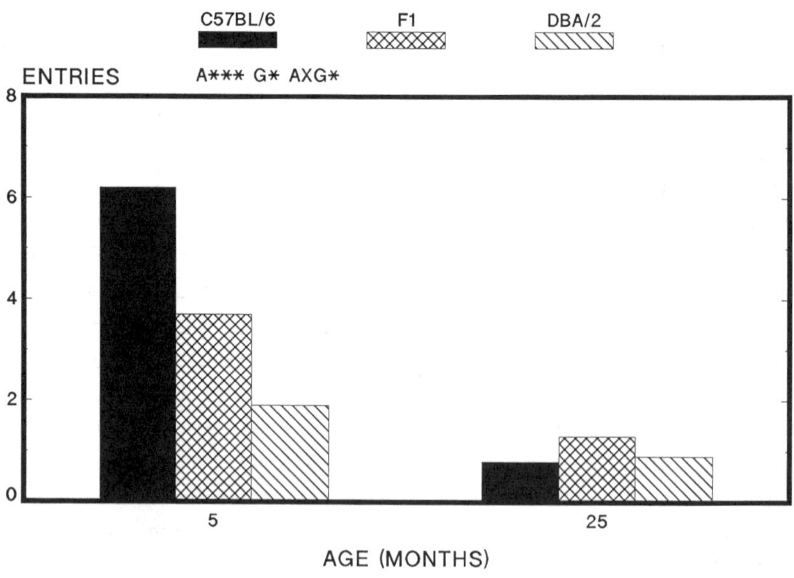


**Figure 6.** Mean RODACTMX (highest RODACT score from three trials) for two age cohorts of mice, separately by age and genotypic group, sexes combined. Significant effects are indicated for age, genotype and age X genotype.

suggest that, although fitness and "vitality" must be correlated to some extent, the relationships between the concepts may be very complex.

## SUMMARY

Given that these behavioral measures were selected from the literature for age-relevance, the demonstrated age differences and age changes are basically replications, though providing specific information for a heretofore untested sample of genetically heterogeneous mice. However, these studies have revealed that these measures differ greatly in their stability, sensitivity, range and susceptibility to confounding effects of cohort, season, previous measurement or duration of rcsidence in the colony. These differences are further complicated by being dependent upon genotype, sex and age. Insofar as these results are generalizable, biomarkers of universal applicability are unlikely to be found, and neither cross-sectional nor longitudinal designs alone can provide an adequate description of aging processes.

The implication is clear that gerometric properties must be a matter of high priority in selecting variables for research on the genetics of aging, and, indeed, for gerontological research in general.

Although not designed to provide critical tests of our basic assumptions, the results are clearly consistent with the lifespan quantitative genetic model. Certainly, they do not cast into doubt the view that aging is complex.

## ACKNOWLEDGEMENTS

The program of research for which these pilot studies were performed is a collaborative enterprise involving as co-investigators F. Ahern, F. Ferguson, G. McClearn, R. Mitchell, J. Nesselroade, R. Parker, C. Reddy, and T. Stout. Studies I and II were supported by the MacArthur Foundation Research Network on Successful Aging. Study III and the ongoing two-generational longitudinal study are supported by NIA grant AG04948. I am much indebted to John Nesselroade and to two anonynmous reviewers for valuable comments. Remaining errors or obscurities are mine alone, of course.

## REFERENCES

COMMITTEE ON ANIMAL MODELS FOR RESEARCH ON AGING, (1981) *Mammalian Models for Research on Aging*. Washington, DC: National Academy Press.

DEAN, III, R. L., SCOZZAFAVA, J., GOAS, J. A., REGAN, B., BEER, B., and BARTUS, R. T. (1981) Age-related differences in behavior across the life span of the C57Bl/6J mouse. *Exp. Aging Res.* **7**: 427-451

FILE, S. E., and WARDILL, A. G. (1975) Validity of head-dipping as a measure of exploration in a modified hole-board. *Psychopharmacologia (Berl.)* **44**: 53-59

GHISELLI, E. E., CAMPBELL, J. P., and ZEDECK, S. (1981) *Measurement theory for the behavioral sciences*. San Francisco: W.H. Freeman

INGRAM, D. K. (1983) Toward the behavioral assessment of biological aging in the laboratory mouse: Concepts, terminology and objectives. *Exp. Aging Res.* **9**: 225-238

INGRAM, D. K., ARCHER, J. R., HARRISON, D. E., and REYNOLDS, M. A. (1982). Physiological and behavioral correlates of lifespan in aged C57BL/6J mice. *Exp. Geron.* **17**: 295-303

INGRAM, D. K., REYNOLDS, M. A. (1986) Assessing the predictive validity of psychomotor tests as measures of biological age in mice. *Exp. Aging Res.* **12**: 155-162

LOEHLIN, J. C. (1987) *Latent variable models: An introduction to factor, path, and structural analysis*. Hillsdale, NJ: Lawrence Erlbaum.

McCLEARN, G. E. (1988) Strategies for biomarker research: Experimental and methodological design. *Exp. Geron.* **23**: 245-255

McCLEARN, G. E. (1981) Animal models of genetic factors in alcoholism. **In**: *Advances in Substance Abuse* **Vol.2** (Ed. M. K. Mello), pp. 185-217. Greenwich, CT: JAI Press.

MIQUEL, J. and BLASCO, M. (1978) A simple technique for evaluation of vitality loss in aging mice, by testing their muscular coordination and vigor. *Exp. Geron.* **13**: 389-396

NESSELROADE, J. R., PRUCHNO, R., and JACOBS, A. (1986) Reliability vs. stability in the measurement of psychological states: An illustration with anxiety measures. *Psychol. Beitrage* **28**: 255-264

SCHAIE, K. W. (1975) Research strategy in developmental human behavior genetics. **In**: *Developmental Human Behavior Genetics* (Ed. K. W. Schaie, V. E. Anderson, G. E. McClearn, and J. Money), pp. 205-219. Lexington, MA: Lexington Books.

## DISCUSSION

1. Does the tail tendon collagen test become more variable with age? Yes, especially after 400 days of age. How do you recognize a "good" biomarker? For example the tail collagen test correlates very well with age in many strains yet B6 collagen ages more slowly than that in B6D2F1 mice, while B6D2F1 mice live longer than B6. Of course many important effects on aging are not shown by longevities, if that particular strain of mice dies of something else. Thus don't limit biomarkers to those that predict longevities. To get reliable results, the same portion of the tail must be tested, as breaking times are longer in portions that are closer than about halfway towards the body, as these are warmer.

2. A problem with the HS mice is that individuals all differ, so they can't be replicated. RFLP mapping was suggested to define those individuals. A problem with RFLP analysis is that it is a discontinuous variable applied to study changes with age that are continuous. Thus it would be difficult to interpret, especially if you don't know how many genes affecting the aging parameter are segregating in the HS population. An alternate approach is to use many unrelated inbred strains and carry out a variety of crosses making many different but genetically defined and repeatable $F_1$ hybrids. Nevertheless, new methods will make RFLP mapping possible using small amounts of DNA, and increasing knowledge will aid interpretations. Thus, it might be wise to save DNA from genetically undefined individuals for whom aging data are available.

3. Effects of shipping were surprisingly large. Test results in mice of different ages were strongly affected by shipping, season shipped, duration of residence and cohort, all causing major effects. This suggests that gerontobiologists should develop their own animal colonies, as the effects of shipping appear to be so complex and important.

# 15

# THE EFFECT OF DIETARY RESTRICTION ON THE EXPRESSION OF A VARIETY OF GENES

Susan Waggoner, Mao-Zhi Gu, Wen-Hsiu Chiang and Arlan Richardson

## ABSTRACT

The effect of dietary restriction on gene expression was studied in liver tissue from male Fischer F344 rats. The relative levels of four mRNAs ($\alpha_{2u}$-globulin, *c-myc*, apolipoprotein AI and apolipoprotein B) were measured in rats fed either *ad libitum* or a calorie-restricted diet. The age-related decrease in $\alpha_{2u}$-globulin mRNA levels was retarded by dietary restriction. On the other hand, the age-related increase in apolipoprotein AI mRNA levels was reduced by dietary restriction. However, dietary restriction did not have any effect on the age- related change in the levels of either *c-myc* mRNA or apolipoprotein B mRNA. Thus, dietary restriction can affect gene expression at the level of transcription; however, dietary restriction does not affect the expression of all genes.

## INTRODUCTION

Dietary restriction, *i.e.*, the restriction of total calories, is the only experimental manipulation that has been shown to consistently increase the survival of laboratory rodents (Masoro, 1988). Dietary restriction increases the mean and maximum survival of rodents and retards and/or reduces the incidence of most age-related diseases. In addition, dietary restriction has a profound effect on a variety of biological processes that change with age. Thus, it is generally accepted that dietary restriction increases the survival of rodents by retarding the aging process (Masoro, 1988).

Although it is well established that dietary restriction increases the survival of rodents, the molecular mechanism responsible for this increase is not known. McCay *et al.* (1935) initially proposed that dietary restriction increased survival by retarding growth and development. However, studies by Weindruch and Walford (1982) showed that dietary restriction initiated in adult life increased the survival of mice. More recently, Yu *et al.* (1985) observed a similar phenomenon in rats. Thus, studies over the past five years demonstrate conclusively that dietary restriction is able to increase survival when initiated well after growth and development have occurred.

In 1960, Berg and Simms proposed that food restriction enhanced the survival of rodents by reducing their body fat. Although body fat of restricted rodents is less than that of rodents fed *ad libitum*, there is no direct experimental evidence that this difference is actually responsible for increased survival. In 1980, Bertrand *et al.*, showed a correlation between greater body fat and greater length of life for rats fed a restricted diet. In other words, the restricted rats with higher body fat lived longer than restricted rats with less body fat. More recently, Harrison *et al.* (1984) showed that longevity was not correlated to body fat content using normal and genetically obese mice. Thus, while it is generally accepted that greater body fat is correlated to decreased survival in humans, the decrease in body fat does not appear to be responsible for the increase in survival that is observed with dietary restriction.

In reviewing the data on dietary restriction, Sacher (1977) suggested that dietary restriction increased survival by reducing the metabolic rate. On the surface, this suggestion appears logical, and subsequently it gained a great deal of support because of the relationship between metabolism and the generation of free radicals. However, until recently, there was no direct experimental evidence for or against this hypothesis. In 1985, McCarter *et al.* tested this hypothesis by measuring the oxygen consumption of rats fed *ad libitum* or restricted diet over a 24 hour period. The metabolic rate per unit of lean body mass was not significantly different for rats fed *ad libitum* or the restricted diet. Therefore, the reduction in caloric intake does not appear to alter the metabolic rate of rodents.

Several investigators (Barrows, 1972; Lindelly, 1982; Richardson and Cheung, 1982) have proposed that the mechanism of action of dietary restriction involved changes in gene expression. This hypothesis has merit because changes in gene expression can have a profound affect on a cell or organism and because it has been shown that gene expression changes with increasing age (Richardson and Birchenall-Sparks, 1983; Richardson *et al.* 1983; Richardson and Semsei, 1987).

To test this proposal, we asked whether dietary restriction could alter age-related changes in gene expression. In our initial experiments, we measured protein synthesis in a variety of tissues from rats fed *ad libitum* or a restricted diet because research conducted during the 1970s showed that an age-related decline in protein synthesis appeared to be a universal phenomenon (Richardson, 1981). In 1985, Birchenall-Sparks *et al.* showed that the rate of protein synthesis by hepatocytes isolated from rats fed a restricted diet was significantly higher than the rate of protein synthesis for hepatocytes isolated from rats fed *ad libitum*. More recently, Ward (1988) confirmed this observation using perfused liver. Our laboratory also showed that dietary restriction resulted in an increase in the protein synthetic activity of kidney (Ricketts *et al.*, 1985) and mitogen-stimulated spleen lymphocytes (Pahlavani *et al.*, 1988)) from rats. Thus, the data demonstrate that dietary restriction enhances the level of protein synthesis in a variety of tissues from old rats.

More recently, our laboratory has focused its effort on the effect of dietary restriction on gene expression at the level of transcription. In an initial series of experiments, we showed that the transcription of $\alpha_{2u}$-globulin was enhanced by dietary restriction (Richardson *et al.*, 1987). In the experiments described herein, we compare the levels of several mRNA species in liver tissue isolated from rats fed *ad libitum* or a restricted diet. These experiments demonstrate that dietary restriction alters the levels of several mRNA species. Thus, dietary restriction can affect gene expression at the level of transcription. However, dietary restriction does not affect the expression of all genes.

## MATERIALS AND METHODS

### Animals and Diets

Male Fischer F344/NHSD rats were obtained from Harlan Industries (Indianapolis, IN) in September 1984 and were caged individually in a barrier facility at the V.A. Medical Center in St. Louis, MO. A detailed description of the dietary restriction regimen and the housing conditions is given by Armbrecht *et al.* (1988). The rats were fed a semi-synthetic casein diet, and the restriction regimen was initiated at 6 weeks of age. The control group was fed the diet *ad libitum*, and the experimental group (restricted) was fed daily 60% of the diet consumed by the rats fed *ad libitum*. The body weight and the survival of the rats in the two groups is described by Armbrecht *et al.* (1988). The mean and 10% survival of the rats on the restricted diet was approximately 30% higher than rats fed *ad libitum*. The pathology associated with male Fischer F344 rats on similar diets has been described by Maeda *et al.* (1985). Only healthy animals were used in the experiments described herein, *i.e.*, rats showing the presence of tumors or exhibiting a rapid loss of weight were excluded.

### RNA Isolation and RNA/cDNA Hybridization

Rats were killed by decapitation and the livers were immediately removed, frozen in liquid nitrogen, and stored at - 80°C. RNA was isolated from guanidine thiocyanate homogenates of the liver by cesium chloride gradient centrifugation as described by Chirgwin (1979). The RNA was precipitated with ethanol, resuspended in RNase-free water at a concentration of 1 mg/ml, and stored at - 80°C until used for hybridization studies.

The levels of the various mRNAs in the RNA preparations were determined by dot blot hybridization as described by Thomas (1980), using cDNA probes that had been labeled with [$^{32}$P]-radioactivity. Northern blot analysis of the RNA was accomplished as described by Rutherford *et al.* (1986) using the method of Southern to transfer the RNA from the gel to nitrocellulose (Southern, 1975). In all experiments, cDNA probes were used to quantify the mRNA levels except for the experiments on $\alpha_{2u}$-globulin mRNA. In these experiments a cRNA probe was used in the hybridization assay as described by Melton *et al.* (1984).

## Isolation and Labeling of cDNA Plasmids

The cDNA probes for $\alpha_{2u}$-globulin, c-myc, apolipoprotein Al, and apolipoprotein B were obtained from Dr. P. Feigelson (Kulkarni *et al.*, 1985), Dr. P.A. Weinberg (Land *et al.*, 1983), Dr. J. Miller (Miller *et al.*, 1983), and Dr. A.J. Lusis (Lusis *et al.*, 1985), respectively. The cDNA containing plasmids were transformed into *E. coli* RR1 (Maniatis *et al.*, 1975) and were isolated by the methods of Birnboim and Doly (1979). The plasmids containing the cDNA insert were labeled with $\alpha$-[$^{32}$P]-dCTP (2000 Ci/mmol) to a specific activity of 2 to 6 × 10$^8$ cpm/µg DNA using a nick translation kit from Bethesda Research Laboratories (Bethesda, MD). The radioactively labeled probes were separated from the [$^{32}$P]-dCTP by Sephadex G-50 chromatography (Maniatis, 1982).

## RESULTS

$\alpha_{2u}$-Globulin is the major urinary protein of male rats and is of interest because it is under multihormonal control. Androgens, estrogens, glucocorticoids, thyroxin, growth hormone, and insulin have been shown to affect the genetic expression of $\alpha_{2u}$-globulin (Roy and Neuhaus, 1967; Roy, 1973; Roy and Leonard, 1973; Roy *et al.*, 1975). In 1983, Roy *et al.* reported that the synthesis of $\alpha_{2u}$-globulin decreased dramatically with increasing age in male rats. Recently, our laboratory showed that the age-related decrease in the synthesis of $\alpha_{2u}$-globulin was due to a decrease in the transcription of the $\alpha_{2u}$-globulin genes (Richardson *et al.*, 1987). In addition, we showed that the genetic expression of $\alpha_{2u}$-globulin was increased when rats were fed a calorie-restricted diet. At 18 months of age the level of $\alpha_{2u}$-globulin mRNA was approximately 2-fold higher in liver tissue from rats fed a restricted diet than in liver tissue from rats fed *ad libitum*.

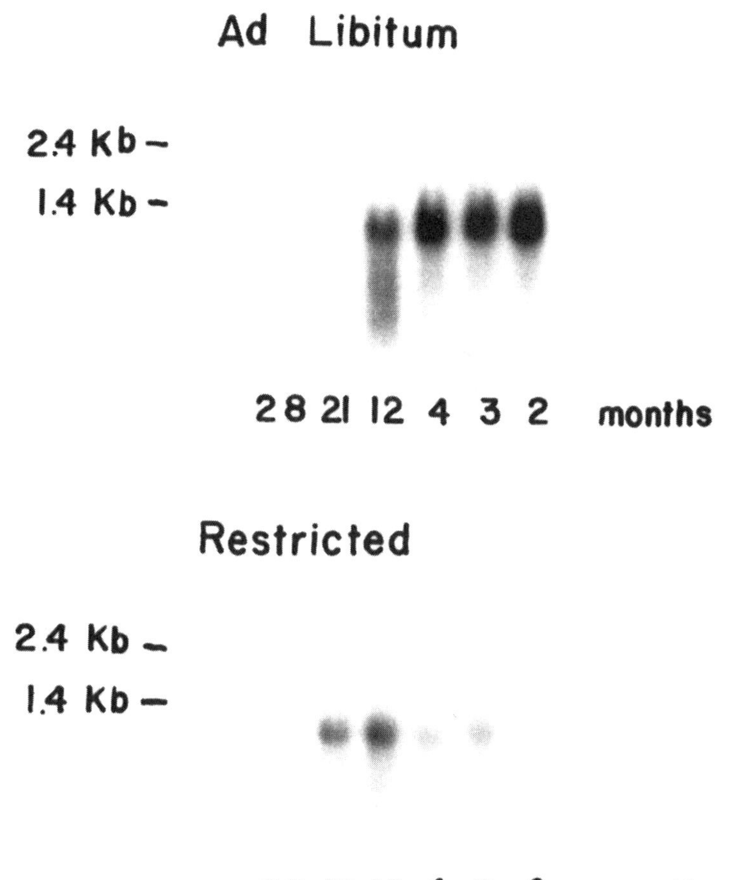


**Figure 1.** Autoradiogram of a Northern Blot for $\alpha_{2u}$-globulin with RNA Isolated from Liver Tissue Obtained from Rats fed *ad libitum* or a restricted Diet. RNA (10 µg/ml lane) was isolated from liver tissue from 2- to 28-month-old rats fed *ad libitum* or the restricted diet. The RNA was fractionated by agarose, transferred to nitrocellulose, and hybridized to a radioactively labeled cDNA probe to $\alpha_{2u}$-globulin. RNA was pooled from 3 to 7 rats for each age, and the migration of RNA standards is shown.

In this study, we measured the levels of $\alpha_{2u}$-globulin mRNA in liver tissue over most of the life span of male Fischer F344 rats fed either *ad libitum* or the restricted diet. Figure 1 shows Northern blot analysis of RNA isolated

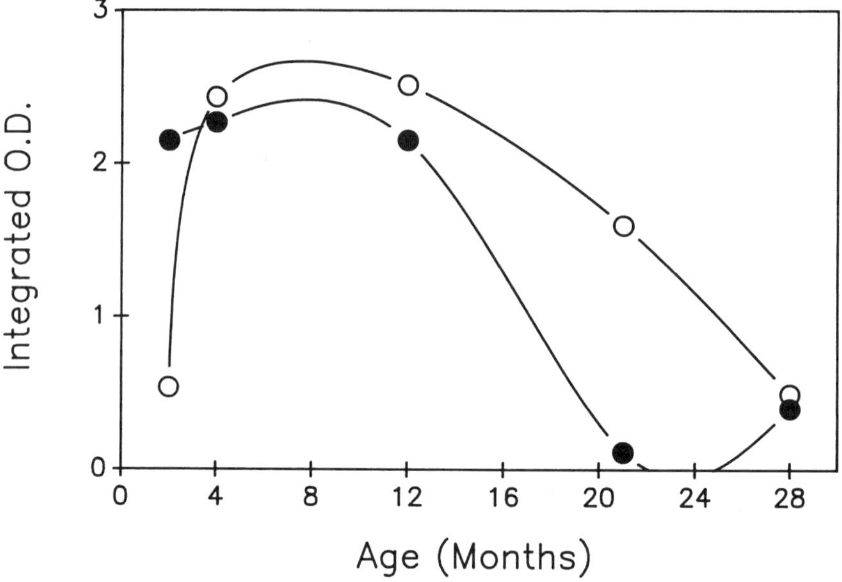


**Figure 2.** Effect of Age and Dietary Restriction on the Expression of $\alpha_{2u}$-Globulin mRNA. The relative levels of $a_{2u}$-globulin mRNA in liver tissue from rats fed *ad libitum* (O) and the restricted diet (●) were determined with pooled samples by dot blot hybridization as described in the Materials and Methods.

from liver tissue of 2- to 28-month-old rats fed *ad libitum* or fed the restricted diet. There was no difference in the size of the $\alpha_{2u}$-globulin mRNA in the rats fed the two diets. However, it is apparent from Figure 1 that the levels of $\alpha_{2u}$-globulin mRNA change with age. Figure 2 shows that the levels of $\alpha_{2u}$-globulin mRNA decreased markedly after 12 months of age in rats fed *ad libitum*, which was shown previously (Richardson *et al.*, 1987). More importantly, Figure 2 shows that the levels of $\alpha_{2u}$-globulin mRNA were altered by dietary restriction. The levels of $\alpha_{2u}$-globulin mRNA were increased by dietary restriction at 21 months of age. However, the levels of $\alpha_{2u}$-globulin mRNA were also altered by dietary restriction in young rats. At 2 months of age, the level of $\alpha_{2u}$-globulin mRNA was almost 80% lower in the restricted rats than in the rats fed *ad libitum*. Roy *et al.* (1983) showed that the levels of $\alpha_{2u}$-globulin in the liver of male rats increases dramatically after puberty (approximately 40 days of age) and reaches a peak level at 3 to 4 months of age. Thus, dietary restriction appears to delay the increase in $\alpha_{2u}$-globulin expression seen at puberty and retard the decline in $\alpha_{2u}$-globulin expression during senescence.

## The Expression of *c-myc*

*myc* is the transforming gene (oncogene) of avian myelocytomatosis virus MC29 (Duesberg *et al.*, 1977). *myc*-containing avian tumor viruses have the ability to cause a broad range of cancers (*e.g.*, acute leukemia, carcinomas, and sarcomas) and to transform fibroblasts and hematopoietic cells in tissue culture (Weiss *et al.*, 1982). It has been found that normal avian and mammalian DNA contains a sequence similar to that of the viral *myc*, *i.e.*, cellular *myc* (Sheiness *et al.*, 1980). In addition, cellular *myc* (*c-myc*) sequences are expressed in normal cells (Eva *et al.*, 1982). For example, Goyette *et al.* (1984) showed that the expression of *c-myc* increased during liver regeneration. The protein produced by the *c-myc* gene is a nuclear, DNA-binding protein (Persson and Leder, 1984). Although the cellular function of this protein is unknown, it is thought to play a role in the proliferation of cells (Kelly *et al.*, 1983). In Figure 3, the levels of *c-myc* mRNA in RNA isolated from normal and regenerating liver were compared. The hybridization of the cDNA probe to various concentrations of RNA isolated from rats before and after $CCl_4$ induced liver regeneration are shown. The levels of *c-myc* mRNA were induced by $CCl_4$ treatment and were at a maximum 24 hours after $CCl_4$ treatment. Goyette *et al.* (1984) has demonstrated a similar time course for the induction of *c-myc* by $CCl_4$.

Figure 4 shows the Northern blot of RNA isolated from 6- to 37-month-old rats. The cDNA probe to *c-myc* mRNA hybridized to a major RNA species of approximately 2.5 Kb. Horikawa *et al.* (1986) reported the size of *c-myc* mRNA in rat liver to be 2.4 Kb. No change in the size of the *c-myc* was observed with increasing age. However, the Northern blot shown in Figure 2 suggests that the level of *c-myc* mRNA changes with age. The relative levels of *c-myc* mRNA in RNA isolated from the livers of 6- to 37-month-old rats was then determined by dot blot analysis, and the data are given in Table 1. The level of *c-myc* mRNA sequences increased 82% between 6 and 24 months of age and then decreased continuously to the level found in the 6 month old rats. These data agree well with the recent study by Matocha *et al.* (1987), who reported that the levels of *c-myc* in liver from male Fischer F344 rats increased continuously between 4 and 24 months of age. However, Matocha *et al.* (1987) did not study rats older than 24 months.

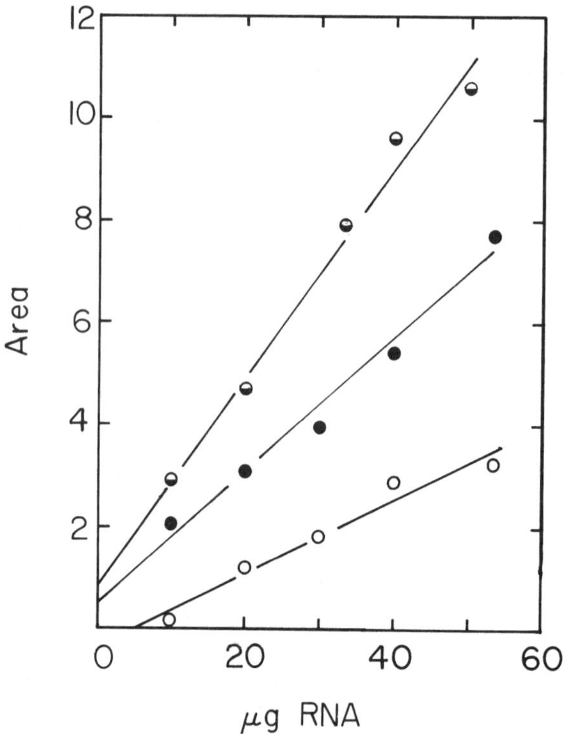



**Figure 3.** Effect of CCl₄ Induced Liver Regeneration on *c-myc* mRNA Levels. The hybridization of the cDNA probe to *c-myc* to 10 to 50 μg of liver RNA isolated from 2-month-old rats before CCl₄ treatment (O) and 24 hours (●) or 48 hours (●) after CCl₄ treatment was determined by dot blot hybridization as described in the Materials and Methods.

Table 2 shows the relative levels of *c-myc* mRNA in RNA isolated from the livers of 18-month-old rats fed *ad libitum* or a restricted diet. Dietary restriction did not retard the age-related increase in *c-myc* mRNA. In fact, the level of *c-myc* was 17% higher in the 18-month-old restricted rats. However, this difference was not statistically significant at the $P < 0.05$ level. Thus, life-long dietary restriction had little, if any, effect on the age-related increase in the expression of *c-myc*.

## The Expression of Apoliproteins

Apolipoproteins are important structural components of lipoprotein particles. They also play a role in lipoprotein metabolism, *e.g.*, they are cofactors for enzymatic reactions and are involved in receptor-mediated uptake of lipoproteins (Nilson-Ehle *et al.*, 1980; Brown and Goldstein, 1976). In this

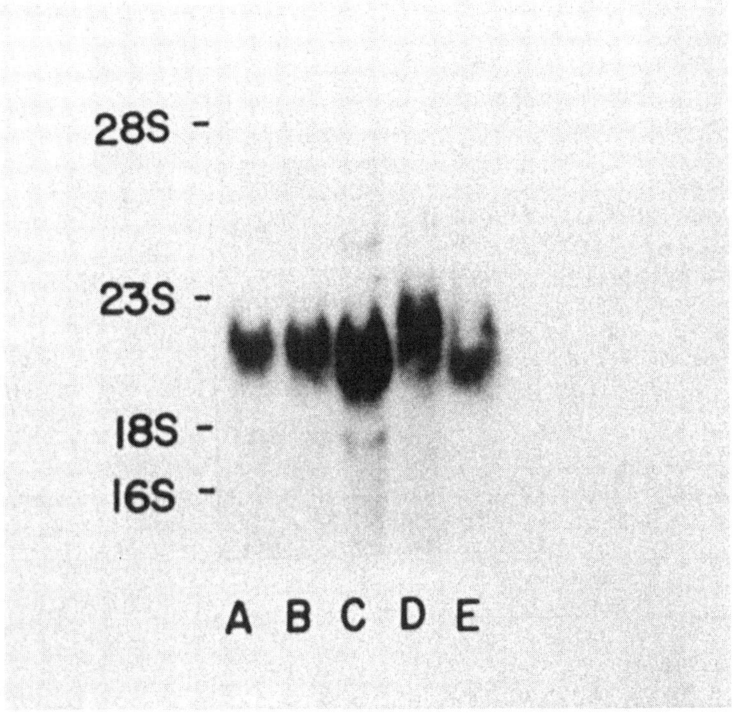



**Figure 4.** Autoradiogram of a Northern Blot for cDNA with RNA from Rats of Various Ages. RNA (40 μg/lane) isolated from liver tissue of 6- (A), 14- (B), 24- (C), 29- (D), and 37- (E) month-old rats was fractionated by agarose gel electrophoresis, transferred to nitrocellulose, and hybridized to a radioactively labeled cDNA probe containing *v-myc*. RNA from four animals of each age was pooled and the migration of rRNA standards from *E. coli* and rat liver is shown.

series of experiments, the effect of age and dietary restriction on the expression of two lipoproteins, apolipoprotein AI (Apo-AI) and apolipoprotein B (Apo-B), were studied in liver tissue. Liver and intestine are the major sites for the synthesis of Apo-AI and Apo-B (Miller *et al.*, 1983).

Apo-AI is the major protein component of high density lipoprotein (HDL) particles; approximately 70% of the protein in HDL is Apo-AI (Archer *et al.*, 1986). In addition, Apo-AI has been found to be the primary activator of lecithin- cholesterol acyltransferase (Fielding *et al.*, 1972). Stein *et al.* (1976) showed that HDL particles are involved in the regulation of cellular membrane cholesterol content as well as the transport of cholesterol from peripheral tissue to the liver. Apo-AI is of medical interest because the levels

**Table 1.** Effect of age on the levels of *c-myc* mRNA in rat liver.

| Age | Relative mRNA Level (area) |
|---|---|
| 6 | 8.17 ± 0.63 |
| 14 | 12.83 ± 0.90 |
| 24 | 14.83 ± 0.75 |
| 29 | 12.26 ± 0.48 |
| 37 | 8.70 ± 0.48 |

Each value represents the mean ± SE of data obtained from four animals for each age. The levels of *c-myc* mRNA were determined by dot blot hybridization as described in Materials and Methods. Forty µg of RNA were used for each dot blot. A significant change ($P < 0.001$) in the level of *c-myc* mRNA with increasing age was observed when the data were analyzed by analysis of variance. Using the Student's T-test it was found that the level of *c-myc* mRNA at 24 months of age was significantly different from the level at 6 months ($P < 0.001$), 29 months ($P < 0.01$), and 37 months ($P < 0.01$). The level of *c-myc* mRNA at 6 months of age was significantly different from the levels at 14 months ($P < 0.05$) and 29 months ($P < 0.01$).

**Table 2.** Effect of dietary restriction on *c-myc* expression in rat liver.

| | Relative mRNA Level (area) |
|---|---|
| *ad libitum* | 0.83 ± 0.17 |
| Restricted | 1.01 ± 0.18 |

The data were obtained from 18-month-old rats fed *ad libitum* or the restricted diet. The data represents the mean SE of four animals for each treatment and were obtained by dot blot analysis as described in Materials and Methods.

of HDL lipoproteins are inversely correlated with the risk of developing atherosclerosis and coronary heart disease (Glueck *et al.*, 1976).

Apo-B is the major protein component of low density lipoprotein (LDL) particles (Huang *et al.*, 1985; Lusis *et al.*, 1985). Apo-B plays an essential role in the assembly and secretion of chylomicrons and very low density lipoproteins. It also functions as a ligand in the removal of LDL from the circulation by receptor-mediated uptake into a variety of cells (Kane, 1983; Innerarity and Mahley, 1978; Brown *et al.*, 1981). Apo-B is a glycoprotein and has been separated into two forms B-45 and B-100. Both B-45 and B-100 are produced by rat liver. B-100 plays a role in the synthesis and secretion of hepatic-derived triglyceride-rich lipoproteins (Kane *et al.*, 1980; Kane, 1983). There is a strong correlation between LDL cholesterol levels and suscep-tibility to coronary heart disease. This same correlation has been found with Apo-B levels (Heiss and Tyroler, 1982).

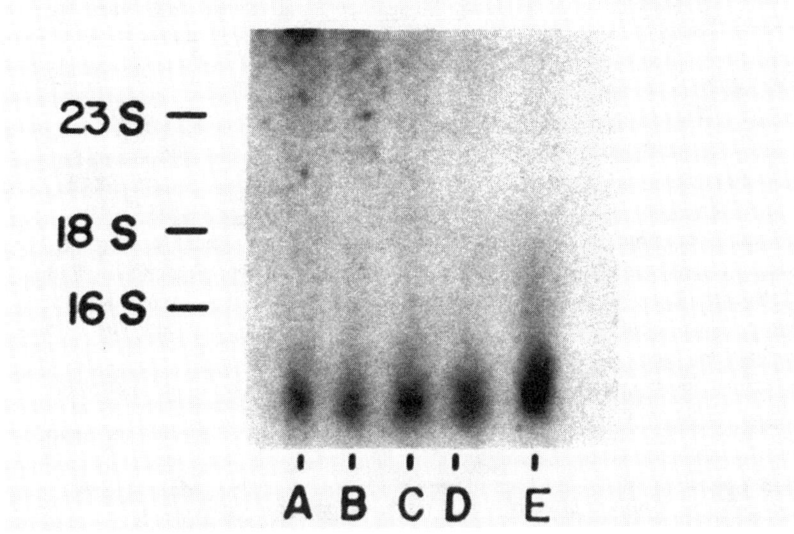


**Figure 5.** Autoradiogram of a Northern Blot for Apo Al with RNA from Rats of Various Ages. RNA (10 μg/lane) isolated from liver tissue of 6- (A), 14- (B), 24- (C), 29- (D), and 37- (E) month-old rats. Northern blot analysis was conducted as described in Figure 4 using a cDNA probe to Apo-Al. RNA from four animals of each age was pooled, and the migration of rRNA standards is shown.

Figure 5 shows the hybridization of the Apo-AI cDNA probe to a Northern blot containing RNA isolated from 6- to 37- month-old rats. The cDNA probe hybridized to an RNA species with a size of 1.0 Kb, which is in good agreement with a previous report by Hamsten *et al.* (1986). It is evident from Figure 3 that the size of the Apo-AI mRNA does not change with age; however, the level appears to increase. Table 4 gives the relative levels of Apo-AI mRNA in liver tissue obtained from 6- to 37-month-old rats. The level of Apo-AI mRNA increased over 30% between 6 and 28 months of age and then increased 40% between 28 and 37 months of age. Table 3 also gives the relative levels of Apo-B mRNA in liver tissue from 6- to 37- month-old rats. The level of Apo-B mRNA increased over 70% between 6 and 24 months of age and decreased dramatically between 28 and 37 months of age.

Next, the effect of dietary restriction on the expression of Apo-AI and Apo-B was measured. Figure 6 shows the hybridization of the Apo-AI probe to a Northern blot containing RNA isolated from 18-month-old rats fed *ad libitum* or the restricted diet. Dietary restriction had no effect on the size of the Apo-AI mRNA; however, it is evident that the level of Apo-AI mRNA was lower in RNA isolated from the rats fed the restricted diet. Table 4 gives the

**Table 3.** Effect of age on Apo-AI and Apo-B mRNA levels in rat liver.

| Age | Relative mRNA Level (area) | |
|---|---|---|
| | Apo-AI | Apo-B |
| 6 | 2.11 ± 0.29 | 1.49 ± 0.61 |
| 14 | 2.26 ± 0.51 | 1.71 ± 0.45 |
| 24 | 3.17 ± 0.27 | 2.58 ± 0.15 |
| 29 | 2.96 ± 0.26 | 2.16 ± 0.11 |
| 37 | 4.19 ± 0.52 | 0.03 ± 0.01 |

Each value represents the mean ± SE of data obtained from five animals for each age. The levels of Apo-AI and Apo-B mRNA were determined by blot hybridization using 8 µg of RNA for each blot. Using analysis of variance, the level of Apo-AI and Apo-B were shown to change significantly with age at the $P < 0.001$ level. Using the Student's T-test, it was found that the values at 37 months of age were significantly different ($P < 0.001$) from the values for all other ages and that the values at 24 months of age were significantly different ($P < 0.05$) from the values at 6 months of age.

**Table 4.** Effect of dietary restriction on Apo-AI and Apo-B

| | Relative mRNA Level (area) | |
|---|---|---|
| | Apo-AI | Apo-B |
| *ad libitum* | 4.89 ± 0.43 | 1.84 ± 0.23 |
| Restricted | 3.44 ± 0.16 | 1.80 ± 0.17 |

The data were obtained from 8 µg of RNA isolated from 18- month-old rats fed *ad libitum* or the restricted diet. The data represent the mean ± SE of four animals for each treatment. Using the Student's T-test, it was found that the level of Apo-AI mRNA was significantly different ($P < 0.05$) for rats fed *ad libitum* and the restricted diet.

relative levels of Apo-AI and Apo-B mRNA in RNA isolated from 18-month-old rats fed *ad libitum* or the restricted diet. The level of Apo-AI mRNA was 30% lower in liver tissue isolated from rats fed the restricted diet. Thus, dietary restriction appears to retard the age-related increase in the level of Apo-AI mRNA (Table 3). However, the level of Apo-B mRNA was essentially the same in liver tissue isolated from rats fed either *ad libitum* or the restricted diet. The data in Table 4 are interesting because the level of both Apo-AI and Apo-B mRNA increased between 6 and 24 months of age. In fact, Apo-B mRNA increased more with age than did Apo-AI mRNA (Table 3).

## DISCUSSION

The data reported herein conclusively demonstrate that gene expression at the level of transcription is altered by dietary restriction. The dramatic age-related decrease in the level of $\alpha_{2u}$-globulin mRNA was markedly reduced by dietary restriction. On the other hand, the age-related increase in

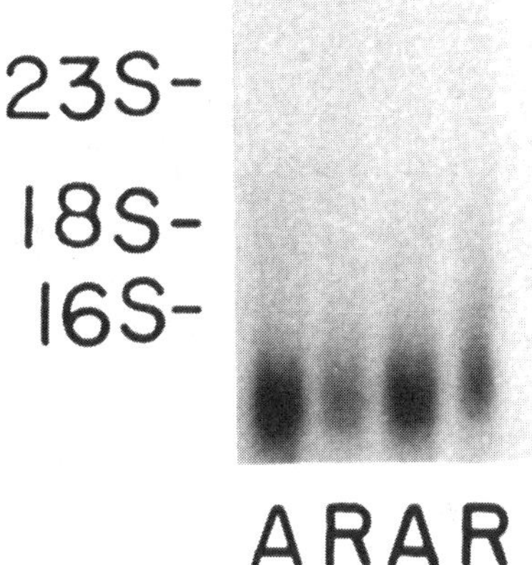


**Figure 6.** Autoradiogram of Northern Blot for Apo AI with RNA from Rats fed *ad libitum* and a Restricted Diet. RNA isolated from liver tissue obtained from 18-month-old rats fed *ad libitum* (A) or a restricted diet (R) was analyzed by a Northern blot as described in Figure 5. RNA was pooled from four rats for each experimental treatment. Two concentrations of RNA were used: 8 µg/ lane (two right lanes) and 16 µg/lane (two left lanes). The migration of rRNA standards is shown.

Apo-AI mRNA levels was retarded by dietary restriction. Thus, dietary restriction enhanced the level of an mRNA species that decreased with age and reduced the level of an mRNA species that increased with age. Although dietary restriction had a significant effect on the levels of $\alpha_{2u}$-globulin mRNA and Apo-AI mRNA, it had no effect on the levels of *c-myc* mRNA or Apo-B mRNA. Thus, the effect of dietary restriction on gene transcription is specific. In other words, not all mRNAs are affected. The selectivity of dietary restriction on mRNA expression shows that the changes in mRNA levels do not arise from general changes in transcription or RNA processing because changes at these levels would affect all mRNA species.

The data obtained in the experiments described herein are consistent with the following hypothesis: the mechanism underlying the increase in survival by dietary restriction involves alterations in gene expression. We have no evidence that the changes in gene expression, which arise through dietary restriction, are responsible for the increase in survival. However, it is reasonable to assume that changes in the transcription of certain genes, and concomitant changes in the levels of the proteins coded by the genes, could have a beneficial effect at the cellular level and consequently could enhance the survival of the organism. For example, dietary restriction has been shown

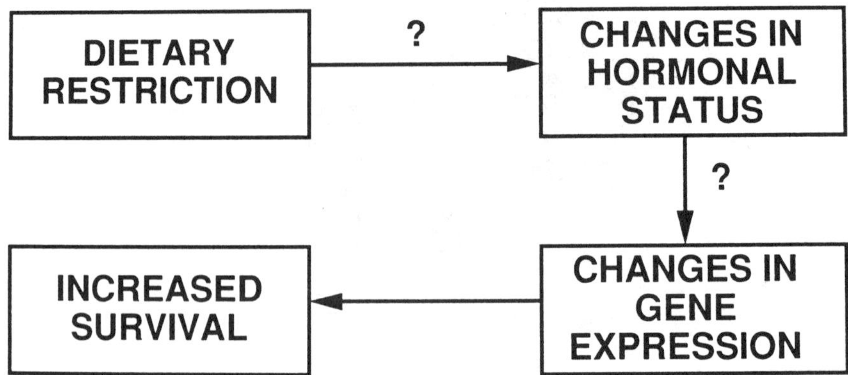


**Figure 7**. A Model Describing the Molecular Mechanism Responsible for Increased Survival by Dietary Restriction.

to increase the expression of several genes involved in free radical detoxification (Semsei and Richardson, 1986). Recently, Pahlavani *et al.* (1988) showed that dietary restriction increased the expression of interleukin-2 by spleen lymphocytes from old rats. Because interleukin-2 plays an essential role in the immune response (Gillis *et al.*, 1978), a change in the expression of interleukin-2 could be an important factor in the reduction of age-associated diseases by dietary restriction. Thus, the current evidence would be compatible with the hypothesis that alterations in gene expression are an important factor in the increase in survival observed for rodents fed calorie-restricted diets.

Although dietary restriction can alter gene expression at the level of transcription, the mechanism responsible for the alteration in gene expression is not known. In Figure 7, we present schematically a model of how dietary restriction might alter gene expression. We propose that dietary restriction alters the expression of specific genes by changing the overall hormonal status of an animal. This mechanism is plausible because research over the past two decades has shown that most hormones can induce or repress the expression of specific genes at the level of transcription. Our data would be consistent with this model. For example, the changes in $\alpha_{2u}$-globulin expression probably result from a change in the hormonal status of the animal because the expression of $\alpha_{2u}$-globulin is sensitive to regulation by a large number of hormones. However, more information is needed on the effect of dietary restriction on hormone levels to prove or disprove the mechanism presented in Figure 7.

Richardson and McCarter (1989) recently presented two models to describe how dietary restriction increases survival and retards the incidence of disease. First, as is generally accepted, dietary restriction would retard the rate of aging at the biological/physiological level. On the other hand, dietary restriction might not have any affect on the aging process or rate of aging. Instead, it would alter the physiological status of an organism in such a way that the levels of those biological processes are enhanced that play an essential role in survival. These models are termed the "rate model" and the "set point model," respectively. Although both models would explain the increased longevity that occurs with dietary restriction, the two models would have quite different consequences (Richardson and McCarter, 1989). For example, the short term affect of dietary restriction would be expected to be quite different for the two models. In the "rate model," dietary restriction would be expected to produce very little change in young rats that are on the restricted diet for a short time. In the "set point model" short term dietary restriction would be expected to produce major physiological changes. The research reported herein cannot prove or disprove either model. However, the effect of dietary restriction on the expression of $\alpha_{2u}$-globulin in young rats would be more compatible with the "set point model" than the "rate model."

## ACKNOWLEDGMENTS

This work was supported by grant AG 01548 from the National Institute on Aging. The authors thank the following investigators for generously supplying the following cDNA probes: $\alpha_{2u}$-globulin from Dr. Philip Fielgleson (Columbia University, New York, NY), c from Dr. Robert A. Weinberg (Whitehead Institute for Biomedical Research, Cambridge, MA), apolipoprotein AI from Dr. Jannette C. Miller (Roswell Park Memorial Institute, Buffalo, NY), and apolipoprotein B from Dr. Aldons J. Lusis (University of California, Los Angeles, CA).

## REFERENCES

ARCHER, T. K., TAM, S. P. and DEELEY, R. G. (1986) Kinetics of estrogen-dependent modulation of apolipoprotein AI synthesis in human hepatoma cells. *J. Biol. Chem.* **261**: 5067-5074.

ARMBRECHT, H. J., STRONG, R., BOLTZ, M., ROCCO, D., WOOD, W. G., and RICHARDSON, A. (1988) Modulation of age-related changes in serum 1,25-dihydroxyvitamin D and parathyroid hormone by dietary restriction of Fisher 344 rats. *J. Nutr.* **118**: 1360-1365.

BARROWS, C. H. (1972) Nutrition, aging and genetic program. *Am. J. Clin. Nutr.* **25**: 829

BERG, B. N. and SIMMS, H. S. (1960) Nutrition and longevity in the rat. II. Longevity and onset of disease with different levels of intake. *J. Nutr.* **71**: 255-263.

BERTRAND, H. A., LYND, F. T., MASORO, E. J. and YU, B. P. (1980) Changes in adipose mass and cellularity through the adult life of rats fed *ad libitum* or a life prolonging restricted diet. *J. Gerontol.* **35**: 827-835.

BIRCHENALL-SPARKS, M. C., ROBERTS, M. S., STAECKER, J., HARDWICK, J. P. and RICHARDSON, A. (1985) Effect of dietary restriction on liver protein synthesis in rats. *J. Nutr.* **115**: 944-950.

BIRNBOIM, H. C. and DOLY, J. (1979) A rapid alkaline extraction procedure for screening recombinant plasmid DNA. *Nuc. Acid Res.* **7**: 1513-1523.

BROWN, M. S. and GOLDSTEIN, J. L. (1976) Receptor mediated control of cholesterol metabolism. *Science* **191**: 150-154.

BROWN, N. S., KOVANEN, P. T. and GOLDSTEIN, J. L. (1981) Regulation of plasma cholesterol by lipoprotein receptors. *Science* **212**: 628-635.

CHIRGWIN, J. W., PRZYBYLA, A. E., MACDONALD, R. J. and RUTTER, W. J. (1979) Isolation of biologically active ribonucleic acid from sources enriched in ribonuclease. *Biochemistry* **18**: 5294-5299.

DUESBERG, P. H., BESTER, K. and VOGT. P. K. (1977) RNA of avian acute-leukemia virus MC29. *Proc. Natl. Acad. Sci. USA* **74**: 4320-4324.

EVA, A., ROBBINS, K. C., ANDERSON, P. R., SRINIVASAN, A., TRONICK, S. R., REDDY, E. P., ELLMORE, N. W., GALEN, A. T., LAUTENBERGER, J. A., PAPAS, T. S., WESTIN, E. H., WONG-STAAL, F., GALLO, R. C. and AARONSON, S. A. (1982) Cellular gene analogous to retroviral *onc* genes are transcribed in human-tumor cells. *Nature* **295**: 116-119.

FIELDING, C. J., SHORE, V. G. and FIELDING, P. E. (1972) A protein cofactor of lecithin: cholesterol acyltransferase. *Biochem. Biophys. Res. Comm.* **46**: 1493-1498.

GILLIS, S., FERM, M. M., OU, W. and SMITH, K. A. (1978) T-cell growth factor: parameters of production and quantitative microassay for activity. *J. Immunol.* **120**: 2027-2037.

GOYETTE, M., PETROPOULOS, C. J., SHANK, P. R. and FAUSTO, N. (1984) Regulated transcription of *c-Ki-ris* and *c-myc* during compensatory growth of rat liver. *Mol. Cell. Biol.* **4**: 1493- 1498.

GLUECK, C. J., GARTSIDE, P., FALLAT, R. W., SIELSKI, J. and STEINER, P. M. (1976) Longevity syndromes: familial hypobeta and familial hyperalpha lipoproteinemia. *J. Lab. Clin. Med.* **88**: 941-957.

HARRISON, D. E., ARCHER, J. R. and ASTOLE, C. M. (1984) Effects of food restriction on aging: separation of food intakes and adiposity. *Proc. Natl. Acad. Sci. USA* **81**: 1835-1838.

HAMSTEN, A., ISELIUS, L., DAHLEN, G. and DE FAIRE, U. (1986) Genetic and cultural inheritance of serum lipids, low and high density lipoprotein cholesterol and serum apolipoproteins A-I, A-II and B. *Atherosclerosis* **60**: 199-208.

HEISS, G. and TYROLER, H. A. (1982) **In:** *Proceedings of the Workshop on Apolipoprotein Quantifications.* pp. 7-24. NIH - DHHS Publication No. (NIH)83-1266. Bethesda, MD: U.S. Government Printing Office.

HORIKAWA, S., SAKATA, K., HATANAKA, M. and TSUKADA, K. (1986) Expression of *c-myc* oncogene in rat liver by a dietary manipulation. *Biochem. Biophys. Res. Comm.* **140**: 574-580.

HUANG, L. S., BACK, S. C., FEINSTEIN, S. I. and BRESLOW, J. L. (1985) Human apolipoprotein B cDNA clone isolation and demonstration that liver apolipoprotein B mRNA is 22 kilobases in length. *Proc. Natl. Acad. Sci. USA* **82**: 6825-6829.

INNERARITY, T. L. and MAHLEY, R. W. (1978) Enhanced binding by cultured human fibroblasts of Apo-E-containing lipoproteins as compared with low density lipoproteins. *Biochemistry* **17**: 1440-1447.

KANE, J. P. (1983) Apolipoprotein B: Structural and metabolic heterogeneity. *Ann. Rev. Physiol.* **45**: 637-650.

KANE, J. P., HARDMAN, D. A. and PAULUS, H. E. (1980) Heterogeneity of apolipoprotein B: isolation of a new species from human chylomicrons. *Proc. Natl. Acad. Sci. USA* **77**: 2465-2469.

KELLY, K., COCHRAN, B. H., STILES, C. H. and LEDER, P. (1983) Cell specific regulation of *c-myc* gene by lymphocyte mitogens and platelet derived growth factor. *Cell* **35**: 603-610.

KULKARNI, A. B., GUBITS, R. M. and FEIGELSON, P. (1985) Developmental and hormonal regulation of $\alpha_{2u}$-globulin gene transcription. *Proc. Natl. Acad. Sci. USA* **82**: 2579-2582.

LAND, H., PARADA, L. F. and WEINBERG, R. A. (1983) Tumorigenic conversion of primary embryo fibroblasts requires at least two cooperation oncogenes. *Nature* **304**: 596-602.

LINDELL, T. J. (1982) Molecular aspects of dietary modulation of transcription and enhanced longevity. *Life Sciences* **31**: 625

LUSIS, A. J., WEST, R., MEHRABIAN, M., REUBEN, M. A., LEBOEUF, R. C., KAPTEIN, J. S., JOHNSON, D. F., SCHUMAKER, V. N., YUHASZ, M. P., SCHOTZ, M. C. and ELOVSON, J. (1985) Cloning and expression of apolipoprotein B, the major protein of low and very low density lipoproteins. *Proc. Natl. Acad. Sci. USA* **82**: 4597-4601.

MAEDA, H., GLEISER, C. A., MASORO, E. J., MURATA, I., McMAHAN, C. A., and YU, B. P. (1985) Nutritional influences on aging of Fischer 344 rats: II. Pathology. *J. Gerontol.* **40**: 671-688.

MANIATIS, T., FRITSCH, E. F. and SAMBROCK. (1982) *Molecular Cloning: A Laboratory Manual.* New York: Cold Spring Harbor Laboratory.

MANIATIS, T., JEFFEREY, A. and KLEID, D. G. (1975) Nucleotide sequence of the rightward operator of phage A. *Proc. Natl. Acad. Sci.* **72**: 1184-1188.

MASORO, E. J. (1988) Food restriction in rodents: an evaluation of its role in the study of aging. *J. Gerontol. Bio. Sc.* **43**: B59-B64.

MATOCHA, M. F., COSGROVE, J. W., ATACK, J. R. and RAPAPORT, S. I. 1987. Selective elevation of *c-myc* transcript levels in the liver of the aging Fischer-344 rat. *Biochem. Biophys. Res. Comm.* **147**: 1-7.

McCARTER, R., MASORO, E. J. and YU, B. P. (1985) Does food restriction retard aging by reducing the metabolic rate? *Am. J. Physiol.* **248**: E488-E490.

McCAY, C., CROWELL, M. and MAYNARD, L. (1935) The effect of retarded growth upon the length of life and upon ultimate size. *J. Nutr.* **10**: 63-79.

MELTON, D. A., KIREG, P. A., REBAGLIATI, M. R., MANIATIS, T., ZINN, K. and GREEN, M. R. (1984) Efficient *in vitro* synthesis of biologically active RNA and RNA hybridization probes from plasmids containing a bacteriophage SP6 promoter. *Nuc. Acid Res.* **12**: 7035-7055.

MILLER, J. C., BARTH, R. K., SHAW, P. H., ELLIOT, R. W. and HASTIE, N. D. (1983) Identification of a cDNA clone for mouse apoprotein A-1 (apo A-1) and its use in characterization of apo A-1 mRNA expression in liver and small intestine. *Proc. Natl. Acad. Sci. USA* **80**: 1511-1515.

NILSON-EHLE, P., GARFINKEL, A. S. and SCHOTZ, M. D. (1980) Lipolytic enzymes and plasma lipoprotein metabolism. *Ann. Rev. Biochem.* **49**: 667-693.

PAHLAVANI, M. A., CHEUNG, H. T., CAI, N. S. and RICHARDSON, A. (1988) Influence of dietary restriction and aging on gene expression in the immune system of rats. In: *Biomedical Advances in Aging.* (In Press), (Ed. A. L. Goldstein), New York: Plenum Publishing Corp.

PERSSON, H. and LEDER, P. (1984) Nuclear location and DNA binding properties of a protein expressed by human *c-myc* oncogene. *Science* **225**: 718-721.

RICHARDSON, A. (1981) The relationship between aging and protein synthesis. In: *Biochemistry in Aging.* (Ed. J. R. Florini), pp. 79-101. Boca Raton: CRC Press.

RICHARDSON, A. and BIRCHENALL-SPARKS, M. C. (1983) Age-related changes in protein synthesis. In: *Review of Biological Research in Aging.* Vol. 1. (Ed. M. Rothstein), pp. 255-273. New York: Alan R. Liss, Inc.

RICHARDSON, A., BIRCHENALL-SPARKS, M. C. and STAECKER, J. L. (1983) Aging and transcription. In: *Review of Biological Research in Aging.* Vol. 1. (Ed. M. Rothstein), pp. 275-294. New York: Alan R. Liss, Inc.

RICHARDSON, A., BUTLER, J. A., RUTHERFORD, M. S., SEMSEI, I., GU, M. Z., FERNAN-DES, G. and CHIANG, W. H. (1987) Effect of age and dietary restriction on the expression of $\alpha_{2u}$-globulin. *J. Biol. Chem.* **262**: 12821-12825.

RICHARDSON, A. and CHEUNG, H. T. (1982) The relationship between age-related changes in gene expression, protein turnover, and the responsiveness of an organism to stimuli. *Life Sciences* **31**: 605-613.

RICHARDSON, A. and SEMSEI, I. (1987) Effect of aging on translation and transcription. In: *Review of Biological Research in Aging.* Vol. 3. (ed. M. Rothstein), pp. 467-483. New York: Alan R. Liss, Inc.

RICHARDSON, A. and McCARTER, R. (1989) Mechanism of food restriction: Change of rate or change of set point? In: *The Potential for Nutritional Modulation of the Aging Processes.* (Eds. D. K. Ingram, G. T. Baker, N. W. Shock), in press. West Point: Food and Nutrition Press.

RICKETTS, W. G., BIRCHENALL-SPARKS, M. C., HARDWICK, J. P. and RICHARDSON, A. (1985) Effect of age and dietary restriction on protein synthesis by isolated kidney cells. *J. Cell Physiol.* **125**: 492-498.

ROY, A. K. (1973) Androgen-dependent synthesis of $\alpha_{2u}$-globulin in the rat: role of the pituitary gland. *J. Endocrinol.* **56**: 295- 301.

ROY, A. K. and LEONARD, S. (1973) Androgen-dependent synthesis of $\alpha_{2u}$-globulin in diabetic rats: the role of insulin. *J. Endocrinol.* **57**: 327-328.

ROY, A. K., McMINN, D. M. and BISWAS, N. M. (1975) Estrogenic inhibition of the hepatic synthesis of $\alpha_{2u}$-globulin in the rat. *Endocrinology* **97**: 1501-1508.

ROY, A. K., NATH, T. S., MOTWANI, N. M. and CHATTERJEE, B. (1983) Age dependent regulation of the polymorphic forms of $\alpha_{2u}$-globulin. *J. Biol. Chem.* **258**: 10123-10127.

ROY, A. K. and NEUHAUS, O. W. (1967) Androgenic control of a sex-dependent protein in the rat. *Nature* **214**: 618-620.

RUTHERFORD, H. S., BAEHLER, C. S. and RICHARDSON, A. (1986) Genetic expression of complement factors and $a_1$ acid glycoproteins by liver tissue during senescence. *Mech. Aging Dev.* **35**: 245- 254.

SACHER, G. A. (1977) Life table modifications and life prolongation. In: *Handbook of the Biology of Aging* (Eds. C. E. Finch and L. Hayflick), pp. 582-638. New York: Van Nostrand Reinhold.

SEMSEI, I. and RICHARDSON, A. (1986) Effect of age on expression of genes involved in free radical protection. *Federation Proceedings* **45**: 1543.

SHEINESS, D. K., HUGHES, S. H., VARMERS, H. E., STUBBLEFIELD, E. and BISHOP, J. M. (1980) The veritable homolog of the putative transforming gene of avian myelocytomatosis virus: characteristics of the DNA locus and its RNA transcript. *Virology* **105**: 415-424.

SOUTHERN, E. M. (1975) Detection of specific sequences among DNA fragments separated by gel electrophoresis. *J. Mol. Biol.* **98**: 503-517.

STEIN, O., VANDERHOECK, J. and STEIN, Y. (1976) Cholesterol content and sterol synthesis in human skin fibroblasts and rat aortic smooth muscle cells exposed to lipoprotein-depleted serum and high density apolipoprotein/phospholipid mixtures. *Biochem. Biophys. Acta.* **431**: 347-358.

THOMAS, P. S. (1980) Hybridization of denatured RNA and small DNA fragments transferred to nitrocellulose. *Proc. Natl. Acad. Sci. USA* **77**: 5201-5205.

WARD, W. F. (1988) Enhancement by food restriction of liver protein synthesis in aging Fischer 344 rat. *J. Gerontol. Biol. Sci.* **43**: B50-B53.

WEINDURCH, R. and WALFORD, R. L. (1982) Dietary restriction in mice beginning at 1 year of age: effect on life-span and spontaneous cancer incidence. *Science* **215**: 1415-1418.

WEISS, R. A., TEICH, N. M. and COFFIN, J. M. (1982) *The Molecular Biology of Tumor Viruses: RNA Tumor Viruses. New York: Cold Spring Harbor Laboratory.*

YU, B. P., MASORO, E. J. and McMAHAN, C. A. (1985) Nutritional influences on aging of Fischer 344 rats. I. Physical metabolic and longevity characteristics. *J. Gerontol.* **40**: 657-670.

# 16

## COMMENTARY - NATURAL SELECTION FOR EXTENDED LONGEVITY FROM FOOD RESTRICTION

David E. Harrison and Jonathan R. Archer

(From : *Growth, Development and Aging* **52**: 65
(1988); **53**: 3 (1989), reproduced with permission)

The only treatment that consistently retards aging in mammals is nutritional manipulation, food or caloric restriction. Providing malnutrition is avoided, it extends lifespans of laboratory mice and rats (McCay *et al.*, 1939; Ross 1976; Weindruch *et al.*, 1986). Knowledge of how food restriction retards aging processes might suggest clinically useful treatments.

How did mice and rats develop the ability to retard aging rates when food is in short supply? An essential clue is the general observation that maximum female reproductive lifespans in most species of mammals are about half of the maximum lifespans. Thus there may be important linkages between the mechanisms controlling female reproductive lifespan and those controlling longevity.

Natural selection acts strongly on mechanisms of reproduction. Imagine the enormous selective advantage of mice that could respond to a drought, or other long-term condition that severely reduced food supplies, by delaying reproductive senescence. After a drought outlasting the maximum female reproductive lifespan, a surviving female that is still able to reproduce could repopulate huge areas once weather conditions and food supplies became favorable. Survivors lacking the food restriction response would have reached female reproductive senescence before food supplies became adequate to raise offspring. In this scenario, the reproductive periods of the most long-lived survivors would be the most important, and they might approach, or at least be proportional to, maximum reproductive lifespans in the laboratory.

We hypothesize that the beneficial effects of food restriction on longevities evolved due to the selective advantages for females whose reproductive lifespans were extended by food restriction. This hypothesis predicts that the beneficial effects of food restriction will be greater in species with shorter female reproductive lifespans. This is required because selective pressure for mechanisms that prolong life in response to food restriction is greater for species with shorter reproductive lifespans. The shorter such lifespans are the more droughts would outlast maximum reproductive lifespans.

We believe that this is a unique prediction. It has not yet been tested adequately due to difficulties in doing comparative longevity experiments with long-lived mammals. If it is true, the specific treatment of food restriction would have little beneficial effect on human longevity. However, studies of the underlying mechanisms by which food restriction retards aging in short-lived species would be highly relevant to human health, if the same mechanisms retard aging in man.

A comparison between two types of mice suggests a feasible test of our hypothesis. Sacher and Hart (1978) recommended comparative studies of the two mouse species *Mus musculus* and *Peromyscus leucopus* because the latter live about twice as long as the former, despite their similar sizes and metabolic rates. Our hypothesis predicts that food restriction will have significantly less benefit for *Peromyscus* mice because their female reproductive lifespans are already twice as long as those of *Mus* mice.

This leads to another related hypothesis. We suggest that the same selective pressures that caused prolonged lifespans in response to food restriction in *Mus*, also caused the extremely long lifespan potential in *Peromyscus*. Thus there might be two ways to survive droughts longer than the normal female reproductive period and retain the ability to reproduce. One was to increase maximum potential longevities in response to food restriction. The other, taken by *Peromyscus* mice, was to increase longevities in general, whether or not there is food restriction.

If the above hypotheses are correct, they lead to two important consequences: (i). Female reproductive senescence is regulated by at least some of the same mechanisms that control longevity, and thus is a good model for studies of aging. (ii). The degree of genetic change required to extend longevity in response to food restriction may be similar to that required to extend longevity in general, since at least one species, *Peromyscus*, adapted using the more general mechanism.

## REFERENCES

McKAY, C. M., MAYNARD, L. A., SPERLING, G., and BARNES, L. L. (1939) Retarded growth, life span, ultimate body size and age changes in the albino rat after feeding diets restricted in calories. *J. Nutr.* **18**: 1-13

ROSS, M. H. (1976) Nutrition and longevity in experimental animals. **In**: *Nutrition and Aging*. (Ed. M. Winick), pp. 43-57. New York: Wiley.

SACHER, G. A. and HART, R. W. (1978) Longevity, aging and comparative cellular and molecular biology of the house mouse, *Mus musculus*, and the white-footed mouse, *Peromyscus leucopus. Birth Defects: Orig. Article Series* **14**: 71-96

WEINDRUCH, R., WALFORD, R. L., FLIGIEL, S., GUTHRIE, D. (1986) The retardation of aging in mice by dietary restriction: Longevity, cancer, immunity and lifetime energy intake. *J. Nutr.* **116**: 641-654

# Section 4

## STRAIN AND MUTANT EFFECTS ON NEUROENDOCRINE AND IMMUNE AGING

# 17

# RATE OF OCCURRENCE OF LESIONS IN 20 INBRED AND HYBRID GENOTYPES OF RATS AND MICE SACRIFICED AT 6 MONTH INTERVALS DURING THE FIRST YEARS OF LIFE

Roderick T.Bronson

## ABSTRACT

A wide variety of lesions occurs in rats and mice during the life span. Many of these have not been categorized and their various rates of occurrence with respect to age, sex and genotype have not been well studied. This paper is an analysis of data from a comprehensive histopathologic examination of all tissues from 1562 normal mice of 11 genotypes and from 518 normal rats of 8 genotypes, sacrificed when healthy at approximate 6 month intervals from 1 to 24 and 30 months of age, respectively. The animals were housed under conventional, non-barrier conditions. The mean age of the mice was 14.1 months; for rats it was 19.4 months. The more numerous genotypes of mice studied included C57 BL/6 (465), BALB/c (269), CBA/CaH (108), CFW (77), CB6F1 (239) and B6D2F1 (108). The rats were of several inbred and hybrid genotypes, including Fischer 344, Buffalo, Wistar-Lewis and Brown Norway and the F1 cross between F-344 females and males of the other genotypes. Approximately 70 rats of each genotype were studied. Altogether 186 separate lesions were observed in the mice, including 23 types of neoplasms. Lesions such as amyloidosis, lymphoid nodules and various kinds of inflammation were observed in many organs. Some of these lesions may have been due to incidental viral and bacterial infections present in the animals from time to time. The rate of occurrence of lesions varied markedly between genotypes but not between the sexes. In the rats 178 lesions were observed, including 35 types of neoplasms. Of these, many were adenomas of endocrine glands. Various inflammatory lesions were quite common. Radiculoneuropathy, retinal atrophy, degenerative glomerulonephropathy and myocardial degeneration were very common age-related lesions in most genotypes. Brown Norway and BN × F344 hybrids had significantly fewer lesions than did albino genotypes. The total number of lesions present in both species increased with age. This paper is an initial attempt at formulating a strict classification of lesions in aging rats and mice.

## INTRODUCTION

This paper is offered as a contribution to the Gerontology of rodents. It describes the morphologically apparent processes, lesions, that were observed in some 2000 rodents killed at fixed time points throughout the first portion of their life spans. It is a data base to be used by investigators who use such animals in research and wonder what abnormal processes may be going on in them. To understand the complex data to be presented, some issues must be considered.

As animals age they are affected by deleterious structural and functional processes. Ordinarily, some are viewed as normal concommitants of the aging process; others are viewed as disease processes not necessarily related to aging. The distinction tends to be based on 1. the effects of the change on morbidity and mortality, 2. its prevalence in the population, and 3. whether it is ordinarily presumed to be preventable. Thus cancer is considered an abnormal process since it causes severe morbidity and mortality, affects many but not all individuals, and is often considered preventable through changes in life style. Greying of hair is usually considered normal since it is of only cosmetic importance, is nearly universal, and is usually accepted as inevitable. This distinction is obviously arbitrary, self-serving, and of little biological validity. It really depends on the setting in which the change occurs. A 10% reduction in physical stamina, which most people would accept as normal aging in humans, might be as fatal as cancer in a migrating bird. A reasonable approach to describing the processes of aging, then, is to report them all, regardless of their emotional or apparent health significance.

Most, or arguably all, changes in structural and functional parameters that deviate from values measured in robust young adults can be considered lesions. Lesions differ from one another conceptually only in that some are worse than others, some have a greater variability in prevalence than others and some can be modified in expression more than others by genetic and environmental factors. Aging can be defined, then, as the progressive accumulation of lesions, leading inevitably to increased morbidity and death. Aging is not a disease. The term "disease" is clinically useful, being a set of clinical, pathologic, epidemiologic, etiologic and other factors that accompany one another and are recognized for diagnostic, therapeutic and prognostic purposes. A disease itself is never directly observable or measurable; only the structural and functional abnormalities, the lesions that comprise it, can be observed and evaluated.

The theoretical difference between "mechanism" and "process" as they relate to aging is important here. One must discover and characterize a process before it is possible to study its mechanism. Mechanisms explain the causation and course of development of processes. Lesions are processes, and each has its own mechanism. Some lesions and their mechanisms have been quite thoroughly studied, because they are important lesions of man. Atherosclerosis is an example. Other lesions are less well characterized. What about "aging" itself? Aging is not a single process; it is comprised of many processes. Its processes are lesions, each with its own mechanism. Aging itself, being simply the summation of many deleterious processes resulting from innately imperfect homeostatic and repair mechanisms, has no mechanism of its own.

If one sacrifices many animals assumed to be healthy at various time points during life (a cross sectional study), as was done here, and studies all tissues grossly and microscopically, one is certain to find lesions. (One will not observe diseases.) More lesions of more kinds will be present in older than in younger animals. In some animals potentially fatal lesions in an early stage of development will be found. Since most animals in such studies can be presumed to be clinically healthy, there may be no functional organic change associated with the lesions. Similar lesions will be present in animals studied after spontaneous death (a longitudinal experiment), though usually one or more advanced lesions will be present that can be presumed to have killed. "Incidental lesions", those presumed by pathologists not to have participated in the fatality, will also be found. They are entirely analogous to all of the lesions observed in cross sectional studies.

Lesions, both structural and functional, can be classified into two groups. Some occur suddenly, progress rapidly and either kill, regress completely or leave various kinds of scars. Infectious and traumatic lesions tend to have this pattern, but genetic lesions could have the same pattern. Others develop slowly, becoming more and more severe as life progresses. The classic degenerative lesions of aging, such as wrinkled skin, follow this pattern. These lesions should not be expected necessarily to progress linearly with time. Some may progress rapidly and then level off for example. Others may eventually kill unless the individual dies from something else first. Nor should lesions be expected to begin at any one time in life. Some may begin in youth, others in midlife and still others late in life.

In considering the lesions observed in aging animals there is an under-standable tendency to want to distinguish "environmental" and "genetic" lesions from "aging" ones. Indeed, considerable amounts of money have been spent to raise experimental rodents under conditions of environmental uniformity, free from pathogens, to insure that most lesions will not be environmentally determined. Removing genetic lesions is much more difficult, and perhaps impossible, since aging may be closely bound up with genetically controlled mechanisms. Often in experimental gerontology one attempts to control genetic variability, but not genetic factors, by using inbred genotypes or the F1 hybrid offspring of two inbred genotypes. Under these admittedly unnatural conditions, each genotype represents one genetic individual replicated many times; another genotype represents another genetic individual replicated many times. One expects that this disadvantage of unnaturalness is outweighed by gains in reduced variability between animals. In fact, however, there remains a disconcerting variability in the rate of occurrence and severity of lesions between individuals even of the same genotype, as is apparent in the data to be presented here. Some of these variably expressed phenotypic traits in mice have been listed by Staats (1985), but no definitive compilation of such lesions in rats and mice is available at this time.

It is not clear where this variability comes from, particularly in animals maintained under environmental conditions which are assumed to be uniform. Possibly the conditions are not really uniform. Pathogens are often present despite precautions, as occurred in the colonies of animals studied for this paper. Animals are housed in different places in the room; group housed animals stand in various places in the dominance order. Maternal factors such as the birth order of infants in a litter and the supply of milk might result in variation between individuals of the same litter and of different litters.

There may be genetic as well as environmental reasons for variability within a genotype. First, some degree of residual heterozygosity may be present in inbred genotypes. Second, even in genetically uniform animals, some phenotypic traits may be expressed variably as a function of an intrinsic threshold mechanism. When the threshold is exceeded the trait is expressed. Whether the threshold is exceeded or not is presumed to be dependent on environmental factors, but pure chance might be proposed as a factor. Indeed, contemporary genetic theory does admit the role of random chance in the determination of phenotype, in addition to nature and nurture (Suzuki *et al.*, 1986).

We have considered the problems of variability within a genotype in the rate of occurrence of lesions. These problems are exacerbated when one studies the pathology of aging in various genotypes of one or several species, as will be shown in the data included in this paper. Some lesions occur in all genotypes of a species, but with variable rates of occurrence. Others, for which there is no evidence of single gene control, occur in one or in several, but not in others. Between-species variability is much more extreme; some lesions may be very common in one species and rare or non-existent in another. The pathology of aging differs in most details even between quite closely related species such as rats and mice. Bewildering variability, apparently due to genetics, predominates. What one supposes to be "aging" lesions are often not shared by inbred genotypes within one species and are rarely shared between species. Different genotypes and different species seem to have entirely different patterns of functional and structural deterioration as they age. And even genetically uniform animals raised under very uniform condition can differ from one another profoundly as they age. A tentative way of distinguishing genetic, environmental and age-related lesions can be proposed. Within a species, any lesion that occurs in one or more genotypes but not in others, maintained under any or most environmental conditions, can be designated as a "genetic" lesion. Any lesion that occurs in all or most genotypes maintained under one set of environmental conditions but not under another can be designated an "environmental lesion". Any lesion that occurs in all or most genotypes of a species regardless of genotype and under all normal environmental conditions can be designated as an "age- related" lesion.

Actually, one should not expect that such clear distinctions could be made easily. Some "genetic lesions", requiring a certain environmental threshold to be exceeded for their phenotypic expression, could not be distinguished easily from purely "environmental lesions". Certainly, no matter how good these above stated rules hold for one species, there is no certainty that data generated from study of one species will hold for another. It should be added that this reductive exclusionary process of designating all lesions as "age-related" if they do not fall into "genetic" or "environmental" classes, begs a major question. If they truly can be shown not to have a causation in nature or nurture, where do they come from? If there is no causality outside of nature and nurture, anything that happens outside of the controls of knowable genetic and environmental mechanisms is purely accidental or chaotic. This is scientifically abhorrent, except, perhaps, to "chaosists". Yet, one must not, for that reason alone, refuse to consider that some or many of the lesions of aging may, in fact, be the result simply of failed control mechanisms. Thus the true lesions of aging may have no mechanisms at all, since the very term "mechanism" implies organization, control, regulation, homeostasis, positive feed back etc.

True age-related lesions may be uncaused; they may result only from chaos, an absence of any controlling mechanism.

Several practical problems are encountered in the analysis of lesions seen in animals throughout the lifespan. Many lesions occur sporadically at low rates of occurrence, as will be shown. Some investigators of a reductionist bent might be tempted to ignore such lesions as simple noise. However, altogether they constitute quite a large number of events that occur during aging and they cannot be ignored arbitrarily only because they individually occur infrequently. Including them in a data base, admittedly, is difficult since one must report a plethora of seemingly trivial random events. The low number of each such lesion makes its statistical analysis unrewarding, even when quite large numbers of animals are included in the study. In this paper all lesions are included regardless of their rates of occurrence in order that the full range of lesions can be appreciated.

Another practical problem one must confront in such studies is that of classifying lesions. As will be shown, both rats and mice have approximately 200 possible spontaneous lesions. Some of the lesions, particularly neoplasms, have been described and many references are included in the bibliography to this paper. However, many of the less interesting ones have not. Only recently have there been attempts to classify all of the lesions of rats and mice (Jones, Mohr & Hunt, 1983, 1985a, 1985b, 1986, 1987, 1988, 1989; Frith & Ward, 1988; Burek, 1978), although many hundreds of thousands of rodents have been studied by pathologists in the course of toxicologic evaluations of drugs and chemicals.

Most such toxicological investigations are designed to answer specific questions about the particular agent being studied. The emphasis of long term studies has been on the potential carcinogenicity of the tested agent, hence neoplasms have received most attention. Each investigation has stood alone, with no particular reason to use terms that are consistent between studies. This is revealed in a recent compilation of pathology data of control animals used in many such studies (Altman, 1985).

Most toxicologic studies have been considered proprietary information, not available to the scientific community. An outstanding exception to this is the "megamouse" $ED_{01}$ study (Cairns, 1980). In many such studies, minor common lesions observed in both control and experimental animals are ignored. This is satisfactory for toxicology but not for gerontology, which comprises all life processes, no matter how trivial they may seem. The classification presented here is an attempt to design a comprehensive classification of all the lesions of laboratory rats and mice that occur during the greater part of the life span.

The study has an important limitation intrinsic to all cross sectional studies. The true rate of occurrence of some important lesions in an age cohort of animals cannot be reflected in data derived from such studies. Consider a lesion that develops and kills rapidly. Some animals sacrificed at, say, 18 months of age will have the lesion. But others, even many others, may have died with the lesion at 16 or 17 months old and still others may die at 19 and 20 months old. Only by combining data from animals that have died in the period before and after each cross sectional time point can one derive a reasonable estimate of the rate of occurrence of the lesion. This was not done in this study and is seldom done in cross sectional studies. An example of an under-represented fatal lesion of mice and rats is thrombosis of the atria of the heart, quite commonly observed in previously reported longitudinal studies (Yunis *et al.*, 1984) but not observed here.

This raises the issue of how data are to be presented. Strictly speaking, in epidemiological parlance, "prevalence" refers to the number of all cases of a disease extant at any one time divided by the total population at risk, and "incidence" refers to the total of all new cases diagnosed in any period divided by the total population at risk. Neither term applies to data on lesions derived from cross sectional studies, so the term "occurrence rate" is used here. It simply refers to the number of animals with the lesion divided by the total number of animals of like kind or of all kinds in the sacrificed sample. No assumptions can be made necessarily as to what is happening in the animals that are still living, nor is the number of such animals relevant. The extent to which the occurrence rate of a lesion in the sample represents that of the group and thereby becomes more like the true prevalence depends on how large the sample is, how common the lesion is and how long it persists. The larger the sample, the more common the lesion and the longer it persists the more representative is the sample of the lesion's true prevalence in the population.

## MATERIALS AND METHODS

The animals studied here were bred and maintained at the Charles River Breeding Laboratory, South Wilmington, Massacchussetts for the National Institute on Aging of the National Institutes of Health. They were multiply, polycarbonate caged virgin males and females, fed Purina rodent chow 5012 pelleted rations, bedded on hardwood shavings and maintained under putative barrier conditions. Periodically during the 6 year long period, 1978 through 1983, mice of various genotypes, ages and sexes were selected from the colonies and sent, live, to the Tufts Veterinary Diagnostic Laboratory, Boston for comprehensive disease surveillance for pathogenic microorganisms and complete pathologic analysis. The rats were not studied for disease surveillance purposes but rather to characterize the lesions of aging in certain genotypes.

Table 1 lists all 1577 mice studied. They were of 5 inbred genotypes: A/HeNNia (A/He), BALB/cNNia (C), C57BL/6NNia (B6), CBA/CaHNNia (CBA/C) and DBA/2NNia (D2); two congenic genotypes: B10.129/JNNia (B10) and CBA/CaHNNia-T6; an outbred stock, Crl:COBS® CFW® (CFW); three hybrid stocks: C57BL/6NNia × C3H/NNia (B6C3), C57BL/6NNia × DBA/2NNia (B6D2) and Balb/cNNia × C57BL/6NNia (CB6). Some mice with an outbred albino background were homozygous for the nude gene (nu/nu). Although some genotypes were represented by a relatively small number of mice, data were available and are included here for comparative purposes. Most mice were 6, 12, 18, and 24 months old. Some 341 were sacrificed at odd times, usually one or, rarely, two months before or after the usual 6 month intervals. Mice of these age groups were grouped with the animals killed at 6 month intervals, on the assumption that variation of one or rarely two months to either side of the 6 month interval would not be significant. The mean age and standard deviation of mice of each genotype and of the overall sample are also given.

Table 2 lists the 518 rats of 8 genotypes studied. Two strains of Brown Norway rats were studied, one from the National Institutes of Health (BN) and one from the Institute for Experimental Gerontology, Rifswijk, The Netherlands (BN/Biry). Three other inbred genotypes were studied: Fischer 344 rats of the specific genotype, COBS® CDF® F344/Crl (F344), Buffalo (Buf) and Wistar-Lewis (Lewis). The study included $F_1$ hybrids of crosses between F344 female rats and male Buf, Lewis and BN rats. The table shows that some genotypes were under-represented at some ages. Only two genotypes were represented at 36 months of age, BN/Biry and Lewis.

All animals were sampled in approximately the same way. After deep surgical anesthesia was induced by intraperitoneal injection of sodium pentobarbitol, blood samples were taken before sacrifice for serological analysis of possible viral pathogens. Samples from the rats were taken for complete blood count and serum chemistry analysis. Nasopharyngeal washes and ceca were cultured for pathologic bacteria and mycoplasma, and ceca and perineum were examined for metazoal parasites such as pinworms. After sacrifice by exsanguination, the animals were thoroughly dissected. Gross lesions were described and representative samples of lesions and organs were sampled, fixed in 10% neutral buffered formalin, embedded in paraffin, sectioned and stained with hematoxylin and eosin. Organs sampled included lungs, heart, thymus, spleen, lymph nodes, kidneys, urinary bladder, liver, colon, pancreas, thyroid-esophagus-trachea in one section often including

**Table 1.** Genotypes, ages and sexes of mice used in pathology characterization study

| Genotype | Age in Months | | | | | | | | | | | Mean Age ± S.D. | | |
| | 6 | | 12 | | 18 | | 24 | | Totals | | Grand | | | |
| | M | F | M | F | M | F | M | F | M | F | Total | M | F | Total |
|---|---|---|---|---|---|---|---|---|---|---|---|---|---|---|
| A/He | 9 | 15 | 9 | 9 | 9 | 9 | 11 | 7 | 38 | 40 | 78 | 15.69 ± 7.16 | 12.92 ± 6.86* | 14.31 ± 7.01 |
| Balb/c | 64 | 17 | 50 | 11 | 52 | 5 | 59 | 11 | 225 | 44 | 269 | 14.92 ± 6.96 | 13.50 ± 7.43* | 14.59 ± 7.20 |
| B6C3F1 | 6 | 0 | 6 | 0 | 8 | 0 | 6 | 0 | 26 | 0 | 26 | – | - | 15.23 ± 7.56 |
| B6D2F1 | 18 | 18 | 6 | 18 | 12 | 12 | 12 | 12 | 48 | 60 | 108 | 13.80 ± 6.77 | 14.00 ± 7.03 | 14.00 ± 7.55 |
| B10.129 | 6 | 6 | 6 | 6 | 6 | 6 | 8 | 5 | 26 | 23 | 49 | 14.18 ± 6.72 | 15.00 ± 6.93 | 15.18 ± 7.16 |
| C57BL/6 | 116 | 40 | 94 | 34 | 63 | 30 | 68 | 20 | 341 | 124 | 465 | 13.50 ± 6.83 | 13.60 ± 6.82 | 13.46 ± 6.94 |
| CBA/CaH | 18 | 18 | 18 | 6 | 12 | 12 | 18 | 6 | 66 | 42 | 108 | 14.72 ± 7.28 | 13.50 ± 6.68 | 14.00 ± 6.86 |
| CBA/CaH-T6 | 6 | 6 | 6 | 6 | 9 | 6 | 5 | 5 | 26 | 23 | 49 | 15.00 ± 6.91 | 14.61 ± 6.70 | 14.75 ± 6.60 |
| CB6F1 | 65 | 0 | 63 | 0 | 54 | 0 | 57 | 0 | 239 | 0 | 239 | - | - | 14.59 ± 6.63 |
| CFW | 13 | 5 | 6 | 11 | 8 | 10 | 4 | 20 | 31 | 46 | 77 | 12.37 ± 6.74 | 17.87 ± 6.39* | 15.74 ± 7.11+ |
| DBA/2 | 24 | 12 | 18 | 6 | 6 | 5 | 7 | 6 | 55 | 29 | 84 | 11.33 ± 6.07 | 13.20 ± 7.24* | 12.07 ± 6.50+ |
| nu/nu | 7 | 0 | 7 | 0 | 7 | 0 | 4 | 0 | 25 | 0 | 25 | - | - | 13.92 ± 6.41 |
| Totals | 352 | 137 | 289 | 107 | 246 | 95 | 259 | 92 | 1146 | 431 | 1577 | 14.13 ± 6.91 | 13.98 ± 7.12 | 14.06 ± 6.86 |

*The mean age of the males and females of the genotype differed significantly, P < 0.05

+ The mean age of all mice of the genotype differed significantly from the mean age of all mice in the sample p < 0.05

**Table 2.** Genotypes, Ages and Sexes of Rats Used in Pathology Characterization Study

| Age | Brown Norway | | | BN/ Biry | | | F344 × BN | | | Buffalo | | | F344 × Buf | | | F344 M | | | Wistar Lewis | | | F344 Lewis | | | Total | | |
|---|---|---|---|---|---|---|---|---|---|---|---|---|---|---|---|---|---|---|---|---|---|---|---|---|---|---|---|
| | M | F | T | M | F | T | M | F | T | M | F | T | M | F | T | M | F | T | M | F | T | M | F | T | M | F | T |
| 6 | 5 | 5 | 10 | 0 | 0 | 0 | 5 | 5 | 10 | 5 | 5 | 10 | 5 | 5 | 10 | 5 | 5 | 10 | 5 | 5 | 10 | 5 | 5 | 10 | 35 | 35 | 70 |
| 12 | 6 | 6 | 12 | 0 | 0 | 0 | 6 | 6 | 12 | 6 | 6 | 12 | 6 | 6 | 12 | 6 | 6 | 12 | 6 | 6 | 12 | 6 | 0 | 6 | 42 | 42 | 84 |
| 18 | 8 | 8 | 16 | 0 | 0 | 0 | 8 | 8 | 16 | 8 | 8 | 16 | 8 | 8 | 16 | 8 | 8 | 16 | 8 | 8 | 16 | 8 | 8 | 16 | 56 | 56 | 112 |
| 24 | 8 | 8 | 16 | 0 | 0 | 0 | 8 | 8 | 16 | 8 | 8 | 16 | 8 | 8 | 16 | 8 | 8 | 16 | 8 | 8 | 16 | 8 | 8 | 16 | 56 | 56 | 112 |
| 30 | 8 | 0 | 8 | 0 | 8 | 8 | 8 | 8 | 16 | 6 | 8 | 14 | 8 | 8 | 16 | 8 | 8 | 16 | 8 | 5 | 13 | 8 | 8 | 16 | 54 | 53 | 107 |
| 36 | 0 | 0 | 0 | 8 | 8 | 16 | 0 | 0 | 0 | 4 | 1 | 5 | 0 | 0 | 0 | 0 | 0 | 0 | 16 | 2 | 18 | 0 | 0 | 0 | 28 | 11 | 39 |
| Total | 35 | 27 | 62 | 8 | 16 | 24 | 35 | 35 | 70 | 37 | 36 | 73 | 35 | 35 | 70 | 35 | 35 | 70 | 51 | 34 | 85 | 35 | 29 | 64 | 271 | 247 | 518 |

Overall Mean Age ± S.D. 20.43 ± 8.02

Excluding 36 Month Old Rats Mean Age ± S.D. 19.43 ± 8.91

parathyroid, salivary glands, adrenals, gonads, accessary sex organs, and skin plus mammary gland . Sections of duodenum, jejunum, ileum, and stomach were taken from rats. Unfortunately, the mouse disease surveillance contracts did not call for the s: all bowel and stomach to be studied. These were studied in only several dozen mice. The heads were processed differently in mice and rats. For mice the entire head was demineralized after fixation in 5% nitric acid for 3 to 4 days. Three cross sections of head were sampled to include pituitary, ears, eyes, Harderian gland, nose, mouth, teeth, cerebrum, thalamus, cerebellum and medulla. For rats, the eyes, Harderian gland, brain and pituitary were dissected and sampled before the skull was demineralized and sampled. In addition to heads, a longitudinal section of a knee joint with skeletal muscle was included for all animals. Sternum and lumbar spine with spinal cord were included for all rats but only for several dozen mice. The tissues from each animal were examined and lesions described by a single pathologist. The author studied approximately 80% of both rats and mice; four other pathologists examined some tissues collected during the first 3 years of the study, 1978 to 1981. Although all pathologists were instructed to report all major and minor lesions, it is not clear to what extent the pathologists attempted to insure concordance between themselves. For this data analysis some diagnoses of each pathologist were checked to eliminate synonyms, but few slides were restudied.

Each distinct diagnosis was assigned a three letter code, the first digit of which referred to the organ system, the second to the type of disease process and the third to the specified lesion. The details are given in footnotes to tables 3 and 4. A numeric code was used for the rats, a naturally more complete alphabetic one for the mice. The codes are retained in this presentation of the data to serve as an index to the lesions.

The chi square test on two by two contingency tables was used to test for the statistical significance of differences between each genotype and all animals in the study in the ratios of animals with and without certain common lesions. Differences between the totals for males and totals for females were studied in the same way. For the analysis of rat data, data for 36 month old animals were left out, since only two genotypes, BN/Biry and Lewis, were represented at that age.

## RESULTS

### General Health Status of the Animals

The animals were generally in good health when shipped to the diagnostic laboratory. They were shipped in batches of one or two dozen each month. The data collected from disease surveillance testing were available for study for this paper, but will not be described in detail. In summary, the colonies from which the animals came must be described as conventional and not specific pathogen free. Many mice had antibodies to such viruses as Sendai virus, mouse hepatitis virus, pneumonia virus of mice, and minute virus of mice. Many rats had serological titers to Sendai virus, sialodacyroadenitis virus, Killam rat virus, Toolan H-1 virus and mouse adenovirus. Many nasophyrangeal cultures from rats and some cecal cultures from both rats and mice grew *Pseudomonas aeruginosa*; other potentially pathogenic bacteria were rarely reported. Mycoplasma were not cultured from nasophyrangeal cultures of any mouse or rat. A few mice had pinworms.

### Lists of Lesions Found

Tables 3 and 4 list all of the lesions encountered, the codes used to designate them, the numbers of male, female and total animals affected, and the mean age and standard deviation of animals with the lesions. Data are included for mice without lesions (ccde NON). Many listed lesions occurred in only a few animals. These will not be dealt with further in this paper. The more numerous lesions, and particularly those that occurred at relatively old mean ages, are described on pages 292 to 313. For many of these lesions and others listed in Tables 3 and 4, further references are given in the bibliography. If any lesion was found to occur significantly more commonly in one or another genotype, that result is presented with its description below and on pages 313 to 318.

### Lesions in Mice

#### *Malignant Lymphoma (ABA)*

Most lymphomas in this study occurred in multiple organs, including lymph nodes, liver and spleen. No attempt was made to classify the tumors according to such systems as that of Pattengale and Taylor (1983) so it is likely that diverse neoplasms are lumped together here. These tumors occurred at a comparatively advanced mean age and significantly more commonly in B6 and D2 mice.

| Lesion Code* | Lesion | No. Males | No. Female | Total | Mean Age | S.D. |
|---|---|---|---|---|---|---|
| | **Table 3.** Lesions Observed in 1577 Mice of 12 Genotypes killed at 6 Monthly Intervals And Mean + S.D. Age of Occurrence of Each Lesion | | | | | |
| AAA | Spleen: hemorrhagic, infarct, focal necrosis | 2 | 0 | 2 | 24.00 | 0.00 |
| ABA | One or more organs: malignant lymphoma | 28 | 21 | 49 | 21.48 | 3.86 |
| ABB | One or more organs: myelogenous leukemia | 2 | 0 | 2 | 18.00 | 8.49 |
| ABC | One or more organs: reticulum cell sarcoma | 5 | 0 | 5 | 24.00 | 0.00 |
| AHB | Spleen: pyogranulomatous splentitis | 1 | 0 | 1 | 12.00 | - |
| AIA | Spleen: amyloidosis | 18 | 1 | 19 | 19.89 | 4.03 |
| AIB | Spleen: hemosiderosis | 2 | 1 | 3 | 16.00 | 9.17 |
| AOA | Spleen: lymphoid hyperplasia | 21 | 15 | 36 | 18.94 | 5.54 |
| BDA | Lymph node: extramedullary hematopoiesis | 2 | 0 | 2 | 15.00 | 4.24 |
| BGH | Lymph node: focal purulent lymphadenitis | 1 | 0 | 1 | 18.00 | - |
| BHC | Lymph node: pyogranulomatous lymphadenitis | 1 | 0 | 1 | 18.00 | - |
| BLA | Lymph node:medullary hemorrhage | 1 | 0 | 1 | 24.00 | - |
| BOA | Lymph node: lymphoid hyperplasia | 9 | 9 | 18 | 20.00 | 5.82 |
| DCA | Brain: cholesteatoma | 0 | 1 | 1 | 18.00 | - |
| DCB | Meninges: meningioma | 5 | 0 | 5 | 19.60 | 5.37 |
| DEA | Spinal roots: degenerative radiculopathy | 1 | 0 | 1 | 18.00 | - |
| DJA | Meninges: meningeal inclusion cyst | 0 | 1 | 1 | 12.00 | - |
| DKE | Brain: mineralization of thalamus | 12 | 2 | 14 | 21.43 | 3.38 |
| EFA | Eye: retinal atrophy | 30 | 48 | 78 | 16.31 | 6.97 |
| EGA | Eye: suppurative keratitis | 3 | 0 | 3 | 22.00 | 3.46 |
| FAB | Harderian gland: focal necrosis | 5 | 2 | 7 | 11.14 | 5.40 |
| FCA | Harderian gland: adenoma | 22 | 10 | 32 | 20.06 | 4.47 |
| FJD | Harderian gland: focal lobular ectasia | 9 | 2 | 11 | 20.18 | 4.85 |
| FOB | Nasolacrimal duct: lymphocytic nodules | 6 | 0 | 6 | 12.00 | 6.57 |
| FOC | Harderian gland: lymphocytic nodules | 38 | 7 | 45 | 18.40 | 4.32 |
| GGK | Ear: suppurative otitis media/interna | 45 | 28 | 73 | 15.45 | 6.84 |
| GHA | Middle ear: polyp with cholesterol clefts | 3 | 0 | 3 | 20.00 | 3.46 |
| GKE | Middle ear: mineralization of epithelium | 1 | 0 | 1 | 6.00 | - |
| HFD | Sublingual salivary gland: atrophy | 2 | 1 | 3 | 20.00 | 6.93 |
| HHA | Salivary gland: chronic fibrosing sialoadenitis | 1 | 1 | 2 | 21.00 | 4.24 |
| HIA | Parotid salivary gland: amyloidosis | 34 | 23 | 57 | 20.74 | 4.64 |
| HOA | Submaxillary salivary gland: lymphocytic nodules | 137 | 41 | 178 | 18.19 | 6.01 |
| IGA | Tongue: suppurative glossitis | 1 | 0 | 1 | 6.00 | - |
| IGB | Lingual glands: purulent sialoadenitis | 1 | 2 | 3 | 6.00 | 0.00 |
| IHA | Oral ulcers | 1 | 1 | 2 | 21.00 | 4.24 |
| IHC | Tongue: focal fibrosis with mast cells | 1 | 2 | 3 | 14.00 | 6.93 |
| IHD | Tongue: foreign body granuloma | 3 | 1 | 4 | 12.00 | 6.93 |
| IKA | Lingual gland: calcification | 3 | 2 | 5 | 8.40 | 5.37 |
| JBD | Nonglandular stomach: squamous cell carcinoma Stomach: squamous epithelial inclusion cyst | 0 | 1 | 0 | 24.00 | - |
| JDA | Stomach: dilatation of crypts | 1 | 0 | 1 | 18.00 | - |
| JJA | Colon: lymphoid hyperplasia | 1 | 0 | 1 | 24.00 | - |
| KAA | Small intesstine: amyloidosis of lamina propria | 3 | 0 | 4 | 22.00 | 3.46 |
| KIA | Colon: dilatation and mineralization of crypts | 7 | 12 | 19* | 21.16 | 4.63 |
| KKA | | 1 | 0 | 1 | 24.00 | - |

| Lesion Code* | Lesion | No. Males | No. Females | Total | Mean Age | S.D. |
|---|---|---|---|---|---|---|
| KNA | Colon: pin worm infection | 7 | 0 | 7 | 19.71 | 6.68 |
| KNB | Colon: Hexamita sp. infection | 1 | 0 | 1 | 24.00 | - |
| LAA | Liver: focal necrosis | 25 | 6 | 31 | 15.68 | 6.13 |
| LAB | Liver: torsion of lobe with infarction | 1 | 0 | 1 | 24.00 | - |
| LBA | Liver: hepatocellular carcinoma | 9 | 0 | 9 | 21.33 | 3.16 |
| LCA | Liver: hepatoma | 28 | 3 | 31 | 18.44 | 5.75 |
| LDB | Liver: atypia of hepatocyte nuclei | 17 | 0 | 17 | 18.35 | 6.17 |
| LDC | Liver: bild duct hyperplasia | 1 | 0 | 1 | 18.00 | - |
| LDD | Liver: inclusion bodies in hepatocytes | 3 | 0 | 3 | 18.00 | 6.00 |
| LGA | Liver: purulent necrotizing hepatitis | 10 | 1 | 11 | 14.18 | 6.16 |
| LHA | Liver: focal leukocytic nodules | 55 | 78 | 133 | 14,51 | 7.88 |
| LHC | Liver: chronic hepatitis, regenerative nodules | 1 | 0 | 1 | 24.00 | - |
| LHD | Liver: granulomatous cholangiohepatitis | 2 | 0 | 2 | 18.00 | 8.49 |
| LIA | Liver: amyloidosis | 9 | 3 | 12 | 19.50 | 4.52 |
| LIB | Liver: fatty change | 42 | 5 | 47 | 16.72 | 5.86 |
| LIC | Liver: glycogen accumulation in hepatocytes | 5 | 0 | 5 | 12.00 | 4.24 |
| LJA | Liver: biliary cysts | 2 | 0 | 2 | 18.00 | 0.00 |
| LJB | Liver: serosal cysts | 1 | 0 | 1 | 18.00 | 0.00 |
| LMA | Liver: telangiectasis | 2 | 0 | 2 | 24.00 | 0.00 |
| LOA | Liver: periportal lymphocytic nodules | 65 | 34 | 99 | 18.67 | 4.99 |
| MAA | Pancreas: focal necrosis | 0 | 1 | 1 | 12.00 | - |
| MCA | Pancreas: cystadenoma of pancreatic ducts | 1 | 0 | 1 | 24.00 | - |
| MDA | Pancreas: hypertrophy of islets | 4 | 0 | 4 | 18.00 | 4.90 |
| MOA | Pancreas: chronic inflammation of ducts | 3 | 1 | 4 | 15.00 | 6.00 |
| NEB | Multifocal myocardial degeneration | 33 | 11 | 44 | 18.95 | 5.78 |
| NHA | Heart: focal chronic myocarditis | 6 | 1 | 7 | 17.14 | 6.41 |
| NIA | Heart: focal myocardial amyloidosis | 56 | 17 | 73 | 20.71 | 4.13 |
| NKA | Heart: epicardial calcification | 62 | 25 | 87 | 11.30 | 5.85 |
| NLA | Heart: vegetative valvular thrombosis | 5 | 1 | 6 | 19.00 | 7.01 |
| NON | No lesion in any organ | 207 | 114 | 321 | 9.15 | 4.82 |
| OCA | Any organ: hemangioma, hemangiosarcoma | 3 | 1 | 4 | 21.00 | 3.46 |
| OLA | Any organ: thromobosis of blood vessels | 2 | 0 | 2 | 21.00 | 4.24 |
| OMA | Any organ: vascular malformation | 1 | 0 | 1 | 24.00 | - |
| PAA | Nose: necrotizing rhinitis | 0 | 1 | 1 | 6.00 | - |
| PCA | Nasal septal glands: adenoma | 1 | 0 | 1 | 24.00 | - |
| PDA | Nasal cavity:squamous metaplasia | 1 | 0 | 1 | 12.00 | - |
| PGA | Nose: purulent rhinitis | 12 | 8 | 20 | 17.40 | 6.99 |
| PGB | Nasopharynz: subacute diffuse pharyngitis | 1 | 0 | 1 | 18.00 | - |
| PGC | Tracea: peritracheal acute cellulitis | 0 | 1 | 1 | 24.00 | - |
| PIA | Trachea: submucosal pigmentation | 3 | 0 | 3 | 16.00 | 3.46 |
| PIB | Nasal septum: hyalinization of interstitium | 421 | 81 | 502 | 15.38 | 6.69 |
| PJA | Nasal gland: dilatation | 2 | 0 | 2 | 15.00 | 12.7 |
| PMA | Nasal septum: deviation | 2 | 1 | 3 | 20.00 | 6.93 |
| POA | Trachea: chronic adenitis of tracheal glands | 2 | 1 | 3 | 22.00 | 3.46 |

**Table 3.** (Continued) Lesions Observed in 1577 Mice of 12 Genotypes killed at 6 Monthly Intervals And Mean + S.D. Age of Occurrence of Each Lesion

| Lesion Code* | Lesion | No. Male | No. Female | Total | Mean Age | S.D. |
|---|---|---|---|---|---|---|
| QAA | Lung: necrotizing alveolitis | 1 | 0 | 1 | 6.00 | - |
| QBA | Lung: bronchoalveolar adenocarcinoma | 55 | 26 | 81 | 20.74 | 4.65 |
| QBC | Lung: metastic hepatocellular carcinoma | 1 | 0 | 1 | 24.00 | - |
| QCA | Lung: adenoma | 7 | 3 | 10 | 17.60 | 6.02 |
| QDA | Lung: alveolar epithelial cell hyperplasis | 21 | 7 | 28 | 16.50 | 7.05 |
| QGA | Lung: purulent pneumonia | 2 | 0 | 2 | 12.00 | 8.49 |
| QHA | Lung: focal chronic pneumonia | 6 | 3 | 9 | 18.00 | 7.94 |
| QHB | Lung: alveolar histiocytosis | 24 | 30 | 54 | 19.11 | 5.48 |
| QHC | Lung: focal or diffuse proliferative pneumonia | 6 | 7 | 13 | 19.38 | 3.59 |
| QHD | Lung: acute bronchitis | 2 | 1 | 3 | 18.00 | 6.00 |
| QKA | Lung: focal mineralization | 4 | 1 | 5 | 16.80 | 5.02 |
| QLA | Lung: hemorrhage | 10 | 3 | 13 | 12.38 | 7.21 |
| QOA | Lung: peribronchial lymphocytic nodules | 130 | 44 | 174 | 15.59 | 7.16 |
| QOB | Lung: perivascular lyphocytic infiltrates | 55 | 2 | 57 | 13.58 | 7.31 |
| QOC | Lung: subpleural lymphocytic infiltrates | 5 | 4 | 9 | 18.00 | 7.94 |
| RBA | Adrenal: pheochromocytoma | 0 | 1 | 1 | 24.00 | - |
| RCA | Pituitary: adenoma | 0 | 6 | 6 | 23.00 | 2.45 |
| RCB | Thyroid: adenoma, cystic papillary adenoma | 1 | 1 | 2 | 18.00 | 8.49 |
| RDA | Adrenal: cortical adenomatous hyperplasia | 1 | 1 | 2 | 21.00 | 4.24 |
| RDB | Thyroid: C cell adenomatous hyperplasia | 14 | 0 | 13 | 18.43 | 6.85 |
| RIA | Thyroid: amyloidosis | 12 | 6 | 18 | 22.24 | 2.82 |
| RIB | Thyroid: focal fatty infiltrate | 1 | 0 | 1 | 12.00 | - |
| RIC | Adrenal: amyloidosis | 5 | 0 | 5 | 21.60 | 3.29 |
| RID | Adrenal: fatty infiltrate into capsule | 0 | 3 | 0 | 6.00 | 4.00 |
| RJA | Thyroid: cystic follicles | 10 | 18 | 28 | 18.86 | 5.59 |
| RJB | Adrenal: cystic medulla | 1 | 0 | 1 | 24.00 | - |
| RJC | Parathyroid cyst | 2 | 0 | 2 | 12.00 | 0.00 |
| ROA | Thyroid: lymphocytic nodules | 1 | 1 | 2 | 21.00 | 4.24 |
| SGA | Bladder: chronic suppurative cystitis | 5 | 1 | 6 | 22.00 | 3.10 |
| SHA | Bladder: chronic cystitis | 10 | 2 | 12 | 13.00 | 5.62 |
| SKA | Bladder: focal perivascular mineralization | 5 | 0 | 5 | 13.20 | 5.02 |
| SOA | Bladder: lymphocytic nodules | 12 | 13 | 25 | 18.72 | 5.00 |
| TAA | Kidney: focal tubular necrosis | 3 | 0 | 3 | 18.00 | 10.39 |
| TAB | Kidney: papillary necrosis | 1 | 0 | 1 | 24.00 | - |
| TDA | Kidney: tubular regeneration | 1 | 0 | 1 | 6.00 | - |
| TDB | Kidney: hypoplasia | 1 | 1 | 2 | 12.00 | 8.49 |
| TEA | Kidney: fatty change of proximal tubules | 10 | 0 | 10 | 6.60 | 1.90 |
| TFA | Kidney: focal cortical atrophy | 23 | 7 | 30 | 20.63 | 5.86 |
| TGA | Kidney: pyelonephritis | 2 | 1 | 3 | 14.00 | 6.93 |
| THA | Kidney: glomerulonephritis | 32 | 13 | 45 | 19.9 | 4.80 |
| TIA | Kidney: amylolidosis of glomeruli | 89 | 41 | 130 | 20.70 | 4.11 |
| TJA | Kidney: hydronephrosis | 18 | 13 | 31 | 19.93 | 5.67 |
| TJB | Kidney: tubular dilatation | 3 | 3 | 6 | 18.00 | 6.57 |
| TKA | Kidney: calcified nodules in cortex | 31 | 13 | 44 | 16.64 | 6.19 |
| TMA | Ureter: malformation | 1 | 0 | 1 | 6.00 | - |

Table 3. (Continued) Lesions Observed in 1577 Micc of 12 Genotypes killed at 6 Monthly Intervals And Mean + S.D. Age of Occurrence of Each Lesion

**Table 3.** (Continued) Lesions Observed in 1577 Mice of 12 Genotypes killed at 6 Monthly Intervals And Mean + S.D. Age of Occurrence of Each Lesion

| Lesion Code* | Lesion | No. Male | No. Female | Total | Mean Age | S.D. |
|---|---|---|---|---|---|---|
| TMB | Ureter: polyp | 2 | 0 | 2 | 24.00 | 0.00 |
| TOA | Kidney: interstitial lymphocytic nodules | 127 | 27 | 154 | 18.56 | 5.78 |
| TOB | Kidney: lymphocytic nodules in medulla | 32 | 1 | 33 | 16.90 | 5.70 |
| UCA | Testis: lydig cell adenoma | 2 | - | 2 | 21.00 | 4.24 |
| UDA | Testis: hyperplasia of interstitial cells | 19 | - | 19 | 14.00 | 4.71 |
| UFA | Testis, epididymus: atrophy | 112 | - | 112 | 19.50 | 5.49 |
| UHA | Testis: epididymus: sperm granuloma | 8 | - | 8 | 16.50 | 5.32 |
| UIA | Testis: lipofuscin deposition | 5 | - | 5 | 21.60 | 3.29 |
| UKA | Testis: mineralization of seminiferous tubules | 4 | - | 4 | 13.50 | 7.55 |
| VCA | Preputial gland: cystic adenoma | 1 | - | 1 | 18.00 | - |
| VDA | Seminal vesicle: adenomatous hyperplasia | 1 | - | 1 | 12.00 | - |
| VFA | Prostate: atrophy | 4 | - | 4 | 21.00 | 6.00 |
| VGA | Seminal vesicles: pyogranulomatous adenitis | 11 | - | 11 | 15.50 | 7.59 |
| VGB | Prostate: purulent prostatitis | 8 | - | 8 | 16.50 | 7.69 |
| VHA | Prostate: chronic fibrosing prostatitis | 15 | - | 15 | 16.8 | 6.09 |
| VJA | Seminal vesicles: dilatation | 18 | - | 18 | 20.67 | 4.70 |
| VKA | Epididymus: focal mineralization of interstitium | 1 | - | 1 | 18.00 | - |
| VOA | Prostate: lymphocytic nodules | 3 | 0 | 3 | 18.00 | 6.00 |
| VOB | Epididymus: lymphocytic nodules | 3 | - | 3 | 24.00 | 0.00 |
| VOC | Vas Deforams: lymphocytic infiltrates | 1 | - | 1 | 12.00 | 0.00 |
| WBA | Ovary: granulosa cell tumor | - | 6 | 6 | 20.00 | 4.90 |
| WCA | Ovary: cystadenoma | - | 3 | 3 | 24.00 | 0.00 |
| WFA | Ovary: atrophy | - | 7 | 7 | 22.30 | 2.93 |
| WIA | Ovary: amyloidosis | - | 34 | 34 | 17.82 | 5.62 |
| WJA | Ovary: parovarian cyst | - | 11 | 11 | 16.90 | 7.00 |
| WJB | Ovary: cystic follicles | - | 26 | 26 | 19.15 | 5.63 |
| WIB | Ovary: lipofuscin deposition | - | 2 | 2 | 24.00 | 0.00 |
| XCA | Uterus: adenomatous polyps | - | 11 | 11 | 22.36 | 2.80 |
| XDA | Endometrial glands: hyperplasia | - | 22 | 22 | 18.00 | 6.96 |
| XGA | Uterus: acute endometritis | - | 12 | 12 | 16.00 | 6.93 |
| XGB | Vagina: eosinophilic and suppurative vaginitis | - | 36 | 36 | 14.33 | 6.13 |
| XIA | Uterus: perivascular amyloidosis | - | 3 | 3 | 16.00 | 3.46 |
| XJA | Uterus: dilatation of endometrial glands | - | 110 | 110 | 18.46 | 5.68 |
| XJB | Uterus: hydrometra | - | 44 | 44 | 17.76 | 5.33 |
| XJC | Fallopian tube: cystic dilatation | - | 5 | 5 | 24.00 | 1.41 |
| XJD | Uterus: subserosal cyst | - | 1 | 1 | 12.00 | - |
| YAA | Peritoneal adipose tissue: necrosis | 3 | 4 | 7 | 14.57 | 680 |
| YAB | Skeletal muscle: necrosis | 2 | 1 | 3 | 16.00 | 9.17 |
| YBA | Any organ: leiomyoma, leiomyosarcoma | 1 | 3 | 4 | 22.50 | 3.00 |
| YBB | Mesentery, pleura: mesothelioma | 0 | 1 | 1 | 24.00 | - |
| YBC | Mammary gland: adenocarcinoma | 0 | 1 | 1 | 18.00 | - |
| YBD | Mammary gland: fibrosarcoma | 0 | 1 | 1 | 18.00 | - |
| YCB | Skin: hair matrix tumor | 0 | 1 | 1 | 24.00 | - |
| YGA | Skin, any site: chronic suppurative dermatitis | 26 | 0 | 26 | 13.67 | 6.88 |

| Lesion Code* | Lesion | No. Male | No. Fe-male | Total | Mean Age | S.D. |
|---|---|---|---|---|---|---|
| | **Table 3.** (Continued) Lesions Observed in 1577 Mice of 12 Genotypes killed at 6 Monthly Intervals And Mean + S.D. Age of Occurrence of Each Lesion | | | | | |
| YHA | Subcutis: pyogranuloma | 2 | 0 | 2 | 21.00 | 4.24 |
| YHB | Peritoneum: focal pyogranulomatous peritontitis | 2 | 1 | 3 | 20.00 | 6.93 |
| YHC | Skin: chronic dermatitis due to implanted hair | 1 | 0 | 1 | 18.00 | - |
| YMA | Skeletal muscle: regeneration | 1 | 0 | 1 | 18.00 | - |
| YOA | Mesentery, omentum: focal lymphocytic infiltrates | 4 | 16 | 22 | 18.00 | 6.68 |
| ZBA | Any site: osteosarcoma | 0 | 1 | 1 | 24.00 | 0.00 |
| ZBB | Petrous temporal bone: osteochrondroma | 0 | 2 | 2 | 18.00 | 8.49 |
| ZHA | Gingiva, tooth root: purulent inflammation | 19 | 13 | 32 | 18.72 | 6.50 |
| ZHB | Alveolar gingiva of incisors: implanted hair | 0 | 6 | 6 | 19.71 | 2.93 |

*DESIGN OF THREE DIGIT CODE

First Digit: Organ

Second Digit: Disease Process

| First Digit: Organ | Second Digit: Disease Process |
|---|---|
| A - spleen | A - necrosis |
| B - lymph node | B - malignant neoplasm |
| C - bone marrow | C - benign neoplasm |
| D - brain | D - abnormal growth, hyperplasia |
| E - eye | E - degeneration |
| F - lacrimal and Harderian gland | F - atrophy |
| G - ear | G - acute inflammation |
| H - salivary glands | H - chronic inflammation |
| I - mouth and tongue | I - tissue storage of abnormal material |
| J - esophagus and stomach | J - cystic change |
| K - intestines | K - mineralization of tissue |
| L - liver | L - hemorrhage, thrombosis |
| M - pancreas | M - malformation |
| N - heart | N - infectious organisms |
| O - vessels | O - lymphoid nodules |
| P - nose and trachea | |
| Q - lungs | Third Digit: Specific Lesion |
| R - endocrine organs | |
| S - bladder and urethra | |
| T - kidney and ureters | |
| U - testis | |
| V - male accessory sex organs | |
| W - ovary | |
| X - uterus. cervox. vagina | |
| Y - skin, mammary glands, connective tissue, adipose tissue pritoneum | |
| Z - skeleton, dentition. | |

**Table 4.** Lesions Observed in 512 Rats of 9 Genotypes Killed at 6 Monthly Intervals and Mean + S.D. Age of Occurrence of Each Lesion

| CODE | LESION[a] | M | F | T | $\bar{X}$ | SD |
|---|---|---|---|---|---|---|
| 011 | ERYTHROLEUKEMIA | 0 | 1 | 1 | 30 | - |
| 012 | MALIGNANT LYMPHOMA | 4 | 1 | 5 | 30 | 4 |
| 015 | MYELOGENOUS LEUKEMIA | 0 | 1 | 1 | 24 | - |
| 031 | LYMPHOID HYPERPLASIA | 2 | 6 | 8 | 24 | 8 |
| 032 | HYPERPLASIA OF PEYER'S PATCHES | 2 | 1 | 3 | 28 | 3 |
| 033 | EXTRAMEDULLARY HEMATOPOIESIS OF SPLEEN | 2 | 2 | 4 | 32 | 3 |
| 034 | HISTIOCYTOSIS OF VERTEBRAL BONE MARROW | 1 | 0 | 1 | 36 | - |
| 041 | ATROPHY OF THYMUS | 45 | 47 | 92 | 17 | 4 |
| 061 | GRANLOMATOUS LYMPHADENITIS | 0 | 1 | 1 | 30 | - |
| 062 | SINUS HISTIOCYTOSIS OF LYMPH NODES | 1 | 4 | 5 | 28 | 3 |
| 063 | HEMOSIDEROSIS OF LYMPH NODES | 5 | 6 | 11 | 26 | 4 |
| 081 | LYMPH NODE CYST | 4 | 0 | 4 | 27 | 6 |
| 112 | MALIGNANT GLIOMA | 3 | 0 | 3 | 30 | 0 |
| 113 | GRANULAR CELL MYOBLASTOMA | 2 | 1 | 3 | 30 | 6 |
| 115 | CHOROID PLEXUS PAPILLARY ADENOCARCINOMA | 0 | 1 | 1 | 36 | - |
| 131 | NEURONAL ECTOPIA OF CEREBRAL CORTEX | 1 | 0 | 1 | 18 | - |
| 132 | ECTOPIC GRANULE CELLS OF CEREBELLAR CORTEX | 3 | 2 | 5 | 24 | 0 |
| 141 | DEGENERATIVE RADICULONEUROPATHY | 61 | 57 | 118 | 31 | 3 |
| 142 | RETINAL ATROPHY | 29 | 50 | 79 | 26 | 7 |
| 143 | OLD CEREBRAL INFARCT | 0 | 1 | 1 | 24 | - |
| 144 | FOCAL GLIOSIS | 0 | 1 | 1 | 24 | - |
| 161 | CHRONIC KERATITIS | 2 | 1 | 3 | 20 | 15 |
| 162 | CHRONIC VENTRICULITIS OF THIRD VENTRICLE | 1 | 0 | 1 | 36 | - |
| 163 | CONJUNCTIVAL GRANULOMA | 1 | 0 | 1 | 18 | - |
| 164 | CHRONIC IRIDOCYCLITIS | 1 | 1 | 2 | 24 | 0 |
| 165 | PITUITARY GRANULOMA | 0 | 1 | 1 | 24 | 0 |
| 171 | CALCIFICATION OF GLOBUS PALLIDUS OR THALAMUS | 9 | 5 | 14 | 28 | 4 |
| 181 | HYDROCEPHALUS | 1 | 0 | 1 | 30 | - |
| 213 | HEPATOCELLULAR CARCINOMA | 1 | 1 | 2 | 36 | - |
| 214 | LEIOMYOSARCOMA OF INTESTINE | 0 | 1 | 1 | 36 | - |
| 221 | HEPATOCELLULAR ADENOMA | 7 | 2 | 9 | 31 | 5 |
| 222 | ADENOMA OF SALIVARY GLAND | 1 | 0 | 1 | 30 | - |
| 223 | ADENOMATOUS HYPERPLASIA OF SALIVARY GLAND | 1 | 1 | 2 | 18 | 7 |
| 224 | ADENOMA OF HARDERIAN GLAND | 1 | 0 | 1 | 24 | - |
| 225 | LEIOMYOMA OF INTESTINES | 2 | 3 | 5 | 31 | 5 |
| 226 | ADENOMA OF BILE DUCT | 1 | 1 | 2 | 30 | 8 |
| 231 | BILE DUCT HYPERPLASIA AND PORTAL FIBROSIS | 123 | 90 | 213 | 25 | 4 |
| 232 | BASOPHILIC HEPATOCYTE NODULES | 26 | 52 | 78 | 27 | 6 |
| 234 | NODULAR HYPERPLASIA OF LIVER | 5 | 2 | 7 | 31 | 2 |
| 235 | HARDERIAN GLAND METAPLASIA OF EXORBITAL GLAND | 23 | 3 | 26 | 15 | 4 |
| 241 | FOCAL OR DIFFUSE ATROPHY OF SALIVARY GLAND | 2 | 2 | 4 | 23 | 6 |
| 242 | FOCAL CENTRILOBULAR NECROSIS OF LIVER | 1 | 2 | 3 | 26 | 3 |
| 243 | EXTRAMEDULLARY HEMATOPOIESIS OF LIVER | 13 | 11 | 24 | 7 | 5 |

**Table 4.** (Continued) Lesions Observed in 512 Rats of 9 Genotypes Killed at 6 Monthly Intervals and Mean + S.D. Age of Occurrence of Each Lesion

| CODE | LESION[a] | M | F | T | $\bar{X}$ | SD |
|---|---|---|---|---|---|---|
| 251 | PURULENT CHOLANGITIS | 1 | 0 | 1 | 30 | - |
| 252 | FOCAL ACUTE HEPATITIS | 1 | 1 | 2 | 28 | 3 |
| 253 | HEPATIC MICROABSCESSES | 39 | 21 | 60 | 24 | 0 |
| 254 | FOCAL ULCERATION OF LARGE BOWEL | 1 | 1 | 2 | 24 | 0 |
| 255 | ULCERATION OF STOMACH | 2 | 0 | 2 | 21 | 4 |
| 261 | CHRONIC DACRYOADENITIS OF HARDERIAN GLAND | 97 | 150 | 247 | 19 | 8 |
| 262 | CHRONIC SIALOADENITIS OF SALIVARY OR EXORBITAL GLAND | 43 | 39 | 82 | 16 | 6 |
| 263 | MICROGRANULOMA OF LIVER | 11 | 11 | 22 | 22 | 7 |
| 264 | CHRONIC ENTEROCOLITIS | 0 | 3 | 3 | 24 | 0 |
| 265 | CHRONIC PERICHOLANGITIS | 32 | 33 | 65 | 15 | 6 |
| 271 | FOCAL VACUOLATION OF HEPATOCYTES | 17 | 4 | 21 | 30 | 5 |
| 272 | FOCAL FATTY CHANGE OF LIVER | 30 | 10 | 40 | 27 | 6 |
| 281 | PELIOSIS HEPATIS | 31 | 6 | 37 | 30 | 5 |
| 282 | CYSTIC DILATATION OF GASTRIC GLANDS | 20 | 22 | 42 | 25 | 7 |
| 283 | CYSTIC DILATION OF BILE DUCTS | 1 | 3 | 4 | 24 | 5 |
| 284 | DILITATION OF DUCTS OF SALIVARY OR HARDERIAN GLAND | 1 | 4 | 5 | 30 | 13 |
| 341 | ARTERIAL SCLEROSIS | 1 | 0 | 1 | 30 | - |
| 342 | FOCAL MYOCARDIAL FIBROSIS AND DEGENERATION | 78 | 55 | 133 | 25 | 7 |
| 344 | SCATTERED MYOCARDIAL FIBER NECROSIS | 36 | 27 | 63 | 18 | 8 |
| 361 | CHRONIC MYOCARDITIS | 56 | 52 | 108 | 25 | 7 |
| 363 | PERIARTERITIS NODOSA | 4 | 4 | 8 | 26 | 10 |
| 367 | FOCAL GRANULOMATOUS EPICARDITIS | 3 | 1 | 4 | 20 | 9 |
| 368 | VEGETATIVE ENDOCARDITIS | 0 | 1 | 1 | 24 | - |
| 371 | FOCAL CALCIFICATION OF WALL OF AORTA | 2 | 1 | 3 | 24 | 12 |
| 411 | BRONCHOALVEOLAR ADENOCARCINOMA | 1 | 2 | 3 | 28 | 3 |
| 431 | ADENOMATOUS HYPERPLASIA OF ALVEOLAE | 5 | 1 | 6 | 26 | 5 |
| 461 | PERIVASCULAR LYMPHOID HYPEPLASIA OF LUNG | 44 | 44 | 88 | 17 | 5 |
| 462 | CHRONIC RHINITIS | 3 | 1 | 4 | 11 | 9 |
| 463 | ALVEOLAR HISTOCYTOSIS | 12 | 35 | 47 | 20 | 8 |
| 464 | CHRONIC FOCAL INTERSTITIAL PNEUMONIA | 34 | 34 | 68 | 14 | 9 |
| 465 | PYOGRANULOMATOUS SUBPLEURAL PNEUMONIA | 3 | 3 | 6 | 18 | 11 |
| 466 | PERIBRONCHIAL LYMPHOID HYPERPLASIA | 22 | 21 | 43 | 20 | 11 |
| 467 | FOCAL ATELECTASIS | 25 | 14 | 39 | 18 | 7 |
| 471 | FOCAL CALCIFICATION OF PULMONARY VESSELS | 73 | 45 | 118 | 16 | 7 |
| 481 | CYSTIC DILATATION OF TRACHEAL GLANDS | 19 | 17 | 36 | 23 | 7 |
| 511 | ISLET CELL ADENOCARCINIMA | 2 | 0 | 2 | 33 | 4 |
| 512 | PHEOCHROMOCYTOMA OF ADRENAL | 13 | 20 | 33 | 30 | 6 |
| 513 | PITUITARY ADENOCARCINOMA | 9 | 9 | 18 | 29 | 4 |
| 514 | ADENOCARCINOMA OF ADRENAL CORTEX | 0 | 2 | 2 | 30 | 0 |
| 515 | ADENOCARCINOMA OF THYROID | 2 | 0 | 2 | 30 | 0 |
| 517 | ADENOCARCINOMA OF THYROID C CELLS | 1 | 0 | 1 | 36 | - |
| 521 | ADENOMA OF PITUITARY | 44 | 73 | 117 | 26 | 6 |
| 522 | ADENOMA OF C CELLS OF THYROID | 14 | 12 | 26 | 30 | 4 |
| 523 | ADENOMA OF ISLET CELLS | 11 | 3 | 14 | 33 | 3 |

**Table 4.** (Continued) Lesions Observed in 512 Rats of 9 Genotypes Killed at 6 Monthly Intervals and Mean + S.D. Age of Occurrence of Each Lesion

| CODE | LESION[a] | M | F | T | $\bar{X}$ | SD |
|---|---|---|---|---|---|---|
| 524 | ADENOMA OF ADRENAL CORTEX | 7 | 8 | 15 | 27 | 4 |
| 525 | ADENOMA OF THYROID | 2 | 2 | 4 | 27 | 3 |
| 526 | ADENOMA OF PARATHYROID | 1 | 0 | 1 | 36 | - |
| 527 | ADENOMA OF PANCREATIC ACINAR CELLS | 2 | 0 | 2 | 30 | 8 |
| 528 | GANGLIONEUROMA OF ADRENAL | 1 | 1 | 2 | 30 | 8 |
| 531 | NODULAR CORTICAL HYPERPLASIA OF ADRENAL | 7 | 4 | 11 | 25 | 10 |
| 532 | HYPERPLASIA OF C CELLS OF THYROID | 12 | 14 | 26 | 24 | 6 |
| 533 | HYPERPLASIA OF PARATHYROID | 9 | 5 | 14 | 29 | 4 |
| 534 | LOBULAR ECTASIA AND ATROPHY OF EXOCRINE PANCREAS | 18 | 15 | 33 | 22 | 6 |
| 536 | HYPERPLASIA OF ISLET CELLS | 46 | 2 | 48 | 18 | 2 |
| 542 | DEGENERATION OF THYROID | 6 | 0 | 6 | 34 | 3 |
| 544 | ATROPHY OF ADRENAL CORTEX | 1 | 3 | 4 | 30 | 7 |
| 561 | CHRONIC INFLAMMATION OF ISLETS OF PANCREAS | 8 | 2 | 10 | 25 | 6 |
| 562 | GRANULOMA OF PANCREAS | 0 | 1 | 1 | 30 | - |
| 563 | CHRONIC PANCREATITIS | 9 | 18 | 27 | 12 | 6 |
| 571 | NODULAR VACUOLATION OF ADRENAL CORTICAL CELLS | 43 | 38 | 81 | 28 | 6 |
| 572 | SUBCAPSULAR VACUOLATION OF ADRENAL CORTICAL CELLS | 18 | 13 | 31 | 28 | 4 |
| 573 | PIGMENT DEPOSITION AROUND PANCREATIC ISLETS | 6 | 6 | 12 | 18 | 6 |
| 581 | CYSTIC PITUITARY | 5 | 1 | 6 | 20 | 5 |
| 582 | TELANGIECTASIA OF ADRENAL CORTEX | 2 | 31 | 33 | 32 | 4 |
| 583 | CYSTIC ADRENAL | 1 | 0 | 1 | 30 | - |
| 584 | COLLOID CYSTS OF THYROID | 13 | 8 | 21 | 22 | 7 |
| 613 | ADENOCARCINOMA OF KIDNEY | 0 | 1 | 1 | 24 | - |
| 621 | ADENOMA OF KIDNEY | 2 | 1 | 3 | 20 | 3 |
| 631 | ADENOMATOUS HYPERPLASIA OF UROTHELIUM | 0 | 0 | 1 | 30 | - |
| 632 | RENAL TUBULAR HYPERPLASIA | 1 | 1 | 2 | 24 | 0 |
| 641 | CHRONIC PROGRESSIVE GLOMERULONEPHROPATHY, MILD | 138 | 85 | 223 | 21 | 7 |
| 642 | CHRONIC GLOMERULONEPHROPATHY, MODERATE TO SEVERE | 25 | 8 | 33 | 29 | 4 |
| 643 | INFARCTS OF KIDNEY | 1 | 0 | 1 | 36 | - |
| 644 | INTERSTITIAL FIBROSIS OF KIDNEY | 1 | 0 | 1 | 24 | - |
| 651 | PYELONEPHRITIS | 2 | 2 | 4 | 18 | - |
| 661 | CHRONIC FOCAL INTERSTITIAL NEPHRITIS | 14 | 8 | 22 | 11 | 8 |
| 662 | MICROGRANULOMA OF KIDNEY | 3 | 0 | 3 | 30 | 10 |
| 664 | CHRONIC CYSTITIS | 1 | 5 | 6 | 15 | 7 |
| 671 | TRANSITIONAL CELL HYPERPLASIA OF RENAL PELVIS | 16 | 53 | 69 | 25 | 7 |
| 681 | HYDRONEPHROSIS | 16 | 31 | 47 | 24 | 8 |
| 682 | CYSTIC KIDNEY CORTEX | 4 | 2 | 6 | 17 | 13 |
| 712 | MESOTHELIOMA OF TUNICA VAGINALIS OR PERITONEUM | 2 | 1 | 3 | 24 | 0 |
| 721 | ADENOMA OF LEYDIG CELLS | 38 | 0 | 38 | 28 | 6 |
| 722 | ADENOMA OF PROSTATE | 1 | 0 | 1 | 12 | - |
| 723 | LIPOMA OF SCROTAL ADIPOSE TISSUE | 1 | 0 | 1 | 36 | - |

Table 4. (Continued) Lesions Observed in 512 Rats of 9 Genotypes Killed at 6 Monthly Intervals and Mean + S.D. Age of Occurrence of Each Lesion

| CODE | LESION[a] | M | F | T | $\bar{X}$ | SD |
|---|---|---|---|---|---|---|
| 731 | HYPERPLASIA OF LEYDIG CELLS | 7 | 0 | 7 | 19 | 2 |
| 741 | ATROPHY OF PROSTATE | 75 | 0 | 75 | 29 | 4 |
| 742 | ATROPHY OF TESTIS | 66 | 0 | 66 | 26 | 7 |
| 743 | ATROPHY OF EPIDIDYMUS | 11 | 0 | 11 | 28 | 4 |
| 744 | INFARCTION OF TESTIS | 1 | 0 | 1 | 24 | - |
| 751 | FOCAL SUPPURATIVE PROSTATISIS | 23 | 0 | 23 | 19 | 8 |
| 761 | CHRONIC PROSTATISIS | 17 | 0 | 17 | 19 | 9 |
| 762 | SPERM GRANULOMAS OF EPIDIDYMUS | 4 | 0 | 4 | 23 | 9 |
| 763 | SPERM GRANULOMAS OF TESTIS | 7 | 0 | 7 | 27 | 8 |
| 764 | CHRONIC INFLAMMATION OF PREPUTIAL GLAND | 1 | 0 | 1 | 6 | - |
| 771 | HEMOSIDERIN IN TESTIS, OLD HEMORRHAGE | 1 | 0 | 1 | 30 | - |
| 811 | LEIOMYSARCOMA OF UTERUS | 0 | 3 | 3 | 24 | 6 |
| 812 | ADENOCARCINOMA OF UTERUS | 0 | 1 | 1 | 24 | - |
| 813 | GRANULOSA CELL ADENOCARCINOMA | 0 | 1 | 1 | 24 | - |
| 821 | HEMANGIOMA OF CERVIX | 0 | 1 | 1 | 30 | - |
| 822 | LEIOMYCOMA OF UTERUS | 0 | 1 | 1 | 12 | - |
| 823 | GRANULOSA OR GRANULOSA-THECA CELL TUMOR | 0 | 13 | 13 | 28 | 5 |
| 831 | ENDOMETRIAL POLYP | 0 | 11 | 11 | 29 | 2 |
| 833 | HYPERPLASIA OF ENDOMETRIAL GLANDS | 0 | 2 | 2 | 27 | 4 |
| 841 | ATROPHY OF OVARY | 0 | 17 | 17 | 24 | 7 |
| 851 | ACUTE VAGINITIS | 0 | 8 | 8 | 23 | 9 |
| 861 | ENDOMETRIAL FIBROSIS | 0 | 39 | 39 | 18 | 6 |
| 862 | FOCAL PYOGRANULOMATOUS METRITIS | 0 | 1 | 1 | 30 | - |
| 871 | PIGMENTATION OF ENDOMETRIUM | 0 | 2 | 2 | 24 | 0 |
| 881 | CYSTIC ENDOMETRIUM | 0 | 31 | 31 | 23 | 7 |
| 882 | CYSTIC FOLLICLES OR PAROVARIAN CYST | 0 | 9 | 9 | 19 | 10 |
| 883 | UTERUS: HYDROMETRA | 0 | 1 | 1 | 12 | - |
| 911 | ADENOCARCINOMA OF MAMMARY GLAND | 0 | 7 | 7 | 27 | 3 |
| 913 | FIBROSARCOMA, ANY SITE | 4 | 1 | 5 | 34 | 3 |
| 914 | MYXOSARCOMA, ANY SITE | 1 | 0 | 1 | 30 | - |
| 915 | SQUAMOUS CELL CARCINOMA OF SKIN | 1 | 0 | 1 | 36 | - |
| 921 | CYSTIC FIBROADENOMA OF MAMMARY GLAND | 0 | 11 | 11 | 30 | 3 |
| 922 | FIBROADENOMA OF MAMMARY GLAND | 0 | 23 | 23 | 30 | 7 |
| 923 | FIBROMA OF MAMMARY GLAND | 3 | 2 | 5 | 31 | 7 |
| 924 | KERATOCANTHOMA OF SKIN | 1 | 0 | 1 | 36 | - |
| 925 | ADENOMA OF MAMMARY GLAND | 2 | 4 | 6 | 19 | 2 |
| 931 | ADENOMATOUS HYPERPLASIA OF MAMMARY GLAND | 0 | 2 | 2 | 30 | 0 |
| 932 | PAPILLARY HYPERPLASIA OF SYNOVIUM | 7 | 4 | 11 | 28 | 3 |
| 933 | HYPERPLASIA OF PERIOSTEUM | 1 | 0 | 1 | 24 | - |
| 941 | INDIVIDUAL SKELETAL MUSCLE FIBER NECROSIS | 22 | 16 | 38 | 15 | 9 |
| 942 | NEUROGENIC ATROPHY OF SKELETAL MUSCLE | 28 | 18 | 46 | 33 | 5 |
| 943 | DEGENERATION OF CARTILAGE OF STERNUM | 9 | 12 | 21 | 23 | 5 |
| 944 | NON-UNION FRACTURE OF TARSUS | 1 | 0 | 1 | 18 | - |

**Table 4.** (Continued) Lesions Observed in 512 Rats of 9 Genotypes Killed at 6 Monthly Intervals and Mean + S.D. Age of Occurrence of Each Lesion

| CODE | LESION | M | F | T | $\bar{X}$ | SD |
|---|---|---|---|---|---|---|
| 945 | OSTEOARTHROSIS OF TARSUS | 3 | 0 | 3 | 16 | 3 |
| 961 | GRANULOMATOUS FOLLICULITIS OF SKIN | 0 | 7 | 7 | 28 | 3 |
| 962 | GRANULOMATOUS STEATITIS, ANY SITE | 4 | 3 | 7 | 23 | 4 |
| 963 | PROLIFERATIVE ARTHRITIS | 1 | 1 | 2 | 33 | 4 |
| 964 | HEMATOMA IN PERITONEAL ADIPOSE TISSUE | 0 | 1 | 1 | 30 | - |
| 965 | GRANULOMA OF MAMMARY GLAND | 1 | 3 | 4 | 20 | 6 |
| 981 | CYSTIC DILATION OF MAMMARY GLANDS AND DUCTS | 7 | 73 | 80 | 26 | 6 |

[a] The first digit of the code represents the organ system in order 0-9 as follows: hemolymphatic, nervous, gastroenteric, cardiovascular, respiratory, endocrine, urinary, male genital, female genital, other. The second digit represents the disease process, in order 1-9, as follows: malignant neoplasm, benign neoplasm, abnormal growth, degeneration and atrophy, acute inflammation, chronic inflammation, tissue storage, cystic change. The third didgit is the particular disease.

[b] F = female, M = male, T = total, X = mean age of occurence in months, SD = standard deviation. The data include 36 month old rats.

*Lymphoid Nodules in Various Organs*

(See codes with "O" as the middle letter)

These aggregations and infiltrations of lymphocytes without germinal centers were very common in all genotypes, usually occurred in several organs in the same individuals, and were probably of little clinical significance. Perhaps they represented reactions to the presence of one or another virus that infected the animals at various times. The mean age of occurrence of the lesions in various organs ranged from 15 to 20 months of age, and there was considerable variability between genotypes. In lung, lymphoid nodules and infiltrates were observed around small blood vessels (QOA), around bronchi (QOB), and just beneath the pleura (QOC). Often lymphocytic infiltrates in two or three of these locations occurred in the same animal. The nodules were also observed in the interstitium of the renal cortex (TOA) and beneath the transitional epithelium of the renal papilla (TOB). Lymphocytic nodules of the Harderian gland (FOC) and kidney (TOA) occurred significantly more often in CB6 mice; nodules in the submaxillary gland (HOA) and portal areas of liver (LOA) occurred significantly more frequently in B6 mice.

*Degenerative Radiculoneuropathy (DEA)*

This lesion was characterized by swelling of one or more spinal roots observed in cross sections of lumbar spinal cord. The swelling was due to gliosis, fibrosis or apparent hypertrophy of nerve sheaths. Although rarely observed in this study, since spinal cord was sampled only in a few mice, this lesion is quite common in older mice of various genotypes and will be described elsewhere.

*Retinal Atrophy (EFA)*

This well known degenerative change of albino rodents was most common in older CFW mice at mean age of 16.2 months and rarely in other genotypes. The photoreceptor layer was the first and most severely affected.

*Adenomatous Hyperplasia/Adenoma of Harderian Gland (FDA)*

The distinction between the two terms is unclear and they are considered synonymous here. The lesion occurred in relatively older mice. It is characterized by nodular proliferations of hypertrophied but differentiated glandular cells. It occurred significantly more often in the two CBA genotypes.

*Suppurative Otitis Media/Interna (GGK)*

This common lesion was present predominantly in B6 mice. It probably had a bacterial etiology, though in these studies the middle ears were not cultured. Polyps of the middle ears, which sometimes had cholesterol clefts (GHA) may have resulted from chronic inner ear infections.

*Amyloidosis of Various Organs (HIA, NIA, TIA, WIA)*

This common age related lesion occurred in older animals of approximately 20 months of age, and usually affected several organs in the same individuals. Amyloidosis occurred significantly more commonly in B6, B6D2 and D2 mice, but occurred in other genotypes as well. Hyalinization of the nasal septum, PIB, the most common lesion reported, was demonstrated by Congo red staining to be amyloid in a few individuals only; special stains were not performed on most such lesions. Interestingly, amyloidosis occurred in this location at a younger mean age than it did elsewhere and in genotypes not otherwise susceptible to amyoidosis, suggesting that it may be a different kind of lesion. The lesions of amyloidosis were tabulated separately by organ in this data analysis. Those interested in how many animals of each genotype had amyloidosis, regardless of organ distribution, should concentrate on amyloidosis of renal glomeruli, TIA. With few exceptions any mouse with amyloidosis had amyloidosis of kidney. From other studies (Yunis *et al.*, 1984) it seems likely that the small intestine may be as likely as the renal glomeruli to develop amyloidosis, but that organ regrettably was under-represented in this study.

*Liver, Focal Necrosis (LAA)*

This consisted of areas of coagulative necrosis scattered at random in the parenchyma without orientation with respect to the lobules. The etiology is obscure. It is commonly observed in animals sacrificed after being shipped.

*Hepatoma (LCA)*

Tumors of hepatic origin were among the most common neoplasms in the study, occurring in older mice and being particularly common in CBA/C mice. Hepatomas were nodular proliferations of well differentiated hepatocytes.

### Hepatocarcinoma (LCB)

These, by contrast to hepatomas, were pleomorphic. Since all histological gradations between malignant and benign tumors were observed, it may be that the distinction is more a matter of histologic grade of malignancy than of fundamental biologic difference. One tumor had metastasized to lung (QBC).

### Focal Leukocyte Nodules in Liver (LHA)

These were small collections of several dozen mononuclear cells and/or neutrophils scattered in the parenchyma. Sometimes neutrophils predominated, giving the lesions the appearance of microabscesses. It is possible that some of these lesions represented extramedullary hematopoieses, though the megakaryocytes characteristic of that lesion were not present.

### Liver, Fatty Change (LIB)

This consisted of vacuolization of hepatocytic cytoplasm, characteristic of lipid accumulation. Usually the lesion involved only a few dozens or hundreds of cells scattered in random patches in the parenchyma. It occurred significantly more commonly in CB6 mice.

### Multifocal Degeneration of Myocardium (NEB)

This lesion was characterized by areas of fibrosis, loss of myocardial cells, proliferation of Anitchkow myocytes and sometimes mild chronic inflammation. It often accompanied myocardial amyloidosis (NIA), and may have been secondary to it in some cases, but was present without it in other cases. The lesion occurred at approximately 20 months of age, as did amyloidosis, but varied with respect to genotype in a different fashion. Both lesions were significantly more common in D2 mice. However degeneration occurred in 14% of CBA/H mice which were not prone to amyloidosis.

### Epicardial Mineralization (NKA)

This well known lesion of certain genotypes of mice was characterized by deposition of mineral in the epicardium. It occurred significantly more commonly in D2 and C mice.

### No Lesions in Any Organ (NON)

As might be expected, mice without any lesions had a very low mean age. A significantly greater proportion of A/He mice than of other genotypes had no lesions.

*Bronchoalveolar Adenocarcinoma (QBA) and Adenoma (QCA)*

Most of these tumors, believed to be of Clara cell origin, were solitary, well circumscribed but never encapsulated. The cells were hyperchromatic, usually uniform in size or pleomorphic. A few invaded adjacent lung parenchyma. Very rarely distant metastasis to other areas of the lung were observed. The tumors occurred significantly more commonly in C, CB6 and CFW mice. A few lung tumors were diagnosed as adenomas. These consisted of epithelial cells that had less hyperchromasia and apparent invasiveness than that characteristic of carcinomas. Since histologic gradations between benign and malignant lung tumors were observed, it is possible that the distinction is a matter of tumor grade and not of basic biology.

*Lung, Alveolar Cell Hyperplasia (QDA)*

This lesion consisted of patches of alveoli lined by large epithelial cells with abundant cytoplasm. There was no disorganization of alveolar architecture and no displacement of adjacent parenchyma.

*Lung, Alveolar Histiocytosis (QHB)*

This was characterized by the accumulation of many large macrophages with abundant brightly eosinophilic cytoplasm, sometimes with crystalline material. This was probably hematoidin which accumulated following phagocytosis of erythrocytes following episodes of hemorrhage (Shultz *et al.*, 1984). The lesion often occurred around lung tumors, but was counted as a separate lesion only if it occurred at a distance from them. It was particularly common in B6, B10 and CFW mice.

*Thyroid, Cystic Follicles (RJA)*

In this lesion at least a few thyroid follicles were markedly dilated and contained pale staining colloid. This occurred at significantly greater rates in CBA/C and CFW mice.

*Renal Cortical Atrophy (TFA)*

This lesion of older mice was characterized by tubular and glomerular atrophy, mild interstitial fibrosis and an overall appearance of collapse of stroma. Usually only a part of the cortex was affected, and often the borders of the lesions were sharp, suggesting that the lesions resulted from partial infarction.

*Glomerulonephritis (THA)*

This lesion was characterized by a uniform thickening of basement membranes of renal glomeruli. Some glomeruli were enlarged and some sclerotic. Protein casts were observed more often in kidneys with this lesion than in those with glomerular amyloidosis (TIA). No genotype had a particular predilection to develop this lesion.

*Hydronephrosis (TJA)*

In nearly all cases only one kidney had a mild to moderately dilated pelvis. Often the cortex was atrophic and sometimes chronically inflamed. CFW mice were particularly prone to develop this lesion.

*Calcified Nodules in Renal Cortex (TKA)*

This was characterized by a few small concretions of mineral scattered in the medulla and less often in the cortex. It occurred most commonly in the CBA/C and CBA/H mice.

*Atrophy of Testis and Epididymus (UFA)*

This common lesion was characterized by atrophy of seminiferous tubules, with little spermatogenesis. Many tubules were lined only by Sertoli cells. The epithelium of the epididymus was atrophic. The two lesions usually went together, and occurred commonly in B6 and CB mice.

*Ovary, Cystic Follicles (WJB)*

This lesion was characterized by cystic dilatation of follicles. It was easily confused with cysts of the ovary not clearly associated with the ovarian parenchyma, parovarian cysts (WJA).

*Endometrial Gland Hyperplasia (XDA)*

The endometrium was thickened with proliferative glands lined by hyperchromatic epithelium. Often the hyperplasia resulted in the formation of polyps (XCA).

*Vagina, Eosinophilic and Suppurative Vaginitis (XGB)*

This change was characterized by a mild to moderately severe infiltration of inflammatory cells in the epithelium and lamina propria of the vagina. Probably in most cases it was related physiologically to the estrus cycle. In this sample it occurred commonly in CBA/C, CFW and D2 mice.

*Dilatation of Endometrial Glands (XJA) and Hydrometra (XJB)*

Often these lesions went together, and in older mice were often accompanied by endometrial hyperplasia (XDA) and endometrial polyps (XCA). XJA occurred significantly more often in B6D2, CFW and DBA mice and XJB in A/HE, CBA/C and CBA/H mice.

*Suppurative Dermatitis (YGA)*

This lesion occurred in younger Balb/c mice and may have been due to fighting, to which that genotype of mouse is particularly prone.

*Purulent Gingivitis and Periodontitis (ZHA)*

This lesion was characterized by various degrees of inflammation around the alveoli of molar teeth. Often in these mice there were frank tooth root abscesses. CBA/C and D2 mice were particularly susceptible.

## Lesions in Rats

*Degenerative Radiculoneuropathy (141)*

This lesion was characterized in early stages by the presence of large vacuoles in both dorsal and ventral roots containing lipid-laden macrophages. In more severe lesions there was complete dissolution of some rootlets, and cholesterol clefts were present. Whether this lesion is responsible for neurogenic atrophy of skeletal muscles (942) was not established. This lesion is somewhat analogous to degenerative radiculopathy (DEA) of mice. All genotypes were equally susceptible to this lesion at 30 months of age.

*Retinal Atrophy (142)*

This consisted of variable loss of retinal layers, apparently starting with the photoreceptor layer and progressing to the bipolar layer. It is analogous to lesion EFA of mice. Buf rats were particularly susceptible.

*Bile Duct Hyperplasia and Portal Fibrosis (231)*

This was histologically variable, characterized by proliferation of bile ducts and fibrosis in portal areas occurring together or alone in each portal area. Some degree of chronic inflammation of portal areas (265) was often present.

*Basophilic Hepatocyte Nodules (232)*

Liver nodules in rats were quite variable, ranging from discrete aggregations of hepatocytes that differed from normal hepatocytes in subtle cytological details, to large nodules with pleomorphic hepatocytes that displaced surrounding parenchyma. In basophilic nodules hepatocytes of normal size had what appeared to be endoplasmic reticulum displaced to the edges of the cytoplasm, leaving a pale perinuclear cytoplasmic clearing. Other types of proliferative lesions were 213, 221 and 234. Basophilic nodules occurred significantly more commonly in F344 rats.

*Focal Vacuolation of Hepatocytes (271) and Fatty Change (272)*

These lesions were characterized by clusters of several hundred hepatocytes with vacuolated cytoplasm. In some lesions the hepatocyte nuclei were centrally located, suggesting accumulation of glycogen (271) and in others the nuclei were displaced, suggesting accumulation of lipid (272). Many rats had both kinds of lesions. Since both lesions had similar mean age of occurrence, and both occurred more often in males than in females, they may have been synonymous.

*Peliosis Hepatis (281)*

Cavernous vascular channels and ectatic sinuosids filled with fibrin and occasional erythrocytes were characteristic of this lesion. Often the areas of telangiectasis were quite large. This lesion occurred significantly more commonly in males than in females.

*Cystic Dilatation of Gastric Glands (282)*

This mild lesion was characterized by occasional dilated gastric crypts, some of which contained proteinaceous droplets. It occurred particularly often in Buf rats.

*Focal Myocardial Fibrosis and Degeneration (342)*

This lesion consisted of quite large patches of fibrosis in the left ventricle and septum, usually most severely in the papillary muscles and adjacent myocardium. In the fibrotic areas there were degenerating myocardial fibers, Anitschkow myocytes and sometimes chronic inflammation.

*Chronic Myocarditis (361)*

This lesion consisted of multiple, variably sized foci of chronic inflammatory cells in the interstitium. Often degenerating cardiac fibers were present within the lesions. This lesion was particularly common in F344 rats.

*Alveolar Histiocytosis (463)*

This lesions in rats was similar to that of mice (QHB).

*Pheochromocytoma (521)*

These tumors were composed of small nests of cells separated by a delicate fibrovascular stroma. Tumor cells contained large vesicular nuclei and moderate amounts of cytoplasm. Often the tumor cells appeared to invade the cortex. These tumors occurred significantly more commonly in Buf rats than in rats of other genotypes.

*Adenoma of Pituitary (521)*

These neoplasms consisted of quite uniform round cells. Cells in some tumors had more cytoplasm than in others. Large vascular spaces were often present. Rare tumors of the pituitary were pleomorphic and appeared to invade leptomeninges. These were diagnosed as adenocarcinomas *(513)*. Adenomas were particularly common in Buf rats. It is possible that cystic dilatation of mammary glands (981) occurred in response to the known secretion of prolactin by these tumors. Perhaps the cystic form of fibroadenoma of mammary gland (921) was due to the same process.

*C Cell Adenoma of Thyroid (522)*

The cells of these tumors had uniform round nuclei and moderately large amounts of eosinophilic cytoplasm. They were arranged as small nests separated by a delicate stroma. The tumors were differentiated from adenomas of the parathyroid (526), which they closely resembled, only by the certain location of the latter within the parathyroid.

*Lobular Ectasia and Atrophy of Exocrine Pancreas (534)*

This lesion usually involved only segments of the pancreas in which there was loss of exocrine tissue and replacement with adipose and fibrous tissue. Often remaining acini had atrophic epithelium and dilated lumens.

*Hyperplasia of Islet Cells (536)*

This lesion was characterized by enlarged pancreatic islets. The numbers of islets appeared increased in some cases. The islet cells themselves were histologically normal, at least at the light microscopic level. This lesion occurred more commonly in males than in females.

*Nodular Vacuolation of Adrenal Cortical Cells (571)*

This lesion consisted of areas in adrenal cortex with cortical cells that had vacuolated cytoplasm. The affected areas did not have rounded contours, suggesting that the lesion was not a variety of nodular hyperplasia or adenoma. This lesion was particularly common in BN rats.

*Subcapsular Vacuolation of Adrenal (572)*

This lesion consisted of small foci under the capsule in the zona glomerulosa that contained vacuolated cells. The lesion was morphologically distinct from 571. It occurred in significantly more F344 × Lewis rats than in other genotypes.

*Telangiectasia of Adrenal Cortex (582)*

These lesions were variably sized areas in which dilated cortical sinusoids displaced normal adrenal. Sometimes the vascular spaces were cavernous. This lesion was very common in Buf rats.

*Colloid Cysts of Thyroid (584)*

Large cystic follicles, ranging in size up to many times the normal follicular diameter, characterized this lesion. It was similar to Lesion RJA of mice.

*Chronic Progressive Glomerulonephropathy (641, 642)*

This common lesion was given two codes, one for the mildly severe lesions and one for the more severe lesions. The most striking feature of the lesion was cystic dilatation of renal tubules which contained proteinaceous casts. Often glomeruli were sclerotic. Occasional foci of hypertrophic tubular epithelial cells suggested regeneration. There were varying degrees of interstitial fibrosis and chronic inflammation. The severe form of this lesion occurred significantly more commonly in F344 rats than in other genotypes.

### Transitional Cell Hyperplasia of Renal Pelvis (671)

In this lesion the transitional cells often extended as finger-like processes into pelvic stroma. Nodules of mineralization were associated with the epithelial changes. This was most common in Buf rats.

### Hydronephrosis (681)

This lesion occurred unilaterally in one of the kidneys or bilaterally. The gross necropsy descriptions did not mention the presence of uroliths as possible etiologic agents. It occurred significantly more commonly in BN and Buf rats.

### Leydig Cell Adenoma (721)

This common testicular tumor was highly vascular in many cases and was composed of sheets of large cells with voluminous eosinophilic cytoplasm. Some tumors had large numbers of lymphocytes at the periphery, sometimes suggesting a diagnosis of lymphoma. This tumor was particularly common in F344 rats.

### Atrophy of Prostate (741)

In this lesion portions of the prostate had dilated glands lined by flattened epithelium.This was particularly common in BN rats.

### Atrophy of Testis (742)

Seminiferous tubules in this lesion had little or no spermatogenesis and were lined by Sertoli cells. In some cases portions of affected testes were normal, and often only one testis was affected. The lesion is analogous to lesion UFA of mice. This was most common in BN rats.

### Cystic Endometrium (881)

This lesion. characterized by dilatation of endometrial glands, resembled that of mice, XJA. It occurred significantly more commonly in Lewis and F344 × Lewis rats than in other genotypes.

### Fibroadenoma of Mammary Gland (922)

This benign neoplasm, of which 921 was a variant, consisted of well differentiated mammary acini, usually with vacuolated cytoplasm, in a stroma composed of collagen of variable density.

### Individual Skeletal Muscle Fiber Necrosis (941)

This lesion was observed as single scattered fibers undergoing phagocytosis by macrophages. Remaining sarcoplasm of affected fibers tended to be hypereosinophilic. Usually no more than one affected fiber per high power field was observed.

### Neurogenic Atrophy of Skeletal Muscle (942)

This consisted of groups of small fibers, often adjacent to fibers of normal size.

### Degeneration of Cartilage of Sternum (943)

This lesion was characterized by focal caseative necrosis of cartilage. Seldom was there any inflammatory reaction. This lesion was very common in Buf rats.

### Cystic Dilatation of Mammary Glands (981)

This common lesion was characterized by large cystic spaces of variable size lined by low cuboidal epithelium and filled with droplets of secretion.

## Genotypic Variation in the Rate of Occurrence of Lesions in Mice

The more numerous lesions were studied statistically to see if any occurred more often in any genotype than in the entire sample of each species. The results are presented in Table 5. In this table the raw numbers of occurrences of each lesion in each genotype are included to make it more convenient for readers to perform any chi square test of interest. Here significant differences, $P < 0.001$, between the proportion of animals of a genotype with and without a lesion and that proportion for all the other animals in the sample are indicated by asterisks. Many of the significant differences were discussed under each specific lesion above. Some readers might find it of interest to perform chi square tests to see if their data for any lesion differs significantly from these. Analysis of these data for mice to find differences between genotypes has several potential pitfalls. First, there is great disparity in the numbers of mice of the various genotypes, ranging from 25 *nu/nu* to 465 B6 mice. The number of B6 mice, in fact, is so large that comparison of any genotype against the entire sample (as was done in Table 5) is to a large extent a comparison of the genotype against B6 mice. Second, disparities in mean age between certain genotypes and in mean age between sexes of the same genotype, some of which were statistically significant as shown in Table 1, can also lead to spurious conclusions. A lesion may have occurred significant-

**Table 5.** Numbers of occurences of each of 44 lesions in each of 12 genotypes of mice

| Lesion Code | Tot-al | Genotypes and Numbers of Mice | | | | | | | | | | | |
|---|---|---|---|---|---|---|---|---|---|---|---|---|---|
| | | A/ He (78) | C (269) | B6C3 (26) | B6D2 (108) | B10.1 29 (49) | B6 (465) | CBA/ CA (108) | CBA/ T-6 (49) | CB6 (239) | CFW (77) | DBA( 84) | nu/ nu (25) |
| ABA | 49 | 1 | 2 | 0 | 2 | 0 | 26* | 1 | 4 | 2 | 2 | 7* | 2 |
| AOA | 36 | 1 | 4 | 0 | 3 | 0 | 11 | 4 | 3 | 3 | 3 | 4 | 0 |
| EFA | 78 | 4 | 3 | 0 | 0 | 0 | 0 | 0 | 0 | 0 | 71* | 0 | 0 |
| FDA | 32 | 3 | 7 | 1 | 0 | 0 | 1 | 12* | 6* | 2 | 0 | 0 | 0 |
| FOC | 44 | 0 | 8 | 1 | 0 | 0 | 16 | 2 | 0 | 14* | 0 | 0 | 3 |
| GGK | 73 | 0 | 4 | 0 | 0 | 5 | 56* | 0 | 0 | 3 | 1 | 4 | 0 |
| HIA | 56 | 0 | 0 | 0 | 15* | 5 | 20 | 0 | 0 | 1 | 1 | 15* | 0 |
| HOA | 178 | 5 | 15 | 2 | 3 | 0 | 99* | 2 | 4 | 26 | 6 | 15 | 1 |
| LAA | 31 | 4 | 9 | 0 | 1 | 0 | 5 | 2 | 0 | 3 | 5* | 1 | 1 |
| LCA | 31 | 1 | 2 | 1 | 3 | 0 | 2 | 13* | 3 | 5 | 1 | 0 | 0 |
| LHA | 133 | 13 | 10 | 2 | 17 | 7 | 46 | 6 | 1 | 9 | 15* | 6 | 1 |
| LIB | 47 | 0 | 7 | 0 | 0 | 0 | 11 | 2 | 0 | 21* | 6 | 0 | 0 |
| LOA | 99 | 0 | 22 | 0 | 0 | 2 | 58* | 1 | 0 | 3 | 13 | 1 | 1 |
| NEB | 44 | 5 | 1 | 0 | 2 | 1 | 6* | 5 | 7* | 3 | 5 | 8* | 1 |
| NIA | 73 | 0 | 0 | 0 | 16* | 5 | 29 | 2 | 0 | 3 | 2 | 16* | 0 |
| NKA | 87 | 1 | 24* | 0 | 0 | 0 | 4 | 7 | 2 | 0 | 0 | 48* | 0 |
| NON | 321 | 27* | 76 | 2 | 17 | 15 | 73 | 31 | 13 | 55 | 1 | 7 | 4 |
| PIB | 502 | 0 | 35 | 20* | 52* | 14 | 212* | 17 | 5 | 122* | 8 | 14 | 3 |
| QBA | 81 | 4 | 24* | 1 | 1 | 2 | 1 | 6 | 2 | 20* | 17 | 0 | 3 |
| QDA | 28 | 3 | 2 | 0 | 0 | 0 | 10 | 4 | 1 | 6 | 2 | 0 | 0 |
| QHB | 54 | 2 | 3 | 0 | 1 | 5* | 30* | 1 | 1 | 1 | 8* | 2 | 0 |
| QOA | 174 | 3 | 38 | 0 | 1 | 1 | 86* | 2 | 0 | 31 | 12 | 0 | 0 |
| QOB | 57 | 0 | 11 | 0 | 0 | 0 | 33 | 0 | 0 | 13 | 0 | 0 | 0 |
| RJA | 28 | 3 | 3 | 0 | 0 | 0 | 1 | 13* | 2 | 0 | 5* | 1 | 0 |
| SOA | 25 | 1 | 2 | 0 | 1 | 0 | 8 | 1 | 0 | 3 | 2 | 7* | 7* |
| TFA | 30 | 2 | 10 | 0 | 4 | 1 | 8 | 0 | 0 | 2 | 1 | 1 | 1 |
| THA | 45 | 2 | 3 | 0 | 2 | 1 | 4 | 11 | 4 | 14 | 1 | 3 | 0 |
| TIA | 130 | 0 | 2 | 0 | 27* | 11* | 57* | 1 | 0 | 2 | 3 | 27* | 0 |
| TJA | 31 | 0 | 3 | 0 | 3 | 3 | 6 | 4 | 0 | 1 | 8* | 3 | 0 |
| TKA | 44 | 1 | 0 | 0 | 0 | 0 | 0 | 28* | 15* | 0 | 0 | 0 | 0 |
| TOA | 154 | 8 | 35 | 0 | 6 | 0 | 48 | 3 | 1 | 36* | 12 | 5 | 0 |
| TOB | 33 | 1 | 13 | 0 | 2 | 0 | 10 | 0 | 0 | 7 | 0 | 0 | 0 |
| UFA | 112 | 1 | 21 | 0 | 3 | 3 | 52* | 17* | 4 | 5 | 1 | 4 | 1 |
| WIA | 34 | 1 | 0 | 0 | 8* | 3 | 0 | 0 | 0 | 0 | 0 | 22* | 0 |
| WJB | 26 | 3 | 2 | 0 | 2 | 0 | 5 | 6 | 3 | 0 | 2 | 3 | 0 |
| XDA | 22 | 1 | 3 | 0 | 4 | 0 | 3 | 1 | 2 | 0 | 4 | 4 | 0 |
| XGB | 36 | 2 | 4 | 0 | 2 | 2 | 3 | 6 | 0 | 0 | 6* | 11* | 0 |
| XJA | 110 | 2 | 9 | 0 | 20* | 2 | 34 | 7 | 4 | 0 | 16* | 16* | 0 |
| XJB | 44 | 12* | 4 | 0 | 0 | 0 | 4 | 10* | 8* | 0 | 5 | 1 | 0 |
| YGA | 26 | 0 | 19* | 0 | 0 | 0 | 5 | 0 | 0 | 0 | 0 | 0 | 2 |
| YOA | 22 | 2 | 1 | 0 | 2 | 1 | 10 | 3 | 0 | 0 | 3 | 0 | 0 |
| ZHA | 32 | 1 | 3 | 0 | 2 | 0 | 5 | 6* | 0 | 3 | 2 | 8* | 2 |

*Indicates that the ratio of mice of the genotype with the lesion to those without was significantly different from the ratio for the entire sample as determined by the Chi Square test on four fold contingency tables. P < 0.001.

ly more often in one genotype or sex than in another only because the mice of the first were older than those of the second.

In addition to variation between genotypes with respect to the rate of occurrence of specific lesions, there was variation with respect to the overall tendency of a genotype to develop lesions. A simple count of asterisks in Table 5 shows that B6, DBA, and CFW mice had significantly more of at least 9 lesions that did all the other mice in the entire sample. A/HE, C, *nu/nu* and B6C3 mice had significantly more of only one or 2 lesions. The two hybrid genotypes, B6D2 and CB6, had significantly more of 5 lesions, suggesting that hybrid vigor was not necessarily protective. Only the A/He genotype had significantly more animals without lesions (NON) than did other genotypes, but this may have been due to the fact that females of that genotype were significantly younger than animals of other genotypes. Interestingly, two similar genotypes, CBA/C and CBA/H differed significantly with respect to lesions LCA, NEB, RJA, UFA and ZHA. (See Table 5.)

The data shed a little light on the mechanism of the well known difference between long lived B6 and shorter lived D2 mice (Russel, 1979). Both genotypes were more prone to develop a larger number of lesions than many other genotypes. Both were susceptible to amyloidosis of one or another organ. Perhaps the difference between them is that the D2 mice were significantly younger than the B6 mice yet were prone to develop as many lesions.

## Genotypic Variation in the Rate of Occurrence of Lesions in Rats

Data for the more common lesions as they occurred in the various genotypes of rats are presented in Table 6. As in Table 5 the significant differences, $P < 0.0001$, between genotypes in rates of occurrence of lesions are designated by asterisks. Some of the problems that stem from comparing groups of widely different sizes and of different mean age do not apply here since the groups of rats were quite uniform with respect to sample size, age and sex. Table 6, like Table 5, can be used to demonstrate which genotypes were more or less susceptible than the others to develop lesions. Seven and six lesions, respectively, occurred more commonly in F344 and Buf rats than in the overall sample. In BN rats, four lesions occurred more commonly; Lewis rats developed only one lesion more commonly. The F344 × BN rats appeared most resistant to lesions since they developed none more frequently than did the overall sample. The other two hybrid rat genotypes each developed 2 lesions more commonly than the other genotypes.

Roderick T.Bronson

**Table 6.** Numbers of Occurrences of Each of 50 Lesions in 8 Genotypes of Rats

| Lesion # | Brown Norway | | | BN/Biry | | | F344 × BN | | | Buffalo | | | F344 × Buf | | | F344 | | | Wistar Lewis | | | Lewis × F344 | | | Lewis 36 mo. | | | Total | | |
|---|---|---|---|---|---|---|---|---|---|---|---|---|---|---|---|---|---|---|---|---|---|---|---|---|---|---|---|---|---|---|
| **Total rats** | M | F | T | M | F | T | M | F | T | M | F | T | M | F | T | M | F | T | M | F | T | M | F | T | M | F | T | M | F | T |
|  | 35 | 27 | 62 | 8 | 16 | 24 | 35 | 35 | 70 | 37 | 36 | 73 | 35 | 35 | 70 | 35 | 35 | 70 | 35 | 29 | 64 | 35 | 29 | 64 | 8 | 2 | 10 | 271 | 247 | 518 |
| 041 | 0 | 0 | 0 | 0 | 0 | 0 | 0 | 0 | 0 | 0 | 0 | 0 | 6 | 8 | 14 | 12 | 8 | 20 | 5 | 7 | 12 | 5 | 6 | 11 | 1 | 0 | 1 | 45 | 47 | 92 |
| 141 | 8 | 0 | 8 | 8 | 16 | 24 | 8 | 6 | 14 | 6 | 13 | 19 | 8 | 8 | 16 | 8 | 8 | 16 | 3 | 1 | 4 | 5 | 4 | 9 | 7 | 1 | 8 | 61 | 57 | 118 |
| 142 | 0 | 0 | 0 | 0 | 0 | 0 | 0 | 0 | 0 | 14 | 26 | 40* | 4 | 5 | 9 | 3 | 4 | 7 | 5 | 5 | 10 | 1 | 9 | 10 | 2 | 1 | 3 | 29 | 50 | 79 |
| 231 | 0 | 0 | 0 | 7 | 3 | 10 | 19 | 6 | 25 | 19 | 22 | 41 | 23 | 21 | 44 | 24 | 15 | 39 | 0 | 4 | 4 | 22 | 18 | 40 | 8 | 1 | 9 | 123 | 90 | 213 |
| 232 | 0 | 1 | 1 | 2 | 3 | 5 | 0 | 1 | 1 | 4 | 5 | 9 | 5 | 7 | 12 | 4 | 18 | 22* | 6 | 2 | 8 | 2 | 13 | 15 | 3 | 2 | 5 | 26 | 52* | 78 |
| 235 | 2 | 0 | 2 | 0 | 0 | 0 | 0 | 0 | 0 | 8 | 0 | 8 | 1 | 3 | 4 | 0 | 0 | 0 | 0 | 0 | 0 | 12 | 0 | 12* | 0 | 0 | 0 | 23* | 3 | 26 |
| 243 | 0 | 0 | 0 | 0 | 0 | 0 | 0 | 0 | 0 | 0 | 0 | 0 | 0 | 1 | 1 | 5 | 2 | 7 | 4 | 4 | 8 | 4 | 4 | 8 | 0 | 0 | 0 | 13 | 11 | 24 |
| 253 | 0 | 0 | 0 | 0 | 1 | 1 | 3 | 0 | 3 | 3 | 1 | 4 | 16 | 6 | 22* | 12 | 11 | 23* | 1 | 0 | 1 | 4 | 2 | 6 | 0 | 0 | 0 | 39 | 21 | 60 |
| 261 | 13 | 19 | 32 | 5 | 12 | 17 | 16 | 21 | 37 | 23 | 28 | 51 | 12 | 14 | 26 | 7 | 20 | 27 | 12 | 11 | 23 | 9 | 25 | 34 | 0 | 0 | 0 | 97 | 150* | 247 |
| 262 | 3 | 1 | 4 | 0 | 0 | 0 | 1 | 2 | 3 | 16 | 10 | 26* | 9 | 9 | 18 | 3 | 6 | 9 | 8 | 8 | 16 | 3 | 2 | 5 | 0 | 1 | 1 | 43 | 39 | 82 |
| 263 | 1 | 3 | 4 | 0 | 0 | 0 | 1 | 0 | 1 | 4 | 2 | 6 | 0 | 0 | 0 | 4 | 3 | 7 | 1 | 2 | 3 | 0 | 1 | 1 | 0 | 0 | 0 | 11 | 11 | 22 |
| 265 | 6 | 6 | 12 | 2 | 0 | 2 | 2 | 2 | 4 | 4 | 4 | 8 | 6 | 9 | 15 | 5 | 4 | 9 | 7 | 8 | 15 | 0 | 0 | 0 | 0 | 0 | 0 | 32 | 33 | 65 |
| 271[a] | 1 | 2 | 3 | 11 | 4 | 15 | 14 | 0 | 14 | 5 | 2 | 7 | 3 | 0 | 3 | 3 | 0 | 3 | 4 | 6 | 10 | 4 | 0 | 4 | 2 | 0 | 2 | 47* | 14 | 61 |
| 281 | 0 | 1 | 1 | 1 | 0 | 1 | 1 | 0 | 1 | 2 | 2 | 4 | 9 | 1 | 10 | 4 | 0 | 4 | 2 | 0 | 2 | 5 | 1 | 6 | 6 | 0 | 6 | 31* | 6 | 37 |
| 282 | 0 | 1 | 1 | 1 | 1 | 2 | 0 | 0 | 0 | 1 | 13 | 14* | 5 | 6 | 11 | 4 | 2 | 6 | 5 | 0 | 5 | 1 | 0 | 1 | 1 | 1 | 2 | 20 | 22 | 42 |
| 342 | 3 | 3 | 6 | 5 | 7 | 12 | 15 | 10 | 25 | 2 | 5 | 7 | 10 | 3 | 13 | 15 | 10 | 25 | 11 | 8 | 19 | 12 | 10 | 22 | 5 | 0 | 5 | 78 | 55 | 133 |
| 344 | 4 | 0 | 4 | 0 | 0 | 0 | 3 | 1 | 4 | 3 | 1 | 4 | 3 | 9 | 12 | 11 | 12 | 23* | 4 | 1 | 5 | 8 | 2 | 10 | 0 | 1 | 1 | 36 | 27 | 63 |
| 361 | 11 | 4 | 15 | 4 | 8 | 12 | 7 | 4 | 11 | 6 | 9 | 15 | 2 | 5 | 7 | 16 | 13 | 29* | 3 | 3 | 6 | 6 | 6 | 12 | 1 | 0 | 1 | 56 | 52 | 108 |
| 461 | 8 | 7 | 15 | 0 | 1 | 1 | 3 | 2 | 5 | 4 | 7 | 11 | 8 | 6 | 14 | 4 | 2 | 6 | 9 | 8 | 17 | 8 | 11 | 19 | 0 | 0 | 0 | 44 | 44 | 88 |
| 463 | 0 | 13 | 13 | 0 | 2 | 2 | 0 | 2 | 2 | 4 | 8 | 12 | 0 | 2 | 2 | 0 | 5 | 5 | 4 | 1 | 5 | 2 | 0 | 2 | 0 | 1 | 1 | 12 | 35* | 47 |
| 464 | 1 | 4 | 5 | 0 | 0 | 0 | 3 | 1 | 4 | 6 | 2 | 8 | 10 | 8 | 18* | 3 | 9 | 12 | 7 | 7 | 14 | 4 | 3 | 7 | 0 | 1 | 1 | 12 | 35* | 47 |
| 466 | 10 | 2 | 12 | 0 | 4 | 4 | 4 | 4 | 8 | 2 | 7 | 9 | 0 | 0 | 0 | 3 | 0 | 3 | 0 | 4 | 4 | 0 | 0 | 0 | 3 | 0 | 3 | 22 | 21 | 43 |
| 471 | 4 | 2 | 6 | 1 | 1 | 2 | 10 | 5 | 15 | 17 | 7 | 24 | 14 | 8 | 22 | 10 | 13 | 23 | 5 | 2 | 7 | 10 | 7 | 17 | 2 | 0 | 2 | 73 | 45 | 118 |
| 481 | 4 | 4 | 8 | 0 | 0 | 0 | 2 | 1 | 3 | 0 | 2 | 2 | 0 | 3 | 3 | 2 | 0 | 2 | 6 | 3 | 9 | 4 | 4 | 8 | 1 | 0 | 1 | 19 | 17 | 36 |
| 512 | 0 | 0 | 0 | 2 | 3 | 5 | 0 | 0 | 0 | 4 | 10 | 14* | 0 | 2 | 2 | 3 | 2 | 5 | 0 | 2 | 2 | 0 | 1 | 1 | 4 | 0 | 4 | 13 | 20 | 33 |
| 521 | 0 | 0 | 0 | 3 | 4 | 7 | 4 | 7 | 11 | 15 | 16 | 31* | 9 | 13 | 22 | 2 | 5 | 7 | 2 | 16 | 18 | 7 | 11 | 18 | 2 | 1 | 3 | 44 | 73* | 117 |
| 522 | 0 | 0 | 0 | 2 | 1 | 3 | 1 | 0 | 1 | 3 | 2 | 5 | 2 | 1 | 3 | 2 | 4 | 6 | 0 | 0 | 0 | 2 | 3 | 5 | 2 | 1 | 3 | 14 | 12 | 26 |
| 532 | 1 | 0 | 1 | 1 | 0 | 1 | 0 | 1 | 1 | 1 | 5 | 6 | 3 | 2 | 5 | 4 | 1 | 5 | 2 | 3 | 5 | 0 | 1 | 1 | 0 | 1 | 1 | 12 | 14 | 26 |

**Table 6.** (Continued) Numbers of Occurrences of Each of 50 Lesions in 8 Genotypes of Rats

| Total rats | Brown Norway | | | BN/ Biry | | | F344 × BN | | | Buffalo | | | F344 × Buf | | | F344 | | | Wistar Lewis | | | Lewis × F344 | | | Lewis 36 mo. | | | Total | | |
|---|---|---|---|---|---|---|---|---|---|---|---|---|---|---|---|---|---|---|---|---|---|---|---|---|---|---|---|---|---|---|
| | M | F | T | M | F | T | M | F | T | M | F | T | M | F | T | M | F | T | M | F | T | M | F | T | M | F | T | M | F | T |
| | 35 | 27 | 62 | 8 | 16 | 24 | 35 | 35 | 70 | 37 | 36 | 73 | 35 | 35 | 70 | 35 | 35 | 70 | 35 | 29 | 64 | 35 | 29 | 64 | 8 | 2 | 10 | 271 | 247 | 518 |
| Lesion # | | | | | | | | | | | | | | | | | | | | | | | | | | | | | | |
| 534 | 6 | 4 | 10 | 2 | 2 | 4 | 3 | 2 | 5 | 1 | 2 | 3 | 1 | 1 | 2 | 5 | 3 | 8 | 0 | 0 | 0 | 0 | 1 | 1 | 0 | 0 | 0 | 18 | 15 | 23 |
| 536 | 2 | 0 | 2 | 8 | 0 | 8 | 0 | 0 | 0 | 10 | 0 | 10 | 8 | 0 | 8 | 5 | 0 | 5 | 8 | 2 | 10 | 5 | 0 | 5 | 0 | 0 | 0 | 46* | 2 | 48 |
| 563 | 0 | 1 | 1 | 1 | 0 | 1 | 3 | 2 | 5 | 0 | 5 | 5 | 2 | 4 | 6 | 2 | 4 | 6 | 0 | 1 | 1 | 1 | 1 | 2 | 0 | 0 | 0 | 9 | 18 | 27 |
| 571 | 13 | 6 | 19* | 2 | 11 | 13 | 11 | 4 | 15 | 1 | 2 | 3 | 4 | 1 | 5 | 2 | 3 | 5 | 5 | 5 | 10 | 3 | 4 | 7 | 2 | 2 | 4 | 43 | 38 | 81 |
| 572 | 9 | 6 | 15 | 2 | 0 | 2 | 2 | 4 | 6 | 0 | 1 | 1 | 1 | 2 | 3 | 0 | 0 | 0 | 3 | 0 | 0 | 18 | 13 | 31* | 0 | 0 | 0 | 35 | 26 | 61 |
| 582 | 1 | 0 | 1 | 0 | 0 | 0 | 0 | 1 | 1 | 1 | 12 | 13* | 0 | 2 | 2 | 0 | 0 | 0 | 0 | 9 | 9 | 0 | 7 | 7 | 0 | 0 | 0 | 2 | 31* | 33 |
| 584 | 1 | 2 | 3 | 1 | 0 | 1 | 3 | 3 | 6 | 2 | 2 | 4 | 2 | 1 | 3 | 1 | 0 | 1 | 1 | 0 | 1 | 1 | 0 | 1 | 1 | 0 | 1 | 13 | 8 | 21 |
| 641 | 7 | 7 | 14 | 3 | 1 | 4 | 16 | 9 | 25 | 17 | 25 | 42 | 19 | 10 | 29 | 20 | 15 | 35 | 20 | 8 | 28 | 22 | 8 | 30 | 7 | 0 | 7 | 138 | 85 | 223 |
| 642 | 0 | 0 | 0 | 1 | 0 | 1 | 0 | 0 | 0 | 2 | 2 | 4 | 2 | 2 | 4 | 10 | 4 | 14* | 6 | 0 | 6 | 0 | 0 | 0 | 1 | 0 | 1 | 25 | 8 | 33 |
| 661 | 2 | 0 | 2 | 0 | 0 | 0 | 3 | 1 | 4 | 1 | 1 | 2 | 1 | 0 | 1 | 0 | 4 | 4 | 2 | 1 | 3 | 2 | 1 | 3 | 0 | 0 | 0 | 14 | 8 | 22 |
| 671 | 5 | 3 | 8 | 0 | 6 | 6 | 0 | 7 | 7 | 9 | 19 | 28* | 0 | 7 | 7 | 0 | 3 | 3 | 2 | 0 | 2 | 0 | 7 | 7 | 0 | 0 | 0 | 16 | 53* | 69 |
| 681 | 12 | 6 | 18 | 0 | 10 | 10 | 0 | 1 | 1 | 3 | 12 | 15* | 0 | 0 | 0 | 1 | 0 | 1 | 0 | 2 | 2 | 0 | 0 | 0 | 0 | 0 | 0 | 16 | 31 | 47 |
| 721 | 0 | 0 | 0 | 1 | 0 | 1 | 3 | 0 | 3 | 1 | 0 | 1 | 1 | 0 | 1 | 18 | 0 | 18* | 0 | 0 | 0 | 6 | 0 | 6 | 8 | 0 | 3 | 38 | 0 | 38 |
| 741 | 18 | 0 | 18* | 8 | 0 | 8 | 8 | 0 | 8 | 7 | 0 | 7 | 6 | 0 | 6 | 11 | 0 | 11 | 8 | 0 | 8 | 6 | 0 | 6 | 3 | 0 | 3 | 75 | 0 | 75 |
| 742 | 20 | 0 | 20* | 5 | 0 | 5 | 7 | 0 | 7 | 10 | 0 | 10 | 7 | 0 | 7 | 4 | 0 | 4 | 1 | 0 | 1 | 4 | 0 | 4 | 8 | 0 | 8 | 66 | 0 | 66 |
| 751 | 0 | 0 | 0 | 0 | 0 | 0 | 0 | 0 | 0 | 4 | 0 | 4 | 1 | 0 | 1 | 5 | 0 | 5 | 4 | 0 | 4 | 7 | 0 | 7 | 2 | 0 | 2 | 23 | 0 | 23 |
| 881 | 0 | 1 | 1 | 0 | 0 | 0 | 0 | 0 | 0 | 0 | 1 | 1 | 0 | 2 | 3 | 0 | 2 | 2 | 0 | 12 | 12* | 0 | 12 | 12* | 0 | 1 | 1 | 0 | 31 | 31 |
| 922 | 0 | 1 | 1 | 0 | 4 | 4 | 0 | 0 | 0 | 0 | 5 | 5 | 0 | 9 | 9 | 0 | 5 | 5 | 0 | 3 | 3 | 0 | 5 | 5 | 0 | 2 | 2 | 0 | 33 | 33 |
| 941 | 0 | 0 | 0 | 0 | 1 | 1 | 3 | 1 | 4 | 3 | 3 | 6 | 3 | 6 | 9 | 3 | 0 | 3 | 6 | 2 | 8 | 4 | 3 | 7 | 0 | 0 | 0 | 22 | 16 | 38 |
| 942 | 1 | 2 | 2 | 7 | 6 | 13 | 0 | 2 | 2 | 4 | 7 | 11 | 1 | 0 | 1 | 5 | 0 | 5 | 2 | 1 | 3 | 1 | 0 | 1 | 7 | 1 | 8 | 28 | 18 | 46 |
| 943 | 1 | 0 | 1 | 0 | 0 | 0 | 0 | 0 | 0 | 6 | 6 | 12* | 1 | 1 | 2 | 0 | 4 | 4 | 1 | 0 | 1 | 0 | 1 | 1 | 0 | 0 | 0 | 9 | 12 | 21 |
| 981[b] | 0 | 6 | 6 | 0 | 10 | 10 | 0 | 6 | 6 | 1 | 14 | 15 | 0 | 6 | 6 | 4 | 6 | 10 | 0 | 11 | 11 | 0 | 12 | 13 | 1 | 2 | 3 | 7 | 73* | 80 |

*The starred total occurrences of the lesion in the breed was significantly greater than expected, P < 0.0001 compared to the total occurrences of the lesion in all the rats of the sample, determined by Chi square analysis on 2x2 contingency tables. Similar stars in the columns for total male and female rats indicate that the lesion occurred significantly more often in the sex whose total is starred, P < 0.0005. The 36 month old BN, buffalo and Wistar rats were not included in the statistical analysis. The eight 30 month old BN/Biry rats were grouped with the BN for the analysis.
[a] Lesion # 271 is grouped with # 272 here  (See description of lesions)
[b] Lesion # 921 is grouped with # 922 here.

### Species Specific Variation in the Patterns of Lesions in Rats and Mice

In comparing the data for the two species it must be kept in mind that the rats were older on average than the mice, approximately 20 and 14 months old respectively. Clear differences between the two species were apparent in the data. Some but not all genotypes of mice very commonly developed amyloidosis as they aged; rats did not. Rats commonly developed degenerative glomerulonephropathy (641, 642), degenerative radiculoneuropathy (141), portal fibrosis with bile duct hyperplasia (231) and basophilic hepatic nodules (232); mice never developed any of these lesions, with the exception of degenerative radiculopathy in mice (DEA).

Neoplasia played a quite different role in the two species. Mice of the genotypes studied were prone to develop four neoplasms, lymphoma (ABA), adenoma/adenocarcinoma of the lung (QBA,QCA), hepatocellular carcinoma/hepatoma (LBA,LCA) and adenoma of Harderian gland (FCA). Pituitary adenoma occurred in only 6 mice. (Had older mice at 30 months of age been studied, it is possible that pituitary adenoma would have been more common, as was the case in another study, Yunis *et al.*, 1984). Several genotypes of rats, particularly F344 and Buf, by contrast, commonly developed pituitary and other endocrine adenomas. Rats, like mice, were prone to various liver tumors but, unlike mice, were resistant to lung tumors. Fibroadenoma of the mammary gland (922) was common in rats but never occurred in mice. It should be mentioned that although lymphoma (012) occurred infrequently in rats in this study, F344 rats in other colonies have been shown to be quite susceptible to a form of this cancer, large granular lymphocyte leukemia (Ward & Reynolds, 1983). A strikingly apparent difference between the species was the difference in the ratios of all malignant and all benign tumors. The ratio in mice was 157:72; in the rats it was 101:253. The ratios would be very similar, however, if the 81 carcinomas of lung in mice had been diagnosed as adenomas.

### Sex Specific Variation in the Rate of Occurrence of Lesions in Rats and Mice

Few differences between the two sexes of mice were found. Focal leukocytic nodules (LHA) occurred in 0.05% of males and 18% of females. Hyalinization of the nasal septum (PIB) occurred in 37% of males, 19% of females. No lesions (NON) occurred in 18% of males and 26% of females. These differences were marginally significant, $p < 0.05$, but conceivably were due to differences in mean age of males and females in the entire sample or in mean age of males and females of one or another genotype in which they commonly occurred. Thus retinal atrophy was significantly more common in females than males, but the females of the genotype in which this lesion was most common, CFW, were approximately 5 months older, on average, than the males (Table 1).

Significant differences, p < 0.0005, between the two sexes of rats in the frequency of occurrence of some lesions in non-sex organs are presented in Table 6. Four lesions occurred more often in males than females: focal vacuolation of hepatocytes (271), peliosis hepatis (281), hyperplasia of pancreatic islets (536) and Harderian gland metaplasia of the exorbital gland (235). (This last is characterized by areas in the exorbital gland which resemble Harderian gland histologically, as originally pointed out by a collaborating pathologist in this study, S. Schelling.) Female rats had significantly more basophilic hepatic nodules (232), pituitary adenomas (521), and transitional cell hyperplasia of renal pelvis (671).

## Age Specific Variation in the Rate of Occurrence of Lesions in Rats and Mice

That some lesions occurred in younger animals and some in older ones is expected. The details of the mean age of occurrence of lesions in the overall samples of mice and rats are to be found in Tables 3 and 4. As stated previously, the lesions described in detail above were those which tended to occur in older animals. Although data from all genotypes were lumped in calculating the mean ± S.D. age of occurrence of these lesions, the tables do show which lesions occurred later and which earlier in life. Clearly, some of those occurring later in life might be viewed as biomarkers of aging.

Enough data for B6 mice were available to make it worthwhile to include data on the age specific rate of occurrence of common lesions in that genotype in Table 7. The table shows, as might be expected, that many lesions occurred more frequently in older than in younger mice. The data are descriptively useful, but the dispersion of data into many cells of the table makes statistical analysis of differences between the age-related rate of occurrence of any lesion unrewarding even for a very large sample such as this. Even less rewarding was statistical comparison of the age related rate of occurrence of any lesion between genotypes, most of which were quite poorly represented.

An important but not unexpected result is that the number of lesions increased with the age of the animals. For example, in the overall sample of mice the percentage of mice at 6 months of age with more than three lesions was 7.3. The percentages were 20.4, 41.7 and 75.9 at 12, 18 and 24 months respectively.

| Table 7. Age specific distributuion of lesions in B6 mice | | | | | | | | |
|---|---|---|---|---|---|---|---|---|
| Lesion Code | Age (Months) | | | | | | | |
| | 6 | | 12 | | 18 | | 24 | |
| Sex | M | F | M | F | M | F | M | F |
| Total | 116 | 0 | 94 | 34 | 63 | 30 | 68 | 20 |
| ABA | 0 | 0 | 1 | 0 | 7 | 2 | 9 | 7 |
| AOA | 0 | 0 | 3 | 0 | 4 | 1 | 2 | 1 |
| FOC | 0 | 0 | 2 | 1 | 8 | 1 | 2 | 2 |
| GGK | 10 | 6 | 4 | 1 | 13 | 8 | 7 | 7 |
| HIA | 0 | 0 | 0 | 0 | 4 | 1 | 12 | 3 |
| HOA | 5 | 1 | 0 | 1 | 28 | 6 | 23 | 11 |
| LAA | 0 | 0 | 0 | 0 | 5 | 0 | 0 | 0 |
| LCA | 0 | 0 | 0 | 0 | 0 | 0 | 0 | 2 |
| LHA | 7 | 9 | 2 | 9 | 4 | 6 | 3 | 5 |
| LIB | 3 | 0 | 1 | 0 | 6 | 0 | 1 | 0 |
| LOA | 1 | 0 | 11 | 2 | 15 | 9 | 12 | 8 |
| NEB | 2 | 0 | 0 | 0 | 2 | 0 | 2 | 0 |
| NIA | 0 | 0 | 0 | 0 | 12 | 1 | 14 | 2 |
| NKA | 2 | 0 | 0 | 0 | 1 | 0 | 1 | 0 |
| NON | 34 | 19 | 14 | 5 | 1 | 1 | 1 | 0 |
| PIB | 43 | 5 | 44 | 6 | 56 | 14 | 36 | 8 |
| QBA | 0 | 0 | 0 | 0 | 0 | 0 | 0 | 0 |
| QDA | 5 | 1 | 0 | 1 | 1 | 0 | 1 | 0 |
| QHB | 2 | 2 | 0 | 3 | 7 | 7 | 4 | 5 |
| QOA | 24 | 5 | 13 | 1 | 16 | 4 | 11 | 12 |
| QOB | 14 | 0 | 9 | 0 | 6 | 0 | 4 | 0 |
| RJA | 0 | 0 | 0 | 0 | 0 | 0 | 1 | 0 |
| SOA | 0 | 0 | 0 | 1 | 0 | 6 | 0 | 1 |
| TFA | 0 | 1 | 0 | 0 | 2 | 0 | 5 | 0 |
| THA | 0 | 1 | 0 | 0 | 3 | 0 | 1 | 1 |
| TIA | 0 | 0 | 0 | 0 | 19 | 2 | 30 | 5 |
| TJA | 1 | 0 | 0 | 0 | 1 | 2 | 2 | 0 |
| TOA | 2 | 1 | 10 | 0 | 18 | 3 | 11 | 3 |
| TOB | 1 | 0 | 5 | 0 | 1 | 0 | 3 | 0 |
| UFA | 1 | 0 | 16 | 0 | 16 | 0 | 19 | 0 |
| XDA | 0 | 0 | 0 | 0 | 0 | 1 | 0 | 2 |
| XGB | 0 | 1 | 0 | 0 | 0 | 2 | 0 | 0 |
| XJA | 0 | 0 | 0 | 6 | 0 | 18 | 0 | 10 |
| XJB | 0 | 1 | 0 | 0 | 0 | 2 | 0 | 1 |
| YGA | 0 | 0 | 0 | 0 | 0 | 0 | 0 | 0 |
| YOA | 1 | 1 | 0 | 1 | 0 | 2 | 0 | 5 |
| ZHA | 1 | 0 | 0 | 0 | 0 | 3 | 0 | 1 |

The relative homogeneity in numbers of rats of each genotype studied at each age made possible an analysis of the extent to which rats of the various genotypes developed certain lesions earlier or later in life than did other genotypes. The results are presented in Table 8. Some of the differences were

**TABLE 8.** Age of occurence of 5 pathologically significant lesions and groups of lesions in 7 genotypes of rats.

| Genotypes | Lesions | | | | | |
|---|---|---|---|---|---|---|
| | Radiculo-neuropathy | Retinal atrophy | Glomerulo-nephropathy | Cardio-myopathies[a] | Benign neoplasms | Malignant neoplasms |
| BN | 116:30±0[b] | 0: | 15:15±6 | 33:26±5 | 6:28±3 | 4:27±3 |
| F344 × BN | 14:30±0 | 0: | 26:18±5 | 40:24±6 | 20:27±4 | 6:28±3 |
| Buf | 14:30±2 | 37:25±5 | 44:20±6 | 22:21±7 | 59:25±5 | 19:26±4 |
| F344 × Buf | 16:30±0 | 9:24±9 | 42:23±7 | 31:21±7 | 42:25±6 | 15:27±4 |
| F344 | 16:30±0 | 8:29±2 | 52:21±7 | 51:24±6 | 60:25±6 | 10:28±4 |
| F344 × Lewis | 9:30±0 | 10:22±8 | 27:22±6 | 29:24±6 | 37:27±4 | 9:29±3 |
| Lewis | 4:30±0 | 9:23±9 | 34:23±6 | 25:23±7 | 12:27±4 | 10:28±3 |

[a] Cardiomyopathies = Focal myocardial fibrosis and degeneration # 342; individual myocardial fiber necrosis, # 344; chronic myocarditis, #361.

[b] Number of rats : mean age ± S.D.. The 36 month old rats were not included in the analysis.

significant, p < 0.01. Lewis and F344 × Lewis rats developed retinal atrophy (142) significantly earlier than Buf rats; glomerulonephropathy (641,642) occurred significantly earlier in several genotypes than in others without correlation with the rate of occurence. Three forms of cardiomyopathy (342, 344, 346) occurred significantly later in BN rats than in Buf and F344 × Buf rats. The genotypes were very uniform with respect to the mean age of occurrence of radiculoneuropathy at 30 months (141). The differences between genotypes in mean age of occurrence of benign and malignant neoplasms were not significant.

## DISCUSSION

Characterization of any phenomenon such as aging is non-analytical and nonreductive. It is a descriptive exercise that must be carried out before mechanisms can be explored. Here, characterization of the lesions of aging rodents was comprehensive; no detail was deemed too unimportant to be left out since there were no criteria to determine what was or was not important. In cross sectional studies like this one, most animals are clinically normal; they have few or no lesions that can be considered clinically significant. The significance of any particular lesion in such studies can only depend on the questions asked in any particular experiment. Clearly these results are presented because a fuller description of the cross-sectional lesions of aging in rodents, and particularly better description of the variability in the rate of occurrence of lesions between species, genotypes, ages and sexes, was believed to be useful. The baseline data presented here should be useful in future experimental cross sectional gerontologic studies of rodents.

Most experimental gerontologic studies have three kinds of end points. First, biomarkers of aging, once identified, can be used in cross sectional studies to find if an experiment has affected the rate of aging. Some of the more commonly occurring lesions in aging animals can be treated as biomarkers of aging and evaluated for rate of occurrence and severity in the animals. When lesions are viewed as biomarkers of aging, they are best studied in cross sectional experiments. Second, longevity of the animals is an obvious and critical end point. It can never be a sufficient end point in itself, however. If the experimental manipulation results in longer or shorter life span, the issue immediately arises as to the mechanism of the change in longevity. Post mortem evaluation is the simplest, and probably the only, way of discovering the mechanism, and is the third kind of end point. For example, it might be found that the rate of occurrence of a particular lethal lesion is lower in treated animals than in controls, or that a common potentially lethal lesion occurs later or to a less severe degree. When lesions are viewed as explanations for mortality, obviously they must be studied in longitudinal studies.

The data set from any experimental gerontologic study, cross sectional or longitudinal, will necessarily resemble the data set presented here, though perhaps without the same degree of detail. In a longitudinal study one might concentrate only on "significant" lesions, those that explain why the animals died. Even then, one often finds a number of potentially lethal lesions in a dead or dying rodent, as was the case in previously reported longitudinal studies (Yunis *et al.*, 1984, Gelman *et al.*, 1987.) In the usual absence of clinical data on rodents, one must still decide which of several "significant" lesions to report. In the opinion of the author, even in longitudinal studies one should first record all lesions, regardless of apparent significance. Practically, once one has developed a sound data base in a computer, recording many lesions is only marginally more difficult than recording only the major ones. Next, the investigator can evaluate the entire data set and decide which lesions to report. That will depend on the questions being asked in the study. For example, carcinogenicity studies will find even the smallest, earliest malignancy significant, even though at that stage of development the tumor was of no health significance to the animal, which probably died from some other disease. In the author's opinion too many published gerontological studies have focussed too narrowly on lesions deemed to be clinically significant, and have not provided readers with a sufficiently wide array of the available data.

This paper does not include data on two other dimensions of variability, the severity of lesions and the interaction between lesions. Severity can be evaluated semiquantitatively quite easily and reproducibly but, except for glomerulonephropathy of rats, was not attempted here. The difficulty in analyzing data for interactions between lesions is very great since the total number of possible interactions is enormous. Most single lesions occur so infrequently that they cannot be evaluated statistically unless "n" is sufficiently large; finding sufficiently large numbers of animals with each of two or more specified lesions becomes exponentially more unlikely. Yet such interactions may be important. Perhaps, for example, glomerulo-nephropathy in rats is significantly associated with cardiomyopathy. Such possible associations were not sought here.

The issue of interactive events is raised in this report, as it would be in others, by the question of how to report lesions of the same type occurring in several organs, such as systemic amyloidosis and malignant lymphoma. One can report the disease once for each animal in which its characteristic lesion is observed, regardless of the organ in which it occurs, as was done here for lymphoma. Alternatively, one can report each occurrence of the lesion in each organ in which it is seen, as was done here for amyloidosis. In the author's opinion it is always best to collect data on lesions as they occur in each organ. After analyzing the data to see if the various experimental groups differ with respect to organ distribution of a particular kind of lesion, one can decide whether or not to lump lesions of the same kind into a single diagnosis. In this study it happens that, by chance, the arbitrary decision to report amyloidosis by organ led to the finding that what was believed to be amyloidosis of the nasal septum was likely to be a different kind of lesion from the amyloidosis of other organs. It was observed in several genotypes not prone to amyloidosis of other organs. Perhaps if the lesions of lymphoma had not been lumped, differences between the genotypes in organ distribution of that disease would have been discovered.

Some important issues regarding the classification of lesions are raised here. The coding system was retained through this paper, not only for its use as an index, but also to stress the point that each lesion in a study, and it is hoped in all rodent studies, should have one single designation. For statistical purposes it actually is of less importance that the name be correct than that all like lesions be called the same thing. A code is as useful as a name for this purpose. Which particular code is used is inconsequential. Interestingly, a three digit code, particularly an alphabetic one, is fully capable of describing all possible lesions of a rodent species.

Not all pathologists would agree that lesions can be classified in the rigid way used here. Many would argue that tissues react to various insults in limited stereotypic fashions, that various pathologic processes often occur simultaneously in the same tissue, and that the processes change and evolve over time. They would argue, therefore, that each individual lesion in each individual is a unique entity that should be diagnosed using whatever appropriate term one chooses from the full set of available pathologic terms, as listed, for instance, in the Standardized Nomenclature of Medicine (College of American Pathologists, 1978). In effect, most pathologists reserve the right to diagnose lesions as they see them. If a term such as "acute bronchopneumonia" comes to mind and seems appropriate to describe a lesion, it will be used, even though the particular form of acute bronchopneumonia may be morphologically distinct from another form. It should be added in fairness that pathologists tend to try to be very precise and consistent in diagnosing tumors, but terms for other lesions tend to be used less precisely.

Indeed, adherence to a strict classification system is an oversimplification and can lead to serious errors, particularly in clinical practice, where each case must be viewed as unique. However in experimental pathology, particularly when only spontaneously occurring lesions are studied as here, the advantages of adhering to a strict classification scheme outweigh any disadvantages. The principal advantage is that different studies of the same kinds of animals can be compared. Another critical advantage is that the data analysis is kept within the control of the pathologists. In many other studies the pathologists diagnose lesions as they see them; it is left up to non-pathologists such as toxicologists and statisticians to computerize and analyze the data. It is always certain that someone, eventually, will reduce all the descriptions and diagnoses in a pathologist's reports to tables and numbers, much as was done here. In the process, dissimilar lesions may be lumped or similar ones may be split unless clear distinctions are made at the outset. In this study it proved very difficult to avoid these kinds of errors, even though the person who made most of the original diagnoses and the person who finally reduced the data to tables was one and the same! In fact more than 400 distinct diagnostic terms were used in the original reports on the mice studied here. Half of these turned out to be synonyms for the final list of lesions. The same problems can be seen in another large retrospective study which attempted to integrate data derived from a wide variety of separate pathologic studies performed by many different pathologists (Altman et. al, 1985). In that report a number of terms appear to be synonymous, but one cannot be sure exactly what each pathologist meant by each diagnosis. Classifications should be viewed as dynamic intellectual constructs, rather like the taxonomy of species. It is appropriate for experts to argue about lumping and splitting and it is expected that the classification will change over time. What is necessary is that at any time everyone agrees to a single system. It is likely that the classification presented here has controversial elements. For example different kinds of lymphoma were lumped together erroneously. Some diagnoses, particularly of some neoplasms, might be unacceptable to some other pathologists.

The classification, moreover, is incomplete. It did not include lesions of very old animals, lethal lesions and lesions of genotypes not represented or poorly represented in the data base. The quite comprehensive literature search presented in the bibliography disclosed approximately 50 additional lesions of each species that were not included in this classification. Many of these were neoplasms. An important lesion that in the more recent experience of the author is present in almost all older mice is small cell hyperplasia of adrenal cortex (Goodman, 1983); it was overlooked in this study. It is hoped that this and other recent efforts to classify the lesions of rodents will result in more comprehensive reporting of lesions according to a generally accepted "taxonomy", particularly in gerontologic studies.

## ACKNOWLEDGEMENTS

The author would like to thank the Tufts veterinary pathologists who originally diagnosed some of the lesions included here. These were Drs. Joseph Alroy, Stephan Engler, Scott Schelling and Rosemary Williams. Ruth Lipman Ph.D. coded many of the diagnoses in mice for computer entry. The Principal Investigator of the original surveillance and characterization contracts, from which the data presented here were derived, was Albert Jonas D.V.M., to whom I owe many thanks. This research was supported by contract Order 263-MD-627770 from the National Institute on Aging, NIH.

## REFERENCES

ALTMAN, P. L. and BIOLOGY DATABOOK EDITORIAL BOARD (1985) *Pathology or Laboratory Mice and Rats.* McLean, VA.: FASEB, Pergamon Infoline.

BUREK, J. D. (1978) *Pathology of Aging Rats.* West Palm Beach, Fl: CRC Press.

CAIRNS, T. (1980) The Ed01 study: introduction, objectives and experimental design. *J. Environ. Path. Tox.* 3: 1-7

COTE, R. A. and COLLEGE OF AMERICAN PATHOLOGISTS, COMMITTEE ON NOMENCLATURE AND CLASSIFICATION OF DISEASE. (1979) *Systematized Nomenclature of Medicine.* Skokie, Il.: College of American Pathologists.

FRITH, C. H., PATTENGALE, P. K., WARD, J. M. (198-) *A Color Atlas of the Hematopoietic Pathology of Mice.* Little Rock, AR.: Toxicology Pathology Associates.

GELMAN, R. WATSON, A. BRONSON, R. and YUNIS, R. (1987) Murine chromosomal regions correlated with longevity. *Genetics* 35: 47-61

GOODMAN, D. G. (1983) Subcapsular-cell hyperplasia, adrenal, mouse. 1983. In: *Monographs on Pathology of Laboratory Animals, Endocrine System* (Eds. T.C. JONES, U. MOHR, and R.D. HUNT) pp. 66-68. Berlin: Springer-Verlag

JONES, T. C., MOHR, U.and HUNT, R. D. (1983) *Monographs on Pathology of Laboratory Animals, Endocrine System.* Berlin: Springer-Verlag

JONES, T. C., MOHR, U.and HUNT, R. D. (1985a) *Monographs on Pathology of Laboratory Animals. Respiratory System.* Berlin: Springer-Verlag

JONES, T. C., MOHR, U.and HUNT, R. D. (1985b) *Monographs on Pathology of Laboratory Animals, Digestive System.* Berlin: Springer-Verlag

JONES, T. C., MOHR, U.and HUNT, R. D. (1986) *Monographs on Pathology of Laboratory Animals, Urinary System.* Berlin: Springer-Verlag

JONES, T. C., MOHR, U.and HUNT, R. D. (1987) *Monographs on Pathology of Laboratory Animals, Genital System.* Berlin: Springer-Verlag.

JONES. T. C., MOHR, U.and HUNT, R. D. (1989) *Monographs on Pathology of Laboratory Animals, Nervous System.* Berlin: Springer-Verlag.

PATTENGALE, P. K. and TAYLOR, C. R. (1983) Experimental models of lymphoproliferative disease. The mouse as a model for human non-Hodgkin's lymphomas and related leukemias. *Am J. Path.* **113**: 237-264

RUSSEL, E. S. (1979) Lifespan and aging patterns. In: *The Biology of the Laboratory Mouse* (Ed. E.L. Green) 511-523, New York: Dover Publ

STAATS, J. (1985) Standardized nomenclature for inbred strains of mice, eighth listing. *Cancer Res.* **45**: 945-977

SUZUKI, D. T, Griffiths, A. J. MILLER, J. H. and Lewontin, R. C. (1985) *An Introduction to Genetic Analysis*, 3rd Ed. New York, W.H. Freeman

WARD, J. M. and REYNOLDS, C. W. (1983) Large granular lymphocyte leukemia: A heterogeneous lymphocytic leukemia in F344 rats. *Am. J. Pathol.* **111**: 1-10

YUNIS, E. J., WATSON, A. L. M., GELMAN, R. S., SYLVIA, S. J. and BRONSON, R. T. (1984) Traits that influence longevity in mice. *Genetics* **108**: 999-1011

## BIBLIOGRAPHY

This bibliography is included as a guide to many of the lesions listed in Tables 3 and 4, and described on pages 292 to 313. It is divided into three sections. The first section includes reports listed alphabetically describing several or many lesions in rodents of various genotypes. The second and third sections include reports describing specific lesions in mice and rats, respectively. The papers are presented in the same order as are the lesions in Tables 3 and 4. Each subsection is headed by the lesion name. The code used throughout this paper is included for its index value. In many instances, where the references discuss lesions not observed in this study or where several lesions of one type are discussed, only the first two digits of the code are included.

## A. GENERAL REFERENCES

AMATO, D. A. and LAGAKOS, S. W. in press. Agreement between pathologists in the $ED_{01}$ experiment. In: *Proceedings of the interdisciplinary group in carcinogenicity experiments*, New York, Springer Verlag.

ANISIMOV, V. N. (1976) Spontaneous tumors in rats of different lines. *Vopr. Onkol.* **22**: 98-110

ANVER, M. R. and COHEN, B. J. (1979) Lesions associated with aging. In: *The Laboratory Rat*, **vol. 1** (Eds. H. J. Baker, J. R. Lindsey and S. H. Weishroth), pp. 149-159, New York: Academic Press.

Bailey, D. W. (1978) Sources of subline divergence and their relative importance for sublines of six major strains of mice. In: *Origins of Inbred Mice* (Ed. H.C. Morse), pp. 197-215, New York: Academic Press.

BENIRSCHKE, K., JONES, T. C. and GARNER, F. M. (1978) *Pathology of Laboratory Animals*. New York: Springer-Verlag.

BERG, B. N. (1967) Longevity studies in rats II. Pathology of aging rats. In: *Pathology of Laboratory Rats and Mice* (Eds. E. Cotchin and E.J.C. Roe), pp. 749-786. Oxford: Blackwell.

BILLUPS, L. H. (1976) Naturally occurring neoplastic disease II. Rat. In: *Handbook of Laboratory Animal Science*, **Vol. 3** (Ed. E.C. Melby and N.H. Altmann), pp. 230-247, West Palm Beach, FL: CRC Press.

BODE, G., HARTIG, F., HEBOLD G. and CZERWEK, H. (1985) Incidence of spontaneous tumors in laboratory rats. *Exp. Pathol.* **28**: 235-243

BUREK, J. D. and HOLLANDER, C. F. (1977) Incidence patterns of spontaneous tumors in BN/Bi rats. *J. Natl. Cancer Inst.* **58**: 99-105

CLAPP, N. K. (1973) *An Atlas of RF Mouse Pathology: Disease Descriptions and Incidences.* U.S. Atomic Energy Commission. pp. 125.

COHEN, B. J. and ANVER, M. R. (1976) Pathological changes during aging in the rat. In: *Special Review of Experimental Aging Research; Progress in Biology* (Eds. M. F. Elias, B. E. Eleftheriou and P. K. Elias), pp. 379-404, Bar Harbor, Maine: E.A.R.

COLEMAN, G. L., BARTHOLD, S. W., OBALDISTAN, S. J. FOSTER, S. J. and JONAS, A. M. (1977) Pathological changes during aging in barrier-reared Fischer 344 male rats. *J. Gerontol.* **32**: 258-278

CONTI, C. J., CLAPP, N., KLEIN-SZANTO, A. J., NESNOW, S. and SLAGA, T. J. (1985) Survival curves and incidence of neoplastic and non-neoplastic disease in SENCAR mice. *Carcinogenesis* **6**: 1649-1652

CONYBEARNE, G. (1980) Effect of quality and quantity of diet on survival and tumour incidence in outbred Swiss mice. *Food Cosmet. Toxicol.* **18**: 65-75

COTCHIN, E., ROE, E. J. C. (1967) *Pathology of Laboratory Rats and Mice.* Oxford: Blackwell Scientific Publications.

CZARNOMSKA, A. (1969) Spontaneous lung and mammary gland cancers in C3H-W, C3H-AW, A-W and DBA-2W inbred strains of mice. *Nowotwory* **19**: 85-92

DEERBERG, F., RAPP, K. G. and KASPAREIT, J. (1987) (Spontaneous diseases as limiting factors in life expectancy of laboratory rats). **94**: 53-55

DEERBERG, F., RAPP. K. G., PITTERMANN, W. and REHM, S. (1980) (Tumor spectrum of the Han: WIST rat). *Z. Versuchstierkd.* **22**: 267-280

DERINGER, M. K. (1965) Occurrence of mammary tumors, reticular neoplasms and pulmonary tumors in stain Balb/c AnDe breeding female mice. *J. National Cancer Inst.* **35**: 1047-1052

EVERETT, R. (1984) Factors affecting spontaneous tumor incidence rates in mice: a literature review. *CRC Crit. Rev. Toxicol.* **13**: 235-251

FESTING, M. F. and BLACKMORE D. K. (1971) Life span of specified-pathogen free (MRC category 4) mice and rats. *Lab. Anim.* **5**: 179-192

FESTING, M. F. W. (Ed.) (1986) Inbred strains of mice, 9th listing. *Mouse News Letter* No. 14: Oxford University Press

FESTING, M. F. W. (Ed.) (1987) Inbred strains of mice, 10th listing. *Mouse News Letter* No. 79: Oxford University Press.

FINOGENOVA, M. A., KOZLOVA, I. N., ANDRIANOVA, M. M. and BELOSHAPKO, A. A. (1980) (Frequency of spontaneous tumors in rats from the Planernaia breeding nursery of the Academy of Medical Sciences of the USSR). *Vopr. Pitan.* **6**: 68-70

FITZGERALD, J. E., SCHARDEIN J. L. and KURTZ, S. M. (1974) Spontaneous tumors of the nervous system of albino rats. *J. Natl. Cancer. Inst.* **52**: 265-273

FOSTER, H. L., SMALL, J. D. and FOX, J. G. (1981) *The Mouse in Biomedical Research, Vol. II, Diseases.* New York: Academic Press.

FRITH, C. H. 198-. *Incidence of Neoplastic and Non-neoplastic Lesions in Several Strains of Mice.* Little Rock, AR: Toxicology Pathology Associates.

FRITH, C. H., HIGHMAN, B. BURGER, G. and SHELDON, W. D. (1983) Spontaneous lesions in virgin and retired breeder BALB/c and C57BL/6 mice. *Lab. Anim. Sci.* **33**: 273-286

GAYLOR, D. W., CHEN, J. J., GREENMAN, D. L.and THOMPSON, C. H. (1985) Occurrence of tumors among litters of BALB/c female mice. *J. Natl. Cancer. Inst.* **74**: 803-809

GOODMAN, D. G., ANVER, M. R., SAUER, R. M., SEELY, J. C., STRANDBERG, J. D., HILDEBRANDT, P. K., VONDERFECHT, S. L., INES JR., C. D, WARD, J. M., PARKER, G. D, BOORMAN, G. A. and URIAH, L. (1986) *Experimentally induced and other proliferative neoplastic lesions of mice.* Washington D.C.: Armed Forces Institute of Pathology.

GOODMAN, D. G., BATES, R. R., WARD, J. M., FRITH, C. H. SAUER, R. M., JONES, S. R., STRANDBERG, J. D., SQUIRE, R. A. MONTALI, R. J.and PARKER, G. A. (1981) *Common lesions in aged B6C3F1 and BALB/cStCrlfC3h/Nctr mice.* Washington D.C.: Armed Forces Institute of Pathology.

GOODMAN, D. G., WARD, J. M., SQUIRE, R. A., PAXTON, M. B. REICHARDT W. D., CHU, K. C.and LINHART M. S. (1980) Neoplastic and nonneoplastic lesions in aging Osborne-Mendel rats. *Toxicol. Appl. Pharmacol.* **55**: 433-437

GOODMAN, D. G., WARD, J. M., SQUIRE, R. A., CHU, K. C.and LINHART M. S. (1979) Neoplastic and non-neoplastic lesions in aging F344 rats. *Toxicol. Appl. Pharmacol.* **48**: 237-248

GOODRICH, C. L. (1975) Life span and inheritance of longevity. *J. Gerontol.* **30**: 257-263

GREAVES, P., RABEMAMPIANINA, Y. (1982) Choice of rat strain: a comparison of the general pathology and the tumor incidence of 2 year old Sprague-Dawley and Long-Evans rats. *Arch. Toxicol.* **5**: 298-303

GREEN, E. L. (1965) *Biology of the Laboratory Mouse,* New York:Dover Publ.

GREEN, M. C. (1981) *Genetic Variants and Strains of the Laboratory Mouse.* Stuttgart: Gustav Fischer Verlag.

HOMBERGER, F., RUSSFIELD, A. B., WEISBURGER, J. H., LIM, S., CHAK, S. P. and WEISBURGER, E. K. (1975) Aging changes in CD-1 HaM/ICR mice reared under standard laboratory conditions. *J. Natl. Cancer Inst.* **55**: 37-45

IWASAKI, K., GLEISER, C. A., MASARO, E. J., McMAHON C. A., SEO, E. J. and YU, B. P. (1988) The influence of dietary protein source on longevity and age-related disease processes of Fischer rats. *J. Gerontol. Biolog. Sci.* **43**: B-5-12

KAWADA, K. and OJIMA, A. (1978) Various epithelial and non-epithelial tumors spontaneously occurring in long-lived mice of A/St, CBA, C57BL/6 and their hybrid mice. *Acta. Pathol. Jpn.* **28**: 25-39

KASPAREIT, J. and DEERBERG, F. (1987) Tumour incidence and tumour spectrum of male Han:NMRI mice - short communication. *Z. Ver-suchstierkd.* **30**: 105-109

KASPAREIT-RITTINGHAUSEN, J., DEERBERG, F. and RAPP, K. (1987) Mortality and incidence of spontaneous neoplasms in BDII/Han rats. *Z. Versuchstierkd.* **30**: 209-216

KIHLSTRUM, J. M. and CLEMENTS, G. R. (1969) Spontaneous findings in Long-Evans rats. *Lab. Anim. Sci.* **19**: 710-715

KINKEL, H. J. (1971) (Spontaneous tumors in Sprague-Dawley rats). *Z. Versuchstierkd.* **13**: 97-100

LOHRKE, H., HESSE, B. and GOERTTLER, K. (1982) Spontaneous tumours in male and female specified pathogen-free Sprague-Dawley rats (outbred stock Sut:SDT). *Z. Versuchstierkd.* **24**: 255-30

MAEDA, H., GLEISER, C.A., MASARO, E. J., MURATA, I., McMAHAN, C. A.and Yu, B. P. (1985) Nutritional influence on aging of Fischer 344 rats II., Pathology. *J. Gerontol.* **40**: 471-488

MAEKAWA, A., KUROKAWA, Y., TAKAHASHI, M., KOKUBO, T., OGIU, T., ONODERA, H., TANIGAWA, H., OHNO, Y., FURUKAWA, F. and HAYASHI, Y. (1983) Spontaneous tumors in F-344/DuCrj rats. *Gann.* **74**: 365-372

MAEKAWA, A. ONODERA, H., TANIGAWA, H., FURUTA, K., KODAMA, Y., HORIUCHI, S. and HAYASHI, Y. (1983) Neoplastic and non-neoplastic lesions in aging sic:Wistar rats. *J. Toxicol. Sci.* **8**: 279-90

MAITA, K., MATSUNUMA, N., MASUDA and H. SUZUKI, Y. (1979) The age-related tumor incidence in Wistar-Imamichi rat. *Jikken Dobutsu* **28**: 555-560

MAITA, K., HIRANO, M., HARADA, T., MITSUMORI, K., YOSHIDA, A., TAKAHASHI, K., NAKASHIMA, N., KITAZAWA, T., ENOMOTO, A. INUI, K. *et al.* (1987) Spontaneous tumors in F344/DuCrj rats from 12 control groups of chronic and oncogenicity studies. *J. Toxicol. Sci.* **12**: 111-126

MYERS, D. D. (1978) Disease patterns in aging inbred mouse strains. Interaction of genetics and environment. **In:** *Genetic Effects of Aging*, vol XIV. (eds. D. Bergsma and D. Harrison) New York: Alan R. Liss.

NATIONAL RESEARCH COUNCIL, COMMITTEE ON ANIMAL MODELS FOR AGING. (1981) *Mammalian Models for Research on Aging.* Washington D.C,: National Academy Press.

NUNZIATA, A. and STORINO, A. A. (1982) Spontaneous neoplastic pathology in control rats - a review. *Vet. Hum. Toxicol.* **24**: 243-247

PETERS, R. L., RABSTEIN, L. S., SPAHN, G. J., MADISON, R. M. and HUEBNER, R. J. (1972) Incidence of spontaneous neoplasms in breeding and retired breeder BALB/c Cr mice throughout the natural life span. *Int. J. Cancer.* **10**: 273-282

POLLARD, M. (1971) Senescence in germfree rats. *Gerontologia* **17**: 333-338

PREJEAN, J. D., PECKHAM, J. C., CASEY, A. E. GRISWALD, D. P. WEISBERGER, E. K. and WEISBERGER, J. H. (1973) Spontaneous tumours in Sprague-Dawley rats and Swiss mice. *Cancer Res.* **33**: 2768-2773

REHM, S., DEERBERG, F. and RAPP, K. G. (1984) A comparison of life-span and spontaneous tumor incidence of male and female Han:WIST virgin and retired breeder rats. *Lab. Anim. Sci.* **34**: 458-464

REHM, S., NITSCHE, B. and DEERBERG, F. (1985) Non-neoplastic lesions of female virgin Han:NMRI mice. Incidence and influence of food restriction throughout life span I. Thyroid. *Lab Anim.* **19**: 214-223

REHM, S., RAPP, K. G. and DEERBERG, F. (1985) Influence of food restriction and body fat on life span and tumor incidence in female outbred Han:NMRF mice in two sublines. *Z. versuchtierk.* **27**: 249-283

REHM, S., SOMMER, R. and DEERBERG, F. (1987) Spontaneous non-neoplastic gastric lesions in female Han:NMRI mice and influence of food restriction throughout life. *Vet. Pathol.* **24**: 216-225

REHM, S., WCISLO, A. and DEERBERG, F. (1985) Non-neoplastic lesions of female virgin Han:NMRI mice. Incidence and influence of food restriction throughout life span. II Respiratory Tract. *Lab Anim.* **19**: 224-235

REUBER, M. D. (1971) Morphologic and biologic correlation of hyperplastic and neoplastic lesions occurring spontaneously in C3H × y hybrid mice. *Br. J. Cancer* **25**: 538-543

ROWLATT, C., CHESTERMAN, F. C. and SHERIFF, M. U. (1976) Lifespan, age changes and tumor incidence in an aging C57BL mouse colony. *Lab. Anim.* **10**: 419-442

SASS, B., PETERS, R. L. and KELLOFF, G. J. (1976) Differences in tumor incidence in two substrains of Claude BALB/c (BALB/cfC) mice, emphasizing renal, mammary, pancreatic and synovial tumors. *Lab. Anim. Sci.* **26**: 736-741

SASS, B., RABSTEIN, L. S., MADISON, R., NIMS, R. M., PETERS, R. L. and KELLOFF, G. J. (1975) Incidence of spontaneous neoplasms in F344 rats throughout the natural lifespan. *J. Natl. Cancer Inst.* **54**: 1449-1456

SASS, B., VERNON, M. L., PETERS, R. L. and KELLOFF, G. J. (1978) Mammary tumors, hepatocellular carcinomas and pancreatic islet cell changes in C3H mice. *J. Nat. Cancer Inst.* **60**: 611-621

SHELDON, W. G. and GREENMAN, D. L. (1980) Spontaneous lesions in control BALB/C female mice. *J. Environ. Pathol. Toxicol.* **3**: 155-167

SHER, S. P. (1982) Tumors in control hamsters, rats and mice: literature tabulation. *CRC Crit. Rev. Toxicol.* **10**: 49-79

SHER, S. P., JENSON, R. D. and BOKELMAN, D. L. (1982) Spontaneous tumors in control F344 and Charles River-CD rats and Charles River CD-1 and B6C3HF1 mice. *Toxicol. Lett.* **11**: 103-110

SMITH, G. W., WALFORD, R. L. and MICKET, M. R. (1973) Lifespan and incidence of cancer and other diseases in selected long-lived inbred mice and their $F_1$ hybrids. *J. Natl. Cancer Inst.* **50**: 1195-1213

SPARROW, S. (1980) Diseases of pet rodents. *J. Small Anim. Pract.* **21**: 1-16

STAATS, J. (1980) Standardized nomenclature for inbred strains of mice: seventh listing. *Canc. Res.* **40**: 2083-2128

STAFFA, J. A. and MEHLMAN, M. A. (1979) *Innovations in Cancer Risk Assessment (ED01 study)*. National Center for Toxicologic Research, American College of Toxicology, Park Forest South, IL: Pathotox Publications, Inc.

STEWART, H. L. (1975) Comparative aspects of certain cancers. **In:** *Cancer, A Comprehensive Treatise*, **Vol. IV** (Ed. F.F. Becker). New York: Plenum Press, pp. 303-367.

Society of Toxicology. 1981. Re-examination of the ED01 study: audit of pathology. *Food and Appl. Toxicol.* **1**: 64-66

STORER, J. B. (1966) Longevity and gross pathology at death in 22 inbred mouse strains. *J. Gerontol.* **21**: 404-409

STORER, J. B. (1978) Effect of aging and radiation in mice of different genotypes. **In:** *Genetic Effects of Aging*, **Vol. XIV.** (eds. D. Gergsma and D. Harrison), pp. 55-70. New York: Alan R. Liss.

SUMI, N., STAVROU, D., FROHBERG, H. and JOCHMANN, G. (1976) The incidence of spontaneous tumors of the central nervous system of Wistar rats. *Arch. Toxicol.* **35**: 1-13

SUZUKI, S., MATSUOKA, A., NIKI, R. and Takagaki, Y. (1981) Pathological studies on spontaneous tumors in mice (author's translation). *Jikken Dobutssu* **30**: 407-420

TAKIZAWA, S. and MIYAMOTO, M. (1976) Observations on spontaneous tumors in Wistar-Furth strain rats. *Hiroshima J. Med. Sci.* **25**: 89-98

TARONE, R. E., CHU, K. C. and WARD, J. M. (1981) Variability in the rates of some common, naturally occurring tumors in Fischer 344 rats and (C57BL/6N × C3H/HeN)F1 (B6C3F1) mice. *J. Nat. Cancer Inst.* **66**: 1175-1181

TURUSOV, V. S., (Ed.) (1973) Tumors of the rat. **In:** *Pathology of Tumours in Laboratory Animals*, Vol. I, Part 1. Lyon: IARC Sci. Publ.

TURUSOV, V. S., (Ed.) (1976) Tumors of the Rat. **In:** *Pathology of Tumours in Laboratory Animals*, Vol. I, Part 2. Lyon: IARC Sci. Publ.

TURUSOV, V. S., (Ed.) (1979) Tumors of the Mouse. **In:** *Pathology of Tumours in Laboratory Animals*, Vol. II. Lyon: IARC Sci. Publ.

UEBERBERG, H. and LUTZEN, L. (1979) The spontaneous rate of tumors in the laboratory rat: strain Chbb: THOM (SPF). *Arzneimittelforschung* **29**: 1876-1879

WAGNER, B. M. (1979) Neoplastic and non-neoplastic lesions in aging F344 rats (letter). *Toxicol. Appl. Pharmacol.* **51**: 384-385

WARD, J. M. (1983) Background data and variations in tumor rates of control rats and mice. *Prog. Exp. Tumor Res.* **26**: 241-258

WARD, J. M., GOODMAN, D. G., SQUIRE, R. A., CHU, K. C. and LINHART, M. S. (1979) Neoplastic and non-neoplastic lesions in aging (C56BL/6N × C3H/HeN)F1 (B6C3F1) mice. *J. Nat. Cancer Inst.* **63**: 849-854

WEISSE, I., KOLLMER, H., TILOV, T. and STOTZER, H. (1975) Spontaneous tumors in a strain of NMRI mice. *Z Versuchtierkd* **17**: 91-98

WEST, J. D., PETERS, J. and LYON, M. F. (1984) Genetic differences between two substrains of the inbred 101 mouse strain. *Genet. Res.* **44**: 343-346

YU, B. P., MASORO, E. J., MURATA, I., BERTRAND, H. A. and LYND, F. T. (1982) Life span study of SPF Fischer male rats fed ad libitum on restricted diets: Longevity, growth, lean body mass and disease. *J. Gerontol.* **37**: 130-141

## B. LESIONS IN MICE

### ABA, Any organ: malignant lymphoma

ABE, C., OKADA, T., SHIOKAWA, Y. and TANAKA, K. (1971) Spontaneous development of lymphoma in New Zealand mice (NZB-W F1 mice). *Arerugi* **20**: 866-872

BORTIN, M. and TRUITT, R. L. (1977) AKR T-cell acute lymphoblastic leukemia: a model for human T-cell leukemia. *Biomedicine* **26**: 309-311

DELLA PORTA, G., CHIECO-BIANCHI, L. and PENNELLI, N. (1979) Tumors of the haematopoietic system. *IARC Sci. Publ.* **23**: 527-576

FREDERICKSON, T. N., MORSE III, H. C., YETTER, R. A., ROWE, W. A., HARTLEY, J. W. and PATTENGALE, P. K. (1985) Multiparameter analysis of spontaneous nonthymic lymphomas occurring in NFS/N mice con-genic for ecotropic murine leukemia viruses. *Am. J. Pathol.* **121**: 349-360

FRITH, C. H., PATTENGALE, P. K. and WARD, J. M. (1985) *A Color Atlas of Hematopoietic Pathology in Mice.* Little Rock: Toxicology Pathology Associates

FRITH, C. H. and WILEY, L. D. (1981) Morphologic classification and correlation of incidence of hyperplastic and neoplastic hematopoietic lesions in mice with age. *J. Gerontol.* **36**: 534-545

LUNDE, M. N. and GELDERMAN, A. H. (1971) Resistance of AKR mice to lymphoid leukemia associated with a chronic protozoan infection, *Besnootia jellisoni. J. Natl. Cancer Inst.* **47**: 485-488

PATTENGALE, P. K. and FRITH, C. H. (1983) Immunomorphologic classification of spontaneous lymphoid cell neoplasms occuring in female BALB/c mice. *J. Natl. Cancer Inst.* **70**: 169-179

PATTENGALE, P. K. and FRITH, C. H. (1986) Contributions of recent research to the classification of spontaneous lymphoid cell neoplasms in mice. *CRC Crit. Rev. Toxicol.* **16**: 185-212

PATTENGALE, P. K. and TAYLOR, C. R. (1983) Experimental models of lymphoproliferative disease: The mouse as a model for human non-Hodgkin's lymphomas and related leukemias. *Am. J. Pathol.* **113**: 237-265

SWAEN, G. J. (1971) The murine leukemias. *Rev.Roum. Inframicrobiol.* **8**: 247-261

### ABC, Any Organ: Reticulum Cell Sarcoma

DUNN, T. B. (1954) Normal and pathologic anatomy of the reticular tissue in laboratory mice. *J. Nat. Cancer Inst.* **14**: 1281-1433

DUNN, T. B. and DERINGER, N. K. (1968) Reticular cell Neoplasms, Type B, or the Hodgkins-like disease of the mouse. *J. Nat. Cancer Inst.* **40**: 771-820

FRITH, C. H., DAVIS, T. M., ZOLOTOR, L. A. and TOWNEND, J. W. (1981a) Histiocytic lymphoma in the mouse. *Leukemia Res.* **4**: 651-662.

PAI, S. R. and RANADIVE, K. J. (1973) Histopathology of spontaneous neoplasms of reticular tissues in inbred line of albino ICRC mouse. *Indian J. Cancer* **10**: 172-182

TALMADGE, J. E. and HART, T. R. (1983) Morphologic studies on a murine reticulum cell sarcoma (histiocytic sarcoma) of histiocytic origin and its metastases. *Vet. Pathol.* **20**: 342-352

## AB-, Any Organ: Mast Cell Tumor

DERINGER, M. K. and DUNN, T. B. (1947) Mast cell neoplasia in mice. *J. Nat. Cancer Inst.* **7**: 289-298
DUNN, T. B. (1969) Mast cell neoplasia in mice. *Nat. Cancer Inst. Monogr.* **32**: 285-287
FRITCH, C. H., SPROWLS, R. W. and BREEDEN, C. R. (1976) Mast cell neoplasia in mice. *Lab. Anim. Sci.* **26**: 478-481

## DB-, DC-, Brain Tumors

HEIDER, K. (1986) Spontaneous craniopharyngioma in a mouse. *Vet. Pathol.* **23**: 522-523
MORGAN, K. T., FRITH, C. H., CROWDER, D. and SWEENBERG, J. (1984) Incidence of primary neoplasms of the nervous system in control mice. *J. Nat. Cancer Inst.* **72**: 151-160
STEWART, H. L., DERINGER, M. K., DUNN, T. B. and SNELL, K. C. (1974) Malignant schwannomas of nerve roots, uterus and epididymis in mice. *J. Nat. Cancer. Inst.* **53**: 1749-1758
WARD, J. M. and RICE, J. M. (1982) Naturally occurring and chemically induced brain tumors of rats and mice in carcinogenesis bioassays. *Ann. NY Acad. Sci.* **381**: 304-319
ZIMMERMAN, H. M. and INNES, J. R. M. (1979) Tumors of the central and peripheral nervous system. *IARC Sci. Publ.* **23**: 629-654

## DJ-, Brain: Hydrocephalus, Cysts

NOBEL, T. A., NYSKA, A., PIRAK, M., SKOLNIK, M. and MESHORER, A. (1987) Epidermoid cysts in the central nervous system of mice. *J. Comp. Pathol.* **97**: 357-359
SPOERRI, O. and ALEXY, H. J. (1974) The subfornical organ in murine hydrocephalus: A light-microscopic study. *Dev. Med. Child. Neurol.* **16**: 91-94
TARASZEWSKA, A. and ZALESKA-RUTCZYNSKA, Z. (1970) Congenital hydrocephalus in mice of strains BN (Sic.) and C57BL. *Pol. Med. J.* **9**: 187-195

## DKE, Brain: Mineralization of Thalamus

MORGAN, K. T., JOHNSON, B. P., FRITH, C. H. and TOWNEND, J. (1983) An ultrastructural study of spontaneous mineralization in the brains of aging mice. *Acta. Neuropathol.* **58**: 120-124
YANAI, T., KUDO, K., MANABE, J. and MATSUNUMA, N. (1984) Spontaneous vascular mineralization in the brain of aged B6C3F1 mice. *Nippon Juigaku Zasshi* **46**: 761-765
YANAI, T., YAMOTO, T., MANABE, J., TAKAOKA, M. and MATSUNUMA, N. (1987) X-ray microanalysis of mineralization in the thalamus of aged mice. *Nippon Juigaku Zasshi* **49**: 920-922

## EFA, Eye: Retinal Atrophy

GREENMAN, D. L., BRYANT, P., KODELL, R. L. and SHELDON, W. (1982) Influence of cage shelf level on retinal atrophy in mice. *Lab. Anim. Sci.* **32**: 353-356

## EM-, Eye: Malformation

RUBIN, L. F. and DALY, I. W. (1982) Ectopic pupil in mice. *Lab. Anim. Sci.* **32**: 64-65

## FCA, Harderian Gland: Adenoma

SHELDON, W. G., CURTIS, M., KODELL, R. L. and WEED, L. (1983) Primary Harderian gland neoplasms in mice. *J. Nat. Cancer Int.* **71**: 61-68

TUCKER, M. J. (1979) Tumors of the Harderian gland. *IARC Sci. Publ.* **23**: 135-146

## GE-, Ear: Degeneration

EHRET, G. (1974) Age-dependent hearing loss in normal hearing mice. *Naturwissenschaften* **61**: 506-507

YAMASAKI, K. and ITAKURA, C. (1985) Osteosclerosis in aged ICR mice. *Nippon Juigaku Zasshi* **47**: 799-802

## GGK, Ear: Otitis Media/Interna

EDIGER, R. D., RABSTEIN, M. M. and OLSON, L. D. (1971) Circling in mice caused by *Pseudomonas aeruginosa. Lab. Anim. Sci.* **21**: 845-848

KOHN, D. F. and MacKENZIE, W. F. (1980) Inner ear disease characterized by rolling in C3H mice. *J. Am. Vet. Med. Assoc.* **177**: 815-817

## HB-, HC-, Salivary Gland: Tumors

CAPUTO, A. and FLORIDI, A. (1971) A transplantable adenocarcinoma of salivary glands of the mouse. *Tumori.* **57**: 75-86

DAWE, C. J. (1979) Tumors of the salivary and lachrymal glands, nasal fossa and maxillary sinuses. *IARC Sci. Publ.* **23**: 91-133

DELANEY, W. E. (1977) Transplantable murine salivary gland carcinomas (myoepithelioma): Biologic behavior and ultrastructural features. *J. Nat. Cancer Inst.* **58**: 61-65

FRITH, C. H. and HEATH, J. E. (1985) Adenoma, adenocarcinoma, salivary gland, mouse. In: *Digestive System* (Eds. T.C.Jones *et al.*) pp. 190, op. cit.

LEIFER, C. L., MILLER, A. S., PUTONG, P. B. and HARWICK, R. (1974) Myoepithelioma of the parotid gland. *Arch. Pathol.* **98**: 312-319

MESFIN, G. M. and PIPER, R. C. (1986) Cystadenoma lymphomatosum-like lesion in the parotid salivary gland of a mouse. *Vet. Pathol.* **23**: 538-539

## IKA, Tongue: mineralization

IMACKA, K., HONJO, K., DOI, K. and MITSUOKA, T. (1986) Development of spontaneous tongue calcification and polypid lesions in DBA/2NCrj mice. *Lab. Anim.* **20**: 1-4

MATSUSHIMA, Y., IMAI, T., WATANABE, O., KAWAHARA, H., OHNE, M. and TAKAI, H. (1984) Spontaneous calcified tongue lesions in DBA mice. *Jikken Dobutsu* **33**: 539-542

## JB-, JC-, Stomach: Tumors

ODASHIMA, S. (1979) Tumors of the oral cavity, pharynx, oesophagus and stomach. *IARC Sci. Publ.* **23**: 147-167

REHM, S., SOMMER, R. and DEERBERG, F. (1987) Spontaneous nonneoplastic gastric lesions in female Han:NMRI mice, and influence of food restriction throughout life. *Vet. Pathol.* **24**: 16-225

## JD-, Stomach: Mucosal Hyperplasia

GREAVES, P. and BOIZIAU, J. L. (1984) Altered patterns of mucin secretion in gastric hyperplasia in mice. *Vet. Pathol.* **21**: 224-228

## JJ-, Esophagus: megaesophagus

RANDELIA, H. P. and LALITHA, V. S. (1988) Megaoesophagus in ICRC mice. *Lab. Anim.* **22**: 23-26

## KB-, KC-, Intestine: Tumors

ROWLATT, C. and CHESTERMAN, F. C. (1979) Tumours of the intestines and peritoneum. *IARC Sci. Publ.* **23**: 169-191

## LBA, LCA, LC-, Liver: Tumors

ANDREW, W. (1962) An electron microscopic study of the age changes in the liver of the mouse. *Am. J. Anat.* **110**: 1-18

BUTLER, W. H. and NEWBERNE, P. M., (Eds.) (1975) *Mouse hepatic neoplasia.* Amsterdam: Elsevier.

FRITH, C. H. and WARD, J. M. (1980) A morphologic classification of proliferative and neoplastic hepatic lesions in mice. *J. Environ. Pathol. Toxicol.* **3**: 329-351

FRITH, C. H. and WILEY, L. (1982) Spontaneous hepatocellular neoplasms and hepatic hemangiosarcomas in several strains of mice. *Lab. Anim. Sci.* **32**: 157-162

GELLATLY, J. B. M. (1975) The natural history of hepatic parenchymal nodule formation in a colony of C57BL mice with reference to the effect of diet. In: *Mouse hepatic neoplasia* (Eds. W. H. Butler and P. W. Newberne), pp. 77-108, Amsterdam: Elsevier.

HOOVER, K. L., WARD, J. M. and STINSON, S. F. (1980) Histopathologic differences between liver tumors in treated (C57BL/6 × C3H)F1 (B6C3F1) mice and nitrofen treated mice. *J. Nat. Cancer Inst.* **65**: 937-948

HRUBAN, Z., KIRSTEN, W. H. and SLESERS, A. (1966) Fine structure of spontaneous hepatic tumors of male C3HfGs mice. *Lab. Invest.* **15**: 577-588

JONES, G. and BUTLER, W. H. (1975) Morphology of spontaneous and induced neoplasia. In: *Mouse hepatic neoplasia* (Eds. W. H. Butler and P. M. Newberne) pp. 21-40, Amsterdam: Elsevier.

JONES, J. C. (1967) Pathology of the liver of rats and mice. In: *Pathology of Laboratory Rats and Mice* (Eds. E. Cotchin and F. J. C. Roe), pp. 1-23, op. cit.

NONOYAMA, T., FULLERTON, F., REZNIK, G., BUCCI, T. J. and WARD, J. M. (1988) Mouse hepatoblastomas: a histologic ultrastructural and immunohistochemical study. *Vet. Pathol.*, in press.

REUBER, M. D. (1967) Poorly differentiated cholangiocarcinomas occurring spontaneously in C3H and C3H × y hybrid mice. *J. Nat. Cancer Inst.* **38**: 901-907

STINSON, S. F., HOOVER, K. L. and WARD, J. M. (1981) Quantitation of differences between spontaneous and induced liver tumors in mice with an automated image analyzer. *Cancer Lett.* **14**: 143-150

TURUSOV, V. S. and TAKAYAMA, S. (1979) Tumors of the liver. *IARC Sci. Publ.* **23**: 193-233

VESELINOVITCH, S. D., MIHAILOVICH, N. and RAO, K. V. (1978) Morphology and metastatic nature of induced hepatic nodular lesions in C57BL × C3H F1 mice. *Cancer Res.* **38**: 2003-2010

VLAHAKIS, G. and HESTON, W. E. (1971) Spontaneous cholangiomas in strain C3H-AXy-fB mice and their hybrids. *J. Nat. Cancer Inst.* **46**: 677-683

WARD, J. M. (1985a) Focal carcinoma in hepatocellular adenoma, liver, mouse. In: *Digestive System* (Eds T.C. Jones *et al.*) pp. 76-78, op. cit.

WARD, J. M. (1984) Morphology of potential preneoplastic hepatocyte lesions and liver tumors in mice and a comparison with other species. In: *Current perspectives in mouse liver neoplasia* (Ed. J.A. Popp), pp. 1-26, Washington, DC: Hemisphere Press.

WARD, J. M. and VLAHAKIS, G. (1978) Evaluation of hepatocellular neoplasms in mice. *J. Nat. Cancer Inst.* **61**: 807-811

WHARTON, F. P. and WRIGHT, D. J. (1977) Observations on a new liver inclusion in the mouse. *Lab. Anim.* **11**: 109-111

YOSHITOMI, K., ALISON, R. H. and BOORMAN, G. A. (1986) Adenoma and adenocarcinoma of the gallbladder in aged laboratory mice. *Vet. Pathol.* **23**: 523-527

## LDD, Liver: Inclusion Bodies in Hepatocytes

HERBST, M. (1976) Glycogenic hepatonuclear inclusions in the aged mouse: An electron microscopical study of the histogenesis of nuclear inclusion. *Pathol. Eur.* **11**: 69-79

LIEBELT, A. G., LIEBELT, R. A. and DMOCHOWSKI, L. (1971) Cytoplasmic inclusion bodies in primary and transplanted hepatomas of mice of different strains. *J. Natl. Cancer Inst.* **47**: 413-427

TOTH, K. and SUGAR, J. (1985) Intranuclear and intracytoplasmic inclusions in normal and neoplastic hepatocytes, mouse. In Jones, T. C. *et al.* Monographs, Digestive, Op. Cit. p. 92.

## LE-, LJA, Liver: Miscellaneous Degenerative and Cystic

GUTTNER, J. (1980) Spontaneous atresia of the common bile duct and secondary biliary liver cirrhosis in two ABD2F1 mice. *Z. Versuchstierkd* **22**: 135-137

LEWIS, D. J. (1984) Spontaneous lesions of the mouse biliary tract. *J. Comp. Pathol.* **94**: 263-271

WARD, J. M. (1985) Cirrhosis, mouse. **In:** *Digestive System* (Eds. T.C. Jones *et al.*) pp. 107-109, op. cit.

## MB- MC-, Pancreas: Tumors

CARDESA, A., BULLON-RAMIREZ, A. and LEVITT, M.H. (1979) Tumours of the pancreas. *IARC Sci. Publ.* **23**: 235-249

CAVALIERE, A., BACCI, M. and FRATINI, D. (1981) Spontaneous pancreatic adenocarcinoma in a mouse (*Mus musculus*). *Lab. Anim. Sci.* **31**: 502-503

## ME-, Pancreas: Degeneration

EPPIG, J. J. and LEITER, E. H. (1977) Exocrine pancreatic insufficiency syndrome in CBA/J mice: Ultrastructural study. *Am. J. Pathol.* **86**: 17-30

LEITER, E. H., DEMPSEY, E. C. and EPPIG, J. J. (1977) Exocrine pancreatic insufficiency syndrome in CBA/J mice: Biochemical study. *Am. J. Pathol.* **86**: 31-46

## NB-, Heart: Tumors

GREGSON, R. L. (1984) A metastasizing cardiac rhabdomyosarcoma in a CD1 strain mouse. *J. Comp. Pathol.* **94**: 477-480

## NKA, Heart: Epicardial Mineralization

BROWNSTEIN, D. G. (1983) Genetics of dystrophic epicardial mineralization in DBA/2 mice. *Lab. Anim. Sci.* **33**: 247-248

DiPAOLA, J. A., STRONG, L. C. and MOORE, G. E. (1964) Calcareous pericarditis in mice of several genetically related strains. *Proc. Soc. Exp. Biol. Med.* **115**: 496-497

DOI, K., MAEDA, N., DOI, C., ISEGAWA, N., SUGANO, S. and MITSUOKA, T. (1985) Distribution and incidence of calcified lesions in DBA/2NCrj and BALB/cAnNCrj mice. *Nippon Juigaku Zasshi* **47**: 479-482

FRITH, C. H., HALEY, T. J. and SEYMORE, B. W. (1975) Spontaneous epicardial mineralization in BALB/cStCr1 mice. *Lab. Anim. Sci.* **25**: 787

RINGS, R. W. and WAGNER, J. E. (1972) Incidence of cardiac and other soft tissue mineralized
    lesions in DBA/2 mice. *Lab. Anim. Sci.* **22**: 344-352
YAMATA, J., TAJIMA, M., MARUYAMA, Y. and KUDOW, S. (1987) Observations on soft
    tissue calcification in DBA/2NCrj mice in comparison with CRJ:CD-1 mice. *Lab. Anim.* **21**:
    289-298

## OCA, Any Organ: Hemangioma, Hemangiosarcoma

FRITH, C. H. and WILEY, L. D. (1982) Spontaneous hepatocellular neoplasms and hepatic
    hemangiosarcomas in several strains of mice. *Lab. Anim. Sci.* **32**: 157-162
GIDDENS, W. E., Jr. and RENNE, R. A. (1985) Hemangiosarcoma, nasal cavity, mouse. In:
    *Respiratory* (Ed. T. C. Jones *et al.*) pp. 72-74, op. cit.
INADA, O. and YUMOTO, T. (1978) Naturally occurring angiosarcoma of the tibia in an NZB
    mouse. *Acta. Pathol. Jpn.* **28**: 99-109

## OH-, Blood Vessels: Periarteritis Nodosa

KYOGOKU, K., KUBOTA, A., NOSE, M., MIMURA, R. and UKAI, K. (1976) Animal model
    for periarteritis nodosa — SL/Nishizuka mice. *Nippon Rinsho* **34**: 655-658

## QB-, QC-, Lung: Adenoma, Adenocarcinoma

DEERBERG, F., PITTERMAN, W. and RAPP, K. (1974) Lung tumor in the mouse: a progressive
    tumor. *Vet. Pathol.* **11**: 430-441
HEATH, J. E., FRITH, C. H. and WANG, P. M. (1982) A morphologic classification and
    incidence of alveolar-bronchiolar neoplasms in control BALB/c female mice. *Lab. Anim.
    Sci.* **32**: 638-647
KAUFFMAN, S. L., ALEXANDER, L. and SASS, L. (1979) Histologic and ultrastructural
    features of the Clara cell adenoma of the mouse lung. *Lab. Invest.* **40**: 700-716
KAUFFMAN, S. L. and SATO, T. (1985) Alveolar Type II cell adenoma, lung, mouse. In:
    *Respiratory System* (Eds T.C. Jones *et al.*) pp. 102-106, op. cit.
KAUFFMAN, S. L. and SATO, T. (1985) Bronchiolar adenoma, lung, mouse. In: *Respiratory
    System* (Eds. T.C. Jones *et al.*) pp. 107, op. cit.
PALMER, K. C. (1985) Clara cell adenoma of the mouse lung: Interaction with alveolar Type II
    cells. *Am. J. Pathol.* **120**: 455-463
STEWART, H. L., DUNN, T. B., SNELL, K. C. and DERINGER, M. K. (1979) Tumors of the
    respiratory tract. *IARC Sci. Publ.* **23**: 251-287

## QHB, Lung: Alveolar Histiocytosis

EMI, Y. and KONISHI, Y. (1985) Endogenous lipid pneumonia in female B6C3F1 mice. In:
    *Respiratory System* (Eds. T.C. Jones *et al.*) pp. 166-168, op. cit..
GREEN, E. U. (1942) On the occurrence of crystalline material in the lungs of normal and
    cancerous Swiss mice. *Cancer Res.* **2**: 210-217
SCHULTZ, L. D., Coman, D. R., Bailey, C. L., Beamer, W. G., Sidman, C. L. (1984) "Viable
    motheaten", a new allele at the motheaten locus. I. Pathology. *Am. J. Path.* **116**: 179-192
WARD, J. M. (1978) Pulmonary pathology of the motheaten mouse. *Vet. Pathol.* **15**: 170-178
YAMASAKI, K. (1985) Pathology of aspiration pneumonia in mice. *Jikken Dobutsu* **34**: 261-265
YANG, Y. H. and CAMPBELL, J. S. (1964) Crystalline excrements in bronchitis and cholecys-
    titis of mice. *Am. J. Pathol.* **45**: 337-345
YASUBA, M., IIDA, M. and ITAKURA, C. (1982) Histopathology of pulmonary alveolar
    proteinosis spontaneously occurring in aged KK mice. *Jikken Dobutsu* **31**: 265-270

## QI-, Lung: Hair Emboli

KAST, A. (1985) Pulmonary hair embolism. **In:** *Respiratory System* (Eds. T.T. Jones *et al.*) pp. 186-194, op. cit.

## QOA, QOB, Lung: Lymphocytic Infiltrates

LINDSEY, J. R., CASSELL, G. H. and DAVIDSON, M. K. (1982) Mycoplamal and other bacterial diseases of the respiratory system. **In:** *The Mouse in Biomedical Research*, Vol. II: Diseases. (H. L. Foster, J. D. Small and J. G. Fox, Eds.), pp. 21-41, New York: Academic Press.

## RB-, RC-, Endocrine Organs: Tumors

BIANCIFIORI, C. (1979) Tumors of the thyroid gland. *IARC Sci. Publ.* **22**: 451-468

DUNN, T. B. (1979) Tumors of the adrenal gland. *IARC Sci. Publ.* **22**: 475-486

DUNN, T. B. (1979) Tumors of the parathyroid gland. *IARC Sci. Publ.* **22**: 469-474

DUNN, T. B. (1970) Normal and pathologic anatomy of the adrenal gland of the mouse, including neoplasms. *J. Nat. Cancer Inst.* **44**: 1323-1389

FELICIO, L. S., NELSON, J. F. and FINCH, C. E. (1980) Spontaneous pituitary tumorigenesis and plasma oestradiol in aging female C57BL/6J mice. *Exp. Gerontol.* **15**: 139-143

FRITH, C. H. (1983) Pheochromocytoma, adrenal medulla, mouse. **In:** *Endocrine System.* (Eds. T. C. Jones *et al.*). p. 27, op. cit.

FRITH, C. H. (1983) Adenoma and carcinoma, adrenal cortex, mouse. **In:** *Endocrine System* (Eds. T. C. Jones *et al.*) pp. 49-56, op. cit.

FRITH, C. H. and HEATH, J. E. (1984) Morphological classification and incidence of thyroid tumors in untreated aged mice. *J. Gerontol.* **39**: 7-10

FRITH, C. H. and HEATH, J. E. (1983) Carcinoma, thyroid, mouse. **In:** *Endocrine System.* (Eds. T.C. Jones *et al.*) p. 188. op. cit.

FRITH, C. H. and SHELDON, W. D. (1983) Hyperplasia, adenoma and carcinoma of pancreatic islets, mouse. **In:** *Endocrine System* (Eds. T.C. Jones *et al.*), pp.297-303, op. cit.

LIEBELT, A. G. (1979) Tumors of the pituitary gland. *IARC Sci. Publ.* **23**: 411-450

MURRAY, A. B. and LUZ, A. (1988) Unusual pelvic endocrine tumors of APUD cell origin in CBA mice. *Vet. Pathol.* **25**: 89-90

ONYEKABA, C. O. (1986) Spontaneous thyroid follicular adenoma in a laboratory mouse (*Mus musculus*). *Jikken Dobutsu* **35**: 471-473

SCHECHTER, J. E., FELICIO, L. S., NELSON, J. F. and FINCH, C. E. (1981) Pituitary tumorigenesis in aging female C57BL/6J mice: A light and electron microscopic study. *Anat. Rec.* **199**: 423-432

VAN ZWIETEN, M. J., FRITH, C. H., NOOTEBOOM, A. L., WOLFE,H. J. and DELELLIS, R. A. (1983) Medullary thyroid carcinoma in female BALB/c mice: A report of 3 cases with ultrastructural, immunohistochemical and transplantation data. *Am. J. Pathol.* **110**: 219-229

## -RD-, Endocrine Organs: Abnormal Growth, Hyperplasia

FRITH, C. H. (1983) Ectopic thyroid, mouse. **In:** *Endocrine System* (Eds. T. C. Jones, U. Mohr, R. D. Hunt) p.171 op. cit.

FRITH, C. H. and FETTERS, J. (1983) Ectopic Parathyroid, Mouse. **In:** *Endocrine System.* (Eds. T.C. Jones, U. Mohr and R.D. Hunt) pp. 263, op. cit.

GOODMAN, D. G. (1983) Subcapular-cell hyperplasia, adrenal, mouse. **In:** *Endocrine System,* (Eds. T. C. Jones, U. Mohr and R. D. Hunt) p. 66, op. cit.

### RE-, Endocrine Pancreas: Degeneration

LIKE, A.A., STEINKE, J., JONES, E. E. and CAHILL, G. F., Jr. (1965) Pancreatic studies in
mice with spontaneous diabetes mellitis. *Am. J. Pathol.* **46**: 621-644

### RI-, Endocrine Organs: Tissue Storage, Amyloidosis

FRITH, C.H. (1983) Lipogenic pigmentation, adrenal cortex, mouse. **In**: *Endocrine System* (Eds.
T.C. Jones *et al.*) p. 60, op. cit.
SAMORAJSKI, T. and ORDY, J.M. (1967) The histochemistry and ultrastructure of lipid
pigment in the adrenal glands of aging mice. *J. Gerontol.* **22**: 253-267
SASS, B. (1983) Amyloidosis, adrenal, mouse. **In**: *Endocrine System* (Eds. T.C. Jones *et al.*) pp.
57-59, op. cit.

### RJ-, Endocrine System: Cystic Change

POUR, P. M., WILSON, J. T., Qureshi S. R. and SALMASI, S. (1983) Cysts, parathyroid,
hamster, rat, mouse. **In**: *Endocrine System* (Eds. T.C. Jones *et al.*) pp. 288, op. cit.
CAMERON, A. M. and SHELDON, W. (1983) Cystoid degeneration, anterior pituitary, mouse.
**In**: *Endocrine System* (Eds. T.C. Jones *et al.*) pp. 165, op. cit.

### SB-, Urinary Bladder: Tumors

FRITH, C. H. (1986) Transitional cell carcinoma, urinary tract, mouse. **In**: *Urinary System* (Eds.
T. C. Jones *et al.*), pp. 331-336, op. cit.
WOOD, M. and BONSER, G. M. (1979) Tumors of the urinary bladder. *IARC Sci. Publ.* **23**:
301-304

### S—, Bladder: Miscellaneous

FRITH, C. H. (1979) Morphologic classification of inflammatory, degenerative and proliferative
lesions of the urinary bladder of mice. *Invest. Urol.* **16**: 435-444

### TB-,TC-, Kidney: Tumors

SASS, B. (1986) Adenoma, adenocarcinoma, kidney, mouse. **In**: *Urinary System*, (Eds. T.C.
Jones *et al.*) pp. 87, op. cit.
SHINOHARA, Y. and FRITH, C. H. (1980) A morphologic classification of benign and malig-
nant renal cell tumors in aged BALB/c mice. *Am. J. Pathol.* **100**: 455-457
TERRACINI, B. and CAMPOBASSO, O. (1979) Tumors of the kidney, renal pelvis and ureter.
*IARC Sci. Publ.* **23**: 289-299

### TFA, Kidney: Focal Cortical Necrosis

GUTTNER, J. and KLAUS, S. (1983) Spontaneously occurring progressive tubular degeneration
of unknown origin in the kidneys of mice. *Z. Versuchstierkd* **25**: 339-342
MONTGOMERY, C. A., Jr. (1986) Infarction, kidney, rat, mouse. **In**: *Urinary System* (Eds. T.
C. Jones *et al.*), pp. 179-183, op. cit.
RUDOFSKY, U. H. (1978) Renal tubulointerstitial lesions in CBA/J mice. *Am. J. Pathol.* **92**:
333-348

### TGA, Kidney: Pyelonephritis

MONTGOMERY, C. A., Jr. (1986) Suppurative nephritis, pyelonephritis, mouse. **In**: *Urinary
System* (Eds. T. C. Jones *et al.*) pp. 215-218, op. cit.

## THA, Kidney: Glomerulonephritis

DIXON, F. J., OLDSTONE, M. B. and TONIETTI, G. (1971) Pathogenesis of immune complex glomerulonephritis of New Zealand mice. *J. Exp. Med.* **134**: 65s-71s

HEWICKER, M. and TRAUTWEIN, G. (1986) Glomerular lesions in MRL mice: A light and immunofluorescence microscopic study. *Zentralbl Veterinarmed* **33**: 727-739

SASS, B. (1986) Glomerulonephritis, mouse. **In**: *Urinary System* (Eds. T. C. Jones *et al.*) pp. 192-206, op. cit.

WIGLEY, R. D., CRAIG, A. S., WILLIAMSON, K. I. and COUCHMAN, K. G. (1975) Spontaneous arteritis and glomerulitis in mice: A comparison of light and electron microscopic renal changes in PN/n, NZB/BL, 101/MAC and CBA/MAC mice. *Lab. Invest.* **33**: 8-15

## TIA, Kidney: Amyloidosis

JAKOB, W. (1971) Spontaneous amyloidosis of mammals. *Vet. Pathol.* **8**: 292-306

KOEGER, A. C., BRANELLEC, A., HIRBEC, G., BLOUQUIT, Y., MOURIQUAND, C., SOBEL, A. and LAGRUE, G. (1984) Biological study of spontaneous amyloidosis in PS mice. *Pathol. Biol. (Paris)* **32**: 959-964

POWERS, J. M., WISNIEWSKI, H. and TERRY, R. D. (1976) Lack of amyloidosis and renal disease in A strain mice. *Arch. Pathol. Lab. Med.* **100**: 69-73

## TI-, Kidney: Pigmentation

BROWN, R. Pigment deposition, kidney, mouse. (1986) **In**: *Urinary System* (Eds. T. C. Jones *et al.*) pp. 244-245, op. cit.

## TJA, Kidney: Hydronephrosis

NAKAJIMA, Y. and GOTO, N. (1982) Hydronephrosis in DDD strain mice. *Jikken Dobutsu* **31**: 320-323

HSU, H. H. (1986) Hereditary hydronephrosis, mouse. **In**: *Urinary System* (Eds. T. C. Jones *et al.*) pp. 273- op. cit..

WALLACE, M. E. (1976) Hydronephrosis in the mouse: The effects of the short-ear gene, sex and ureteral vascular system. *Am. J. Anat.* **147**: 1932

WERDER, A. A., AMOS, M. A., NIELSEN, A. H. and WOLFE, G. H. (1984) Comparative effects of germfree and ambient environments on the development of cystic kidney disease in CFWwd mice. *J. Lab. Clin. Med.* **103**: 399-407

## TJ-, Kidney: Cystic Change

GIALAMAS, J., HOGER, H. and ADAMIKER, D. (1987) Polycystic kidney disease in infant mice. *Z. Versuchstierkd* **30**: 217-222

## TKA, Kidney: calcification

CLAPP, M. J., WADE, J. D. and SAMUELS, D. M. (1982) Control of nephrocalcinosis by manipulating the calcium:phosphorus ration in commercial rodent diets. *Lab. Anim.* **16**: 130-132

MORRISSEY, R. (1986) Renal calcification, mouse. **In**: *Urinary System* (Eds. T. C. Jones *et al.*) pp. 361-363, op. cit.

HIGHMAN, B. and DAFT, F. S. (1951) Calcified lesions in C3H mice given purified low-protein diets. *A.M.A. Arch. Pathol.* **52**: 221-229

YAMATA, J., TAJIMA, M., MARUYAMA, Y. and KUDOW, S. (1987) Observations on soft tissue calcification in DBA/2NCrj mice in comparison with CRJ:CD-1 mice. *Lab. Anim.* **21**: 289-298

## TOA, Kidney: Interstitial Lymphoid Nodules

MONTGOMERY, C. A., Jr. (1986) Interstitial nephritis, mouse. **In:** *Urinary System* (Eds. T. C. Jones *et al.*) pp. 210-214, op. cit.

## UB-, UC-, Testis: Tumors

MOSTOFFI, F. K. and BRESLER, V. M. (1979) Tumors of the testis. *IARC Sc. Publ.* **23**: 325-349
DAMJANOV, I., SOLTER, D. and SKREB, N. (1979) Teratomas. *IARC Sci. Publ.* **23**: 655-661

## VB-, VC-, Male Accessary Sex Organs: Tumors

FRANKS, L. M. (1979) Tumors of the accessory male sex glands. *IARC Sci. Publ.* **23**: 351-368
KASPAREIT, J. and DEERBERG, F. (1987) Spontaneous tumors of the seminal vesicles in male Han:NMRI mice. *Z. Versuchstierkd* **29**: 277-281

## VG-, Male Accessory Sex Organs: Acute Inflammation

HONG, C. C. and EDIGER, R. D. (1978) Perputial gland abscess in mice. *Lab. Anim. Sci.* **28**: 153-156
NEEDHAM, J. R. and COOPER, J. E. (1976) Bulbourethral gland infections in mice associated with *Staphylococcus aureus*. *Lab. Anim. Sci.* **10**: 311-315

## WBA, Ovary: Granulosa Cell Tumor

ALISON, R. H. and MORGAN, K. T. (1987) Granulosa cell tumor, ovary, mouse. **In:** *Genital System* (Eds. T. C. Jones *et al.*) pp. 22-29, op. cit.
BEAMER, W. G., HOPPE, P. C. and WHITTEN, W. K. (1985) Spontaneous malignant granulosa cell tumors in ovaries of young SWR mice. *Cancer Res.* **45**: 5575-5581
BIELSCHOWSKY, M. and DATH, E. F. (1973) Spontaneous granulosa cell tumors in mice of strains NZC-B1, NZO-B1, NZY-B1 and NZB-B1. *Pathol.* **5**: 303-310
LEMON, P. G. and GUBAREVA, A. V. (1979) Tumors of the ovary. *IARC Sci. Publ.* **23**: 385-409

## WB-, WC-, Ovary: Other Tumors

ABBOTT, D. P., GREGSON, R. L. and IMM, S. (1983) Spontaneous ovarian teratomas in laboratory mice. *J. Comp. Pathol.* **93**: 109-114
ALISON, R. H., LEWIS, D. J. and MONTGOMERY, C. A. (1987) Ovarian choriocarcinoma in the mouse. *Vet. Pathol.* **24**: 226-230
ALISON, R. H. and MORGAN, K. T. (1987) Teratoma, ovary, mouse. **In:** *Genital System* (Eds. T. C. Jones *et al.*) pp. 46-52, op. cit.
FRITH, C. H., ZUNA, R. E. and MORGAN, K. (1981) A morphologic classification and incidence of spontaneous ovarian neoplams in three strains of mice. *J. Nat. Cancer Inst.* **67**: 693-702
LEMON, P. G. and GUBAREVA, A. V. (1979) Tumors of the ovary. *IARC Sci. Publ.* **23**: 385-410
MAJEED, S. K., ALSION, R. H., BOORMAN, G. A. and GOPINATH, C. (1986) Ovarian yolk sac carcinoma in mice. *Vet. Pathol.* **23**: 776-778
MORGAN, K. T. and ALISON, R. H. (1987) Cystadenoma, ovary, mouse. **In:** *Genital System* (Eds. T. C. Jones *et al.*) pp. 42-45, op. cit.
MORGAN, K. T. and ALISON, R. H. (1987) Tubular adenoma, ovary, mouse. **In:** *Genital System* (Eds. T. C. Jones *et al.*) pp. 36-41, op. cit.
REHM, S., DIERKSEN, D. and DEERBERG, F. (1984) Spontaneous ovarian tumors in Han:NMRI mice: Histologic classification, incidence and influence of food restriction. *J. Nat. Cancer Inst.* **72**: 1383-1395

SCHUELER, R. L. and EDIGER, R. (1975) Murine ovarian teratoma. *Am. J. Vet. Res.* **36**: 341-342

## XB-, XC-, Uterus, Cervix, Vagina: Tumors

CHOUROULINKOV, I., GUILLON, J. and GUERIN, M. (1969) Endometrial sarcomas in mice: A survey of 130 cases. *J. Nat. Cancer Inst.* **42**: 593-603

DAWSON, P. I., BROOKS, R. E. and FIELDSTEEL, A. H. (1974) Unusual occurrence of endometrial sarcomas in hybrid mice. *J. Nat. Cancer Inst.* **52**: 207-211

GUTTNER, J. (1980) Adenomyosis in mice. *Z. Versuchstierkd* **22**: 249-251

KLEIN-SZANTO, A. J., CONTI, C. J. and CARTAGENOVA, R. E. (1974) Ultrastructure of a vaginal myxoma of a rat. *Vet. Pathol.* **11**: 289-296

MUNOZ, N., DUNN, T. B. and TURUSOV, V. S. (1979) Tumors of the vagina and uterus. *IARC Sci. Publ.* **23**: 359-383

SASS, B. (1981) Mixed mesenchymal tumors of the mouse uterus. *Lab. Anim.* **15**: 365-369

REUBER, M. D., VLAHAKIS, G. and HESTON, W. E. (1981) Spontaneous hyperplastic and neoplastic lesions of the uterus in mice. *J. Gerontol.* **36**: 663-673

STEWART, H. L., SASS, B., DERINGER, M. K., DUNN, T. B., LIOTTA, L. A. and TOGO, S. (1984) Pure yolk sac carcinoma of the mouse uterus: Report of 8 cases. *J. Nat. Cancer Inst.* **73**: 115-122

## XJB, Uterus: Hydrometra

KUNSTYR, I., MATTHIESEN, T., GARTNER, K., MAESS, J. and HEIMANN, W. (1982) Post-mating non-infectious hydrometra in BALB/c:Bom mice. *Lab. Anim.* **16**: 51-55

## XM-, Vagina: Atresia

MATSUSHITA, S. and MATSUMOTO, T. (1984) Pathology of vaginal atresia in BALB/cA-nu/+ and BALB/cA- mice. *Jikken Dobutsu* **33**: 365-368

## YBC, Mammary Gland: Mammary Adenocarcinoma

DUNN, T. B. (1959) Morphology of mammary tumors in mice. In: *The Pathology of Cancer* (Ed. F. Homburger), pp. 38-84. New York: Hoeber-Harper.

FAULKIN, L. J., MITCHELL, D. J., YOUNG, L. J. T., MORRIS, D. W., MALONE, R. W., CARDIFF, R. D. and GARDNER, M. B. (1984) Hyperplastic and neoplastic changes in the mammary glands of feral mice free of endogenous mouse mammary tumor virus provirus. *J. Nat. Cancer Inst.* **73**: 971-982

MEDINA, D. (1973) Pre-neoplastic lesions in mouse mammary tumorigenesis. *Methods of Canc. Res.* **7**: 3-53

MORII, S., TSUBARA, A., FUJII, T. and OISHI, Y. (1984) Histopathology of mammary tumors in mice and rats. *Jikken Dobutsu* **33**: 47-59

PAI, S. R. (1973) Influence of oxytocin on pituitary-adrenal-gonad relationship and on the development of mammary tumors in C3H mice. *Indian J. Med. Res.* **61**: 1810-1817

SASS, B., VLAHAKIS, G. and HESTON, W. E. (1982) Precursor lesions and pathogenesis of spontaneous mammary tumors in mice. *Toxicol. Pathol.* **10**: 12-21

SASS, B. and DUNN, T. B. (1979) Classification of mouse mammary tumors in Dunn's miscellaneous group, including recently reported types. *J. Nat. Cancer Inst.* **62**: 1287-1293

SQUARTINI, F. (1979) Tumors of the mammary gland. *IARC Sci. Publ.* **23**: 43-90

## YBD, Mammary Gland, any Organ: Fibrosarcoma

SOMVANSHI, R. and IYER, P. K. (1978) Mammary fibrosarcoma in a mouse (*Mus musculus*). *Indian Vet. J.* **55**: 993-994

Stewart, H. L. (1979) Tumors of soft tissues. *IARC Sci. Publ.* **23**: 487-505

## YB-, YC-, Skin: Tumors

BOGOVSKI, P. (1979) Tumors of the skin. *IARC Sci. Publ.* **23**: 1-41.

WARD, J. M., QUANDER, R., DEVOR, D., WENK, M. L. and SPANGLER, E. F. (1986) Pathology of aging female SENCAR mice used as controls in skin two-stage carcinogenesis studies. *Environ. Health Perspect.* **68**: 81-89

## YGA, Skin: Suppurative Dermatitis

McBRIDE, D. F., STARK, D. M. and WALBERG, J. A. (1981) An outbreak of staphylococcal furunculosis in nude mice. *Lab. Anim. Sci.* **31**: 270-272

STOWE, H. D., WAGNER, J. L. and OICK, J. R. (1971) A debilitating fatal murine dermatitis. *Lab. Anim. Sci.* **21**: 892-897

WEISBROTH, S. H., SCHER, S. and BOMAN, I. (1969) *Pasteurella pneumotropica* abscess syndrome in a mouse colony. *J. Am. Vet. Med. Assoc.* **155**: 1206-1210

## YH-, YA-, Skin: Chronic Inflammation, Necrosis

BELL, J. F., MOORE, G. J., CLIFFORD, C. M. and RAYMOND, G. H. (1970) Dry gangrene of the ear in white mice. *Lab. Anim.* **4**: 245-254

HONG, C. C. and EDIGER, R. D. (1978) Self-mutilation of the penis in C57BL/6N mice. *Lab. Anim.* **12**: 55-57

KOOPMAN, J. P., VAN DER LOGT, J. T., MULLINK, J. W., HEESSEN, F. W., STAD-HOUDERS, A. M., KENNIS, H. M. and VAN DER GULDEN, W. J. (1984) Tail lesions in C3H/He mice. *Lab. Anim. Sci.* **18**: 106-109

LITTERST, C. L. (1974) Mechanically self-induced muzzle alopecia in mice. *Lab. Anim. Sci.* **24**: 806-809

## ZA-, Bone: Necrosis

YAMASAKI, K. and ITAKURA, C. (1988) Aseptic necrosis of bone in ICR mice. *Lab. Anim.* **22**: 51-53

## ZBA, Any Site: Osteosarcoma

FRITH, C. H., JOHNSON, B. P. and HIGHMAN, B. (1982) Osteosarcomas in BALB/c female mice. *Lab. Anim. Sci.* **32**: 60-63

FRITH, C. H., JOHNSON, B. P. and HIGHMAN, B. (1982) Osteosarcomas in control and 2-acetylaminofluorene treated mice. *Lab. Anim. Sci.* **32**: 60-63

GOSSNER, W. and LUZ, A. Tumors of the jaws. *IARC Sci. Publ.* **23**: 611-628

STANTON, M. F. Tumors of the bone. *IARC Sci. Publ.* **23**: 577-610

## Z—, Teeth, Bone: Miscellaneous Lesions

ROBINS, M. W. and ROWLATT, C. (1971) Dental abnormalities in aged mice. *Gerontologia* **17**: 261-272

SASS, B. and MONTALI, R. J. (1980) Spontaneous fibroosseous lesions in aging female mice. *Lab. Anim. Sci.* **30**: 907-909

## C. LESIONS IN RATS

### 012, Malignant Lymphoma


ABBOTT, D. P., PRENTICE, D. E. and CHERRY, C. P. (1983) Mononuclear cell leukemia in aged Sprague-Dawley rats. *Vet. Pathol.* **20**: 434-439

ALLEN, J. and ASHBY, R. (1982) Preliminary communication investigations on leukemia in the F344 rat. *Arch. Toxicol.* **5**: 307-309

BECKERS, A. and BAZIN, H. (1978) Incidence of spontaneous ileocecal immunocytomas in hybrids of LOU/C rats and rat strains with low spontaneous tumor incidence. *J. Natl. Cancer Inst.* **60**: 1505-1508

HINSULL, S. N. and BELLAMY, D. (1977) Spontaneous thymoma in an inbred strain of rat. *J. Natl. Cancer Inst.* **58**: 1609-1614

KUSEWITT, D. F., HAHN, F. F. and PICKRELL, J. A. (1982) Hematologic and serum chemical characteristics of mononuclear leukemia in Fischer 344 rats. *Lab. Anim. Sci.* **32**: 275-277

STROMBERG, P. C. and VOGTSBERGER, L. M. (1983) Pathology of the mononuclear cell leukemia of Fischer Rats, Part I: Morphologic studies. *Vet. Pathol.* **20**: 698-708

STROMBERG, P. C., VOGTSBERGER, L. M., MARSH, L. R. and WILSON, F. D. (1983) Pathology of the mononuclear cell leukemia of Fischer rats, Part II: Hematology. *Vet. Pathol.* **20**: 709-717

STROMBERG, P. C., VOGTSBERGER, L. M. and MARSH, L. R. (1983) Pathology of the mononuclear cell leukemia of Fischer rats, Part III: Clinical chemistry. *Vet. Pathol.* **20**: 718-726

STROMBERG, P. C., ROJKO, J. L., VOGTSBERGER, L. M., CHENEY, C. and

BERMAN, R. (1983) Immunologic, biochemical and ultrastructural characterization of the leukemia cell in F344 rats. *J. Nat. Cancer Inst.* **71**: 173-181

WARD, J. M. and REYNOLDS, C. W. (1983) Large granular lymphocyte leukemia: A heterogeneous lymphocytic leukemia in F344 rats. *Am. J. Pathol.* **111**: 1-10


### 015, Myelogenous Leukemia


HEATH, J. E. (1981) Granulocytic leukemia in rats: a report of two cases. *Lab. Anim. Sci.* **31**: 504-506


### 01-, Histiocytic Sarcoma


BARSOUM, J. N., HANNA, W., GOUGH, A. W., SMITH G. S., STURGESS, J. M. and DE LA IGLESIA. F. A. (1984) Histiocytic sarcoma in Wistar rats: a light microscopic, immunochemical and ultrastructural study. *Arch. Pathol. Lab. Med.* **108**: 802-807

MAJEED, S. K. and GOPINPATH, C. (1985) Hodgkins disease-like lesion in a rat. *J. Comp. Pathol.* **95**: 123-126

GREAVES, P. and FACCINI, J. M. (1981) Spontaneous fibrous histiocytic neoplasms in rats. *Br. J. Cancer* **43**: 402-411

PORT, C. D., VAN PELT, L. F. and WILLIAMS, R. M. (1982) Histiocytic sarcoma of the scrotum in a rat. *Lab. Anim. Sci.* **32**: 74-77

YAMAMOTO, H. and IMAI, S. (1986) Two cases of spontaneous malignant fibrous histiocytoma in Wistar rats. *Jikken Dobutsu* **35**: 97-100


### 041, Atrophy of Thymus


KUPER, C. F., BEEMS, R. B. and HOLLANDER, V. M. (1986) Spontaneous pathology of the thymus in aging Wistar (Cpb:WU) rats. *Vet. Pathol.* **23**: 270-277

## 112, Brain Tumors

ADAMS, S. W. and CROWLEY, A. M. (1987) Posterior paralysis due to spontaneous oligodendroglioma in the spinal cord of a rat. *Lab. Anim. Sci.* **37**: 345-347

ABBOTT, D. P. (1982) Malignant schwannomaa of the dorsal spinal nerve root in a laboratory rat. *Lab. Anim.* **16**: 224-229

AIUCHI, M., UTSUMI, F., KOBAYASHI, K., KUROSAKI, E. and SAKUMA, S. (1984) A case of astrocytoma in an aged rat. *Nippon Juigaku Zasshi* **46**: 233-237

AIUCHI, M., UTSUMI, F., KOBAYASHI, K. KUROSAKI, E. and SAKUMA, S. (1985) Oligodendroglioma in a aged rat. *Nippon Juigaku Zasshi* **47**: 453-457

AL ZUBAIDY, A. J. and MALINOWSKI, W. (1984) Spontaneous pineal body tumors (pinealomas) in Wistar rat: A histological and ultrastructural study. *Lab. Anim.* **18**: 224-229

DAGLE, G. E., ZWICKER, G. M. and RENNE, R. A. (1979) Morphology of spontaneous brain tumors in the rat. *Vet. Pathol.* **16**: 318-324

JANISCH, W. and OSSKE, G. (1966) Spontaneous ependymoma of the brain in a rat. *Zdrav. Prac.* **109**: 520-523

KASPAREIT, J. and DEERBERG, F. (1986) Multiple tumors in the brain of a male Han:SPRD rat. *Z. Versuchstierkd.* **28**: 282-283

KRINKE, G., NAYLOR, D. C., SCHMID, S., FROHLICH, E. and SCHNIDER, K. (1985) The incidence of naturally-occurring primary brain tumors in the laboratory rat. *J. Comp. Pathol.* **95**: 175-192

MAEKAWA, A., ONODERA, H., TANIGAWA, H., FURUTA, K., TAKAHASHI, M., KUROKAWA. T., KOKUBO, T., OGIU, T. UCHIDA, O., KOBAYASHI, K. *et al.* (1984) Spontaneous tumors of the nervous system and associated organs and/or tissues in rats. *Gann.* **75**: 784-791

MAJEED, S. K. and GOPINATH, C. (1985) Hodgkin's diease-like lesion in a rat. *J. Comp. Pathol.* **95**: 123-126

MAWDESLEY-THOMAS, L. E. and NEWMAN, A. J. (1974) Some obervations on spontaneously occurring tumors of the central nervous system of Sprague-Dawley derived rats. *J. Pathol.* **112**: 107-116

YAMASAKI, K. and FUKUSHIMA, Y. (1986) Ependymoma in a rat. *Jikken Dobutsu* **35**: 509-510

YAMATE, J., TAJIMA, M., NUNOYA, T. and KUDOW, S. (1987). Spontaneous tumors of the central nervous system of Fischer 344/DuCrj rats. *Nippon Juigaku Zasshi* **49**: 67-75

## 113, Granular Cell Myoblastoma

BERMAN, J. J., RICE, J. M. and STRANDBERG, J. (1978) Granular cell variants in a rat schwannoma: Evidence of neurogenic origin of granular cell tumor (myoblastoma). *Vet. Pathol.* **15**: 725-731

MITSUMORI, K., MARONPOT, R. R.and BOORMAN, G. A. (1987. Spontaneous tumors of the meninges in rats. *Vet. Pathol.* **24**: 50-58

MITSUMORI, K., DITTRICH, K.L., STEFANSKI, S., TALLEY, F. A. and

MARONPOT, R. R. (1987) Immunohistochemical and electron microscopic study of meningeal granular cell tumors in rats. *Vet. Pathol.* **24**: 356-359

## 13-, Degeneration of Brain

CURLES, R. G., NELSON, M. B., BRIMMER, F. and TELLEZ, C. (1977) Brain and spinal cord lesions in the newborn rat. *Lab. Anim.* **11**: 251-255

## 13-, Corneal Dermoid

NICHOLS, C. W. and YANOFF, M. (1969) Demoid of a rat cornea. *Pathol. Vet.* **6**: 214-216

## 14-, Cataract

IBRAHEEM, K. G. (1970) Estimation of the normal distribution of cataract in the rat. *Bull. Ophthalmol. Soc. Egypt* **63**: 195-198

## 141, Degenerative Radiculoneuropathy

UREK, J. D., VAN DER KOGEL, A. J. and HOLLANDER, C. F. (1976) Degenerative myelopathy in three strains of aging rats. *Vet. Pathol.* **13**: 321-331

KRINKE, G., SUTER, J. and HESS, R. (1981) Radicular myelinopathy in aging rats. *Vet. Pathol.* **18**: 335-341

MITSUMORI, K., MAITA, K. and SHIRASU, Y. (1981) An ultrastructural study of spinal nerve roots and dorsal root ganglia in aging rats with spontaneous radiculoneuopathy. *Vet. Pathol.* **18**: 714-726

## 142, Retinal Degeneration

BELLHORN, R. W., RHEINHARDT, J. M., BURNS, M. S. and MATTHES, M. T. Retinal degeneration in the WKY rat. *Prog. Clin. Biol. Res.* **247**: 317-331

SCHARDEIN, J. L., LUCAS, J. A. and FITZGERALD, J. E. (1975) Retinal dystrophy in Sprague-Dawley rats. *Lab. Anim. Sci.* **25**: 323-326

SCHMIDT, R. E. (1983) Diagnostic exercise: retinal degeneration. *Lab. Anim. Sci.* **33**: 433-434

## 181, Hydrocephalus

KOTO, M., MIWA, M., SHIMIZU, A., TSUJI, K., OKAMOTO, M. and ADACHI, J. (1987) Inherited hydrocephalus in Csk:Wistar-Imamichi rats, Hyd strain: A new disease model for hydrocephalus. *Jikken Dobutsu* **36**: 157-162

PARK, A. W. and NOWOSIELSKI-SLEPOWRON, B. J. (1979) Hydrocephalus in the laboratory rat. *Acta. Morphol. Neerl. Scand.* **17**: 191-207

## 21-, Squamous Cell Carcinoma of Tongue, Stomach and Esophagus

CARDESA, A. and OVERLAR, M. Y. (1985) Carcinoma in situ, esophagus, rat. In: *Digestive System* (T. C. Jones *et al.*) pp. 265-267. op. cit.

CARDESA, A. and OVELAR, M. Y. (1985) Squamous cell carcinoma, esophagus,rat. In: *Digestive System* (T. C. Jones *et al.*) pp. 268-271, op. cit.

FUKUSHIMA, S. and ITO, N. (1985) Squamous cell carcinoma, forestomach, rat. In: *Digestive System* (T. C. Jones et. al.) pp. 292-295, op. cit.

KOCIBA, R. J.and KEYES, D. G. (1985) Squamous cell carcinoma, tongue, rat. In: *Digestive System* (Eds. T. C. Jones *et al.*) pp. 255-260, op. cit.

## 21-, Adenocarcinoma of Stomach

SZENTIRMAY, Z.and SUGAR, J. (1985) Adenocarcinoma, glandular stomach, rat. In: *Digestive System* (Eds. T. C. Jones *et al.*) pp. 301-309, op. cit.

## 21-, Colonic Carcinoma

GRASSO, P. and CREASEY, M. (1969) Carcinoma of the colon in a rat. *Eur. J. Cancer* **5**: 415-419

MIWA, M., TAKENAKA, S., ITO, K., FUJIWARA, K. and KOGURE, K. (1976) Spontaneous colon tumors in rats. *J. Natl. Canc. Inst.* **56**: 615-621

NEWBERNE, P. M. and ROGERS A. E. (1985) Adenocarcinoma, colon and rectum, rat. In: *Digestive System* (Eds. T.C. Jones *et al.*), pp. 365-370, op. cit.

BOORMAN, G. A.and EUSTIS, S. L. (1985) Acinar-cell carcinoma, pancreas. **In**: *Digestive System* (Eds. T. C. Jones *et al.*), pp. 213-223, op. cit.

## 21-, Cholangiocarcinoma

BANNASCH, P., BENNER, U.and ZERBAN, H. (1985) Cholangiofibroma and cholangiocarcinoma, liver, rat. **In**: *Digestive System* (Eds. T. C. Jones *et al.*) pp. 52-65, op. cit.

## 21-, Hemangiosarcoma of Liver

POPP, J. A. (1985) Hemangiosarcoma, liver, rat. **In**: *Digestive System* (Eds. T. C. Jones *et al.*) pp. 69-70, op. cit.

## 21-, Kupffer's Cell Sarcoma

POPP, J. A. (1985) Kupffer's cell sarcoma, liver, rat. **In**: *Digestive System* (Eds. T. C. Jones *et al.*) pp. 73-75, op. cit.

## 213, Hepatocellular Carcinoma

IMAI, K., YOSHIMURA, S. and HANJHO, J. (1982) Spontaneous liverneoplasms in Sprague-Dawley rats. *Jikken Dobutsu* **31**: 51-54

Institute of Laboratory Animal Resources, National Research Council. (1979. Histological typing of liver tumors in the rat. *J. Nat. Cancer Inst.* **64**: 180-205

POLLARD, M. and LUCKERT, P. H. (1979) Spontaneous liver tumors in aged germfree Wistar rats. *Lab. Anim. Sci.* **29**: 74-77

POLLARD, M. (1982) Spontaneous liver tumors in laboratory rats(letter). *J. Nat. Cancer Inst.* **68**: 884

POPP, J. A. (1985) Hepatocellular carcinoma, liver, rat. **In**: *Digestive System* (Eds. T. C. Jones *et al.*) pp. 39-46. op. cit.

SQUIRE, R. A. and LEVITT M. H. (1975) Report of a workshop on classification of specific hepatocellular lesions in rats. *Cancer Res.* **35: 3214-3223**

## 214, Leiomyosarcoma

TAKAHASHI, M. (1985) Leiomyoma and leiomyosarcoma, stomach, rat. **In**: *Digestive System* (Eds. T. C. Jones *et al.*) pp. 310-314, op. cit.

## 22-, Hemangioma of Liver

BROOKS, P. N. and ROE, F. J. C. (1985) Hemangioma, liver, rat. 1985. **In**: *Digestive System* (Eds. T. C. Jones *et al.*) pp. 71-72, op. cit.

## 22-, Ameloblastic Odontoma

BARBOLT, T. A. and BHANDARI, J. C. (1983) Ameloblastic odontoma in a rat. *Lab. Anim. Sci.* **33**: 583-584

## 222, Adenoma of Salivary Gland

SASAKI, S. (1982) A primary neoplasm in the submaxillary gland of a rat. *J. Comp. Pathol.* **92**: 437-443

## 22-, Papilloma of forestomach

FUKUSHIMA, S. and ITO, N. (1985. Papilloma, forestomach, rat. **In**: *Digestive System* (Eds. T. C. Jones *et al.*) pp. 289-291, op. cit.

## 22-, Papilloma of Esophagus

OVELAR, M. Y. and CARDESA, A. Squamous cell papilloma, esophagus, rat. **In**: *Digestive System* (Eds. T. C. Jones *et al.*) pp. 263-265, op. cit.

## 22-, Cholangioma

BROOKS, P. N. and ROE, F. J. C. (1985) Cholangioma, liver, rat. **In**: *Digestive System* (Eds. T. C. Jones *et al.*) pp. 66-68.

## 221, Hepatocellular Adenoma

BROOKS, P. N. and ROE, F. J. C. (1985) Hepatocellular adenoma. **In**: *Digestive System* (Eds. T. C. Jones *et al.*) pp. 47-51, op. cit.

## 22-, Adenoma of Exocrine Pancreas

LOVE, L., PELFRENE, A., GARCIA, H. (1977) Acinar adenomas of the pancreas in MRC-Wistar rats. *J. Vomp. Pathol.* **87**: 307-310

## 23-, Oval cell Hyperplasia

HOOVER, K. L. Oval cell hyperplasia, liver, mouse, rat. **In**: *Digestive System* (Eds T. C. Jones et al) pp. 125-126, op. cit.

## 23-, Miscellaneous Lesions in Liver

VAN ZWIETEN, M. J. and HOLLANDER, C. F. (1985) Polyploidy, liver, rat. **In**: *Digestive System* (Eds T. C. Jones *et al.*) pp. 83-85, op. cit.

VAN ZWIETEN, M. J. and HOLLANDER, C. F. (1985) Herniation of liver through esophageal hiatus, rat. **In**: *Digestive System* (Eds. T. C. Jones *et al.*) pp. 127-130, op. cit.

VAN ZWIETEN, M. J. and HOLLANDER, C. F. (1985) Intranuclear and intracytoplasmic inclusions, liver, rat. **In**: *Digestive System* (Eds. T. C. Jones *et al.*) pp. 86-91, op. cit.

MULLINK, J. W., VOS-MAAS, M., BUSSINK, G. P. and HANEVELD, G. T. (1977) Congenital venous hypoplasia in the liver of rats. *Lab. Anim. Sci.* **11**: 149-153

## 232, Basophilic Hepatocyte Nodules

BANNASCH, P., ZERBAN, H. and HACKER, H. J. Foci of altered hepatocytes, rat. **In**: *Digestive System* (Eds. T. C. Jones *et al.*) pp. 10-15, op. cit.

CHIU, T. and CHEN, H. C. (1986) Spontaneous basophilic hypertrophic foci of the parotid glands in rats and mice. *Vet. Pathol.* **23**: 606-609

## 24-, Perisinusoidal Fibrosis, Cirrhosis

BERNAU, D., GUILLOT, R., DURAND-SCHNEIDER, A.M., POUSSIER, P.,MOREAU, A. and FELDMANN, G. (1985) Liver perisinusoidal fibrosis in BB rats with or without overt diabetes. *Am. J. Pathol.* **120**: 38-45

ZAKI, H. (1966) Fatty cirrhosis in the rat, XII The cirrhotic nodules. *Arch. Pathol.* **81**: 536-543

## 243, Extramedullary Hematopoiesis

VAN ZWIETEN, M. J. and HOLLANDER, C. F. Extramedullary hematopoiesis, liver, rat. In: *Digestive System* (Eds. T. C. Jones *et al.*) pp. 97-99, op. cit.

## 244, Atrophy of Exocrine Pancreas with Lobular Ectasia

BOORMAN, G. A. and EUSTIS, S. L. (1985) Atrophy, exocrine pancreas, rat. In: *Digestive System* (Eds. T. C. Jones *et al.*) pp. 239-244, op. cit.

## 255, Ulceration of Stomach

WRIGHT, J. R. Jr., YATES, A. J., SHARMA, H. M. and THIBERT, P. (1981) Spontaneous gastric erosions and ulcerations in BB Wistar rats. *Lab. Anim. Sci.* **31**: 63-66

## 271, Focal Vacuolization of Hepatocytes

BANNASCH, P., ZERBAN, H. and FUGEL, H. J. (1985) Spongiosis hepatis, rat. In: *Digestive System* (Eds. T. C. Jones et. al.) pp 116-122, op.cit.

## 281, Peliosis Hepatis

BANNASCH, P., WAYSS, K. and ZERBAN, H. (1985) Peliosis hepatis, rodents. In: *Digestive System* (Eds. T. C. Jones *et al.*) pp 110-115, op. cit.

LEE, K. P. (1983) Peliosis hepatis-like lesions in aging rats. *Vet. Pathol.* **20**: 410-423

## 28-, Esophageal Impaction

RUBEN, Z., ROHRBACHER, E. and MILLER, J. E. (1983) Esophageal impaction in BHE rats. *Lab. Anim. Sci.* **33**: 63-65

## 31-, Cardiac Neoplasms

HOCH-LIGETI, C., RESTREPO, C. and STEWART, H. L. (1986) Comparative pathology of cardiac neoplasms in humans and in laboratory rodents: A review. *J. Nat. Cancer Inst.* **76**: 127-142

BODE, G. and HARTIG, F. (1981) Primary neoplasms of the heart. *Exp. Pathol.* **19**: 31-36

ROBERTSON, J. L., GARMAN, R. H. and FOWLER, E. H. (1982) Spontaneous cardiac tumors in eight rats. *Vet. Pathol.* **19**: 30-37

YAMATE, J., KUDOW, S. and TAJIMA, M. (1984) Morphology of spontaneous cardiac tumors in F344 rats. *Nippon Juigaku Zasshi* **46**: 381-384

## 341, Arteriosclerosis

JUDD, J. T. and WEXLER, B. C. (1969) The role of lactation and weaning in the pathogenesis of arteriosclerosis in female breeder rats. *J. Atherosclr. Res.* **10**: 153-172

WEXLER, B. C. (1969) Exacerbation of spontaneously occurring arteriosclerosis in breeder rats following chronic treatment with cortisone. *J. Atheroscler. Res.* **8**: 267-277

WEXLER, B. C. (1979) Spontaneous arteriosclerosis in old, male,virgin Sprague-Dawley rats. *Atherosclerosis* **34**: 277-290

ZAHOR, Z., CZABANOVA, V. and KOMARKOVA, A. (1969) The dependence of post-reproduction arteriopathy in rats on diet. *J. Atheroscler. Res.* **9**: 279-282

## 342, Focal Myocardial Fibrosis and Degeneration

LEWIS, D. J. (1980) Sub-endocardial fibrosis in the rat: a light and electron microscopical study. *J. Comp. Pathol.* **90**: 577-583

SAEGUSA, J. and KAWAI, K. (1982) Six cases of endocardial disease in the rat. *Nippon Juigaku Zasshi* **44**: 961-966

## 363, Periarteritis Nodosa

OPIE, E. L., LYNCH, C. J. and TERSHAKOVEC, M. (1970) Sclerosis of the mesenteric arteries of rats: Its relation to longevity and inheritance. *Arch. Pathol.* **89**: 306-313

## 41-, Squamous Cell Carcinoma of nasal mucosa and lung

BOORMAN, G. A. (1985) Squamous cell carcinoma, lung, rat. **In:** *Respiratory System.* (Eds. T. C. Jones *et al.*) pp 124-126. op. cit.

KERNS, W. D. (1985) Squamous cell carcinoma, nasal mucosa, rat. **In:** *Respiratory System.* (Eds. T.C. Jones *et al.*) pp 54-61, op cit.

## 411, Bronchoalveolar Adenocarcinoma

BOORMAN, G. A. (1985) Bronchiolar/alveolar adenoma, lung, rat. **In:** *Respiratory System* (Eds. T. C. Jones *et al.*) pp 99-101, op. cit.

BOORMAN, G. A. (1985) Bronchiolar/alveolar carcinoma, lung, rat. **In:** *Respiratory System* (T. C. Jones *et al.*) pp 112-116, op. cit.

## 43-, Nasal adenoma

KERNS, W. D. (1985) Polypoid adenoma, nasal mucosa, rat. **In:** *Respiratory System* ( Eds. T. C. Jones *et al.*) pp 41-46, op. cit.

## 463, Alveolar Histiocytosis

EMI, Y., HIGASHIGUCHI, R. and KONISHI, Y. (1985) Pulmonary lipidosis, rat. **In:** *Respiratory System* (Eds. T. C. Jones *et al.*) pp 169-170. op. cit.

WELLER, W. (1985) Alveolar lipoproteinosis, rat. **In:** *Respiratory System* (Eds. T. C. Jones *et al.*) pp 171-176, op. cit.

## 46-, Chronic Inflammation of Upper Respiratory Tract

SCHOEB, T. R. and LINDSEY, J. R. (1985) Murine respiratory mycoplasmosis, upper respiratory tract, rat. **In:** *Respiratory System* (Eds. T. C. Jones *et al.*) pp 78-83 op. cit.

## 466, Peribronchial Lymphoid Hyperplasia

GREGSON, R. L., DAVEY, M. J. and PRENTICE, D. E. (1979) Bronchus-associated lymphoid tissue (BALT) in the laboratory-bred and wild rat (*Rattus norvegicus*). *Lab. Anim. Sci.* **13**: 239-243

## 47-, Hair Fragment Emboli in Lung

TEKELI, S. (1974) Occurrence of hair-fragment emboli in the pulmonary vascular system of rats. *Vet. Pathol.* **11**: 483-485

## 51-, Craniopharyngoma

CARLTON, W. W. and GRIES, C. L. (1983) Craniopharyngioma, pituitary gland, **In**: *Endocrine System* (Eds. T. C. Jones *et al.*) pp. 149-152, op. cit.

## 511, Islet Adenocarcinoma

LEWIS, D. J., OFFER, J. M. and PRENTICE, D. E. (1982) Metastasizing pancreatic islet cell tumors in the rat. *J. Comp. Pathol.* **92**: 139-147

## 512, Pheochromocytoma

BOSLAND, M. C. and BAR, A. (1984) Some functional characteristics of adrenal medullary tumors in aged male Wistar rats. *Vet. Pathol.* **21**: 129-140

CHENG, L. (1980) Pheochromocytoma in rats: Incidence, etiology, morphology and functional activity. *J. Environ. Pathol. Toxicol.* **4**: 219-228

MAJEED, S. K. and HARLING, S. M. (1986) Malignant phaeochromocytoma with widespread metastasis in the rat. *J. Comp. Pathol.* **96**: 575-580

STRANDBERG, J. D. (1983) Pheochromocytoma, adrenal medulla, rat. **In**: *Endocrine System* (Eds. T. C. Jones *et al.*) pp. 22-26, op. cit.

## 513, Pituitary Adenocarcinoma

CARLTON, W. W. and GRIES, C. L. (1983) Adenoma and carcinoma, pars distalis, rat. **In**: *Endocrine System* (Eds. T. C. Jones *et al.*) pp. 134-144, op. cit.

MAGNUSSON, G., MAJEED, S. K. and GOPINATH, C. (1979) Infiltrating pituitary neoplasms in the rat. *Lab. Anim. Sci.* **13**: 111-113

## 514, Adenocarcinoma of Adrenal Cortex

STRANDBERG, J. D. (1983) Adenocarcinoma, adrenal cortex, rat. **In**: *Endocrine System* (Eds. T. C. Jones *et al.*) pp. 46-48. op. cit.

## 515, Follicular Cell Adenocarcinoma of Thyroid

BOORMAN, G. A. (1983) Follicular cell carcinoma, thyroid, rat. **In**: *Endocrine System* (Eds. T. C. Jones *et al.*) pp. 180-185, op. cit.

## 517, Adenocarcinoma of Thyroid C Cells

BOORMAN, G. A. and DeLELLIS, R. A. Medullary carcinoma, thyroid, rat.**In**: *Endocrine System* (Eds. T. C. Jones *et al.*) pp. 200-203, op. cit.

BOORMAN, G. A. and HOLLANDER, C. F. (1976) Animal model of human disease: Medullary carcinoma of the thyroid. *Am. J. Pathol.* **83**: 237-240

CAHILL, G. F. (1980) Needs for animal models of human diseases of the endocrine system. *Am. J. Pathol.* **101**: 131s-140s

ROE, F. J. and BAR, A. (1985) Enzootic and epizootic adrenal medullary proliferative diseases of rats: Influence of dietary factors which affect calcium absorption. *Hum. Toxicol.* **4**: 27-52

SUZUKI, H., MOHR, U. and KIMMERLE, G. (1979) Spontaneous endocrine tumors in Sprague-Dawley rats. *J. Cancer Res. Clin Oncol.* **95**: 187-196

## 51-, Neuroblastoma

REZNIK, G. and WARD, J. M. Neuroblastoma, adrenal, rat.**In**: *Endocrine System* (Eds. T. C. Jones *et al.*) pp. 35-36, op. cit.

## 52-, Pinealoma

BUREK, J. D., VAN ZWIETEN, M. J. and SOLLEVELD, H. A. (1983) Pinealoma, rat. **In**: *Endocrine System* (Eds. T. C. Jones *et al.*) pp. 350-354, op. cit.

## 521, Adenoma of Pituitary

CARLTON, W. W. and GRIES, C. L. (1983) Pituicytoma, neurohypophysis, rat. **In**: *Endocrine System* (Eds. T. C. Jones *et al.*) pp. 156-160 op. cit.

CARLTON, W. W. and GRIES, C. L. (1983) Adenoma, pars intermedia, anterior, pituitary, rat. **In**: *Endocrine System* (Eds. T. C. Jones *et al.*) pp. 145-148, op. cit.

FITZGERALD, J. E., SCHARDEIN, J. L. and KAUMP, D. H. (1971) Several uncommon pituitary tumors in the rat. *Lab. Anim. Sci.* **21**: 581-584

HALL, L. B., YOSHITOMI, K. and BOORMAN, G. A. (1987) Pathologic features of abdominal and thoracic paragangliomas in F344/N rats. *Vet. Pathol.* **24**: 315-322

## 521, Adenoma of Pituitary

BARSOUM, N. J., MOORE, J. D., GOUGH, A. W., STURGESS, J. M. and DE LAIGLESIA, F. A. (1985) Morphofunctional investigations on spontaneous pituitary tumors in Wistar rats. *Toxicol. Pathol.* **13**: 200-208

BERRY, P. H. (1986) Effect of diet or reproductive status on the histology of spontaneous pituitary tumors in female Wistar rats. *Vet. Pathol.* **23**: 610-618

KOVACS, K., HORVATH, E., BILBAO, J. M. and ILSE, R. G. (1977) Annulate lamellae in spontaneous prolactin cell adenomas of the rat pituitary. *Anat. Anz.* **141**: 59-65

MAJEED, S. K., GOPINATH, C. and MAGNUSSON, G. (1980) Ultrastructure of spontaneous pituitary neoplasms in the rat. *J. Comp. Pathol.* **90**: 239-246

PICKERING, C. E. and PICKERING, R. G. (1984) The effect of repeated reproduction on the incidence of pituitary tumours in Wistar rats. *Lab. Anim. Sci.* **18**: 371-378

TROUILLAS, J., GIROD, C., CLAUSTRAT, B., CURE, M. and DUBOIS, M. P. (1982) Spontaneous pituitary tumors in the Wistar-Furth/Ico rat strain: An animal model of human prolactin adenoma. *Am. J. Pathol.* **109**: 57-70

## 522, Adenoma of C Cells

BOORMAN, G. A. and DeLELLIS, R. A. (1983) C-cell adenoma, thyroid, rat. **In**: *Endocrine System* (Eds. T. C. Jones *et al.*) pp. 197-199, op. cit.

## 523, Adenoma of Islet Cells

KOVACS, K., HORVATH, E., ILSE, R. G. and ILSE, D. (1976) Spontaneous pancreatic beta cell tumor in the rat: A light and electron microscopic study. *Vet. Pathol.* **13**: 286-294

## 524, Adenoma of Adrenal Cortex

STRANDBERG, J. D. (1983) Adenoma, adrenal cortex, rat.**In**: *Endocrine System* (Eds. T. C. Jones *et al.*) pp. 41-45, op. cit.

## 525, Adenoma of Thyroid

BOORMAN, G. A. (1983) Follicular cell adenoma, thyroid, rat. **In**: *Endocrine System* (Eds. T. C. Jones *et al.*) pp. 177-179, op. cit.

## 526, Adenoma of Parathyroid

POUR, P. M., WILSON, J. T. and SALMASI, S. (1983) Adenoma, carcinoma,parathyroid, rat. In: *Endocrine System* (Eds. T. C. Jones *et al.*) pp. 281-287, op. cit.

## 528, Ganglioneuroma

REZNIK, G. and WARD, J. M. (1983 Ganglioneuroma, adrenal, rat. In: *Endocrine System* (Eds. T. C. Jones *et al.*) pp. 30-34, op. cit.

REZNIK, G., WARD, J. M. and REZNIK-SCHULLER, H. (1980) Ganglioneuromas in the adrenal medulla of F344 rats. *Vet. Pathol.* **17**: 614-621

TODD, G. C., PIERCE, E. C. and CLEVINGER, W. G. (1970) Ganglioneuroma of the adrenal medulla in rats: A report of three cases. *Vet. Pathol.* **7**: 139-144

## 53-, Miscellaneous Growth Abnormalities

BOORMAN, G. A. (1983) Follicular cell hyperplasia, thyroid, rat. In: *Endocrine System* (Eds. T. C. Jones *et al.*) pp. 176-177, op. cit.

PARKER, G. A. and VALERIO, M. G. (1983) Ectopic thymus, thyroid, rat. In: *Endocrine System* (Eds. T. C. Jones *et al.*) pp. 173-175, op. cit.

PARKER, G. A. and VALERIO, M. G. (1983) Ectopic thyroid, rat. In:*Endocrine System* (Eds. T.C. Jones *et al.*) pp. 172-173, op. cit.

## 531, Nodular Cortical Hyperplasia of Adrenal

STRANDBERG, J. D. (1983) Focal hyperplasia, adrenal cortex, rat. In: *Endocrine System* (Eds. T. C. Jones *et al.*) pp. 37-40, op. cit.

## 531, Hyperplasia of Adrenal Medulla

STRANDBERG, J. D. (1983) Hyperplasia, adrenal medulla, rat. In: *Endocrine System* (Eds. T. C. Jones *et al.*) pp. 18-21, op. cit.

## 532, C Cell Hyperplasia

BOORMAN, G. A. and DeLELLIS, R. A. (1983) C-cell hyperplasia, thyroid, rat. In: *Endocrine System* (Eds. T. C. Jones *et al.*) pp. 192-196, op. cit.

533, Hyperplasia of Parathyroid

POUR, P. M., WILSON, J. T. and SALMASI, S. (1983) Hyperplasia, parathyroid,rat. In: *Endocrine System* (Eds. T. C. Jones *et al.*) pp. 263-274, op. cit. 268.

## 56-, Lymphocytic thyroiditis

TODD, G. C. (1983) Lymphocytic thyroiditis, rat. In: *Endocrine System* (Eds. T. C. Jones *et al.*) pp. 212-214, op. cit. 212.

## 57-, Lipogenic Pigmentation of Adrenal

PARKER, G. A. and VALERIO, M. G. (1983) Lipogenic pigmentation, adrenal cortex, rat. In: *Endocrine System* (Eds. T. C. Jones *et al.*) pp. 64-67, op. cit. 64.

## 571, Lipid Hyperplasia of Adrenal Cortex

ZAK, F. (1983) Lipid hyperplasia, adrenal cortex, rat. In: *Endocrine System* (Eds. T. C. Jones *et al.*) pp. 80-84, op. cit.

## 581, Cystic Pituitary

CARLTON, W. W. and GRIES, C. L. (1983) Cysts, pituitary; rat, mouse and hamster. **In**: *Endocrine System* (Eds. T. C. Jones *et al.*) pp. 161-163, op. cit.

## 61-, Transitional Cell Carcinoma

DEERBERG, F., REHM, S. and JOSTMEYER, H. H. (1985) Spontaneous urinary bladder tumors in DA/Han rats: A feasible model of human bladder cancer. *J. Nat. Cancer Inst.* **75**: 1113-1121

PAULI, B. U., COON, J. S. and WEINSTEIN, R. S. (1986) Transitional cell carcinoma, bladder, rat. **In**: *Urinary System* (Eds. T. C. Jones *et al.*) pp. 322-330, op. cit.

BOORMAN, G. A. and HOLLANDER, C. F. (1974) High incidence of spontaneous urinary bladder and ureter tumors in the brown Norway rat. *J. Nat. Cancer Inst.* **52**: 1005-1008

## 61-, Squamous Cell Carcinoma of Urinary Bladder.

ITO, N. and HIROSE, M. (1986) Squamous cell carcinoma, urinary bladder, rat. **In**: *Urinary System* (Eds. T. C. Jones *et al.*) pp. 341-346, op. cit.

## 61-, Adenocarcinoma of Urinary Bladder

STULA, E. F. (1986) Adenocarcinoma, urinary bladder, rat. **In**: *Urinary System* (Eds. T. C. Jones *et al.*) pp. 346-351, op. cit.

STULA, E. F. (1986) Undifferentiated carcinoma, urinary bladder, rat. **In**: *Urinary System* (Eds. T. C. Jones *et al.*) pp. 352-354, op. cit.

## 613, Nephroblastoma

CARDESA, A. and RIBALTA, T. (1986) Nephroblastoma, kidney, rat. **In**: *Urinary System* (Eds. T. C. Jones *et al.*) pp. 71-79, op. cit.

GIALAMAS, J., HOGER, H. and ADAMIKER, D. (1987) Spontaneous nephroblastomas in rats. *Z. Versuchstierkd.* **29**: 65-69

MAGNUSSON, G. (1969) Spontaneous nephroblastomas in the rat. *Z.Versuchstierkd.* **11**: 293-297

PITTERMANN, W. and DEERBERG, F. (1974) Spontaneous nephroblastomas in SPF Han rats. *Berl. Munch. Tierarztl. Wochenschr.* **87**: 178-180

## 61-, 62-, Miscellaneous Kidney Tumors

BANNASCH, P., ZERBAN, H. and HACKER, H. J. (1986) Onocytoma, kidney, rat. 49. **In**: *Urinary System* (Eds. T. C. Jones *et al.*) pp. 49-60, op. cit.

BORDON, L. R. (1986) Spontaneous lipomatous tumors in the kidney of the Crl:CD(SD) rat. *Toxicol. Pathol.* **14**: 175-182

HARD, G. C. (1986) Mesenchymal tumor, kidney, rat. **In**: *Urinary System* (Eds. T. C. Jones *et al.*) pp. 61-70, op. cit.

HARD, G. C. (1986) Lipomatous tumors, kidney, rat. **In**: *Urinary System* (Eds. T. C. Jones *et al.*) pp. 71-79, op. cit. 80.

ITO, N. and SHIRAI, T. (1986) Papilloma, urinary bladder, rat. **In**: *Urinary System* (Eds. T. C. Jones *et al.*) pp. 337-340, op. cit.

GOLDSCHMIDT, R. (1981) Urinary bladder papilloma as a cause of monstrous hydronephrosis. *Z. Versuchstierkd* **23**: 80-83

KUNZE, E. (1986) Hyperplasia, urinary bladder, rat. **In**: *Urinary System* (Eds. T. C. Jones *et al.*) pp. 291-293, op. cit.

## 63-, Persistent Urachus

BORRAS, M. (1983) Three cases of persistent urachus with umbilical abscess in Wistar rats. *Lab. Anim. Sci.* **17**: 55-58

## 63-, Renal Tubular Karyomegaly

RICHARDSON, J. A. and WOODARD, J. C. (1986) Renal tubular karyocytomegaly, rat. **In:** *Urinary System* (Eds. T. C. Jones *et al.*) pp. 189-190, op. cit. 189.

## 641, Chronic Progressive Glomerulonephropathy

BOLTON, W. K., BENTON, F. R., MACLAY, J. G. and STURGILL, B. C. (1976) Spontaneous glomerular sclerosis in aging Sprague-Dawley rats, Part I: Lesions associated with mesangial IgM deposits. *Am. J. Pathol.* **85**: 277-302

BOLTON, W. K. and STURGILL, B. C. (1980) Spontaneous glomerularsclerosis in aging Sprague-Dawley rats, Part II: Ultrastructural studies. *Am. J. Pathol.* **98**: 339-356

GOLDSTEIN, R. J., TURLOFF, J. R. and HOOK, J. D. (1988) Age-related nephropathy in laboratory rats. *FASEB J.* **2**: 2241-2251

GRAY, J. E. (1977) Chronic progressive nephrosis in the albino rat. *CRC Crit. Rev. Toxicol.* **5**: 115-144

GRAY, J. E. (1986) Chronic progressive nephrosis, rat. **In:** *Urinary System* (Eds. T. C. Jones *et al.*) pp. 174-178, op. cit.

HIROKAWA, K. (1975) Characterization of age-associated kidney disease in Wistar rats. *Mech. Aging Dev.* **4**: 301-316

ITAKURA, C., IIDA, M. and GOTO, M. (1977) Renal secondary hyperparathyroidism in aged Sprague-Dawley rats. *Vet. Pathol.* **14**: 463-469

KRAUS, B. and CAIN, H. (1974) A spontaneous nephropathy of Wistar-type rats: The light and electron microscopic changes of the glomerula (author's transl.). *Virchows. Arch. (Pathol. Anat.)* **363**: 343-358

KREISBERG, J. I. and KARNOVSKY, M. J. (1978) Focal glomerularsclerosis in the fawn-hooded rat. *Am. J. Pathol.* **92**: 637-652

OWEN, R. A. and HEYWOOD, R. (1986) Age-related variations in renal structure and function in Sprague-Dawley rats. *Toxicol. Pathol.* **14**: 158-167

PETER, C. P., BUREK, J. D. and VAN ZWIETEN, M. J. (1986) Spontaneous nephropathies in rats. *Toxicol. Pathol.* **14**: 91-100

SOLLEVELD, H.A. and BOORMAN, G.A. (1986) Spontaneous renal lesions in five rat strains. *Toxicol. Pathol.* **14**: 168-174

UCHIDA, K., ONOUE, M., TAKAHASHI, T., KUSANO, N. and MUTAI, M. (1980) Histopathological findings of age-related kidney lesions in inbred strain Fischer-344/Yit rats (author's transl.). *Jiken Dobutsu* **29**: 45-54

WYNDHAM, J. R., EVERITT, A. V. and EVERITT, S. F. (1983) Effects of isolation and food restriction begun at 50 days on the development of age-associated renal disease in the male Wistar rat. *Arch. Gerontol. Geriatr.* **2**: 317-332

## 64-, Papillary Necrosis of Kidney

ELLIOTT, G. A. (1986) Papillary necrosis, rat. **In:** *Urinary System* (Eds. T. C. Jones *et al.*) pp. 184-186, op. cit.

## 651, Pyelonephritis

DUPRAT, P. and BUREK, J. D. (1986) Suppurative nephritis, pyelonephritis, rat. **In:** *Urinary System* (Eds. T. C. Jones *et al.*) pp. 219-224, op. cit.

## 67-, Urolithiasis

IMAI, S., MORIMOTO, J., KIYOZUKA, Y., SHIMA, M., NAKAMORI, K. and KHAN, S.R. and WOODARD, J.C. (1986) Calcium oxalate urolithiasis, rat. **In**: *Urinary System* (Eds. T. C. Jones *et al.*) pp. 355-360, op. cit.

MAGNUSSON, G. and RAMSAY, C. H. (1971) Urolithiasis in the rat. *Lab. Anim. Sci.* **5**: 153-162

PATERSON, M. (1979) Urolithiasis in the Sprague-Dawley rat. *Lab. Anim. Sci.* **13**: 17-20

WOODARD, J. C. and KHAN, S. R. (1986) Phosphate urolithiasis, rat. **In**: *Urinary System* (Eds. T. C. Jones *et al.*) pp. 364-368, op. cit.

## 67-, Amyloidosis

GREEN, C. J. (1974) Amyloidosis as an incidental finding in rats on experiment. *Lab. Anim. Sci.* **8**: 99-101

## 67-, Nephrocalcinosis

IWATA, H., HIROUCHI, Y., INOUE, H. and ENOMOTO, M. (1986) Pathological study on nephrocalcinosis in F344/Du Crj rats. *Jikken Dobutsu* **35**: 299-305

SILVERMAN, J. and RIVENSON, A. (1980) Nephrocalcinosis in two young rats: A case report. *Lab. Anim. Sci.* **14**: 241-242

TSUBURA, Y. (1986) Spontaneous calcification in F344/Slc and F344/JCL rats. *Jikken Dobutsu* **35**: 521-525

## 681, Hydronephrosis

BURTON, D. S., MARONPOT, R. R. and HOWARD, F. L. 3rd. (1979) Frequency of hydronephrosis in Wistar rats. *Lab. Anim. Sci.* **29**: 642-644

FUJITA, K., FUJITA, H. M., OHTAWARA, Y., SUZUKI, K., TAJIMA, A. and ASO, Y. (1979) Hydronephrosis in ACI/N rats. *Lab. Anim. Sci.* **13**: 325-327

MARONPOT, R. R. (1986) Spontaneous hydronephrosis, rat. **In**: *Urinary System* (Eds. T. C. Jones *et al.*) pp. 268-270, op. cit.

O'DONOGHUE, P. N. and WILSON, M. S. (1977) Hydronephrosis in male rats. *Lab. Anim. Sci.* **11**: 193-194

## 71-, Miscellaneous Tumors of Testis

BOORMAN, G. A., REHM, S., WAALKES, M. P., ELWELL, M. R. and EUSTIS, S.L. (1987) Seminoma, testis, rat. **In**: *Genital System* (Eds. T. C. Jones *et al.*) pp. 192-194, op. cit.

KIM, S. N., FITZGERALD, J. E. and DE LA IGLESIA, F. A. (1985) Spermatocytic seminoma in the rat. *Toxicol. Pathol.* **13**: 215-221

BOORMAN, G. A., ABBOTT, D. P., ELWELL, M. R. and EUSTIS, S. L. (1987) Sertoli's cell tumor, testis, rat. **In**: *Genital System* (Eds. T. C. Jones *et al.*) pp. 195-199, op. cit.

## 721, Interstitial Cell Tumor

RAO, M. S. and REDDY, J. K. (1987) Interstitial cell tumor, testis, rat. **In**: *Genital System* (Eds. T. C. Jones *et al.*) pp. 184-191, op. cit.

## 71-, Adenocarcinomas of Accessary Male sex organs

BOSLAND, M. C. (1987) Adenocarcinoma, seminal vesicle/coagulating gland,rat. **In**: *Genital System* (Eds. T. C. Jones *et al.*) pp. 272-274, op. cit.

BOSLAND, M. C. (1987) Adenocarcinoma, prostate, rat.

PARKER, G. A. and GRABAU, J. (1987) Adenoma and adenocarcinoma, preputial gland, rat. **In:** *Genital System* (Eds. T. C. Jones *et al.*) pp. 275-281, op. cit.

SHAIN, S. A., McCULLOUGH, B. and SEGALOFF, A. (1975) Spontaneous adenocarcinomas of the ventral prostate of aged A X C rats. *J. Nat. Cancer Inst.* **55**: 177-180

REZNIK, G. and WARD, J. M. (1981) Morphology of neoplastic lesions in the clitoral and preputial gland of the F344 rat. *J. Cancer Res. Clin. Oncol.* **101**: 249-263

## 712, Mesotheliomas of Tunica Vaginalis etc.

DEERBERG, F. and REHM, S. Spontaneous mesotheliomas in Han:WIST rats. *Z. Versuchstierkd* **23**: 296-302

MAWDESKEY-THOMAS, L. E. and HAGUE, P. H. (1970) Mesothelioma of the tunica vaginalis in a rat. *Lab. Anim. Sci.* **4**: 29-36

NASH, G. and KALINER, G. (1984) Spontaneous pericardial mesothelioma in a rat. *Z. Versuchstierkd* **26**: 185-188

## 722, Adenoma of Prostate

BOSLAND, M. C. (1987) Adenoma, prostate, rat. **In:** *Genital System* (Eds. T. C. Jones *et al.*) pp. 261-266, op. cit.

## 73-, Miscellaneous Hyperplasias of Male Genital Organs

BOSLAND, M. C. (1987) Hyperplasia, prostate, rat. **In:** *Genital System* (Eds. T. C. Jones *et al.*) pp. 267-271, op. cit.

MAEKAWA, A. and HAYASHI, Y. (1987) Adenomatous hyperplasia, rete testis,rat. **In:** *Genital System* (Eds. T. C. Jones *et al.*) pp. 234-236, op. cit.

REZNIK, G. and WARD, J. M. (1981) Morphology of hyperplastic and neoplastic lesions in the clitoral and preputial gland of the F344 rat. *Vet. Pathol.* **18**: 228-238

RESNIK, G. and REZNIK-SCHULLER, H. (1980) Pathology of the clitoral and preputial glands in aging F344 rats. *Lab. Anim. Sci.* **30**: 845-850

## 731, Hyperplasia of Leydig Cells

BOORMAN, G. A., HAMLIN, M. H. Jr. and EUSTIS, S. L. (1987) Focal interstitial cell hyperplasia, testes, rat.**In:** *Genital System* (Eds. T. C. Jones *et al.*) pp. 200-203, op. cit.

## 74-, Degeneration of Epididymis

CARDY, R. H. (1987) Segmental degeneration of the epididymis in aged F344 rats. *Vet. Pathol.* **24**: 361-363

## 744, Atrophy of Testis

WRIGHT, J. R. Jr. (1987) Atrophy, testis, rat. **In:** *Genital System* (Eds. T. C. Jones *et al.*) pp. 218-226, op. cit.

YUAN, Y. D. and McENTEE, K. (1987) Testicular degeneration, rat. **In:** *Genital System* (Eds. T. C. Jones *et al.*) pp. 212-217, op. cit.

## 761, Chronic Prostatitis

PARKER, G. A. and GRABAU, J. (1987) Chronic prostatitis, rat. **In:** *Genital System* (Eds. T.C. Jones *et al.*) pp. 287-289, op. cit.

## 811, Leiomyosarcoma of Uterus

SOLLEVELD, H. A. (1987) Leiomyoma and leiomyosarcoma, uterus, rat.In: *Genital System* (Eds. T. C. Jones *et al.*) pp. 116-119, op. cit.

## 812, Adenocarcinoma of Uterus

DEERBERG, F., REHM, S. and PITTERMANN, W. (1981) Uncommon frequency of adenocarcinomas of the uterus in virgin Han:Wistar
rats. *Vet. Pathol.* **18**: 707-713

ELSINGHORST, T. A., TIMMERMANS, H. J. and HENDRIKS, H. G. (1984) Comparative pathology of endometrial carcinoma. *Vet. Q.* **6**: 200-208

GOODMAN, D. G. and HILDEBRANDT, P. K. (1987) Adenocarcinoma, endometrium, rat. In: *Genital System* (Eds. T. C. Jones *et al.*) pp. 78-79, op. cit.

## 81-, 82-, Miscellaneous Tumors of Uterus, Cervix and Vagina

BUREK, J. D. and HOLLANDER, C. F. (1976) High incidence of spontaneous cervical and vaginal tumors in an inbred strain of brown Norway rats (BN/Bi). *J. Nat. Cancer Inst.* **57**: 549-554

CAMPBELL, J. S. (1987) Adenocanthoma, uterus, rat. In: *Genital System* (Eds. T. C. Jones *et al.*) pp. 110-115, op. cit.

ELCOCK, L. H., STUART, B. P., MUELLER, R. E. and HOSS, H. E. (1987) Deciduoma, uterus, rat. In: *Genital System* (Eds. T. C. Jones *et al.*) pp. 140-145, op. cit.

GOODMAN, D. G. and HILDEBRANDT, P. K. (1987) Squamous cell carcinoma,endometrium/cervix, rat. In: *Genital System* (Eds. T. C. Jones *et al.*) pp. 82-83, op. cit.

GOODMAN, D. G. and HILDEBRANDT, P. K. (1987) Stromal sarcoma, endometrium, rat. In: *Genital System* (Eds. T. C. Jones *et al.*) pp. 70-71, op. cit.

GOODMAN, D. G. and HILDEBRANDT, P. K. (1987) Papillary adenoma, endometrium,rat. In: *Genital System* (Eds. T. C. Jones *et al.*) pp. 78-79, op. cit.

SOBIS, H. (1987) Choriocarcinoma, uterus, rat. In: *Genital System* (Eds. T. C. Jones *et al.*) pp. 138-139, op. cit.

SOBIS, H. (1987) Yolk sac carcinoma, rat. In: *Genital System* (Eds. T. C. Jones *et al.*) pp. 127-133, op. cit.

SOBIS, H. (1987) Embryonal carcinoma, uterus, rat. In: *Genital System* (Eds. T. C. Jones *et al.*) pp. 134-137, op. cit.

SOBIS, H. (1987) Teratoma, uterus, rat.In: *Genital System* (Eds. T. C. Jones *et al.*) pp. 120-126, op. cit.

STOICA, G., CAPEN, C. C. and KOESTNER, A. (1989) Sertoli's cell tumor, ovary, rat. In: *Genital System* (Eds. T.C. Jones *et al.*) pp. 30-36, op. cit.

## 81-, Adenocarcinoma of Clitoral Gland

PARKER, G. A. and GRABAU, J. (1987) Adenoma and adenocarcinoma, clitoral gland, rat.In: *Genital System* (Eds. T. C. Jones *et al.*) pp. 169-176, op. cit.

## 823, Granulosa/Theca Cell Tumor

MAEKAWA, A. and HAYASHI, Y. (1987) Granulosa/theca cell tumor, ovary, rat. In: *Genital System* (Eds. T. C. Jones *et al.*) pp. 15-21, op. cit.

## 831, Endometrial Polyp

GOODMAN, D. G. and HILDEBRANDT, P. K. (1987) Stromal polyp, endometrium, rat.In: *Genital System* (Eds. T. C. Jones *et al.*) pp. 146-147, op. cit.

## 83-, Hermaphroditism

MAGNUSSON, G. (1970) Hermaphroditism in a rat. *Pathol. Vet.* 7: 474-480

## 851, Acute Vaginitis

YUAN, Y. D. and CARLSON, R. G. (1987) Structure, cyclic change and function, vagina and vulva, rat.**In**: *Genital System* (Eds. T. C. Jones *et al.*) pp. 161-168, op. cit.

## 883, Hydrometra

HOMMA, S. and AZUMA, R. (1981) Pathogenesis of hydrometra-endometritis complex in rats. *Nippon Juigaku Zasshi* **43**: 387-398

## 91-, Miscellaneous Soft and Hard Tissue Tumors

COLEMAN, G. L. (1980) Four intrathoracic hibernomas in rats. *Vet. Pathol.* **17**: 634-637

GLAISTER, J. R. (1981) Rhabdomyosarcoma in a young rat. *Lab. Anim. Sci.* **15**: 145-146

GREGSON, R. L. and OFFER, J. M. (1981) Metastasizing chondrosarcoma in laboratory rats. *J. Comp. Pathol.* **91**: 409-413

MINATO, Y., TAKADA, H., YAMANAKA, H., WADA, I., TAKESHITA, M. and OKANIWA, A. (1983) Spontaneous rhabdomyosarcoma in a young rat. *Nippon Juigaku Zasshi* **45**: 837-842

REZNIK, G. and RUSSFIELD, A. (1981) Chordoma of the spinal cord in an F344 rat. *Pathol. Res. Pract.* **172**: 191-195

RUBEN, Z., ROHRBACHER, E. and MILLER, J. E. (1986) Spontaneous osetogenic sarcoma in the rat. *J. Comp. Pathol.* **96**: 89-94

STEFANSKI, S. A., ELWELL, M. R. and YOSHITOMI, K. (1987) Malignant hibernoma in an F344 rat. *Lab. Anim. Sci.* **37**: 347-350

## 942, Neurogenic Atrophy of Skeletal Muscle

VAN STEENIS, G. and KROES, R. (1971) Changes in the nervous system and musculature of old rats. *Vet. Pathol.* **8**: 320-332

## 94-, Miscellaneous Degenerative Lesions of Hard Tissues

CHIU, T. and LEE, K. P. (1984) Auricular chondropathy in aging rats. *Vet. Pathol.* **21**: 500-504

HIJIKATA, S. (1979) Spinal abnormalities and abnormal curvatures in man and their disease model. *Jikken Dobutsu* **28**: 603-605

IWATA, S., NOMURA, Y., TSUHCIYA, A., ISHIBASI, M. and SAITO, Y. (1979) Pathological studies of the spine and the spinal cord in young Ishibashi rats (ISR): Preliminary report. *Jikken Dobutsu* **28**: 605-606

SIMON, M. R. (1984) The rat as an animal model for the study of senile idiopathic osteoporosis. *Acta. Anat. (Basel.)* **119**: 248-250

## 943, Degeneration of Cartilage of Sternum

JASTY, V., BARE, J. J., JAMISON, J. R., PORTER, M. C., KOWALSKI, R. L., CLEMENS, G. R., JACKSON, G. E. and HARTNAGEL, R. E. Jr. (1986) Spontaneous lesions in the sternums of growing rats. *Lab. Anim. Sci.* **36**: 48-51

YAMASAKI, K. and INUI, S. (1985) Lesions of articular, sternal and growth plate cartilage in rats. *Vet. Pathol.* **22**: 46-50

## 945, Osteoarthrosis

KATO, M. and ONODERA, T. (1984) Spontaneous osteochondrosis in rats. *Lab. Anim. Sci.* **18**: 179-187

YAMASAKI, K. (1986) Pathology of degenerative osteoarthrosis of the thoracic vertebrae in rats. *Jikken Dobutsu* **35**: 245-248

## 9—, Miscellaneous Lesions of Integument

BEEMS, R.B., GRUYS, E. and SPIT, B. J. (1978) Amyloid in the corpora amylacea of the rat mammary gland. *Vet. Pathol.* **15**: 347-352

GIALAMAS, J., HOGER, H. and ADAMIKER, D. (1985) Spontaneous skincalcinosis in the rat. *Z. Versuchstierkd* **27**: 155-162

HENDERSON, J. D. Jr. (1975) Cutaneous horn in a laboratory rat. *Vet. Med. Small Snim. Clin.* **70**: 141

## DISCUSSION

1. This paper alone is a small reference book of the pathobiology of aging, including an unusually varied data set and all done by the same pathologist. It demonstrates that Bronson is the leading active student of the pathology of aging in rodents. It includes a unique set of codes to lead the reader through the various lesion types, and offers a view into the pathology of aging for the non-expert, yet includes much of value that can be found nowhere else.

2. These data were not taken from animals tested when dead or moribund. Thay should be thought of as "biomarkers", testing animals while they still appeared healthy, and might have been used for other types of biological studies. Aging seems to be a number of different processes (functions?), which can be pathologically defined as lesions (structure?), specific to the particular genotype and environment of the individual. These processes must be characterized before we can study underlying mechanisms. Flurkey pointed out that changes with age do not have to be dysfunctions; some may be just time-dependent changes. These might be distinguished from senescence, postmature changes causing deterioration. Tutarro suggested that senescence is the increase with age in pathology, while aging is all biological changes with age.

3. The numbers of B6 mice are greatly in excess of those for other strains. Therefore, rare lesions from these are better represented than from other genotypes. Were the cross-sectionally selected animals completely representative of their group, or may there have been inadvertent selection of unusually healthy, or unhealthy, individuals? To avoid this possibility, the animals to be tested should be selected and identified at the beginning of the study, but otherwise treated exactly as the total group.

4. Most aging mouse strains, studied until death, show high percentages of death from lymphomas. Smith disagreed, saying this was 50-60% at most, and that 129 strain mice die with very low incidences of lymphoma or other cancers in his laboratory.

5. Practically, instead of discarding ill-appearing animals in aging studies, both healthy and ill animals should be tested, and the effects of disease defined. This requires excellent pathological information, so as not to confuse age-associated changes and changes caused by lesions.

6. Once sufficient data are available, it is extremely important to define age-incidences for different lesions; this may be an excellent way to show the effects of genetic differences and of treatments such as dietary restriction.

# 18

# DEVELOPMENT OF A GENETIC MODEL FOR ACATALASEMIA: TESTING THE OXYGEN FREE RADICAL THEORY OF AGING


Glenn C. Bewley and William J. Mackay


## ABSTRACT


Activated oxygen species have been demonstrated to be the important agents in oxygen toxicity; they act by disrupting the structural and functional integrity of cells through lipid peroxidation events, DNA damage and protein inactivation. The accumulated effect of oxygen free radical damage is thought to be a contributing factor to aging, carcinogenesis and tumor promotion, and an ever-increasing list of aging-related disorders. Catalase ($H_2O_2$:$H_2O_2$ oxidoreductase; EC 1.11.1.6) and superoxide dismutase (superoxide:superoxide oxidoreductase; EC 1.15.1.1) are two major enzyme systems important in the cellular defense against oxygen free radical damage. Genetic models for acatalasemia should provide an important source of material in assessing the role of oxygen free radical damage in biological aging and whether antioxidant enzymes play a significant role in minimizing these effects. The existing mammalian hypocatalasemics are inadequate for such studies since there is significant catalase activity in many solid tissues. Thus, we have isolated six mutant alleles of the catalase gene in *Drosophila melanogaster*. Complete loss of function alleles exhibit a severe viability effect during early development and shorten mean life span of the adult fly by 75-86%. However, catalase activities above 3% of normal restores viability to wild type levels, suggesting a threshold effect. In contrast, a positive correlation exists between catalase activity levels and mean life span, where a temporal increase in life span is accompanied by a delayed onset of senescence. These results suggest that while genetics may program maximum life span potential, the accumulation of oxygen free radical induced damage may severely restrict life span, resulting in accelerated aging and death. These results also suggest that antioxidant enzymes are likely to play a critical role in the cellular defense system against oxygen free radical damage and in protecting eukaryotic organisms from free radical-induced aging events.

## INTRODUCTION

Activated oxygen species have been demonstrated to be the important agents in oxygen toxicity and the accumulated affect of oxygen free radical damage has been widely postulated to be a contributing factor to aging, carcinogenesis and tumor promotion, and an ever increasing list of aging related disorders (Ames, 1983; Cerutti, 1985, 1987; Halliwell and Gutteridge, 1984; Pryor, 1987). The free-radical theory of aging first proposed by Harman (1956) states that free-radical reactions, arising largely during the course of normal metabolism, are responsible for a progressive, temporal accumulation of cellular changes that are responsible for the ever-increasing likelihood of disease and death that accompanies advancing age. If Harman's theory is tenable, and there is a significant amount of circumstantial evidence to suggest that it is (reviewed by Harman, 1984), then the steadily increasing environmental sources of ionizing radiation, ozone, chemical mutagens and carcinogens, many of which act through activated oxygen species, pose an additional risk with respect to the epidemiology of free radical associated diseases and premature aging events. Thus, free radical damage is likely to be a process that restricts life span, while the maximum life span potential of an organism is set by a genetic program. A corollary to this theory is that agents with oxyradical scavenging properties (*i.e.* antioxidants) should extend life span but not significantly alter maximum life span potential.

The univalent pathway for the complete reduction of dioxygen is illustrated in Figure 1. Three active intermediates that are derived from consecutive univalent reductions are the superoxide anion ($O_2^-$), hydrogen peroxide ($H_2O_2$), and the hydroxyl radical (OH.). Superoxide anions are converted to $H_2O_2$ either by spontaneous dismutation or enzymatic dismutation involving superoxide dismutase (SOD) activity (Fridovich, 1978). According to current dogma, the deleterious effects in aerobic cells associated with endogenously generated prooxidants are due to reactions initiated by the hydroxyl radical, which is produced in a superoxide anion-driven Fenton cycle involving the reduction of $H_2O_2$ in the presence of transition metals (Halliwell and Gutteridge, 1984; Green and Hill, 1984). The hydroxyl radical reacts with very high rate constants and with most organic substrates found in the living cell. The superoxide anion and $H_2O_2$ are less reactive as oxidants. However, $H_2O_2$ molecules are uncharged and can diffuse through cytological membranes to significant distances from their endogenous sites of origin before generating intracellular hydroxyl radicals.

$$(1) \quad O_2 + e^- \longrightarrow O_2^-$$

$$(2) \quad O_2^- + e^- + 2H^+ \longrightarrow H_2O_2$$

$$(3) \quad H_2O_2 + e^- + H^+ \longrightarrow H_2O + OH\cdot$$

$$(4) \quad OH\cdot + e^- + H^+ \longrightarrow H_2O$$

**Figure 1.** The univalent pathway of oxygen reduction. Equations one through four summarize the sequence of single-electron reductions of dioxygen and the major reduction products that are formed. For a more detailed treatment see Green and Hill (1984).

Aerobic organisms have evolved both non-enzymatic and enzymatic defense mechanisms to remove activated oxygen species and to provide protection against the effects of oxygen radical-induced cellular and genetic damage (Fridovich, 1977; Ames, 1983; Halliwell and Gutteridge, 1984; Cerutti, 1985, 1987; Imlay *et al.*, 1988). Two major antioxidant enzymes, superoxide dismutase (SOD;superoxide:superoxide oxidoreductase; E.C. 1.15.1.1) and catalase ($H_2O_2$:$H_2O_2$ oxidoreductase; E.C. 1.11.1.6) are thought to effectively remove activated oxygen species (Figure 2). SOD catalyzes the dismutation of superoxide anion to hydrogen peroxide (Fridovich, 1986), while catalase catalyzes the breakdown of hydrogen peroxide to water and dioxygen (Aebi, 1984). By scavenging both superoxide anion and hydrogen peroxide, formation of the highly reactive hydroxyl radical is limited.

The development of genetic models for antioxidant enzymes in eukaryotic organisms should provide a direct approach to determining the relationship of oxygen free radical damage to biological aging and the role of each enzyme in the protection of organisms from premature aging events. Recent studies have reported the isolation of loss of function SOD and catalase alleles in the bacterium *E. coli* (Carlioz and Touati, 1986; Loewan *et al.*, 1985) and of catalase in the yeast *S. cerevisiae* (Cohen *et al.*, 1985). These mutants are

$$\underline{\text{SUPEROXIDE DISMUTASE}}$$

$$O_2^- \; + \; O_2^- \; + \; 2H^+ \quad\longrightarrow\quad H_2O_2 \; + \; O_2$$

$$\underline{\text{CATALASE}}$$

$$\text{CATALASE} \; - \; Fe^{3+} \; + \; H_2O_2 \longrightarrow \text{COMPOUND I}$$

A) CATALATIC REACTION:

$$\text{COMPOUND I} \; + \; H_2O_2 \longrightarrow \text{CATALASE} \; - \; Fe^{3+} \; + \; 2H_2O \; + \; O_2$$

B) PEROXIDATIC REACTION:

$$\text{COMPOUND I} \; + \; RH_2 \longrightarrow \text{CATALASE} \; - \; Fe^{3+} \; + \; 2H_2O \; + \; R$$

**Figure 2.** Enzymatic reactions involved in scavenging activated oxygen species. Superoxide dismutases catalyze the dismutation of the superoxide anion to $H_2O_2$ and $O_2$. Catalase catalyzes the decomposition of $H_2O_2$ via a two step reaction. The formation of an active complex-I between $H_2O_2$ and the iron of the hematin prosthetic group occurs first. Compound I is decomposed back to free enzyme through the oxidation of a hydrogen donor which can be a second molecule of $H_2O_2$ (catalatic reaction), or other organic molecule such as phenol, formic acid, alcohol, or primary amines (peroxidatic reaction). The predominant reaction depends on the concentration of the H donor and the ratio of $H_2O_2$ generation to enzyme concentration.

viable under standard culture conditions but are hypersensitive to environments containing elevated levels of ionizing radiation, $H_2O_2$, and redox-cycling drugs known to induce oxygen free radicals *in vivo*. The purpose of this study is the development of a genetic model for acatalasemia in a multicellular eukaryotic organism and a subsequent analysis of the phenotypic effects of this condition on life span parameters.

| Table 1. Tissue-specific catalase activities in $Cs^a$ and $Cs^b$ mice | | | |
|---|---|---|---|
| Genotype[1] | Tissue Specific Activity[2] | | |
| | Liver | Kidney | Blood |
| $Cs^a$ | 9.63 (100%) | 11.9 (100%) | 1.31 (100%) |
| $Cs^b$ | 9.27 (96%) | 1.9 (16%) | 0.19 (15%) |

[1] Genotype of congenic mouse strains are as follows: Control (C3H/HeAnl/$Cs^a$) and acatalasemic (C3H/HeAnl/$Cs^b$).

[2] Activity is expressed as mean units per mg. protein of three separate extracts for each tissue.

## Mammalian Acatalasemics

Takahara (1952) first described a genetic defect influencing human catalase expression in Japanese individuals who exhibited a deficiency of blood catalase enzyme activity (acatalasemia). Short term clinical manifestations of human acatalasemia appear predominantly in the mouth. In moderate cases oral ulcerations develop, while more severe forms of the disease are manifested as alveolar gangrene and atrophy resulting in widespread loss of teeth (Takahara, 1968). It should be pointed out that the acatalasemic phenotype is not equally expressed in each individual even though these human acatalasemics have extremely low levels of blood catalase activity, and no long term health effects have been reported. Subsequent studies have revealed that all human acatalasemics actually possess normal or near normal levels of catalase activity in many solid tissues and should be more correctly termed hypocatalasemic (Aebi and Wyss, 1978).

An acatalasemic mouse strain, $Cs^b$, was first described by Feinstein *et al.* (1966). This catalase mutation was identified by screening blood catalase activity levels in a group of "discard mice" from irradiation studies performed at the Oak Ridge National Laboratory during the 1950's and has thus historically been considered an X-ray-induced mutation. The level of catalase activity for kidney, liver, and erythrocytes in the $Cs^a$ (control) and $Cs^b$ (acatalasemic) strains are illustrated in Table 1. These values are in general agreement with earlier reports which demonstrate that there is little reduction in the level of liver catalase activity in the $Cs^b$ strain relative to $Cs^a$ while both $Cs^b$ kidney and erythrocytes have reduced levels of enzymatic activity (Aebi *et al.*, 1968). The $Cs^b$ mutation has been mapped to the region of the catalase structural gene on chromosome 2 and exhibits additive inheritance of catalase activity in erythrocytes from $Cs^a$ (control) × $Cs^b$ F1 hybrid animals (Dickerman *et al.*, 1968; Hoffman and Grieshaber, 1974). Numerous immunological, physical, and molecular studies of catalase from the $Cs^b$ strain have yielded valuable insights into the nature of this genetic defect. Concomitant shifts of both the electrophoretic mobility and heat stability of $Cs^b$-derived catalase from erythrocytes, kidney, and liver strongly suggest that an aberration exists within the protein-encoding sequence of the catalase structural gene (Aebi *et al.*, 1968; Holmes and Duly, 1974; Feinstein *et al.*, 1967; 1968; Feinstein, 1970). In recent studies conducted in our laboratory it has been demonstrated that the level of catalase-specific cross-reactive material (CRM) is diminished in certain $Cs^b$ tissues, in relative concordance with the $Cs^b$ catalase activity levels (Figure 3). The recent isolation of a murine liver cDNA clone and subsequent molecular analyses have revealed that the genetic defect which results in differential expression of catalase in $Cs^b$ tissues does not mediate its effect at the level of transcription, but rather at the level of translation and/or catalase protein turnover (Shaffer *et al.*, 1987). No phenotypic affects have been associated with this mouse strain.

In conclusion, the mammalian hypocatalasemics described in this section are not adequate models for studying the phenotypic affects of acatalasemia since there is significant catalase activity in many solid tissues. Consequently, the development of model systems in other organisms is necessary.

## Isolation of Catalase Mutations in *Drosophila*

*Drosophila melanogaster* provides the best metazoan organism for developing a genetic model for acatalasemia because of the rich source of genetic variants and chromosomal rearrangements available for the design of mutant screening protocols and the ease of manipulating the genome. *Drosophila* catalase has been purified to homogeneity, is tetrameric with a subunit molecular weight of 58,000 daltons and catalase-monospecific antibodies have been raised (Nahmias and Bewley, 1984). Two distinct peaks of catalase activity are observed during *Drosophila* development, with the first peak occurring in late third instar larvae just prior to puparium formation and the second and larger of the two peaks occurring during metamorphosis (Bewley *et al.*, 1983). Upon eclosion of the adult, catalase activity reaches a steady state level which is maintained throughout the life span of the adult fly.

The structural gene, $Cat^+$, for *Drosophila* catalase has been mapped to the cytogenetic interval 75D1-76A3 on the left arm of chromosome 3 by dosage responses to segmental aneuploidy (Figure 4; Lubinsky and Bewley, 1979). In addition, recombination mapping of activity variants places the gene at 3-47.0 which is within the boundaries of this dosage sensitive region (Bewley *et al.*, 1986; Mackay and Bewley, 1989). Figure 4 shows a series of four deficiencies which either flank or include the dosage sensitive region. Two of these deficiencies flank the proximal side of the region, *Df(3L)in$^{61j1}$(76F;77D)* (Arajarvi and Hanna-Alava, 1969) and *Df(3L)VW3(76A3;76B2)* (Ashburner

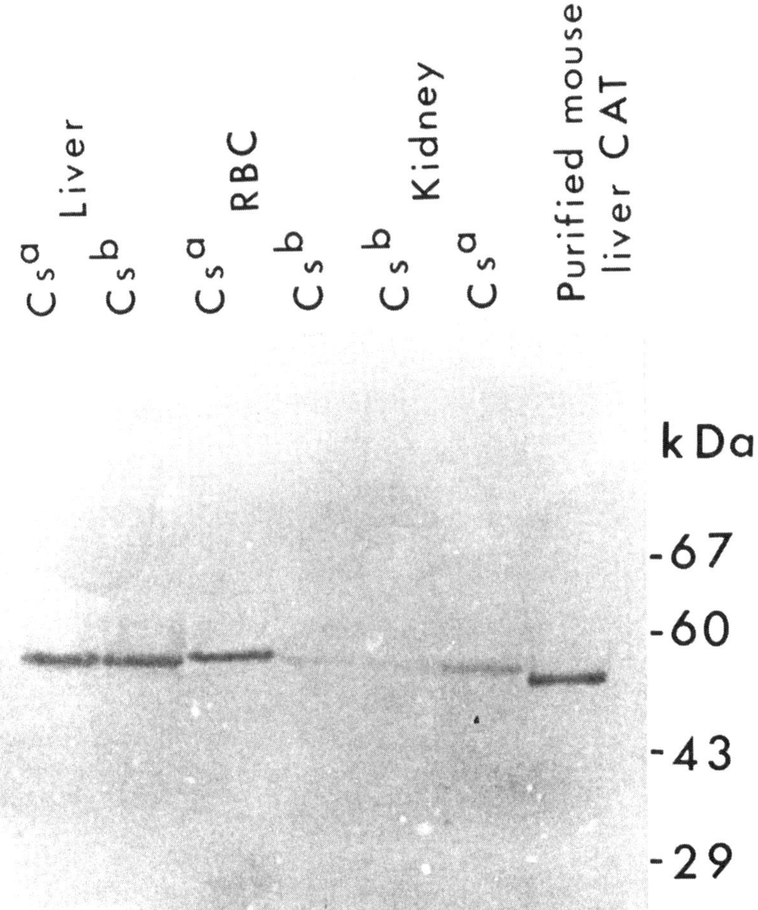


**Figure 3.** Immunoblot of catalase from $Cs^a$ and $Cs^b$ mouse tissue. Total protein from each homogenized tissue was separated by 10% sodium dodecyl sulfate polyacrylamide gel electrophoresis-SDS PAGE and electroblotted onto nitrocellulose as previously described (Bewley, *et al.*, 1986). The filter was overlaid first with purified anticatalase IGg and second with goat-anti rabbit IGg conjugated with horseradish peroxidase and developed according to instructions by the supplier (BioRad). Mouse liver catalase was purified to homogeneity by a combination of organic solvent fractionation, DE52 cellulose and phenyl sepharose chromatography (Nahmias and Bewley, 1984) and antibodies were raised in New Zealand white rabbits. (Modified from Shaffer, *et al.*, 1987).

*et al.*, 1981), while one deficiency flanks the distal side of the region, *Df(3L)W^{r4}(75B8-11;75C5-7)* (Mackay and Bewley, 1989). The fourth deficiency, *Df(3L)Cat^{DH104}(75C1;75F1)* (Mackay and Bewley, 1989), was found to uncover the catalase locus and was subsequently used in a screen for

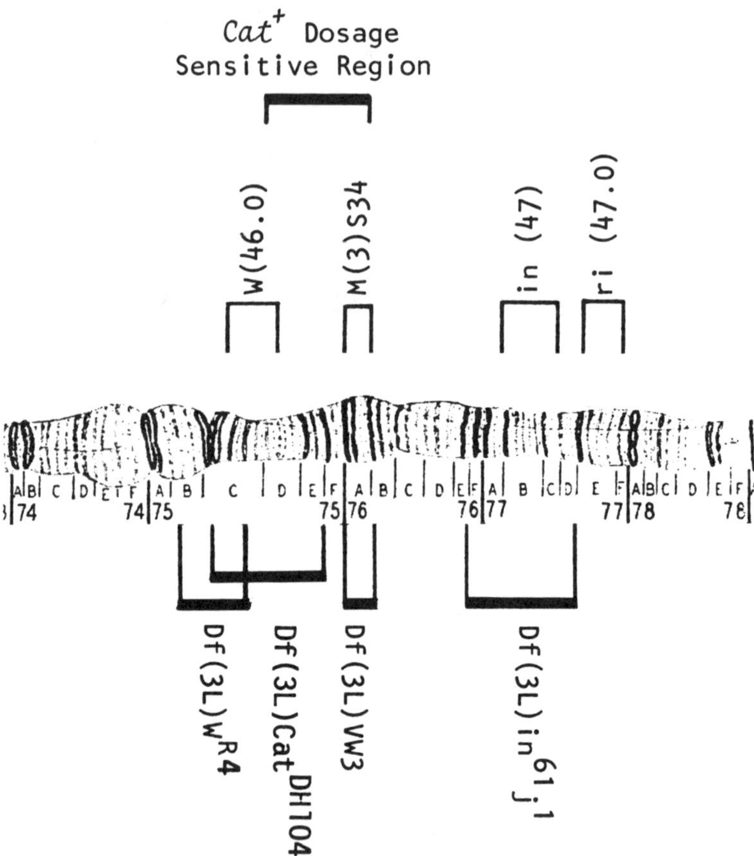


**Figure 4.** Relationship of genetic variants, including both visible markers and chromosome deficiencies, that flank and/or include the catalase dosage sensitive region on the left arm of chromosome three in *Drosophila*. The limits of the dosage sensitive region are from 75D1 to 76A3 as defined by screening the entire *Drosophila* genome using a series of reciprocal translocation stocks with breakpoints in the Y chromosome and the autosomes (Lubinsky and Bewley, 1979). The stable deficiency *Df(3L)Cat*DH104 was found to uncover the catalase locus and was subsequently utilized to screen for ethyl methanesulfonate (EMS) induced mutations within the 75C1-F1 interval delimited by this deficiency. All genetic symbols are defined in Lindsley and Grell (1968) and Mackay and Bewley (1989). (From Mackay and Bewley, 1989).

recessive ethyl methanesulfonate induced mutations within the 75C1-75F1 interval delimited by this deficiency.

Since the phenotype of complete loss of function alleles at the $Cat^+$ locus could not be predicted *a priori*, we designed a standard F2 mutagenesis screen that would allow us to isolate both putative recessive lethal mutations at the $Cat^+$ locus in addition to catalase mutations that would be phenotypically

| Table 2. Catalase and soperoxide dismutase activities of *Drosophila* acatalasemic mutants[a] | | |
|---|---|---|
| Strain [b] | Catalase Activity | Superoxide Dismutase Activities |
| $Cat^+$ Control | 100% | 100% |
| Df(3L)Cat $^{DH104}$/+ | 42% | 100% |
| Df(3L) lxd$^9$/+ | 98% | 52% |
| CAT$^{n1}$ | 0% | 102% |
| CAT$^{n2}$ | 5% | 103% |
| CAT$^{n3}$ | 2% | 100% |
| CAT$^{n4}$ | 0% | 100% |
| CAT$^{n5}$ | 2% | 103% |
| CAT$^{n6}$ | 4% | 103% |

viable. This was done by using a rapid biochemical assay which we call the "fizz" test (see Mackay and Bewley, 1989, for a complete description of the screening protocol). A total of thirty-five independently-derived recessive lethal mutations within the 75C1-75F1 interval, in addition to six independently-derived viable acatalasemic mutants, were recovered from a screen of 4512 F2 chromosomes. Subsequent spectrophotometric assays demonstrated that none of the thirty-five recessive lethal mutations had an effect on the expression of catalase as heterozygotes, while the six viable acatalasemic mutants exhibited catalase activities ranging from 0-5% of the $Cat^+$ control strain (Table 2). Two of these mutants, $Cat^{n1}$ and $Cat^{n4}$, had no detectable levels of catalase activity throughout *Drosophila* development (Mackay and Bewley, 1989). In addition, western-blot analysis demonstrated that the two null catalase activity strains, $Cat^{n1}$ and $Cat^{n4}$, had no detectable levels of catalase- specific cross-reacting material (CRM⁻) while the other four strains, $Cat^{n2}$, $Cat^{n3}$, $Cat^{n5}$, and $Cat^{n6}$, had low but detectable amounts of CRM that generally coincide with the level of enzymatic activity observed for each mutant (Figure 5).

Each of the six catalase mutants were also assayed, as adults, to determine the level of SOD activity. These results show that a loss of catalase activity in *Drosophila* apparently has no effect on SOD activity since all six catalase mutant alleles displayed wild type levels of this enzyme (Table 2).

A complementation matrix for catalase activity among all six mutant alleles is illustrated in Figure 6. Two significant observations can be made from this data. First, no heteroallaelic combination gave rise to complete restoration of catalase activity indicating that there is but one functional gene within the *Drosophila* genome. Second, the 15 heteroallelic combinations exhibited a range of activity levels from 0% to 51% of the $Cat^+$ control strain.

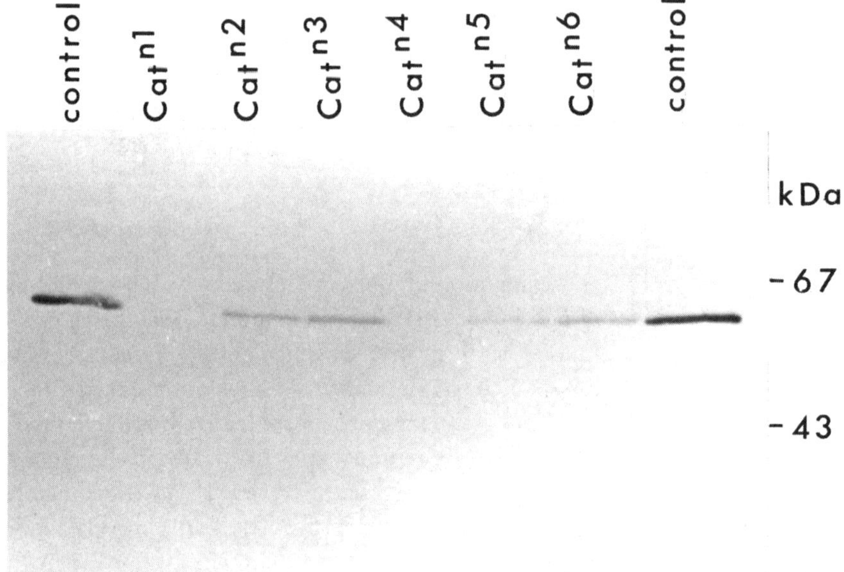



**Figure 5.** Immunoblot of total *Drosophila* protein separated on 12.5% SDS PAGE and electroblotted onto nitrocellulose. The blot was developed as described in Figure 3 except that antibodies elicited against purified *Drosophila* catalase were used (Nahmias and Bewley, 1984). All six *Drosophila* catalase mutants were analyzed relative to the unmutaginized $Cat^+$ control strain containing the recessive markers *cp in ri $p^p$*. (Modified from Mackay and Bewley, 1989).

For the most part, the activity level for each combination can be explained by additive affects for each mutant chromosome. However two combinations, $Cat^{n6}/Cat^{n2}$ and $Cat^{n6}/Cat^{n3}$, display positive complementation yielding activities greater than their predicted additive values. The point here is that these mutant combinations provide a wide spectrum of activity levels which can subsequently be used in studies designed to examine the phenotypic effects of acatalasemia on life span parameters and the role of oxygen free radical damage in biological aging.

|      | n1 | n2 | n3 | n4 | n5 | n6 |
|------|----|----|----|----|----|----|
| n1   |    | 4  | 2  | 0  | 1  | 11 |
| n2   |    |    | 23 | 4  | 10 | 49 |
| n3   |    |    |    | 2  | 1  | 51 |
| n4   |    |    |    |    | 0  | 12 |
| n5   |    |    |    |    |    | 20 |

**Figure 6.** Complementation matrix for all six catalase mutations crossed in all pair-wise combinations. The catalase activity of the *Cat*[+] control strain was 152.4±10.6 units per mg protein (9 determinations) and this value was normalized to 100%. Activity values for each heteroallelic combination are presented as a percent of this control value. (Modified from Mackay and Bewley, 1989).

## Acatalasemia and Viability

A major conclusion stemming from results of the *Drosophila* mutant screen is that the condition of acatalasemia *per se* does not result in a lethal phenotype. Of the 35 recessive lethal alleles recovered within the 75C1-75F1 interval, none demonstrated an effect on catalase expression. On the other hand, the six viable acatalasemic alleles exhibit a range of viability affects during development. To illustrate the relationship of catalase activity to viability, a scatter plot for all 15 heteroallelic combinations of these six mutant alleles is presented in Figure 7A where the activity level for each combination ranges from 0-50% of the *Cat*[+] control strain (Figure 6). While this plot does not demonstrate a statistically significant correlation between viability and catalase activity, it is evident that complete loss of function combinations have a severe negative viability affect, reducing viability to 5-25% of normal. This is better illustrated in Figure 7B where a linear correlation of viability on activity is demonstrated for those heteroallelic combinations exhibiting less than 3% of the control activity. For catalase activity levels above 3% the viability parameter rapidly approaches 100%. This observation suggests a threshold level of activity above which viability is not affected. A possible explanation for a threshold phenomenon is that catalase is well known to be an extraordinarily efficient enzyme where the catalytic rate constant is approximately $10^7$ liter mol$^{-1}$ sec$^{-1}$ (Aebi, 1984), and it has been estimated that one molecule of catalase can decompose approximately 42,000 molecules of $H_2O_2$ per second at 0°C in mammalian tissues (Aebi and Wyss, 1978). This finding is particularly interesting when viewed in the light of reports that describe the genetic defects influencing catalase expression in mammalian systems. The threshold effect described for *Drosophila* acatalasemics provides a reasonable explanation for the general lack of observable phenotypic effects in the mammalian acatalasemics since catalase for both the human and mouse mutations is likely to be expressed at sufficient levels in all tissues to afford protection from the long-term toxic effects of endogenous hydrogen peroxide.

## Acatalasemia and Life Span Modification

The free radical theory of aging as originally proposed by Harman predicts that antioxidants should lengthen the maximum life span of animals. This idea has been tested by feeding animals antioxidant chemicals to see if life span can be experimentally extended (reviewed by Balin, 1982; Melhorne and Cole, 1985; Sohal, 1987). Many conflicting results have resulted from this approach and interpretation of the existing data is difficult. Alternatively, Cutler (1986) has compared the tissue concentration of a number of antioxidant enzymes and organic scavengers of free radical derivatives in different mammals to the life span energy potential for that organism (LEP is defined as the metabolic rate times the maximum life span potential for a species). The rationale here is that longer lived species should have more effective oxygen radical defense mechanisms than shorter lived species when aging is viewed as an accumulation of toxic cellular effects of oxyradical production. Cutler's results provide some support for the free radical theory of aging since there is a strong positive correlation between the tissue concentration of some antioxidants and LEP, but it is also ambiguous in that there is either no correlation or a negative correlation for a number of other antioxidants. Particularly perplexing is the strong positive correlation with SOD activity but a negative correlation for both catalase and glutathione peroxidase. These kind of results have led others to propose a modified free radical theory of aging which states that oxygen free radicals are implicated in processes that shorten or limit life span below the maximum life span potential for an organism, but that the control of free radical reactions cannot lengthen maximum life span (Melhorn and Cole, 1985; Pryor, 1987). We have taken the more direct approach of isolating mutations in genes encoding

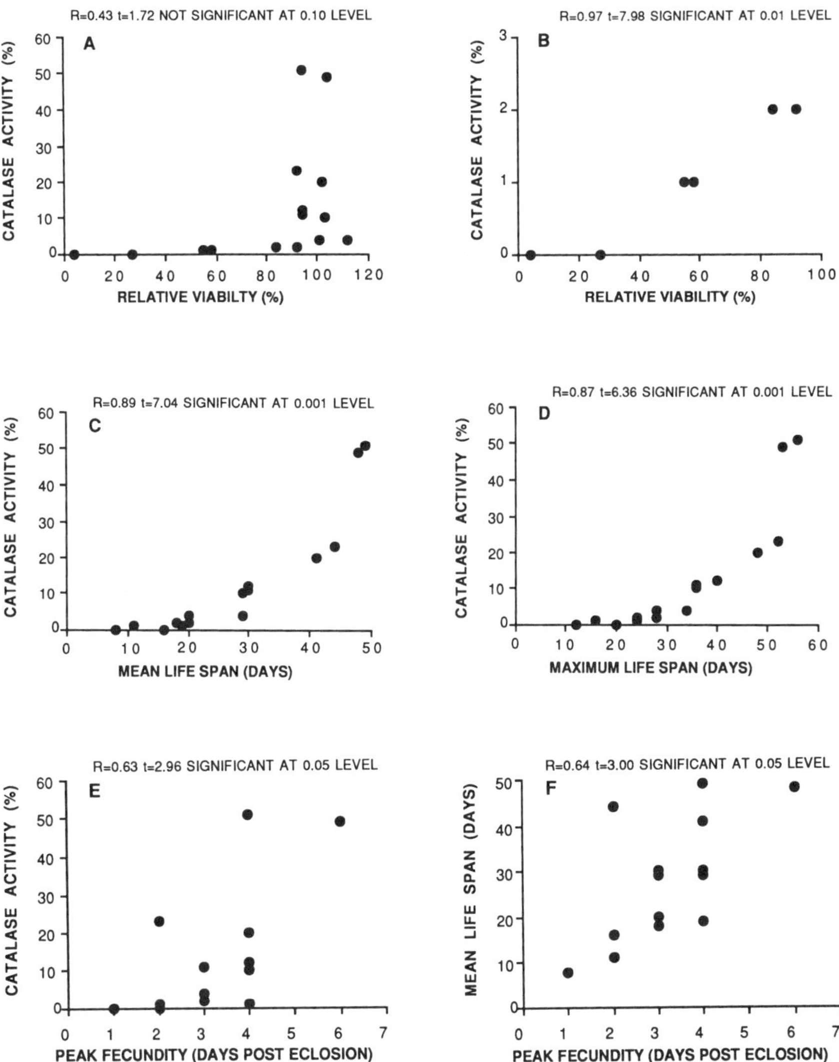



**Figure 7.** Scatter plots illustrating the relationship between catalase activity and life history parameters for the fifteen heteroallelic combinations represented in Figure 6. The statistical analysis corresponding to each plot is depicted at the top of each panel where **R** = the product-moment correlation coefficient, and **t** = the student's **t** test value. Relative viability was determined as a percent of expected segregation frequencies for each heteroallelic combination where the frequency of the homozygous control *Cat*[+] strain was normalized to 100% (Mackay and Bewley, 1989). The data represented in panel B is a subset of the data in panel A illustrating the significance level of catalase activity on viability where the catalase activity is less than 3% of Cat[+] control levels. Peak fecundity was determined by counting the number of eggs laid per day per female and is a measure of the temporal pattern of reproductive capacity. Each determination is the mean of six replicate experiments.

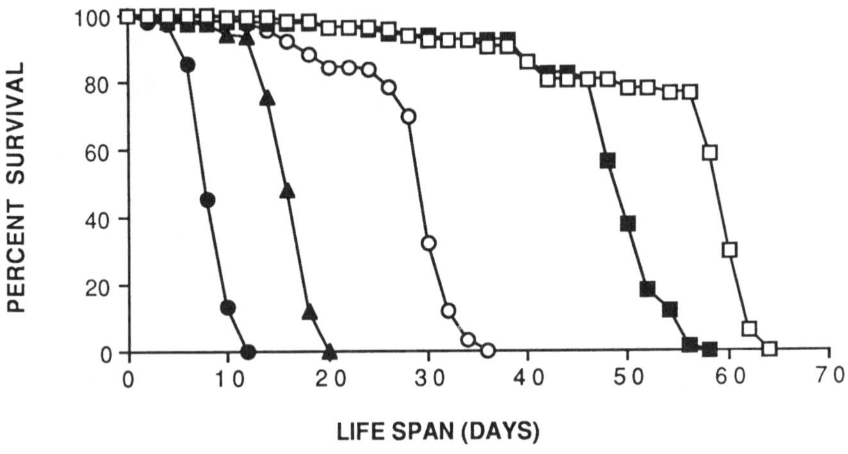


**Figure 8.** Survival curves for six heteroallelic combinations of selected catalase mutants and the $Cat^+$ control strain. Each curve was determined from six independent cultures containing 50 flies and checked every two days for survival. Catalase activity levels for each genotype are as follows: no activity (both ● and ▲), 20% activity (O), 50% activity (■), and 100% activity for the $Cat^+$ control strain (□). The mean and maximum life span of the control strain is 58 and 62 days, respectively. Note the temporal directionality in life span as a function of catalase activity. The increased mean life span for each combination is clearly accompanied by a delayed onset in the time of senescence as determined by changes in locomotor activity, peak fecundity, and accumulation in aging pigment.

specific antioxidant enzymes and then using this material to examine the relationship between levels of antioxidant enzyme activities and life span parameters.

In our collection of catalase mutants, complete loss of function alleles result in a striking reduction of both mean and maximum life span, *i.e.* 75-86% (Figures 7C, D and 8). In addition, a positive linear correlation of catalase activity level with life span modification is demonstrated for the 15 heteroallelic combinations of Figure 6. As catalase activity increases from 0-50%, a temporal shift in both mean and maximum life span occurs toward the value for the $Cat^+$ control strain, while catalase activities above 50% have a rapidly diminishing effect on life span (Figure 8). These results are consistent with a modified version of the free radical theory of aging since complete loss, or reduced levels, of catalase activity severely restrict life span while a progressive increase in the level of activity does not lengthen life span beyond the maximum for the control strain.

It is reasonable to suggest that a reduced capacity to scavenge $H_2O_2$ in the acatalasemic mutants leads to an increased intracellular concentration of $H_2O_2$, thereby putting the mutant flies at greater risk to long term free radical damage, leading in turn to accelerated aging and subsequently a shorter life span. Since superoxide dismutase activity in these same flies is unaffected, an accelerated rate of hydroxyl radical formation could be expected to occur through a superoxide anion-driven Fenton cycle involving the reduction of elevated levels of $H_2O_2$ in the presence of reduced transition metals. Here it is also interesting to speculate on the interrelated role of SOD and catalase activities in this process. Since $H_2O_2$ is the direct product of the dismutation reaction, could a reduction in SOD activity in an acatalasemic background partially rescue the acatalasemic mutants by actually extending life span? In other words, is a metabolic balance between these two enzyme activities important in life span determination? This question becomes relevant with a recent observation in *E. coli* cells transformed with copies of the prokaryotic Fe-SOD gene (Scott *et al.*, 1987). Transformed cells exhibit an 11-fold increase in total SOD activity while other oxidant defense parameters, including catalase, remain at normal levels. Paradoxically, rather than increasing tolerance, these cells are at greater risk to oxygen toxicity and the authors conclude that an effective defense against reactive oxygen species requires a balance between antioxidant enzyme levels that cannot necessarily be improved by increases in activities of single enzymes alone. This observation can be extended to Down's syndrome patients, which results from trisomy of the distal part of the long arm of chromosome 21 and which contains the gene for human Cu/Zn SOD. Here a 50% increase in SOD expression fails to confer anti-aging benefits, while several age-related pathologies are accelerated (Sinet, 1982; Mayes *et al.*, 1984). The relationship of a metabolic balance between antioxidant enzymes to life span determination in eukaryotic organisms is an area worthy of additional investigation. Several phenotypic properties of the acatalasemic mutants in *Drosophila* suggest that they may undergo early senescence. First, all the mutant combinations exhibit an early accumulation of pigmentation on the dorsal thorax and at the base of the wing. This pigmentation pattern is normally observed during the senescence period of wild type strains of *Drosophila* and most likely represents an age dependent accumulation of aging pigment, *i.e.* lipofuscin, which is indicative of the cumulative affects of oxidative damage. Second, all the catalase mutants exhibit a marked decrease in locomotor activity just prior to the exponential mortality phase of their respective life span curves (Figure 8). Each population becomes extremely lethargic leading to an eventual cessation of flight where the flies just sit on the bottom of the culture. This behavioral pattern is not observed in the $Cat^+$ control strain until approximately 50-55 days of adult life. Finally, the temporal pattern for reproductive capacity in each mutant combination is contracted and the timing of peak fecundity is positively correlated with both catalase activity level and life span parameters (Figure 7E and F). Taken together, these phenotypes suggest that a loss of catalase activity accelerates aging in *Drosophila*, leading to premature senescence and death. In addition, we suggest that age dependent pigmentation patterns, locomotor activity and timing of the peak reproductive period can serve as useful biomarkers in defining the onset of senescence in *Drosophila*.

## CONCLUSION

Although there seems to be little doubt that oxygen free radicals are produced in aerobic cells during oxidative metabolism, or that free radicals can cause significant damage to cellular components, numerous uncertainties still exist concerning the oxygen free radical theory of aging (Melhorn and Cole, 1985; Sohal, 1987). This paper describes our efforts to develop a genetic system that will be useful in testing some of the predictions of the free radical theory of aging. Initially, we have isolated six mutations in the gene coding for catalase in *Drosophila* and have used this material to demonstrate that acatalasemia severely restricts life span. In addition, life span is positively correlated with catalase activity levels where a temporal increase in life span is accompanied by a delay in the onset of senescence. These results suggest that oxidative damage is a major component in life span determination of *Drosophila* and that antioxidant enzymes are likely to play a critical role in the cellular defense system against the kind of damage important in aging. In this sense, it is important to examine the properties of loss of function alleles for other genes encoding antioxidant enzymes. Recent work by Phillips, *et al.* (1989) has demonstrated that a null mutation for the gene encoding Cu/Zn SOD in *Drosophila* exhibits a reduction in mean life span from 60 to 12 days. This observation further strengthens the predictions made in this study.

A corroborative approach to testing predictions of the free radical theory of aging would be P-element transformation of *Drosophila* with copies of genes encoding antioxidant enzymes. The gene for *Drosophila* Cu/Zn SOD has been cloned (Seto *et al.*, 1987) and we are currently involved in efforts to clone Mn SOD and catalase. Transgenic flies would provide critical information on the following questions: (1) Are the restricted life spans and early senescence events associated with acatalasemia, and possibly with mutants for other antioxidant enzymes, rescued by the expression of wild type copies of their respective genes in transgenic flies? Rescue would constitute strong evidence indeed for the role of free radical damage in the aging process and in life span determination. (2) Can an overexpression of antioxidant enzymes in transgenic flies lead to an increased tolerance to oxidative stress and/or an extended maximum life span? (3) Do large increases in the expression of a single enzyme, *i.e.* catalase or SOD, enhance tolerance to conditions of oxygen stress or result in an imbalance for oxygen free radical metabolism? These are important questions that may lead to the use of interventive measures to reduce the damage caused by free radicals and therefore the rate of aging.

Finally, the idea that it is damage to DNA, rather than to other macro-molecular structures, that promotes aging is a testable model that we find particularly attractive. Evidence seems to be accumulating that oxidative DNA damage in somatic cells does occur and that the rate of damage to DNA increases with specific metabolic rate where larger animals owe a longer life span to a lower metabolic rate and correspondingly lower rates of oxidative DNA damage (Saul *et al.*, 1987; Adelman *et al.*, 1988). The catalase mutants described in this study should provide a critical approach to examining both germ line and somatic mutation rate in acatalasemic *Drosophila* exhibiting shortened life span parameters.

## ACKNOWLEDGMENTS

We thank Robert Markovsky and R. Brian Sutton for technical assistance. This work was supported by National Institutes of Health Research Grant No. AG01739 to G.C.B. and by National Research Service Award No. AG05380 to W.J.M. This is paper 11968 of the Journal Series of the North Carolina Agricultural Research Service, Raleigh, NC 27695-7601.

## REFERENCES

AEBI, H. E. (1984) Catalase *in vitro*. pp. 121-126. **In:** *Methods of Enzymol.* **105**: Edited by L. Packer, Academic Press, New York

AEBI, H., E. BOSSI, M. CANTZ, S. MATSUBARA and H. SUTER (1968) Acatalasemia in Switzerland. p. 41. **In:** *Hereditary Disorders of Erythrocyte Metabolism* **Vol. I**: Edited by E. Beutler Grune & Stratton, New York

AEBI, H. E. and S. R. WYSS (1978) Acatalasemia. pp. 1792-1807. **In:** *The Metabolic Basis of Metabolic Disease.* Edited by J. B. Stanbury, J. B. Wyngaarden and D. S. Fredrickson. McGraw-Hill Book Company, New York

ADELMAN, R., R. L. SAUL and B. N. AMES (1988) Oxidative damage to DNA: Relation to species metabolic rate and life span. *Proc. Natl. Acad. Sci. USA* **85**: 2706-2708

AMES, B. N . (1983) Dietary carcinogens and anticarcinogens: oxygen radicals and degenerative diseases. *Science* **221**: 1256-1264

ARJARVI, P. and A. HANNA-ALAVA (1969) Cytogenetic mapping of *in* and *ri*. *Drosophila Inform. Serv.* **44**: 73

ASHBURNER, M., P. ANGEL, C. DETWILER, J. FAITHFULL, D. GUBB, G. HARRINGTON, T. LITTLEWOOD, S. TSUBOTA, J. VELLISSARIA and V. WALKER (1981) A report of new mutants. *Drosophila Inform. Serv.* **56**: 186-191

BALIN, A. K. (1982) Testing the free radical theory of aging. In: *Testing the Theories of Aging*: Edited by A.C. Adelman and G.S. Roth, pp. 138-175. CRC Press, Boca Raton, Fl.

BEWLEY, G. C., W. J. MACKAY and J. L. COOK (1986) Temporal variation for the expression of catalase in *Drosophila melanogaster*: correlations between the rates of enzyme synthesis and levels of translatable catalase-messenger RNA. *Genetics* **113**: 919-938

BEWLEY, G. C., J. A. NAHMIAS and J. L. COOK (1983) Developmental and tissue-specific control of catalase expression in *Drosophila melanogaster*: correlations with rates of enzyme synthesis and degradation. *Devel. Genet.* **4**: 49-60

CARLIOZ, A. and D. TOUATI (1986) Isolation of superoxide dismutase mutants in *Escherichia coli*: is superoxide dismutase necessary for aerobic life? *EMBO J.* **5**: 623-630

CERUTTI, P. A. (1985) Prooxidant states and tumor promotion. *Science* **227**: 375-381

CERUTTI, P. A. (1987) The role of DNA damage and its repair in aging; future directions of research. In: *Modern Biological Theories of Aging*: Edited by H. R. Warner, R. N. Butler, L. R. Sprott and E. L. Schneider. Raven Press, New York.

COHEN, G., F. FESSL, A. TRACZYL, J. RYTKA and H. RUIS (1985) Isolation of the catalase A gene of *Saccharomyces cerevisiae* by complementation of the *cta1* mutation. *Mol. Gen. Genet.* **200**: 74-79

CUTLER, R. G. (1986) Aging and Oxygen radicals. pp. 251-285. In: *Physiology of oxygen Radicals*: Edited by A. E. Taylor, S. Matalon, and P. Ward. American Physiological Society. William & Wilkins Co., New York.

DICKERMAN, R. C., R. N. FEINSTEIN and D. GRAHN (1968) Position of the acatalasemic gene linkage group V of the mouse. *J. Heredity* **59**: 177

FEINSTEIN, R. N., J.B. HOWARD, J. T. BRAUN and J. C. SEAHOLM (1966) Acatalalsemic and hypocatalasemic mouse mutants. *Genetics* **53**: 923-933

FEINSTEIN, R. N., J. T. BRAUN and J. B. HOWARD (1967) Acatalasemic and hypocatalasemic mouse mutants. II. Mutational variations in blood and solid tissue catalases. *Arch. Biochem. Biophys.* **120**: 165-169

FEINSTEIN, R. N., H. SUTER and B. N. JAROSLOW (1968) Blood catalase polymorphism: Some immunological aspects. *Science* **159**: 638-640

FEINSTEIN, R. N. (1970) Acatalasemia in the mouse and other species. *Biochem. Genet.* **4**: 135-155

FRIDOVICH, I. (1977) Oxygen is toxic! *Bioscience* **27**: 462-466

FRIDOVICH, I. (1978) The biology of oxygen radicals. *Science* **201**: 875-880

FRIDOVICH, I. (1986) Superoxide dismutases. *Adv. Enzymol.* **58**: 61- 97

GREEN, M. G. and H. A. O. HILL (1984) Chemistry of dioxygen. pp. 3- 21. In: *Methods of Enzymol.* **105**: Edited by L. Packer. Academic Press, New York.

HALLIWELL, B. and J. M. C. GUTTERIDGE (1984) Oxygen toxicity, oxygen radicals, transition metals and disease. *Biochem. J.* **219**: 1-14

HARMAN, D. (1956) A theory based on free radical and radiation chemistry. *J. Geront.* **11**: 298-300

HARMAN, D. (1984) Free radical theory of aging: the free radical diseases. *Age (Omaha)* **7**: 111-131

HOFFMAN, H. A., and C. K. GRIESHABER (1974) Genetic studies of murine catalase: Liver and erythrocyte catalase controlled by independent loci. *J. Hered.* **65**: 277-279

HOLMES, R. S., and J. A. DULEY (1975) Biochemical and genetic studies of peroxisomal multiple enzyme systems: alpha-hydroxyacid oxidase and catalase. pp. 191-225. In: *Isozymes.* **Vol. I**: *Molecular Structure* Edited by C. L. Market Academic Press, New York.

IMLAY, J. A. and S. LINN (1988) DNA damage and oxygen radical toxicity. *Science* **240**: 1302-1309

LINDSLEY, D. L. and E. H. GRELL (1968) *Genetic Variations* of *Drosophila melanogaster. Carnegie Inst. Wash. Publ.* **No. 627**

LOEWEN, P. C., B. L. TRIGGS, C. S. GEORGE and B. E. HRABARCHUK (1985) Genetic mapping of katG, a locus that affects synthesis of the bifunctional catalase-peroxidase hydroperoxide I in *Escherichia coli. J. Bacteriol.* **162**: 661-667

LUBINSKY, S. and G. C. BEWLEY (1979) Genetics of catalase in *Drosophila melanogaster*: rates of synthesis and degradation of the enzyme in flies aneuploid and euploid for the structural gene. *Genetics* **91**: 723-742

MACKAY, W. J. and G. C. BEWLEY (1989) The genetics of catalase in *Drosophila melanogaster*: Isolation and characterization of acatalasemic mutants. *Genetics* (in press).

MAYES, J., R. MUNEER and M. SIFERS (1984) Superoxide dismutase activity and oxygen toxicity in Down syndrome fibroblasts. *Am. V. Hum. Genet.* **36**: 153 A038

MELHORN, R. V. and G. COLE (1985) The free radical theory of aging: A critical review. *Adv. Free Radical Biol. and Med.* **1**: 165-223

NAHMIAS, J. A. and G. C. BEWLEY (1984) Characterization of catalase purified from *Drosophila melanogaster* by hydrophobic interaction chromatography. *Comp. Biochem. Physiol. [B]* **77**: 355-364

PHILLIPS, J. P., S. D. CAMPBELL, D. MICHAUD, M. CHARBONNEAU, and A. J. HILLIKER (1989) A null mutation of cSOD in *Drosophila* confers hypersensitivity to paraquat and reduced longevity. *Proc. Natl. Acad. Sci. USA* (in press).

PRYOR, W. A. (1987) The free-radical theory of aging revisited: A critique and a suggested disease-specific theory. pp. 89-112. In: *Modern Biological Theories*: Edited by H. R. Warner, R. N. Butler, L. R. Sprott and E. L. Schneider. Raven Press, New York.

SAUL, R. L., P. GEE and B. N. AMES (1987) Free radicals, DNA damage, and aging. pp. 113-129. In: *Modern Biological Theories of Aging*: Edited by H. R. Warner, R. N. Butler, L. R. Sprott and E. L. Schneider. Raven Press, New York

SCOTT, M. D., S. R. MESHNICK and J. W. EATON (1987) Superoxide dismutase-rich bacteria: Paradoxical increase in oxidant toxicity. *J. Biol. Chem.* **265**: 3640-3645

SETO, N. O. L., S. HAYOAHI and G. M. TENER (1987) The sequence of the Cu/Zn superoxide dismutase gene of *Drosophila. Nucl. Acids Res.* **15**: 10601

SHAFFER, J. B., R. B. SUTTON and G. C. BEWLEY (1987) Isolation of a cDNA clone for murine catalase and analysis of an acatalasemic mutant. *J. Biol. Chem.* **262**: 12908-12911

SINET, P. M. (1982) Metabolism of oxygen derivatives in Down's syndrome. *Ann. N.Y. Acad. Sci.* **396**:83-94

SOHAL, R. S. (1987) The free radical theory of aging: A critique. pp. 431- 449. In: *Review of Biological Research in Aging*. Vol. 3: Edited by M. Rothstein. Alan R. Liss, Inc., New York.

TAKAHARA, S. (1952) Progressive oral gangrene probably due to lack of catalase in the blood (acatalasemia). *Lancet* **263**: 1101-1104

TAKAHARA, S. (1968) Acatalasemia in Japan. p. 21. In: *Hereditary Disorders of Erythrocyte Metabolism* **Vol. I**: Edited by E. Beutler. Grune & Stratton, New York.

## DISCUSSION

1. This paper uses *Drosophila* rather than mammalian models, and is specifically directed to one type of mutation testing, the free radical hypothesis. It is important to remember that any treatment may cause damage and reduce longevities, but such a result does not suggest that aging acts through the treatment in question. Reducing longevity by reducing catalase activity is consistent with the hypothesis that damage from free radicals is an important aging process. It does not prove the hypothesis because catalase removal may cause damage and reduce longevities in ways entirely unrelated

to normal aging. Strong support for the free radical hypothesis would be provided if a treatment was developed that reduced free radical levels and this extended longevities. Reducing longevities is easy and can have many causes; extending them is difficult and would strongly suggest that aging processes have been retarded.

# 19

# GENETIC RELATIONSHIPS BETWEEN PUBERTY, REPRODUCTION AND LIFESPAN

James F. Nelson

## ABSTRACT

Evidence and theoretical arguments are reviewed which support the hypothesis that genetically specified relationships exist between selected reproductive processes and organismic aging, both within and among species. Three aspects of reproduction are considered: puberty, fecundity, and the age-related decline of fertility. It is proposed that age at puberty is positively correlated with lifespan. Three arguments for this coupling are presented. First, interventions that extend lifespan delay puberty. Second, age-specific mortality begins to increase and several measures of physiological performance begin to decline shortly after puberty. Finally, evolutionary theory indicates that aging is a consequence of the declining force of natural selection once transmission of the germ line is assured (*e.g.*, after sexual maturation); an argument is presented demonstrating how this theory is consistent with a coupling between the determinants of the timing of puberty and those of organismic aging. Genetic relationships between fecundity and aging are also proposed. Although evolutionary arguments predict an inverse relationship between fecundity and lifespan, there are documented instances and a basis for expecting a positive relationship between these two attributes, at least within some species. Finally, data and theoretical arguments are reviewed which suggest that the timing of the age-related loss of fertility may be positively correlated with lifespan, and hence, that age-related infertility and organismic aging may be coupled by common regulatory mechanisms.

## INTRODUCTION

An important question in research on the development and aging of the reproductive system is the extent to which these processes are coupled, either causally or by some common regulatory mechanism, to the aging of the organism as a whole (*i.e.*, organismic aging). Organismic aging is herein defined as the composite of molecular, cellular and physiological changes that increases the probability of death with advancing chronologic age. Although it is generally accepted that better understanding of reproductive aging will lead to improved therapeutic interventions and may even provide insight into other neural- and endocrine-dependent aging processes (Finch *et al.*, 1984; Nelson and Felicio, 1985; 1987; vom Saal and Finch, 1988), little attention has been given to the possibility that the reproductive system may actually be coupled to organismic aging. If reproductive processes are coupled to organismic aging, understanding that coupling should provide insight into fundamental causes of aging. Because such a coupling would be genetically determined, genetic approaches may be useful in establishing its extent and underlying mechanisms. The objective of this paper is to review and evaluate the evidence that genetic relationships exist between reproductive processes and organismic aging. Three aspects of reproduction are considered: puberty, fecundity and the age-related decline of reproductive function.

## The Relationship Between Puberty and Longevity

The age of onset of puberty is positively correlated with longevity across species (Western and Ssemakula, 1982; Calder, 1984). However, correlations between the timing of developmental events across species do not necessarily indicate a causal or regulatory coupling between them. Onset of puberty and length of life may covary across species only because selection pressure has operated on a common factor to which both are linked; under such circumstances, the evolved determinants of the timing of puberty could differ from those influencing lifespan. A common factor linking puberty and lifespan, as noted by Harvey and Zammuto (1985), may be body size, since puberty and longevity are positively correlated with body size (Calder, 1984). Thus, the longer juvenile period of larger animals may reflect the longer time required to reach a larger adult size. The longer overall lifespan of larger animals could in turn reflect the longer time required to reach puberty combined with post-pubertal resistance to organismic aging to permit the longer time required to reproduce and to raise offspring to maturity. In this case the determinants of age at puberty and age at death would be different, and therefore understanding the determinants of the timing of puberty would provide little insight into the determinants of lifespan. It is noteworthy, however, that the relationship between puberty and longevity remains after accounting for differences in body size (Harvey and Zammuto, 1985). Nevertheless, this does not imply that puberty and lifespan are coordinately regulated. From cross species comparisons it is difficult to exclude the possibility that puberty and lifespan, though correlated, are independently regulated.

A regulatory coupling linking puberty and longevity can only be inferred unequivocally if a relationship between these two attributes can be found within a species (*i.e.*, if, as a consequence of environmental manipulation, puberty and lifespan covary). Although the strength and frequency of correlations between puberty and longevity within species has not been extensively studied, limited evidence suggests that at least in some species there is a common regulatory coupling that links the timing of puberty with lifespan. Chronic caloric restriction, which prolongs mean and maximum lifespan in a number of species, delays the onset of puberty if it is begun at weaning (Glass and Swerdloff, 1980; Merry and Holehan, 1979; Bronson, 1986). However, it must be noted that the life extending effect of caloric restriction does not solely depend upon a delay in puberty, since it will also extend lifespan when initiated well after attainment of puberty (Weindruch and Walford, 1982). A positive relation between longevity and age of puberty has even been observed in a wild population of ground squirrels under varying conditions of food abundance (Zammuto and Millar, 1985). Neonatal thyroxine treatment, which produces chronic hypothyroidism in adulthood and which extended mean and maximum lifespan by about 10% in one study (Ooka *et al.*, 1983), also delays the onset of puberty in females (Gellert *et al.*, 1971).

Evidence that organismic aging begins at puberty provides another possible basis for the positive relation between puberty and lifespan. Actuarial studies of human populations indicate that age-specific mortality is at its nadir in the early teens and begins to rise shortly thereafter, although marked increases are not apparent until middle age (Faber, 1982; National Center for Health Statistics, 1983). Further evidence that vulnerability to life-threatening challenge, and hence aging, begins peripubertally is provided by recent evidence that the $LD_{50}$ for surface area burns increases linearly from childhood onward (Ball and Squire, 1949). Sampling intervals were too infrequent to assess whether this measure of vulnerability begins to increase before, during or after puberty. An analogous study in mice showed that their survival time after exposure to a toxic dose of salicylic aldehyde peaked around puberty and declined linearly thereafter (Strong, 1968). These data are consistent with the hypothesis that the physiological, cellular and molecular processes which increase vulnerability to death begin to predominate over those which protect from death in early life, possibly around the time of puberty. Although the identity of those changes is unknown, a number of physiological parameters peak around puberty and begin to decline shortly thereafter. These may play a role in increased vulnerability or at least point to areas of organismic and cellular function that may play initiatory roles in the aging processes. For example, peak physical performance in swimming and sprinting declines significantly within the first decade after puberty (Schulz and Curnow, 1988). Basal metabolic rate in rats exhibits a precipitous decline within the first weeks after puberty (Denckla, 1974). Protein synthesis and turnover also show strikingly early age-related diminution (Richardson and Semsei, 1987), though whether the decline in these functions begins at puberty is not known. While the relationship of these changes to increases in age-specific mortality remains unclear, their potential importance to the maintenance of peak physiological function and repair is apparent, and the cause for their early decline deserves investigation. An understanding of the genetic regulation of these changes as well as genetic differences in such regulation should help to reveal their importance to aging processes as well as the mechanisms responsible for those processes.

That puberty may be related to the onset of aging processes is also consistent with the evolutionary argument which proposes that aging is the inevitable consequence of the deleterious mutations that accumulate within a species as a result of reduced selection pressure with advancing postpubertal chronologic age (Williams, 1957; Charlesworth, 1980; Kirkwood, 1981; Rose and Hutchinson, 1987). According to this hypothesis, the selection pressure against mutations that increase vulnerability to life threatening challenges (or the pressure for mutations that protect against such challenges) begins to decline progressively after a reproductive age has been reached that maximizes the probability of survival of the species. In the simplest formulation of this argument, mutations whose deleterious effects on survival do not become manifest until after some optimal period of reproductive activity will accumulate in a species. Similarly, mutations that potentiate reproductive fitness early in the reproductive lifespan but are deleterious at later ages will also be maintained in a species. These two processes are termed "mutation accumulation" and "antagonistic pleiotropy", respectively. Although their relative importance to the genetic specification of aging is unknown, most evolutionary geneticists agree that together they account for the phenomenon of aging. Undoubtedly, the age at which organismic aging begins, and the rate at which it occurs, will vary among species depending on their natural history. The evidence that aging begins shortly after puberty, though vulnerability is not increased significantly until middle-age (to ensure survival of the offspring), is consistent with these evolutionary arguments.

Several important predictions derive from these arguments. In species with the potential for marked variation in onset of puberty, it would be predicted that natural selection would favor a delayed onset of organismic aging for those individuals whose puberty was delayed, insofar as such aging reduced reproductive fitness. Additionally, the extent that antagonistic pleiotropy contributes to the aging of a species would be expected to affect the degree to which genetic determinants of reproductive fitness play a role in the aging process. As described elsewhere in this book, the fecundity of outbred *Drosophila* early in its lifespan is inversely related to lifespan (see Rose), and at least one mutation that lengthens life in *C. elegans* concomitantly reduces fecundity (Friedman and Johnson, 1988). The pubertal increase of androgen secretion, essential for reproduction in males, yet potentially deleterious for long-term survival (see Nelson, 1988), provides another potential example of antagonistic pleiotropy. Another explanation for the apparent correlation between the timing of puberty and the onset of organismic aging is raised by this example. Since the expression of many genes that potentiate reproductive fitness is initiated or enhanced at puberty, the initiation of their deleterious actions probably also begins at this time.

## The Relationship Between Fecundity and Longevity

According to the evolutionary arguments discussed above and at greater length in the accompanying chapters by Charlesworth, Kirkwood and Rose, tradeoffs between fecundity and longevity may be expected because of limited energy supplies and, also, because of antagonistic pleiotropy. Thus, selection for longer lifespan may reduce fecundity and, conversely, increasing fecundity should shorten lifespan. Some experimental evidence is provided by these authors to support this hypothesis. In selection experiments that extended lifespans of fruit flies, early fecundity was reduced, though it should be noted that cumulative fecundity did not appear to be reduced, since long lived populations also had a longer fecund period (Luckinbill *et al.*, 1984; Rose and Hutchinson, 1987). It is also noteworthy that a single-gene mutation has recently been identified in *C. elegans* which extends longevity but greatly reduces fecundity (Friedman and Johnson, 1988, also see Johnson in this book).

The extent to which an inverse relationship between fecundity and longevity is associated with genetic differences in longevity among closely related mammalian species or among different genotypes within a single species remains unclear. Indeed, there are arguments and data to suggest that a positive relation may exist. For example, one of the strongest correlates of longevity across long-lived inbred mouse strains is litter size (Roderick and Storer, 1961). Litter size, a measure of fecundity, had a strong positive correlation with longevity in this series of inbred strains. Although it is important to note that this relationship may reflect differential levels of inbreeding depression and thus may not be a useful model for understanding the evolutionary basis for aging, it remains an interesting and potentially important phenomenon to explore. Are the differences in fecundity among inbred strains related to differences in ovulation frequency, the ability to support fetuses, or are they intrinsic to the fetus itself? These questions are readily answerable, and could offer direction in pursuing the basis for age differences in the longevity of these relatively long-lived strains. For example, increased viability of embryos from long-lived strains would point to different avenues of investigation from those suggested if differences in ovulation frequency were found to account for the increased fecundity of the longer-lived strains. One means of addressing the question of whether the positive relationship between fecundity and longevity in inbred strains is a consequence of inbreeding depression would be to determine whether the relationship is maintained among a variety of F1 crosses.

## The Relationship Between Reproductive Aging and Longevity

The possibility that declining fertility is coupled with, and thus may be a predictor of, organismic aging has received little attention, despite some evidence suggesting this relationship. Selection for longer reproductive lifespan in *Drosophila* increased longevity in two separate studies (Luckinbill *et al.*, 1984; Rose and Hutchinson, 1987). A recent comparison of duration of fertility among congenic mouse strains differing in MHC loci also showed a positive correlation with longevity (Lerner *et al.*, 1988). However, recombinant inbred lines of *C. elegans* revealed no correlation between duration of fertility and lifespan (Johnson, 1987), indicating that the coupling between reproductive lifespan and longevity is not always present.

Why might the loss of fertility in females be correlated with longevity? One possible explanation is based on the hypothesis that aging involves a progressive loss of the reserve capacity of physiological systems that are needed to respond to internal and external challenges (Strehler, 1977; Masoro, 1985). The energetic and regulatory demands of pregnancy are clearly great, particularly in the latter period of gestation when fetal burden is large. They might therefore overcome the physiologic reserves of a middle-aged organism already beginning its age-related decline. It is noteworthy that, in mice, one of the most well-defined species in terms of reproductive aging, the earliest age-related decline in litter size is predominantly due to losses occurring late in gestation, when energy demands are presumably greatest (Nelson and Felicio, 1985). With advancing chronological aging, losses occur at progressively earlier stages in pregnancy. This could reflect a declining ability with advancing age to meet the growing energy demands of pregnancy and thus account for its postulated coupling to organismic aging.

## Summary and Proposed Research Directions

In this paper hypotheses that puberty, fecundity and reproductive aging are genetically coupled to organismic aging have been outlined. The proposed relationship between puberty and aging involves several aspects. The hypothesis that the timing of puberty is coupled positively to longevity needs to be tested in a number of species under a variety of conditions that modulate the timing of puberty to establish the strength and significance of this relationship. The evidence that organismic aging begins at puberty, as measured by actuarial data and physiological performance, calls attention to the need for greater effort on the part of gerontologists to study this phase of the life cycle and its potential initiatory role in aging processes. Given the evidence that at least some aging processes begin at puberty, more attention should be given to identifying genes whose expression is altered around puberty and their potential role in organismic aging. Further study is needed to establish the strength and nature of the relationship between fecundity and organismic aging, and between reproductive aging and organismic aging - in particular, to identify the circumstances determining whether these relationships are positive or negative (or absent). Testing these hypotheses will focus attention on potentially important aspects of the aging processes that heretofore have received relatively little attention.

## ACKNOWLEDGMENTS

I wish to express my thanks to Dr. Lêda S. Felicio for her critical support of, and intellectual contributions to, the ideas presented herein. This work was supported in part by a grant from the Medical Research Council of Canada.

## REFERENCES

BALL, J. P. and SQUIRE, J. R. (1949) A study of mortality in a Burn Unit. *Ann. Surg.* **130**: 160-169

BRONSON, F. H. (1986) Food-restricted, prepubertal, female rats: Rapid recovery of luteinizing hormone pulsing with excess food, and full recovery of pubertal development with gonadotropin-releasing hormone. *Endocrinology* **118**: 2483-2487

CALDER, W. J., III. (1984) *Size, Function and Life History.* Harvard University Press, Cambridge, MA.

CHARLESWORTH, B. (1980) *Evolution in Age-structured Populations.* Cambridge: Cambridge University Press.

DENCKLA, W. D. (1974) Role of the pituitary and thyroid glands in the decline of minimal $O_2$ consumption with age. *J. Clin. Invest.* **53**: 572-581

FABER, J. F. (1982) *Life Tables for the United States: 1900-2050*; Actuarial Study No. 87, SSA Pub. No. 11-11534 Washington Office of the Actuary, Social Security Administration.

FINCH, C. E., FELICIO, L. S., MOBBS, C. V., and NELSON, J. F. (1984) Ovarian and steroidal influences on neuroendocrine aging processes in female rodents. *Endo. Rev.* **5**: 467-497

FRIEDMAN, D. B. and JOHNSON, T. E. (1988) A mutation in the age-1 gene in *Caenorhabditis elegans* lengthens life and reduces hermaphrodite fertility. *Genetics* **118**: 75-86

GELLERT, R. J., BAKKE, J. L., and LAWRENCE, N. L. (1971) Delayed vaginal opening in the rat following pharmacologic doses of T4 administered during the neonatal period. *J. Lab. Clin. Med.* **77**: 410-416

GLASS, A. R., and SWERDLOFF, R. S. (1980) Nutritional influences on sexual maturation in the rat. *Fed. Proc.* **39**: 2360

HARVEY, P. H. and ZAMMUTO, R. M. (1985) Patterns of mortality and age at first reproduction in natural populations of mammals. *Nature* **315**: 319-320

JOHNSON, T. E. (1987) Aging can be genetically dissected into component processes using long-lived lines of *Caenorhabditis elegans*. *Proc. Natl. Acad. Sci. USA* **84**: 3777-3781

KIRKWOOD, T. B. L. (1985) Comparative and evolutionary aspects of longevity. In: *Handbook of the Biology of Aging, 2nd ed.* (Finch, C. E. and Schneider, E. L., Eds). pp.27-44.

LERNER, S. P., ANDERSON, C. P., WALFORD, R. L., FINCH, C. E. (1988) Genotypic influences on reproductive aging of inbred female mice: Effects of H-2 and non-H-2 alleles. *Biol. Reprod.* **38**: 1035-1043

LUCKINBILL, L. S., ARKING R., CLARE, M. J., CIROCCO, W. C., MUCK, S. A. (1984) Selection for delayed senescence in *Drosophila melanogaster*. *Evolution* **38**: 996-1003

MASORO, E.J. (1985) Metabolism. In: *Handbook of the Biology of Aging, 2nd ed.* (Finch, C.E. and Schneider, E.L., eds). pp. 540-563.

MERRY, B. J., and HOLEHAN, A. M. (1979) Onset of puberty and duration of fertility in rats fed a restricted diet. *J. Reprod. Fert.* **57**: 253-259

NATIONAL CENTER FOR HEALTH STATISTICS. 1983. Advance report of final mortality statistics, 1980. *Monthly vital statistics report* **Vol. 32, No. 4**, Supplement.

NELSON, J. F. (1988) Puberty, gonadal steroids and fertility: potential reproductive markers of aging. *Exper. Geront.* **23**: 359-367

NELSON, J. F. and FELICIO, L. S. (1985) Reproductive aging in the female: an etiological perspective. *Rev. Biol. Res. Aging* **2**: 251-314

NELSON, J. F., and FELICIO, L. S. (1987) Reproductive aging in the female: an etiological perspective updated. *Rev. Biol. Res. Aging* **3**: 359-381

OOKA, H., FUJITA, S., and YOSHIMOTO, E. (1983) Pituitary-thyroid activity and longevity in neonatally thyroxine-treated rats. *Mech. Age. Devel.* **22**: 113-120

RICHARDSON A., and SEMSEI, I. (1987) Effect of aging on translation and transcription. *Rev. Biol. Res. Aging* **3**: 467-483

RODERICK, T. H. and STORER, J. B. (1961) Correlation between mean litter size and mean life span among 12 inbred strains of mice. *Science* **134**: 48-49

ROSE, M. R. and HUTCHINSON, E. W. (1987) Evolution of Aging. *Rev. Biol. Res. Aging* **3**: 23-32

SCHULZ, R., and CURNOW, C. (1988) Peak performance and age among superathletes: track and field, swimming, baseball, tennis, and golf. *J. Gerontol. Psych. Sci.* **43**: P113-120

STREHLER, B. L. (1977) *Time, Cells and Aging, 2nd ed.* Academic Press, New York, NY.

WILLIAMS, G. C. (1957) Pleiotropy, natural selection and the evolution of senescence. *Evolution* **11**: 398-411

VOM SAAL, F. S., and FINCH, C. E. (1988) Reproductive senescence: phenomena and mechanisms in mammals and selected vertebrates. In: *The Physiology of Reproduction* (Eds. E. Knobil and J.D. Neill) Vol. 2, pp 2351-2413. New York, NY: Raven Press.

WEINDRUCH, R., and WALFORD, R. L. (1982) Dietary restriction in mice beginning at 1 year of age: Effect on lifespan and spontaneous cancer incidence. *Science* **215**: 1415-1418

WESTERN, D. and SSEMAKULA, J. (1982) Life history patterns in birds and mammals and their evolutionary interpretation. *Oecologia (Berl)* **54**: 281-290

ZAMMUTO, R. M., and MILLAR, J. S. (1985) Environmental predictability, variability, and *Spermophilus columbianus* life history over an elevational gradient. *Ecology* **66**: 1784-1794

## DISCUSSION

1. Are genetic determinants of fecundity also modulators of longevity? Roderick and Storer (*Science* **134**: 48-9, 1961) found a strong positive correlation (r=0.69, with r=0.90 if the leukemia prone AKR data are removed) between mean litter size and mean lifespan in inbred mouse strains. Perhaps these are due only to inbreeding depression in both longevity and fecundity, yet this was not suggested by Nelson's data. B6C3HF1 cycles occurred earlier than in either parent strain, and cycle times were less variable.

2. Fertility is quantitative, as the initial litter sizes are not as great as later ones, though eventually litter sizes decline with age.

3. Do longer-lived genotypes have better control of cycling? Better neuroendocrine mechanisms? Nelson answered that they seem to cycle more frequently and regularly, and Flurkey referred to data that 8 month old B6CBAF1 mice continued to cycle during stress that caused both parent strains to stop. Charlesworth reminded us that attenuation of selective pressure starts once reproduction starts; he favors the use of $F_1$ over inbred strains.

4. Tutarro notes that a major difference between the long-lived mouse, *Peromyscus*, and the laboratory mouse strains is that the former controls circadian patterns much better. Might this be because they have been less "domesticated" in laboratory environments? Cross-species comparisons only suggest cause and effect, they cannot prove it, as genes controlling mortality may be very different in different species.

# 20

# GENETICS OF ALTERED SIGNAL TRANSDUCTION DURING AGING

George S. Roth

## ABSTRACT

Changes in many signal transduction mechanisms occur during aging. Particular research emphasis has been placed on those hormone and neurotransmitter dependent processes which serve to regulate various physiological functions. Aging affects these mechanisms at both the "receptor" and "post-receptor" levels. A number of genetic models have been employed to examine such alterations, both from the comparative and molecular genetic standpoints.

## INTRODUCTION

The regulation of most physiological functions is dependent on the ability of cells to communicate with each other as well as to receive environmental input. The process by which such information influences cellular functions is called signal transduction. Most common among the substances which provide such signals are hormones, neurotransmitters and related agents (Roth, 1985; Williams, 1981). Usually, hormones *etc.* initiate signal transduction sequences by attaching to very specific proteins called receptors (King and Mainwaring, 1974). These may be located on the surface of, or inside, the cell and sometimes in the nucleus. The interaction of agent and receptor triggers subsequent physico-chemical events, culminating in a particular biological response on the part of the cell. In the process certain chemical agents, termed "second-messengers", may be produced or transported. Most notable among these are cyclic nucleotides, inositol phosphates, and certain ions, including calcium (Cuatrecasas, 1974; Meldolesi and Pozzan 1987).

Optimal function and maintenance of homeostatic balance are dependent upon the ability of cells and tissues to regulate their biological activity through appropriate signal transduction mechanisms at appropriate times. Unfortunately, during senescence such physiological balance becomes disturbed, at least partly as a consequence of altered signal transduction mechanisms. This chapter will focus on these mechanisms, as well as their amenability to analysis in different genetic models of aging and at the molecular genetic level.

## ALTERED SIGNAL TRANSDUCTION DURING AGING IS THE CONSEQUENCE OF BOTH RECEPTOR AND POST-RECEPTOR CHANGES

### Receptors

Numerous articles in recent years have dealt with the subject of age changes in signal transduction mechanisms. These have been broadly grouped into those at the "receptor" and "post-receptor" levels. As previously reviewed, (Roth *et al.*, 1986), the most consistent and best agreed upon receptor change during aging is the loss of $D_2$ dopamine receptors from the corpus striatum. Loss of beta adrenergic receptors from several brain regions is also fairly well established (for a review see Roth and Hess, 1982).

In the case of steroid receptors, a strong consensus concerning the loss of estrogen receptors from aged rodent uterus and selected brain regions as well as for androgen receptor loss in senescent rat prostate has been reached (for a review see Roth and Hess, 1982). However, some recent discrepancies concerning glucocorticoid receptor changes have arisen (Roth, 1985). Possible explanations for these differing results have been discussed elsewhere (Roth and Hess, 1982; Kalimi, 1984). Nevertheless, it is interesting to note that age-related reductions in glucocorticoid receptor levels in liver (Bolla, 1980; Singer *et al.*, 1973), certain brain regions, (Defiore and Turner, 1981; Roth, 1976), skeletal muscle, (Roth, 1974; Mayer *et al.*, 1981; Sharma and Timiras 1987), lymphoid cells and tissues, (Petrovic and Markovic, 1975; Roth, 1975; Joncourt *et al.* , 1985), and cultured lung fibroblasts (Rosner and Cristofalo, 1981; Forciea and Cristofalo, 1981; Kondo *et al.*, 1978; Kalimi and Seifter, 1979) from various species, including humans, have been reported by at least three independent laboratories. In contrast, independent agreement on stable glucocorticoid receptor concentrations during aging exists for rodent liver (Roth, 1974; Latham and Finch, 1976; Kalimi *et al.*, 1983), and several brain regions (Defiore and Turner 1981; Carmickle *et al.* , 1979; Nelson *et al.* , 1976).

Ultimately, the value of such investigations will probably be determined by their generalized relevance to human aging. Thus, it becomes important to focus on areas of basic agreement. Consequently, if results of experimental animal studies mimic findings in specific human hormone/neurotransmitter response systems or serve simply as models of general mechanisms of age changes they would seem to be worthwhile.

Age-related changes in receptors have been closely linked to altered responsiveness in a number of cases (for a review see Roth and Hess, 1982). Probably the greatest agreement exists for loss of striatal dopaminergic receptors and motor responsiveness, cerebellar cortex beta adrenergic receptors and stimulated adenylate cyclase activity, and uterine estrogen receptors and estrogenic regulation of enzymes governing energy metabolism and cell proliferation.

It should be pointed out that not all receptors decrease in concentration during aging. A few have been reported to remain at constant levels but exhibit decreased binding affinity for their respective ligands (Roth and Hess, 1982). In some cases this may be attributable to changes in circulating levels of homologous or heterologous hormones which can alter the coupling of receptors to effector systems such as the G proteins (Feldman *et al.*, 1984). Many others remain unchanged, while several actually increase in concentration during aging (Roth and Hess, 1982). Moreover, even a well documented change in receptor concentration or affinity during aging is no guarantee that such alterations are causally related to changes in responsiveness. In many cases, so-called "spare receptors', are present in concentrations far greater than necessary to effect maximal responsiveness (Cuatrecasas, 1974). Thus, even substantial receptor loss results in a negligible change in response. Most studies of receptors during aging have been performed in mammals. Although some of these have employed human cells and tissues, they have usually been carried out with rodents, including mice, rats, rabbits and hamsters (Roth and Hess, 1982). A few studies have also been performed in lower species such as birds (Boyd-Leinen *et al.*, 1982) and molluscs (Stefano and Leung, 1986). Unfortunately, it is rare for a given receptor system to be examined in more than 2 species. A feeble attempt was made at the time of the first Genetic Effects on Aging Conference in 1978 to compare heterologous steroid receptor changes during the aging of various species having differing maximal lifespans (Roth, 1978). Although the result was a rough correlation between the relative degree of receptor loss and percentage of lifespan completed, a much more satisfactory comparison would have been for the same tissue-receptor system.

Happily, 10 years later, the field has advanced sufficiently to perform such an analysis for the striatal $D_2$ dopamine receptor system. Table 1 compares the rate of this receptor loss in mice, rats, rabbits, monkeys and humans (for exact references see Lai *et al.*, 1987). Unfortunately, it now appears that a decrease in dopamine receptor concentration is not a linear function of age in all species/strains. Nevertheless, it is heartening to note that on average the mean rate of loss is between 5 and 10% per tenth of maximal lifespan in

**Table 1.** Mean Rates Of Change In Concentrations Of Striatal Dopamine Receptors Relative To Maximal Life Spans (mls) Of Several Species

| Species | MLS | Mean change per year | Mean change per 0.1 MLS | Age Range Studied | | Binding ligand/Method/Site |
|---|---|---|---|---|---|---|
| | | | | Time | Range of MLS studied | |
| Human | 115Y | -0.35% | -4% | 2-94Y | 0.02-0.82 | spiroperidol/PM/CN |
| | | -0.61% | -7% | 19-77Y | 0.17-067 | spiroperidol/PM/CN |
| | | NS | NS | 19-59Y | 0.17-0.51 | spiroperidol/PM/CN |
| | | -0.78% | -9% | 20-73Y | 0.17-0.63 | 3-N-methylspiperone /PET/CN |
| Macaque | 37Y | -0.43% | -5% | 16-94Y | 0.14-0.82 | spiroperidol/PM/CN |
| Rabbit | 13Y | -2.1% | -8% | 2-22Y | 0.05-0.59 | spiroperidol/PM/CN |
| Rat | 56m | -6.2% | -8% | 0.4-5.5Y | 0.03-0.42 | spiroperidol/PM/ST |
| | | -34% | -16% | 3-22m | 0.05-0.39 | spiroperidol/PM/ST |
| | | -24% | -11% | 10-30m | 0.18-0.54 | haloperidol/PM/ST |
| | | -23% | -11% | 6-25m | 0.11-0.45 | ADTN/PM/ST |
| | | -23% | -11% | 6-25m | 0.11-0.45 | haloperidol/PM/ST |
| | | -24% | -11% | 4.5-24m | 0.08-0.45 | ADTN/PM/ST |
| | | -17% | -8% | 4-24m | 0.07-0.43 | spiroperidol/PM/ST |
| | | -33% | -15% | 12-30m | 0.21-0.54 | spiroperidol/PM/ST |
| | | -19% | -9% | 3.5-26m | 0.06-0.46 | spiroperidol/PM/ST |
| | | -21% | -10% | 5-25m | 0.09-0.45 | spiroperidol/PM/ST |
| | | -17% | -8% | 4-22m | 0.07-0.39 | spiroperidol/PM/ST |
| Mouse | 48m | -14% | -6% | 6.5-28.5m | 0.13-0.59 | spiroperidol/PM/ST |
| | | -25% | -10% | 3-28m | 0.06-0.58 | spiroperidol/PM/ST |
| | | -19% | -8% | 3-24m | 0.05-0.43 | spiroperidol/PM/ST |

m, month; NS, not significant; PET, positron emission tomography; PM, postmortem; Y, year; CN, caudate nucleus; ST, striatum; MLS, maximal lifespan; Adapted from Lai *et al.* (1987) with permission

essentially all species examined. Thus, despite differences in methodology and laboratory to laboratory variation, loss of striatal $D_2$ receptors appears to be a fairly robust index of the aging of one type of signal transduction mechanism.

## Post-Receptor Events

In many situations in which receptor changes do not occur, or appear to be functionally unimportant during aging, post-receptor mechanisms have been examined. These also have been reviewed extensively elsewhere (Roth, 1985; Roth and Hess, 1982). However, several new trends in this area appear to be emerging.

Various steroid hormone-receptor complexes exhibit an impaired ability to bind to nuclear acceptor sites with high affinity during aging, even in cases where total cellular receptor concentrations may be unaltered. Such reductions have been reported for estrogens in rodent uterus (Chuknyiska *et al.*, 1985; Chuknyiska and Roth, 1985; Chuknyiska, and Roth, 1986; Jiang and Peng, 1981; Belisle and Lehoux, 1983; Belisle *et al.*, 1985; Belisle *et al.*, 1986), liver (Konoplya *et al.* , 1986) and brain (Jiang and Peng, 1981; Wise *et al.* , 1984), for glucocorticoids in rat liver (Bolla, 1980; Parchman, *et al.*, 1978) and cultured human fibroblasts (Forciea and Cristofalo, 1981) and for androgens in rat prostrate (Shain and Boesel, 1977). At least two studies (Chuknyiska *et al.*, 1986; Belisle *et al.*, 1986) have concluded that age-related reductions in the ability of steroid hormone-receptor complexes to bind to nuclei with high affinity are the consequence of alterations at both the receptor and nuclear levels.

Stimulation of cyclic AMP production by various hormones and neurotransmitters also appears to be altered during aging in a number of systems (for reviews see Roth, 1979 and Dax, 1985). In some cases this may be due to an impaired coupling of receptors to adenylate cyclase due to an inability to form high-affinity complexes with ligands (Scarpace and Abrass, 1983; Narayanan and Derby, 1982; and Feldman *et al.*, 1984). However, a variety of possible explanations can be offered for other reports of age-related reductions in stimulation of adenylate cyclase. These include; the loss of the enzyme catalytic or regulatory subunits; increased levels of inhibitory components; changes in membrane fluidity, and/or other chemical alterations which might render the cyclase system less functional.

Probably the most exciting class of post-receptor changes to be identified recently includes those calcium-dependent, hormone/neurotransmitter responses that decline during aging. In general, such dysfunctions appear to be due to impaired stimulation of calcium mobilization, even in the absence of receptor changes. In fact, many of these impaired responses can be at least partially restored if sufficient calcium can be moved to the proper intracellular locations in aged cells. These include beta-adrenergic-stimulated myocardial contraction (Guarnieri *et al.*, 1980), alpha-adrenergic-stimulated parotid cell glucose consumption (Gee *et al.*, 1986) and electrolyte secretion (Ito *et al.*, 1982), alpha-adrenergic- and serotonergic-stimulated aortic contraction (Cohen and Berkowitz, 1976), cholinergic regulation (Peterson and Gibson, 1983; Meyer *et al.*, 1986; Crews *et al.*, 1986; Peterson and Gibson, 1984; Peterson *et al.*, 1985), of cognitive (Davis *et al.*, 1983) and motor function (Peterson and Gibson, 1983), compound 48-80 stimulated histamine release from mast cells (Orida and Feldman, 1982), lectin-stimulated thymic lymphocyte mitogenesis (Wu *et al.*, 1985; Miller, 1986), luteinizing-hormone-releasing-hormone stimulated gonadotropin release from pituitary cells (Chuknyiska *et al.*, 1987), release of beta glucuronidase and elastin-like protease from polymorphonuclear leukocytes (Fulop *et al.* , 1985), and a number of others (see Table 2, and Roth (1988) for references).

Although at first glance it would appear that stimulation of calcium movement, from both extra- and intracellular sites, becomes impaired during aging, elucidation of the precise mechanisms involved is clearly much more difficult. For example, calcium movement may occur through a number of processes involving various cellular components in different cell types (Meldolesi and Pozzan, 1987). While in some cases stimulation of calcium mobilization from these sites is clearly reduced with age (Segal, 1986; Michaelis *et al.*, 1984; Vitorica and Satusgegui, 1986; Gafni and Yuh, 1985; Hansford and Castro, 1982), in other systems calcium movement seems unaffected (Williams, 1984), and actual increases in intracellular calcium content (Peterson and Goldman, 1986; Landfield and Pitler, 1984), or uptake components (Govoni *et al.*, 1985; Battaini *et al.*, 1985) may occur during aging. Moreover, in at least two cases it has been reported that even when directly exposed to relatively high calcium concentrations, aged fibroblasts (Praeger and Cirstofalo, 1984) and cortical synaptosomes (Meyer *et al.*, 1986) exhibit reduced responsiveness.

Some of the apparent inconsistencies in these studies may come from differences in cell types or the categories of calcium mobilization being examined. Timing of calcium movement mechanisms is also critical and the actual relationship between the calcium flux(es) in question and the final biological response must be ascertained. Since responsiveness is usually dependent on free rather than total calcium it is conceivable that high total intracellular calcium concentrations in some aged cells (Meyer *et al.*, 1986; Praeger and Cristofalo, 1984) may actually impede normal fluxes of free calcium, thus resulting in impaired responsiveness. Obviously, such systems need to be examined on a case-by-case basis for precise elucidation of the molecular mechanisms responsible for age-associated decrements in calcium-dependent functions.

Since aging studies of post-receptor events have only become popular in recent years, it is still not possible to compare different genetic models as has been done for striatal dopamine receptors. Nevertheless, the apparently widespread manifestation of these phenomena, especially those involving impaired calcium mobilization in mice, rats and humans (see Roth, 1988) suggests that they will be common to many species.

**TABLE 2.** Systems Exhibiting Impaired Stimulation of Calcium Mobiliation During Aging

| Stimulus | Species | Tissue | Response |
|---|---|---|---|
| alpha adrenergic | rat | parotid | electrolyte secretion |
| alpha adrenergic | rat | parotid | glucose oxidation |
| alpha adrenergic | rat | aorta | contraction |
| beta adrenergic | rat | heart | contraction |
| cholinergic | rat | brain (striatum) | dopamine release |
| depolarization | rat | heart | contraction |
| depolarization | rat | brain (forebrain and cortex) | acetylcholine release |
| depolarization | mouse | brain (forebrain) | acetylcholine release |
| depolarization | mouse | whole animal | motor function |
| depolarization | rat | whole animal | maze learning |
| serotonin | rat | aorta | contraction |
| gonadotropin releasing hormone | rat | pituitary | gonadotropin secretion |
| lectin | rat | lymphocyte | mitogenesis |
| lectin | mouse | lymphocyte | mitogenesis |
| lectin | human | lymphocyte | mitogenesis |
| compound 48-80 | rat | mast cell | histamine release |
| formyl-methionyl leucyl-phenyl-alanine | human | neutrophil | superoxide generation |
| thyroid hormones | human | erythrocyte | activation of calcium ATPase |
| low density lipoprotein | human | polymorphonuclear leukocytes | release of $\beta$-glucuronidase |
| cytochalasin B | human | polymorphonuclear leukocytes | release of $\beta$-glucuronidase |
| immune complexes | human | polymorphonuclear leukocytes | release of $\beta$-glucuronidase |
| phosphatidylserine | rat | brain | protein kinase activation |

Adapted from Roth (1988) with permission.

## MOLECULAR GENETIC APPROACHES TO THE ELUCIDATION OF MECHANISMS OF ALTERED SIGNAL TRANSDUCTION

Gerontologists have only just begun to exploit the explosive proliferation of recombinant DNA technology to examine age changes in gene expression. In fact, the regulation of gene expression through various signal transduction mechanism lags even further behind. For several years, our laboratory has been elucidating those regulatory processes which cause both basal and stimulated luteinizing hormone (LH) production to decrease with age in rats, while prolactin (PRL) production concomitantly increases (Chuknyiska, *et al.*, 1987; Haji *et al.* , 1984; Chuknyiska *et al.* , 1986). This is a particularly intriguing paradigm to examine at the molecular genetic level since each of

**TABLE 3.** Effect of Age on Luteinizing Hormone and Prolactin Concentrations Compared With Their Respective Messenger RNA Levels

| Age (mo.) | PRL | | LH | |
|---|---|---|---|---|
| | ng/ml serum | Relative mRNA OD units | ng/ml serum | Relative mRNA OD units |
| 6-7 | 6.4 ± 1.1 (13)[a] | 0.23 ± 0.03 (12)[d] | 5.7 ± 0.1 (18)[b] | 0.78 ± 0.12 (17)[c] |
| 23-25 | 36.6 ± 11.7 (10)[b] | 0.40 ± 0.08 (9)[d] | 2.7 ± 0.3 (10)[b] | 0.30 ± 0.03 (4)[c] |

Serum PRL and LH concentrations and pituitary homogenate PRL and LH-β mRNA levels were determined for ovariectomized female Wistar rats as previously described (Stewart *et al.*, 1988). Values represent the means ± standard errors for the numbers of rats indicated in parenthesis. Data adapted from Stewart *et al.* (1988) with permission.

[a], [b], [c] Significantly different from the group having the same letter ($p < 0.01$) by unpaired Student's test.

[d] Not significantly different from the group having the same letter ($p > 0.05$) by unpaired Student's test.

these polypeptide hormones is produced by a different population of pituitary cells, although both can be stimulated by estrogen through genomic action. Since estrogen receptors have been reported not to change with age in the pituitary (Haji *et al.*, 1981) differential changes in LH and PRL gene expression with age probably are due to post-receptor changes.

In a preliminary study, we have employed cDNAs to the LH and PRL genes to measure the expression of the mRNAs for these hormones during aging (Stewart *et al.*, 1988). Table 3 summarizes the results of these experiments. Surprisingly, the increased levels of PRL seen during aging are not paralleled by increases in the mRNA for this hormone. Although a trend toward a slight increase in message exists, it is very small (not significant) compared to the increase in PRL release. In contrast, the age related decrease in LH concentration is more closely aligned with a reduction in LH mRNA. Thus, different molecular genetic mechanisms appear to be responsible for differential changes in pituitary hormone expression during aging. It is interesting to note that certain enzymes whose concentrations decrease with age have been reported to parallel changes in the concentrations of their respective mRNAs (*e.g.* Richardson *et al.*, 1987). This phenomenon would seem to be analogous to the changes in LH reported here. To our knowledge, no studies of mRNA levels for enzymes whose concentrations *increase* with age have yet been reported. It will, therefore, be extremely interesting to see whether elevated expression of certain genes during aging may be due to post-transcriptional mechanisms, while reduced expression may be the consequence of reduced mRNA transcription.

## SUMMARY AND CONCLUSIONS

The mechanisms responsible for altered signal transduction during aging have been the focus of intense research interest in recent years. Alterations occur at both the "receptor" and "post-receptor" levels. Two different strategies have been employed to examine these age changes from a genetic standpoint. 1) Various species, having different maximal lifespans, have been examined for alterations in signal transduction during aging. The best comparison has been for the loss of striatal $D_2$ dopamine receptors which occurs at a rate of 5-10% per decile of maximal lifespan in mice, rats, rabbits, monkeys and humans. 2) Recombinant DNA technology has been utilized to examine molecular genetic mechanisms of altered signal transduction. Preliminary studies on differential age changes in LH and PRL production suggest that these may occur at either the transcriptional and translational levels depending on the type of change.

Obviously, a tremendous amount of work remains to be performed using both approaches. Better controlled analyses of "receptor" and "'post-receptor, changes need to be carried out using different genetic models and identical techniques in the same laboratory. The degree to which molecular genetic technology can be applied to these problems is limited only by one's imagination. Clearly then, we stand at the threshold of an unprecedented opportunity for potentially unlimited advances in both biogerontology and the elucidation of basic signal transduction mechanisms through appropriate application of genetic technology.

## REFERENCES

BATTAINI, F., GOVONI, S., RIUS, A. and TRABUCCHI, M. (1985) Age-dependent increase in $^3$H-verapamil binding to rat cortical membranes. *Neurosci. Lett.* **61**: 67-71.

BELISLE, S. BEAUDRY, C. and LEHOUX, J. G. (1983) Endocrine aging in CBA mice: Characterization of uterine cytosolic and nuclear sex steroid receptors. *Exp. . Gerontology* **17**: 417-423.

BELISLE, S. BELLABARBA, D. and LEHOUX, J. G. (1985) On the presence of non-functional uterine estrogen receptors in middle-aged and old C57BL/6J mice. *Endocrinology* **116**: 148-153.

BELISLE, S., BELLABARBA, D., LEHOUX, J. G., ROBEL, P. and BAULIEU, E. E. (1986) Effect of aging on the dissociation kinetics and estradiol receptor nuclear interactions in mouse uteri: correlation with biological effects. *Endocrinology* **118**: 750-758.

BOLLA, R. (1980) Age-dependent changes in rat liver steroid hormone receptor proteins. *Mech. Ageing and Devel.* **12**: 119-122.

BOYD-LEINEN, P. A. FOURNIER, D. and SPELSBERG, T. C. (1982) Nonfunctioning progesterone receptors in the developed oviducts from estrogen-withdrawn immature chicks and aged nonlaying hens. *Endocrinology* **30**: 111-120.

CARMICKLE, L. J., KALIMI, M. and TERRY, R. D. (1979) Aging rat brain: changes in steroid hormone receptors and morphometric characteristics. *Fed. Proc.* **30**: 482.

CHUKNYISKA, R. S., BLACKMAN, M. R., HYMER, W. C. and ROTH, G. S. (1986) Age-related alterations in the number and function of pituitary lactotropic cells from intact and ovariectomized rats. *Endocrinology* **118**: 1856-1862.

CHUKNYISKA, R. S., BLACKMAN, M. R. and ROTH, G. S. (1987) Ionophore A23187 and calcium ions partially reverse the *in vitro* LH secretory defect of pituitary cells from old rats. *Am. J. Physiol.* **253**: E233-E237.

CHUKNYISKA, R. S., HAJI, M., FOOTE, R. H. and ROTH, G. S. (1985) Age associated changes in nuclear binding of rat uterine estradiol receptor complexes. *Endocrinology* **116**: 547-551.

CHUKNYISKA, R. S., JUSTINIANO, C. and ROTH, G. S. (1986) Impaired conversion of rat uterine estradiol receptor during aging. *Exp. Gerontology* **21**: 255-265.

CHUKNYISKA, R. S. and ROTH, G. S. (1985) Decreased estrogenic stimulation of RNA polymerase II in aged rat uterus is apparently due to reduced nuclear binding of receptor-estradiol complexes. *J. Biol. Chem.* **260**: 8661-8663.

COHEN, M. L. and BERKOWITZ, B. A. (1976) Vascular contraction: effect of age and extracellular calcium. *Blood Vessels* **67**: 139-149.

CREWS, F. T., MEYER, E. M., GONZALES, R. A., THEISS, C., OTERO, D. H., LARSEN, K., KARULLI, R. and CALDERINI, G. (1986) Presynaptic and postsynaptic approaches to enhancing central cholinergic neurotransmission. **In**: *Treatment Development Strategies for Alzheimer's Disease* (Eds. T. Crook, R. Bartus, S. Ferris and S. Gershon) pp. 385-419. Madison, CT: Pawley Associates.

CUATRECASAS, P. (1974) Membrane Receptors. *Ann. Rev. Biochem.* **43**: 169-232.

DAVIS, H. P., IDOWU, A. and GIBSON, G. E. (1983) Improvement of 8-arm maze performance in aged Fischer 344 rats with 3, 4 diaminopyridine. *Exp. Aging Res.* **9**: 211-214.

DAX, E. M. (1985) Receptors and associated membrane events in aging. **In**: *Review of Biological Research in Aging* Vol. 2 (Ed. M. Rothstein). pp. 315-336, New York, N.Y.: Academic Press.

DEFIORE, C. H. and TURNER, B. B. (1981) Glucocorticoid binding is decreased in hippocampus but not cortex of aged rats. *Abstr. Soc. Neurosci.* **7**: 947.

FELDMAN, R. D., LIMBIRD, L. E., NADEAU, J., ROBERTSON, D. and WOOD, A. J. J. (1984) Alterations in leukocyte 0-receptor affinity with aging. *N. Engl. J. Med.* **310**: 815-819.

FORCIEA, M. A. and CRISTOFALO, V. J. (1981) Glucocorticoid specific binding in WI-38 cells: confirmation of an age-associated decline in receptors in a cell free preparation. *The Gerontologist* **21**: 179.

FULOP, T., FORIS, G., WOUND, I., PARAGH, G. and LEOVEY, A. (1985) Age related variations of some polymorphonuclear leukocyte functions. *Mech. Ageing and Devel.* **29**: 1-8.

GAFNI, A. and YUH, K. (1985) Age-related deterioration in the sarcoplasmic reticulum $Ca^{2+}$ pump. *The Gerontologist* **25**: 215-216.

GEE, M. V., ISHIKAWA, Y., BAUM, B. J. and ROTH, G. S. (1986) Impaired adrenergic stimulation of rat parotid cell glucose oxidation during aging: the role of calcium. *J. Gerontol.* **41**: 331-335.

GOVONI, S. RUS, A., BATTAINI, F., BIANCHI, A. and TRABUCCHI, M. (1985) Age-related reduced affinity of H-nitrendipine labeling of brain voltage dependent calcium channels. *Brain Res.* **333**: 374-377.

GUARNIERI, T., FILBURN, C. R., ZITNIK, G., ROTH, G. S. and LAKATTA, E. G. (1980) Mechanisms of altered cardiac inotropic responsiveness during aging in the rat. *Am. J. Physiol.* **239**: H501-H508.

HAJI, M., KATO, K., NAWATA, H. and IBAYASHI, H. (1981) Age-related changes in the concentrations of cytosol receptors for sex steroid hormones in the hypothalamus and pituitary gland of the rat. *Brain Res.* **204**: 373-386.

HAJI, M., ROTH, G. S. and BLACKMAN, M. R. (1984) Discordant Age-related alterations in the *in vitro* secretion of luteinizing hormone and prolactin by pituitary cells of ovariectomized rats: effect of 17-β estradiol. *Am. J. Physiol.* **247**: E483-E488.

HANSFORD, R. G. and CASTRO, F. (1982) Effect of senescence on $Ca^{2+}$ ion transport by heart mitochondria. *Mech. Ageing and Devel.* **19**: 5-13.

ITO, H., BAUM, B. J., UCHIDA, T., HOOPES, M. T., BODNER, L. and ROTH, G. S. (1982) Modulation of rat parotid alpha adrenergic responsiveness at a step subsequent to receptor activation. *J. Biol. Chem.* **246**: 9532-9538.

JIANG, M. J. and PENG, M. T. (1981) Cytoplasmic and nuclear binding of estradiol in the brain and pituitary of old female rats. *Gerontology* **27**: 51-57.

JONCOURT, F., WANG, Y., KRISTENSEN, F. and DEWECK, A. L. (1985) Age-related changes in the formation of glucocorticoid and insulin receptors during lectin-induced activation of human peripheral blood lymphocytes. *Gerontology* **31**: 293-300.

KALIMI, M. and SEIFTER, S. (1979) Glucocorticoid receptors in WI-38 fibroblasts: Characterization and changes with population doublings in culture. *Biochim. Biophys. Acta* **583**: 352-361.

KALIMI, M., GUPTA, S. HUBBARD, J. and GREENE, K. (1983) Glucocorticoid receptors in adult and senescent rat liver. *Endocrinology* **112**: 341-347.

KALIMI, M. (1984) Glucocorticoid receptors: from development to aging. A review. *Mech. Aging and Devel.* **24**: 129-138.

KING, R. J. B. and MAINWARING, W. I. P. (1974) *Steroid-Cell Interactions.* Baltimore, MD: University Park Press.

KONDO, H., KASUGA, H. and NOUMORA, T. (1978) *Specific binding of glucocorticoids to human diploid fibroblasts during in vitro* aging. Abstracts of the XII Intl. Congress of Gerontology , 26-27.

KONOPLYA, E. F., LUKSKA, G. L., SAVATEEV, S. K. and NAUMOV, A. D. (1986) Steroid-receptor complexes and their interactions with rat liver nuclei during ontogenesis. *Mech. Aging and Devel.* **35**: 95-107.

LAI, H. BOWDEN, D. M. and HORITA, A. (1987) Age-related decreases in dopamine receptors in the caudate nucleus and putamen of the Rhesus monkey (*Macaca mulatta*). *Neurobiology of Aging* **8**: 45-49.

LANDFIELD, P. W. and PITLER, T. A. (1984) Prolonged $Ca^{2+}$-dependent after hyper-polarizations in hippocampal neurons of aged rats. *Science* **276**: 1089-1091.

LATHAM, K. R. and FINCH, C. E. (1976) Hepatic glucocorticoid binders in mature and senescent C57BL/6J mice. *Endocrinology* **98**: 1480-1489.

MAYER, M., AMIN, R. and SHAFRIR, E. (1981) Effect of age on myofibrillary protease activity and muscle binding of glucocorticoid hormones in the rat. *Mech. Aging and Devel.* **17**: 1-10.

MELDOLESI, J. and POZZAN, T. 1987. Pathways of $Ca^{2+}$ influx at the plasma membrane: voltage-, receptor-, and second messenger- operated channels. *Exp. Cell Res.* **171**: 271-283.

MEYER, E. M., CREWS, F. T., OTERO, H. and LARSON, K. (1986) Aging decreases the sensitivity of rat cortical synaptosomes to calcium ionophore-induced acetylcholine release. *J. Neurochem.* **47**: 1244-1246.

MICHAELIS, M. L., JOHE, K. and KITOS, T. E. (1984) Age-dependent alterations in synaptic membrane systems for calcium regulation. *Mech. Aging and Devel.* **25**: 215-225.

MILLER, R. A. (1986) Immunodeficiency of aging: restorative effects of phorbol ester combined with calcium ionophore. *J. Immunol.* **137**: 805-808.

NARAYANAN, N. and DERBY, J. (1982) Alterations in the properties of β-adrenergic receptors of myocardial membranes in aging: impairments in agonist-receptor interactions and guanine nucleotide regulation accompany diminished catecholamine responsiveness of adenylate cyclase. *Mech. Aging and Devel.* **l9**: 127-139.

NELSON, F. J., HOLINKA, C. F., LATHAM, K. R., ALLEN, J. K., and FINCH, C. E. (1976) Corticosteroid binding in cytosols from brain regions of mature and senescent male C57BL/6J mice. *Brain Res.* **115**: 345-351.

O'MALLEY, B. W. and MEANS, A. R. (1978) *Receptors for Reproductive Hormones.* New York, NY: Plenum Press.

ORIDA, N. and FELDMAN, J. D. (1982) Age related deficiency in calcium uptake by most cells. *Fed. Proc.* **41**: 822.

PARCHMAN, G. L., CAKE, M. H. and LITWACK, G. L. (1978) Functionality of the liver glucocorticoid receptor during the life cycle and development of a low affinity membrane binding site. *Mech. Aging and Devel.* **7**: 227-240.

PETERSON, C. and GIBSON, G.E. 1983. Amelioration of age-related neurochemical and behavioral deficits by 3, 4-diamopyridine. Neurobiol. of Aging **4**: 25-30.

PETERSON, C. and GIBSON, G. E. (1984) Aging and 3, 4 diaminopyridine alter synaptosomal calcium uptake. *J. Biol. Chem.* **258**: 11482-11486.

PETERSON, C. and GOLDMAN, J. E. (1986) Alterations in calcium content and biochemical processes in cultured skin fibroblasts from aged and Alzheimer donors. *Proc. Nat. Acad. Sci. USA* **83**: 2758-2762.

PETERSON, C., NICHOLLS, D. G. and GIBSON, G. E. (1985) Subsynaptosomal distribution of calcium during aging and 3, 4 diaminopyridine treatment. *Neurobiol. of Aging* **6**: 297-304.

PETROVIC, J. S. and MARKOVIC, R. Z. (1975) Changes in cortical binding to soluble receptor proteins in rat liver and thymus during development and aging. *Devel. Biol.* **45**: 176-182.

PRAEGER, F. C. and CRISTOFALO, V. J. (1984) Age-related loss of response to elevated $CaCl_2$ by WI-38 cells. *The Gerontologist* **24**: 226-227.

RICHARDSON, D. A., BUTLER, J. A., RUTHERFORD, M. S., SEMSEI, I., GU, M. Z., FERNANDES, G. and CHIANG, W. H. (1987) Effect of age and dietary restriction on the expression of $\alpha_{2u}$-globulin. *J. Biol. Chem.* **262**: 12821-12825.

ROSNER, B. A. and CRISTOFALO, V. J. (1981) Changes in specific dexamethasone binding during aging in WI-38 cells. *Endocrinology* **108**: 1965-1971.

ROTH, G. S. (1974) Age related changes in specific glucocorticoid binding by steroid responsive tissues of rats. *Endocrinology* **94**: 82-90.

ROTH, G. S. (1975) Reduced glucocorticoid responsiveness and receptor concentration in splenic leukocytes of senescent rats. *Biochem. Biophys. Acta* **399**: 145-156.

ROTH, G. S. (1976) Reduced glucocorticoid binding site concentration in cortical neuronal perikanya from senescent rats. *Brain Res.* **107**: 345-354.

ROTH, G. S. (1978) Hormonal receptor and responsiveness changes during aging: genetic modulations. **In:** *Genetic Effects on Aging* (Eds. D. Bergsma and D. E. Harrison) pp. 365-384. New York, N.Y.: A.R. Liss.

ROTH, G. S. (1979) Hormone action during aging: alterations and mechanisms. *Mech. Aging and Devel.* **9**: 497-514.

ROTH, G. S. (1985) Changes in hormone/neurotransmitter action during aging. **In:** *Homeostatic Function and Aging* (Eds. B. B. Davis and W. G. Wood), pp. 41-58. New York, NY: Raven Press.

ROTH, G. S. (1988) Changes in hormone action with age; altered calcium mobilization and/or responsiveness impaires signal transduction. **In:** *Endocrine Function and Aging* (Ed. H. J. Armbrecht) in press. New York, N.Y.: Springer Verlag.

ROTH, G. S., HENRY, J. M. and JOSEPH, J. A. (1986) The striatal dopaminergic system as a model of altered neurotransmitter action during aging: effects of dietary and neuroendocrine manipulations. *Progr. Brain Res.* **70**: 473-484.

ROTH, G. S. and HESS, G. D. (1982) Changes in the mechanisms of hormone and neurotransmitter action during aging: current status and the role of receptor and post receptor alterations. *Mech. Aging and Devel.* **20**: 175-194.

SAPOLSKY, R. M., KREY, L. C. and McEWEN, B. S. (1983) Corticosterone receptors decline in a site-specific manner in the aged rat brain. *Brain Res.* **289**: 235-240.

SAPOLSKY, R. M, KREY, L. C., McEWEN, B. S. and RAINBOW, T. C. (1984) Do vasopressin-related peptides induce hippocampal corticosterone receptors? Implications for aging. *J. Neurosci.* **4**: 1479-1485.

SCARPACE, P. J. and ABRASS, I. B. (1983) Decreased beta-adrenergic agonist affinity and adenylate cyclase activity in senescent rat lung. *J. Gerontology* **38**: 143-147.

SEGAL, J. (1986) Studies on the age-related decline in the response of lymphoid cells to mitogens: measurement of concanavalin A binding and stimulation of calcium and sugar uptake in thymocytes from rats of varying ages. *Mech. Aging and Devel.* **33**: 295-303

SHAIN, S. A. and BOESEL, R. W. (1977) Aging-associated diminished rat prostrate androgen receptor content concurrent with decreased androgen dependence. *Mech. Aging and Devel.* **6**: 219-232.

SHARMA, R. and TIMIRAS, P. S. (1987) Regulatory changes in glucocorticoid receptors n the skeletal muscle of immature and mature male rats. *Mech. Aging and Devel.* **37**: 249-256.

SINGER, S. H., ITO, H. and LITWACK, G. L. (1973) $^3$H-cortisal binding by young and old human liver cytosol proteins *in vitro*. *Intl. J. Biochem.* **4**: 569-573.

STEFANO, G. B. and LEUNG, M. K. (1986) Opioid aging and seasonal variations in invertebrate ganglia: evidence for an opioid compensatory mechanism. **In:** *Handbook of Comparative Opioid and Related Neuropeptide Mechanisms.* Vol 2. (Eds. G.B. Stefano) pp. 199-209, Boca Raton, FL: CRC Press.

STEWART, D., BLACKMAN, M. R., DANNER, D. P., KOWATCH, M. A., and ROTH, G. S. (1988) Discordant age-related alterations in prolactin and LH-β gene expression in the female rat. *Endocrinology* in press.

VITORICA, J. and SATUSTEGUI, J. (1986) The influence of age on the calcium-efflux pathway and matrix calcium buffering in brain mitochondria. *Biochem. Biophys. Acta.* **851**: 209-216.

WILLIAMS, P. B. (1984) Effect of age upon the uptake and binding of calcium in rat aorta. *Biochem. Pharmacol.* **33**: 3097-3099.

WILLIAMS, R. H. (1981) *Textbook of Endocrinology.* Philadelphia, PA: Saunders.

WISE, P. M., McEWEN, B. S., PARSONS, B. and RAINBOW, T. C. (1984) Age related changes in cytoplasmic estradiol receptor concentrations in microdissected brain nuclei: correlation with changes in steroid induced sexual behavior. *Brain Research* **321**: 119-126.

WU, W., PAHLAVANI, M., RICHARDSON, A. and CHEUNG, H. T. (1985) Effect of age on lymphocyte proliferation induced by A-23187 through an interleukin independent pathway. *J. Leukocyte Biol.* **38**: 531-540.

## DISCUSSION

1. Asked whether the binding constant for dopamine changes with age, Roth replied that there are no overall changes in binding affinities with antagonists, but with agonists there are two states, high and low affinity, and the amount of the high affinity declines with age. With epinephrine receptors the binding of agonists doesn't change, and that of antagonists declines with age. There are no changes with age in the PRL storage pool, either in the serum or within cells. The data are not yet available on synthesis *vs.* removal rates; obviously, balanced changes in these cannot detected from equilibrium levels.

2. E2 levels in females do, of course, change with age. Nelson points out that E2 doesn't simply increase as mice stop cycling, it goes to a less fluctuating pattern, with levels slightly higher than basal during cycling, but less than the most elevated levels reached during cycling. E2 levels during diestrous are similar in cycling 6-7 month olds and in the constant diestrous 25 month olds.

# 21

# GENE EXPRESSION IN T LYMPHOCYTES FROM AGING MICE

Richard A. Miller


## ABSTRACT

The decline in T lymphocyte-dependent immune function in old mice and humans can be modelled convincingly by *in vitro* culture protocols. Recent work on T cell activation has shown that aging leads to a decline in the proportion of T cells that can respond to activating mitogens. Defects in the generation of calcium signals, involving both diminished influx of calcium ions and probably increased activity of cytoplasmic extrusion systems, seem to contribute to sluggish responses, and are especially dramatic in a T cell subset marked by surface expression of the PGP-1 marker, a glycoprotein thought to demark memory T cell populations. Although work on age-dependent losses in expression of T cell activation genes is still in its infancy, early work has revealed defects in expression of the growth factor IL-2 and of its receptor, and alterations in the expression of the c-myc proto-oncogene. In the mouse, the decline in c-myc mRNA expression seems not to reflect any loss in production of primary transcripts, but may instead represent alterations in the processing or stabilization of these transcripts.


The mouse immune system presents many advantages as a model in which to examine age-associated changes in gene expression. T lymphocyte function can be shown to decline with age using a wide variety of *in vivo* and *in vitro* assays, a fair selection of which can also be employed in studies of human aging. The labors of a sizeable cadre of basic immunologists have provided the immunogerontologist with monoclonal antibodies that dissect the interacting lymphocyte populations, and with cloned probes for the interaction molecules that determine immune specificity and amplify immune responses. Indeed, thanks to its fluid anatomical configuration, the immune system is one of the few complex, multicellular systems that can be removed from the body, dissected into its component cellular constituents, and re-assembled, either in culture or in an adoptive host, in a way that will faithfully mimic the function of the original. Age-associated decline in T cell function can be retarded by calorie restriction (Weindruch *et al.*, 1982, Miller and Harrison, 1984), allowing gerontologists to exploit this powerful probe of the aging process. Until recently, assessment of murine immune function almost always required access to spleen cells, making longitudinal studies impractical and direct comparison to human immunology (which is largely a study of peripheral blood cells) invalid. Limiting dilution methods, however, make it feasible to assess murine helper, cytotoxic, and growth factor dependent proliferation on blood samples as small as 5 to 50 microliters (Miller, 1984), and *in situ* hybridization combined with fluorescent cell sorting methods now allows one to examine expression of specific genes in specific subpopulations without sacrificing the donor.

This essay has two goals: (1) to provide a brief overview of our current understanding of immune decline in aging mice; and (2) to review the small amount of information already available about how disordered gene expression contributes to immune dysfunction. More comprehensive reviews of T cell immune function in aging can be found in recent review articles (Gottesman, 1987; Miller, 1989). There are at least two major classes of T lymphocytes, "cytotoxic" cells that can bind to and lyse specific targets (*e.g.* tumor cells, or virally infected cells), and "helper" cells that provide signals required for function by the cytotoxic T cells as well as by B lymphocytes, macrophages, and several types of non-lymphoid cell as well. Helper cells often provide their help in the form of antigen-nonspecific growth and maturation factors called lymphokines, of which interleukin 2 (IL-2), a growth factor for both T and B cells, is among the best characterized. (Most classifications of T cells also mention "suppressor" T cells, thought to regulate immune responses at a variety of levels. Experiments on suppressor T cells are very difficult to interpret, if indeed such cells exist as a distinct class of lymphocytes, and little consensus has emerged about the numbers, specificity, and properties of these cells, or their possible role in the aging process.) Defects have been demonstrated in the production of IL2 by helper T cells from old mice (Gillis *et al.*, 1981; Thoman and Weigle, 1981; Miller and Stutman, 1981), as well as in the response to IL2 (Gillis *et al.*, 1981) and in the production of IL-2 receptors (Vie and Miller, 1986; Nagel *et al.*, 1988).

Although defects can thus be defined in both the helper and cytotoxic subsets, not all T cells within each subset are equally affected by age. This conclusion is supported by several lines of evidence. First, limiting dilution culture assays (Nordin and Collins, 1983; Miller, 1984) have shown that the number of splenic T cells able to respond to a mitogen declines with age, whether the response is detected by IL-2 production, the generation of cytotoxic effectors, or IL-2 dependent clonal proliferation. The amount of functional effect (*e.g.* lymphokine secreted, or cytotoxic clone size generated) by each clonal precursor that does respond, however, seems not to be affected by donor age. Similar findings have emerged from tests of mouse peripheral blood T cells (Miller and Harrison, 1984). Flow cytometric cell cycle studies of human T cells have suggested a decline, with donor age, in the proportion of peripheral blood cells that can leave the resting $G_0$ phase for the $G_1$ and later stages of the mitotic cell cycle (Staiano-Coico *et al.*, 1984; Kubbies *et al.*, 1985). Cell cycle studies of mouse T cell responses, using thymidine incorporation kinetics (Abraham *et al.*, 1977), have reached similar conclusions.

From this perspective, the aging immune system resembles a mosaic of functional and nonfunctional cells, in which nonfunctional cells gradually become an increasing proportion of the population as the animal grows older. Recent work from our laboratory has centered on two questions: what is wrong with the nonfunctional cells, and where do they come from?

We have evidence that some T cells from aging mice exhibit defects in the receptor-coupled activation process detectable within the first 60 seconds of exposure to a mitogen. Con A induces a rapid increase in cytoplasmic calcium concentration ("$[Ca]_i$") from a resting level between 100 and 150 nanomolar to a level between 250 and 400 nanomolar, but the average $[Ca]_i$ is lower in T cells from old mice, and the proportion of T cells that exhibit any increase in $[Ca]_i$ also declines with age (Miller *et al.*, 1987). Both CD4(+) helper and CD8(+) cytotoxic cells are affected (Philosophe and Miller, submitted). In principle, such a defect might represent alterations in either the rate of mitogen-induced $Ca^{2+}$ influx or in the activity of systems that act to buffer rapid changes in $[Ca]_i$, most probably the plasma membrane calcium pump. We have evidence suggesting that alterations in both factors may contribute to the activation defect. The rate of $^{45}Ca$ influx into Con A treated T cells does indeed decline over the first 60 seconds after mitogen addition in T cells from old mice (Lerner, Philosophe, and Miller, 1988). On the other hand, altered influx cannot be the entire story, since T cells from old mice are relatively resistant to changes in $[Ca]_i$ even when such changes are induced by exposure to the calcium ionophore ionomycin, an agent that bypasses receptor-dependent signal transduction pathways by facilitating calcium translocation across the plasma membrane in the direction of the 10,000-fold trans-membrane concentration gradient (Miller *et al.*, 1989). We can show that there is no age-dependent decline in the rate at which ionomycin/calcium complexes enter T cells, and therefore take these results as indirect evidence for an age-dependent increase in the efficiency of the calcium buffering processes. Such an increase could play a major role in blunting the rise in $[Ca]_i$ that is thought to help initiate the T cell activation process.

We also have recent evidence to suggest that the age-related defects in $Ca^{2+}$ signal generation contribute to the decline in the number of functional T cells as measured by limiting dilution culture assays. Using the fluorescence-activated cell sorter to separate those T cells whose [Ca]ᵢ increases after Con A treatment from those that do not, we found (Philosophe and Miller, submitted) that the former cell population was greatly enriched, and the latter greatly depleted, in functionally competent T cells using culture assays for IL-2 production, proliferation, and cytotoxicity. Interestingly, similar degrees of enrichment were obtained whether the T cells were initially stimulated by Con A, by antibody to the CD3 ε chain of the T cell antigen receptor, or even by the receptor-independent stimulator ionomycin. These results suggest that there may exist a population of T cells that are rare in young mice but relatively frequent in old mice, and that are relatively refractory to any agent that tends to increase [Ca]ᵢ. The cells in this population are in fact the ones that fail to proliferate and to mature in the *in vitro* functional assays.

Work in my laboratory has also recently identified a cell surface marker that seems to discriminate functional from hypofunctional cells in mice, and that suggests a developmental origin for the less responsive cells. PGP-1 is a 95 kDa surface glycoprotein widely distributed among lymphoid and nonlymphoid cells within the mouse (Trowbridge *et al.*, 1982). Within the peripheral T cell population, however, evidence is accumulating to suggest (Budd *et al.*, 1987a; Budd *et al.*, 1987b) that virgin T cells, newly emigrating from the thymus, express relatively little PGP1, and that an encounter with antigen may lead to an increase in surface PGP1 expression as a part of the activation process. The $PGP1^{hi}$ phenotype, once acquired, seems to be long lasting, in that most memory T cells are $PGP1^{hi}$ in both mice and humans (Sanders *et al.*, 1988). We reasoned that memory cells were likely to continue to accumulate as new antigens were encountered throughout the lifespan, while the output of new, $PGP1^{lo}$ virgin T cells from thymus was likely to decline with age, and that these factors in combination would increase the relative proportion of $PGP1^{hi}$ T cells in old mice. We have in fact been able to demonstrate (Lerner, Yamada, and Miller, submitted) that the proportion of $PGP1^{hi}$ T cells does indeed increase with age, from about 25% of the T cell pool in young mice to about 60% in 18 - 24 month old animals. Equivalent shifts are seen among helper and cytotoxic subpopulations, and are seen within blood, spleen, and lymph node populations. We have also found that $PGP1^{hi}$ T cells are dramatically less able to respond in functional assays. Interestingly, $PGP1^{lo}$ cells isolated from old mice, though fewer in number than in young mice, are fully as competent to respond to Con A (Lerner, Yamada, and Miller, submitted). Within the helper population, $PGP1^{hi}$ cells, compared to $PGP1^{lo}$ cells, are also less able to generate calcium signals after exposure to Con A, anti-CD3 antibody, or ionomycin (Philosophe and Miller, submitted). Thus PGP1, a marker for previously-activated peripheral T cells, seems to distinguish a population of T cells whose numbers increase in old mice and that are relatively unable to respond to calcium-linked mitogenic agents. The ability to isolate hyporesponsive T cells on the basis of PGP1 and $Ca^{2+}$ signal generation should provide us with useful cellular material in which to examine age-dependent losses in gene activation.

Some activating agents (*e.g.* Con A, some anti-CD3 antibodies) induce all steps of T cell activation through DNA synthesis and mitosis, while others activate only a subset of these transitions. The protein kinase activator phorbol myristate acetate (PMA) and the calcium ionophore ionomycin, used together, are mitogenic for resting mouse T cells, and lead to the sequential activation of the *c-fos* and *c-myc* proto-oncogenes, followed by induction of the genes for the growth factor IL2 and its receptor, and eventually by histone gene activation and DNA replication. PMA in the absence of ionophore, however, induces *c-myc*, *c-fos*, and IL2 receptor activation but not IL2 synthesis; PMA treated cells thus become responsive to added IL2, but do not proceed into S-phase unless IL2 is added. Doses of ionomycin that are co-mitogenic with PMA do lead to activation of *c-fos* and *c-myc*, but to neither IL2 nor IL2 receptor activation. Stimulation of T cells with one or the other of these "partial" mitogens can therefore provide an interesting model with which to investigate activation of the complementary pathways that together lead to full responsiveness.

Very little data is currently available to suggest how aging alters expression of these cell cycle-linked genes. Wu *et al.* (1986) have published data showing a decline, with age, in mRNA accumulation for IL2 in rat spleen cells stimulated with Con A, suggesting that declines in IL2 secretion in this species may be related to underlying defects in expression of the IL2 gene. Holbrook *et al.* (1988), however, using a Northern blotting method less susceptible to cross-reacting species than the dot-blotting method employed by Wu *et al.*, have found no decline in IL2 mRNA accumulation in Con A stimulated rat splenic T cells, and in fact the question of whether aging leads to a decline in IL2 (protein) production in this species is in conflict (Gilman *et al.*, 1982; Wu *et al.*, 1986; Holbrook *et al.*, 1988). In humans, Nagel *et al.* (1988) have found an age-specific decline in the accumulation of mRNA for both IL2 and the IL2 receptor in peripheral blood T cells stimulated with PHA. Our own preliminary data on mouse T cells (Macauley and Miller, unpublished) suggests that aging leads to a consistent decline in mRNA accumulation for the p55 component of the IL2 receptor after Con A stimulation.

It is clear that far more information, using a variety of activating agents, will be needed before a coherent picture emerges.

Changes in expression of these mid-$G_1$ genes are likely to represent the consequences of disordered expression of genes that act much earlier in the activation process, among which the proto-oncogenes are especially good candidates for study. We have shown (Buckler *et al.*, 1988) that Con A induces increased accumulation of c-myc mRNA in T cells of both young and old donors within an hour, levels that peak within 4 - 8 hours before declining. While c-myc mRNA expression is timed identically in T cells from young and old mice, the amount of mRNA accumulation in old T cells is about 2-fold lower. *In situ* hybridization experiments are in progress to determine if, as we expect, this decline represents a 2-fold loss in the number of T cells expressing c-myc. In other cell types, changes in the level of c-myc have in some cases been shown to depend largely on mitogen-induced increases in transcription rates, in some cases supplemented by increases in the stability of this very short-lived mRNA. Our data, surprisingly, were consistent with neither possibility. We found that c-myc mRNA, once formed, was degraded with a $t_{1/2}$ between 10 and 15 minutes in both young and old T cells (Buckler *et al.*, 1988). In three experiments using the nuclear run-on method to measure gene transcription rates, we found that Con A induced a 6-fold increase in transcription rate in T cells from both young and old donor animals. This disparity between the decline in accumulation of the mature mRNA and the unaltered rate of transcription suggests that aging might lead to defects in the processing, stabilization, or export of the primary intranuclear transcripts for c-myc. Such a mechanism would not be entirely unprecedented: interferon treatment of cells of a murine myeloid line inhibits the accumulation of mature, cytoplasmic c-myc mRNA, without a corresponding block in transcription, by causing the accumulation of an unspliced intranuclear precursor of the cytoplasmic species (Harel-Bellan *et al.*, 1988).

Studies of *c-myc* expression in T lymphocytes from human peripheral blood have reached somewhat different conclusions (Gamble, 1987). In good agreement with the murine data, PHA seems to stimulate less c-myc mRNA accumulation in T cells from old donors than from young donors. In contrast to the murine data, however, Gamble was able to document a decline, with donor age, in mitogen induced transcription of the downstream exons of the *c-myc* gene. It remains to be seen whether the differences between the human and mouse results reflect differences in species, cell source (blood *vs.* spleen), mitogen (PHA *vs.* Con A) or a technical artifact. It will also be informative to search for age-dependent processing defects in transcripts of other genes stimulated early in the T cell activation process (*e.g. c-fos*) and to examine the effects of other mitogenic agents. It will be important to apply more sensitive methods that can monitor gene expression in the smaller numbers of T cells available from cell sorter methods, *e.g. in situ* hybridization, or combinations of reverse transcription and the polymerase chain reaction recently shown to be able to quantify lymphokine mRNA extracted from samples as small as a few hundred cells (Rappolee *et al.*, 1988). Ultimately, our goal must be to explain age-associated changes in the activation of specific gene sequences in terms of corresponding changes in the signal transduction pathways that stimulate gene expression, the state of the chromatin controlling the expressibility of specific transcripts, and the processing systems that convert the original transcripts into functional mRNAs.

## ACKNOWLEDGEMENTS

This work was supported by NIH grants AG-03978 and AG-07114, by a Scholar Award from the Leukemia Society of America, and by a Research Career Development Award from the National Institute on Aging.

## REFERENCES

ABRAHAM, C., TAL, Y. and GERSHON, H. (1977) Reduced *in vitro* response to concanavalin A and lipopolysaccharide in senescent mice: a function of reduced number of responding cells. *Eur. J. Immunol.* **7**: 301-304

BUCKLER, A., VIE, H., SONENSHEIN, G. and MILLER, R. A. (1987) Defective T lymphocytes in old mice: diminished production of mature c-myc RNA after mitogen exposure not attributable to alterations in transcription or RNA stability. *J. Immunol.* **140**: 2442-2446

BUDD, R. C., CEROTTINI, J. C., HORVATH, C., BRON, C., PEDRAZZINI, T., HOWE, R. C. and MACDONALD, H. R. (1987a) Distinction of virgin and memory T lymphocytes. Stable acquisition of the PGP1 glycoprotein concomitant with antigenic stimulation. *J. Immunol.* **138**: 3120-3129

BUDD, R. C., CEROTTINI, J. C. and MACDONALD, H. R. (1987b) Phenotypic identification of memory cytolytic T lymphocytes in a subset of Lyt-2$^+$ cells. *J. Immunol.* **138**: 1009-1013

GAMBLE, D. A. (1987) *Analysis of c-myc gene expression in relationship to proliferative capacity in human lymphocytes and the effect of aging.* Ph.D. Thesis Cornell University Medical College.

GILLIS, S., KOZAK, R., DURANTE, M. and WEKSLER, M. E. (1981) Immunological studies of aging. Decreased production of and response to T cell growth factor by lymphocytes from aged humans. *J. Clin. Invest.* **67**: 937-942

GILMAN, S. C., ROSENBERG, J. S. and FELDMAN, J. D. (1982) T lymphocytes of young and aged rats. II. Functional defects and the role of Interleukin-2. *J. Immunol.* **128**: 644-650

GOTTESMAN, S. R. S. (1987) Changes in T-cell-mediated immunity with age: an update. *Rev. Biol. Res. Aging* **3**: 79-111

HAREL-BELLAN, A., BRINI, A. T. and FARRAR, W. L. (1988) IFNγ inhibits *c-myc* gene expression by impairing the splicing process in a colony-stimulating factor dependent murine myeloid cell line. *J. Immunol.* **141**: 1012-1017

HOLBROOK, N. J., CHOPRA, R. K., McCOY, M. T., NAGEL, J. E., ADLER, W. H. and SCHNEIDER, E. L. (1988) Expression of Interleukin 2 and the Interleukin 2 receptor in aging rats. *Cell. Immunol.* in press.

KUBBIES, M., SCHINDLER, D., HOEHN, H. and RABINOVITCH, P. S. (1985) BrdU-Hoechst flow cytometry reveals regulation of human lymphocyte growth by donor-age-related growth fraction and transition rate. *J. Cell. Physiol.* **125**: 229-234

LERNER, A., PHILOSOPHE, B. and MILLER, R. A. (1988) Defective calcium influx and preserved inositol phosphate generation in T cells from old mice. *Aging: Immunol. and Infect. Dis.* **1**: 149-157

MILLER, R. A. (1984) Age-associated decline in precursor frequency for different T cell-mediated reactions, with preservation of helper or cytotoxic effect per precursor cell. *J. Immunol.* **132**: 63-68

MILLER, R. A. (1989) Aging and the immune response. **In**: *Handbook of the Biology of Aging* (Ed. E. L. Schneider), in press.

MILLER, R. A. and HARRISON, D. E. (1984) Delayed reduction in T cell precursor frequencies accompanies diet-induced lifespan extension. *J. Immunol.* **136**: 977-983

MILLER, R. A., JACOBSON, B., WEIL, G. and SIMONS, E. R. (1987) Diminished calcium influx in lectin-stimulated T cells from old mice. *J. Cell. Physiol.* **132**: 337-342

MILLER, R. A., PHILOSOPHE, B., GINIS, I., WEIL, G. and JACOBSON, B. (1989) Defective control of cytoplasmic calcium in T lymphocytes from old mice. *J. Cell. Physiol.* **138**: 175-182

MILLER, R. A. and STUTMAN, O. (1981) Decline, in aging mice, of the anti-TNP cytotoxic T cell response attributable to loss of Lyt-2⁻, IL2 producing helper cell function. *Eur. J. Immunol.* **11**: 751-756

NAGEL, J. E., CHOPRA, R. K., CHREST, F. J., McCOY, M. T., SCHNEIDER, E. L., HOLBROOK, N. J. and ADLER, W. H. (1988) Decreased proliferation, interleukin 2 synthesis, and interleukin 2 receptor expression are accompanied by decreased mRNA expression in phytohemagglutinin-stimulated cells from elderly donors. *J. Clin. Invest.* **81**: 1096-1102

NORDIN, A. A. and COLLINS, G. D. (1983) Limiting dilution analysis of alloreactive cytotoxic precursor cells in aging mice. *J. Immunol.* **131**: 2215-2218

RAPPOLEE, D. A., MARK, D., BANDA, M. J. and WERB, Z. (1988) Wound macrophages express TGF-α and other growth factors *in vivo*: analysis by mRNA phenotyping. *Science* **241**: 708-712

SANDERS, M. E., MAKGOBA, M. W., SHARROW, S. O., STEPHANY, D., SPRINGER, T. A., YOUNG, H. A. and SHAW, S. (1988) Human memory T lymphocytes express increased levels of three cell adhesion molecules (LFA-3, CD2, and LFA-1) and three other molecules (UCHL1, CDw29, and PGP1) and have enhanced IFN-gamma production. *J. Immunol.* **140**: 1401-1407

STAIANO-COICO, L., DARZYNKIEWICZ, Z., MELAMED, M. R. and WEKSLER, M. E. (1984) Immunological studies of aging. IX. Impaired proliferation of T lymphocytes detected in elderly humans by flow cytometry. *J. Immunol.* **132**: 1788-1792

THOMAN, M. L. and WEIGLE, W. O. (1981) Lymphokines and aging: Interleukin-2 production and activity in aged animals. *J. Immunol.* **127**: 2101-2106

TROWBRIDGE, I. S., LESLEY, J., SCHULTE, R., HYMAN, R. and TROTTER, J. (1982) Biochemical characterization and cellular distribution of a polymorphic, murine cell-surface glycoprotein expressed on lymphoid tissues. *Immunogenetics* **15**: 299-312.

VIE, H. and MILLER, R. A. (1986) Decline, with age, in the proportion of mouse T cells that express IL2 receptors after mitogen stimulation. *Mech. Aging and Dev.* **33**: 313-322

WEINDRUCH, R., GOTTESMAN, S. R. S. and WALFORD, R. L. (1982) Modification of age-related immune decline in mice dietarily restricted from or after midadulthood. *Immunology* **79**: 898-902

WU, W., PAHLAVANI, M., CHEUNG, H. T. and RICHARDSON, A. (1986) The effect of aging on the expression of Interleukin 2 messenger ribonucleic acid. *Cellular Immunol.* **100**: 224-231

## DISCUSSION

1. If the only changes with age in this system are in the percentages of T cells with particular receptors, then these are changes in cell populations, and the mechanism may lie at the level of control for T cell populations. Answering the question, is the inability of cells from old mice to respond to calcium ions a change in the cell and not a change in the population, Miller noted that there are no changes in IP3 with age, IP4 is a product of IP3, and there is no loss with age in IP4 producing ability. He also noted that this result is controversial, and that one other group finds less IP3 generation with age, while his group finds no age difference.

2. PGP-1$^{hi}$ T cells appear to be defective in Miller's responses. Does this occur only because the thymus produces fewer PGP-1$^{lo}$ cells? These changes may be adaptive, for example in reducing the chances of T cells causing autoimmune reactions. PGP-1$^{hi}$ cells should respond well to their original antigens, if they are produced after an immune response. However they may gradually lose their ability to respond to anything. Whether membrane fluidity changes has not been tested in this system.

3. Asked to relate the molecular changes in T cells to functions of the organism, Miller noted that these T cells should respond poorly to immune stimuli in general. He noted that transplants of an infant thymus and young marrow were reported to improve T cell responses in old mice, but he has not looked at the PGPI marker in these T cells.

# Section 5

## CHROMOSOME REGIONS AND MUTATIONS AFFECTING AGING

# 22

# AN ANALYSIS OF CLASS I AND CLASS II MAJOR HISTOCOMPATIBILITY ANTIGEN EXPRESSION ON C57BL/6 LYMPHOCYTES DURING AGING

Diane Janick-Buckner and Carol M. Warner

## ABSTRACT

The products of the major histocompatibility complex (MHC) are cell surface glycoproteins which are involved in the recognition of, and response to, foreign antigens. Previous studies have suggested that the density of cell surface MHC antigen influences the immune response. An age-related change in the cell surface expression of these antigens may result in altered immune function. The expression of class I (H-2K$^b$ and H-2D$^b$) and class II (IA$^b$) antigens on the cell surface of peripheral blood and spleen lymphocytes from C57BL/6 mice was analyzed using an indirect immunofluorescence assay. While the relative fluorescence of the class I positive lymphocytes increased with age on both peripheral blood and spleen lymphocytes, the percentage of class I positive lymphocytes did not change in either tissue. In contrast, the percentage of spleen lymphocytes expressing IA$^b$ was significantly decreased in the spleen but not in the peripheral blood of aged mice. The relative fluorescence of IA$^b$ positive lymphocytes did not change with age in either the spleen or peripheral blood. The steady state level of class II mRNA in spleen lymphocytes was analyzed and was shown to decrease in the oldest mice analyzed. The age-related decline of splenic class II mRNA and IA$^b$ positive cells was determined to be due to a decrease in splenic B lymphocytes and a concomitant increase in the T lymphocyte population. These alterations in MHC antigen expression may contribute to the alterations in immune function during aging.

## INTRODUCTION

The age-related decline of immune function in humans and experimental animals has been well documented. Some of the functional changes which occur in lymphocytes during aging include impaired proliferation in response to antigen and mitogen (Weksler and Hutteroth, 1974; Cheung *et al.*, 1983; Negoro *et al.*, 1986, 1987), decreased interleukin-2 (IL-2) synthesis and secretion (Thoman and Weigle, 1983; Cheung *et al.*, 1983; Negoro *et al.*, 1986), decreased expression of IL-2 receptors (Negoro *et al.*, 1986) and alteration of membrane signal transduction (Miller, 1986; Proust *et al.*, 1987). Although both T and B lymphocyte activities are impaired with advancing age, it has been suggested that age-related changes in B lymphocyte function may result from altered T helper or T suppressor cell activity (Nordin and Makinodan, 1974; Krogsrud and Perkus, 1977; Serge and Serge, 1976). However, there is evidence to suggest that B cells from old individuals may be intrinsically defective (Whistler *et al.*, 1985; Ennist *et al.*, 1986; Hara *et al.*, 1987).

The major histocompatibility complex (MHC) antigens are cell surface glycoproteins that are involved in the recognition of, and response to, foreign antigens (McDevitt, 1981; Flavell *et al.*, 1986). The MHC in the mouse is referred to as the histocompatibility-2 or H-2 complex. The genes which encode these glycoproteins are located on chromosome 17 in the mouse and are divided into classes based on structural similarities.

Class I H-2K and H-2D antigens consist of a transmembrane heavy chain (45 kDa) which is noncovalently associated with a light chain, $\beta$-2 microglobulin (12 kDa), on the cell surface. These antigens are expressed on virtually all cells and are involved in graft rejection and cytotoxic T cell mediated lysis (McDevitt, 1981; Flavell *et al.*, 1986). Indeed, a minimum density of class I MHC antigen appears to be necessary on target cells in order for lysis by cytotoxic T cells to occur. Thus, the cell surface density of class I antigens may influence immune responsiveness (Goldstein and Mescher, 1987).

Class II MHC antigens are transmembrane heterodimers consisting of an $\alpha$-chain (33-34 kDa) and a $\beta$-chain (28-29 kDa). In the mouse, two isotypic forms of class II MHC antigens exist: these are IA, comprised of A$\alpha$ and A$\beta$ subunits, and IE, comprised of E$\alpha$ and E$\beta$ subunits. Class II MHC antigens are expressed constitutively on B cells and can be induced on macrophages, endothelial cells and certain epithelial cells (Hammerling *et al.*, 1976; Kearney *et al.*, 1977: Unanue *et al.*, 1984; Manyak *et al.*, 1988). Previous studies have indicated that the cell surface density of class II MHC antigens on macrophages and B cells is important in determining the magnitude of the immune response (Henry *et al.*, 1977; Bottomly *et al.*, 1983; Matis *et al.*, 1983; Bekkoucha *et al.*, 1984).

Since there is evidence to suggest that the cell surface density of class I and class II MHC antigens influences immune responsiveness, an age-related change in MHC antigen expression could result in an alteration in immune function. In this paper, the density of class I and class II antigens on the cell surface of peripheral blood and spleen lymphocytes from C57BL/6 mice of various ages was measured by an indirect immunofluorescence assay. In addition, the percentage of T and B lymphocytes in spleens of C57BL/6 mice at ages between 2 and 22 months was analyzed. Lastly, the steady state level of class II MHC mRNAs in spleen lymphocytes was measured using slot blot hybridization analysis.

## MATERIALS AND METHODS

### Mice

C57BL/6 mice (H-2$^b$ haplotype) were used from our own aging colony. Offspring of mice originally obtained from the Jackson Laboratories (Bar Harbor, Maine) were added to the colony every 6 months and maintained under clean, conventional conditions. Only mice which appeared healthy and displayed no gross visible internal or external abnormalities were used. Both male and female mice were used in each age group in all experiments.

### Spleen Lymphocyte Preparation

Peripheral blood was collected from mice at the ages indicated *via* the orbital venous sinus using heparinized capillary tubes (Allied Corp., Fisher Scientific, Pittsburgh, Pennsylvania). The blood was diluted into phosphate buffered saline, pH 7.0 containing 60 U/ml heparin (Sigma Chemical Co., St. Louis, Missouri) and then centrifuged at 3000 × g for 5 minutes through a Ficoll-Hypaque density gradient (density=1.094) to remove red blood cells. The mononuclear cell layer was removed and washed in RPMI-1640 (Gibco Laboratories, Grand Island, New York), 1% gamma globulin-free fetal calf serum (FCS; Gibco Laboratories), 0.1% NaN$_3$ (Fisher Scientific Co., Fair Lawn, New Jersey).

Spleens were removed after mice had been sacrificed by cervical dislocation. Single cell suspensions were obtained by pressing the spleens through a fine mesh screen. Mononuclear cells were isolated from the single cell suspension as described above.

## Immunofluorescence Staining and Analysis

The density of cell surface MHC antigens on peripheral blood and spleen lymphocytes was determined using an indirect immunofluorescence assay. All washes and incubations were done in RPMI-1640 medium containing 1% FCS and 0.1% NaN3. The intensity of fluorescence associated with cells after labelling should be proportional to the amount of antigen present on the cell surface. Cells were incubated for 1 hour at 4°C with one of the monoclonal antibodies Y-3P, 27-11-13 or B8-24-3, which recognize $IA^b$, $D^b$ and $K^b$, respectively (Janeway *et al.*, 1984; Ozato and Sachs, 1981; Kohler *et al.*, 1981). The cells were then washed and resuspended in medium containing fluorescein isothiocyanate (FITC)-conjugated goat anti-mouse antibodies specific for mouse IgG subclasses (ICN Biomedicals, Inc., Costa Mesa, California). Control cells were labelled with second layer antibodies alone in order to determine background fluorescence. After incubating 1 hour at 4°C, the cells were washed and resuspended in medium containing 1% formaldehyde. The cells were fixed for 12 hours at 4°C, washed and then analyzed on a flow cytometer.

In order to analyze splenic B and T lymphocyte populations, a dual immunofluorescence assay was utilized. MHC antigens were labelled as above, whereas, cell surface IgM or Thy 1.2 were labelled with antibodies specific to either of them (rabbit anti-mouse IgM, Jackson Immuno Research Laboratories, Inc., West Grove, Pennsylvania; or rat anti-mouse Thy 1.2, Becton-Dickinson, Mountain View, California), using an appropriate R-phycoerythrin (PE)-conjugate as a second layer (PE-goat $F(ab')_2$ anti-rabbit IgG, Tago Immunologicals, Burlingame, California; or PE-goat anti-rat IgG, Caltag Laboratories, South San Francisco, California). Cells that were Thy 1.2⁻, IgM⁻ were considered null cells.

Cells were analyzed in an EPICS 752 flow cytometer (EPICS Division, Coulter Corporation, Hialeah, Florida) equipped with an argon ion laser (Coherent, Palo Alto, California) adjusted to emit 488 nm with a power output of 400 mW. Gating was performed according to forward light scatter and right angle light scatter in order to exclude cell debris, red blood cells and monocytes. Green and red fluorescence were monitored using a 525 nm and 575 nm band pass filter, respectively. Fluoresence data was collected on a log scale. For each sample, $10^4$ cells were analyzed. The mean fluorescence channel and percent positive cells were determined for each sample using an EASY88 computer analysis system (EPICS Division, Coulter Corporation).

## Slot Blot Hybridization Analysis of Class II MHC Spleen Lymphocyte mRNA

Steady state levels of class II MHC mRNAs were analyzed by slot blot hybridization analysis using a modified method of Pikó *et al.* (1984). The samples were prepared as described by Pikó *et al.* with modifications only in the DNA digestion step. DNA digestion was performed in the presence of 310 U/ml RNAs in (Promega Biotech, Madison, Wisconsin) and 5 mM dithiothreitol and the digestion time was extended to 1 hour. The RNA samples were blotted onto Zeta-Probe nylon membrane (Bio-Rad, Richmond, California) using a slot blot apparatus (Schleichter and Schuell, Inc., Keene, New Hampshire).

## $^{32}$P-Labelled DNA Probes

The DNA fragments used for making $^{32}$P-labelled probes specific for A$\alpha$, A$\beta$, E$\alpha$ and actin mRNAs were isolated from the following plasmids: 546 bp *Eco*RI-*Pst*I fragment from pcE$\beta$s2 (Mengle-Gaw and McDevitt, 1983, 1985); 683 bp *Pst*I fragment from pA$\alpha^d$ (Davis *et al.*, 1984); 550 bp *Sma*I fragment from pA$\beta^d$ (Malissen *et al.*, 1983); and a 1.5 kbp *Hind*III fragment from pRS$\alpha$A3 (Solomon and Rubenstein, 1987). Cells from C57BL/6 mice (H-2b haplotype) express only IA$^b$, not IE$^b$, on the cell surface (Jones *et al.*, 1981). This is due to a deletion in the promoter and signal peptide region of the E$\alpha$ gene, which is consequently not transcribed (Dembic *et al.*, 1985). However, the E$\beta$ gene is transcribed and its mRNA is present in the cytoplasm of cells which are capable of expressing it. Therefore, we analyzed the steady state levels of E$\beta$ in addition to A$\alpha$ and A$\beta$ class II MHC mRNAs.

The level of actin expression does not change with age in rodent lymphocytes (Cheung *et al.*, 1987); therefore, it was used as a control measure of sample RNA. DNA fragments were labelled with $^{32}$P-dCTP (New England Nuclear, Boston, Massachusetts) using an oligolabelling kit (Pharmacia Fine Chemicals, Piscataway, New Jersey). Filters were prehybridized at 42°C for about 3 hours as described previously (Maniatis *et al.*, 1982). Prehybridization buffer was removed and replaced with fresh buffer and 2-4 $\times$ $10^7$ cpm $^{32}$P-labelled DNA probe. Hybridization was done at 42°C for at least 24 hours. Following hybridization, filters were rinsed as recommended by the manufacturer. The filters were exposed to X-ray film at -70°C with an intensifying screen, and the resulting autoradiograms were scanned with a densitometer. The signal obtained for each sample was normalized to the sample's amount of actin signal. Data is expressed as percent of actin control.

## Statistical Analysis

Statistical analyses were performed using SAS 5.16 computer software (SAS Institute, Inc., Cary, North Carolina). Analysis of variance was applied to all data with $p < 0.05$ chosen as the level of significance.

## RESULTS

The results of the analyses performed on C57BL/6 peripheral blood lymphocytes from mice at 2, 8, 14 and 22 months of age are shown in Figures 1A and B. The cell surface density of class I and class II MHC antigens was measured by indirect immunofluorescence labelling. As can be seen in Figure 1A, there is a small but significant increase in the relative fluorescence of H-2K$^b$ on peripheral blood lymphocytes from mice of increasing ages ($p < 0.05$). This indicates that there is an increase in the density of this class I antigen on peripheral blood lymphocytes during aging. In contrast, the density of the class II antigen IA$^b$ did not change with advancing age since there was no change in the relative fluorescence of IA$^b$ positive peripheral blood lymphocytes ($p = 0.6$). An analysis of the percentage of peripheral blood lymphocytes expressing H-2K$^b$ or IA$^b$ (Figure 1B) indicated that the percentages of these lymphocytes in the peripheral blood were essentially the same at all of the ages analyzed ($p = 0.2$ and $p = 0.6$, respectively). It should be noted that data obtained from male versus female mice did not differ significantly, therefore, all data points are representative of combined male and female values.

The relative fluorescence of H-2K$^b$, H-2D$^b$ and IA$^b$ positive spleen lymphocytes is shown in Figure 2A. While there is an age-related increase in the relative fluorescence of spleen lymphocytes labelled with monoclonal antibodies to H-2K$^b$ and H-2D$^b$ antigens ($p < 0.01$ for both), a similar change does not appear following labelling of spleen lymphocytes with antibody to IA$^b$ ($p = 0.8$). Thus, it appears that the cell surface class I MHC antigen density on spleen lymphocytes increases with age while class II MHC antigen density remains essentially the same. These results are similar to those obtained above with peripheral blood lymphocytes.

It should be noted that although there superficially appears to be a difference in the cell surface density of the various class I and class II antigens analyzed on spleen lymphocytes (*i.e.*, IA$^b$ K$^b$ D$^b$ density) due to differences in relative fluorescence (*e.g.*, Figure 2A), it is not possible to make such a conclusion. This is because the manner in which the first and second layer antibodies interact with their target structures is not known (*i.e.*, number of immunoglobulin molecules per target; see Dower and Segal, 1985).

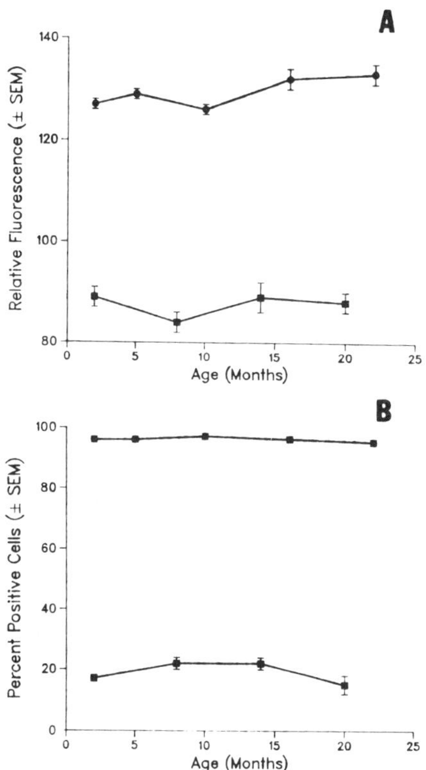


**Figure 1A.** Relative fluorescence of H-2K$^b$ (●) and IA$^b$ (■) positive peripheral blood lymphocytes. Values represents the mean ± SEM of 3 female and 3 male C57BL/6 mice at the ages 2, 8, 14 and 20 months. **Figure 1B.** Percentages of H-2K$^b$ (●) and IA$^b$ (■) lymphocytes in the peripheral blood lymphocyte population. Each point represents the mean ± SEM for the same mice used in Figure 1A.

The percentage of spleen lymphocytes which express class I and class II antigens is shown in Figure 2B. The percentage of H-2K$^b$ or H-2D$^b$ positive spleen lymphocytes does not change with age. However, the percentage of IA$^b$ positive spleen lymphocytes decreases with age (p < 0.01). Thus, the percentage of IA$^b$positive lymphocytes in the spleens of C57BL/6J mice declines with age, although the percentage of these cells in the peripheral blood does not change significantly.

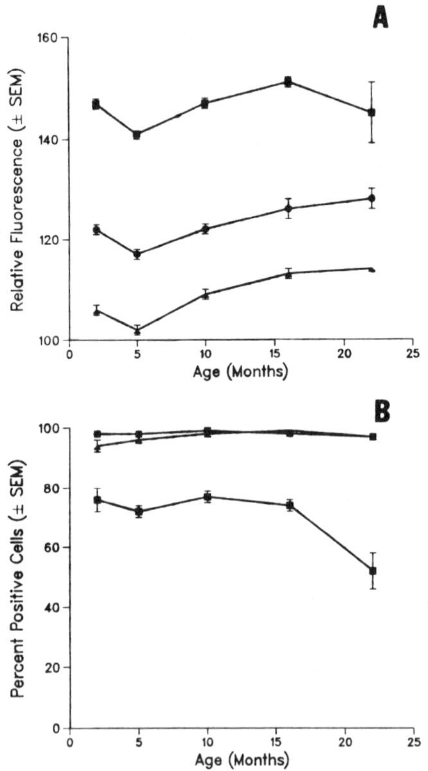



**Figure 2A.** Relative staining intensities of H-2K$^b$ (●), H-2D$^b$ (▲) and IA$^b$ (■) positive C57BL/6 spleen lymphocytes at 2, 5, 10, 16 and 22 months. Values represent the mean ± SEM of 6 mice (3 female and 3 male). **Figure 2B.** Percent H-2K$^b$ (●), H-2D$^b$ (▲) and IA$^b$ (■) positive lymphocytes in spleens of C57BL/6 mice. Each point represents the mean ± SEM for the same mice used in Figure 2A.

The age-related decline in IA$^b$ positive spleen lymphocytes could be due to an increase in a population(s) of cells which have similar light scatter characteristics but lack constitutive expression of IA$^b$ (*i.e.*, T cells or null cells) or to an increase in immature B lymphocytes (sIgM$^+$, IA$^-$) in the spleen (Hammerling *et al.*, 1976; Kearney *et al.*, 1977). In order to distinguish between these possibilities spleen lymphocytes were dual labelled with anti-MHC monoclonal antibodies and a FITC-conjugated second layer, and either anti-IgM or anti-Thy 1.2 antibodies which were labelled with an appropriate second layer PE-conjugate. The percentage of T and B lymphocytes and null cells which comprise the C57BL/6J spleen lymphocyte population at various ages is shown in Figure 3. There is an age-related decrease in the percentage of splenic IgM$^+$ (p < 0.05) cells and a concomitant increase in the percentage of cells that are Thy 1.2$^+$ (p < 0.01). The splenic null cell population did not change with age. In addition, the IgM$^+$, IA$^-$ lymphocyte population did not change with age (data not shown). Therefore, the age-related decline in splenic IA$^b$ positive cells appears to be due to a decrease in IgM$^+$, IA$^{b+}$ lymphocytes.

The steady state levels of A$\alpha$, A$\beta$ and E$\beta$ mRNAs were determined and are shown as percent of actin mRNA in Figures 4A and B. In each case, the steady state level of class II MHC mRNA is decreased in the oldest mice analyzed. This age-related decrease in spleen lymphocyte class II mRNA levels corresponds to the decrease in the percentage of spleen lymphocytes which are capable of expressing class II MHC mRNAs (*i.e.*, B lymphocytes).

## DISCUSSION

Class I and II MHC antigens are central in determining the immune response to foreign antigens (McDevitt, 1981; Flavell *et al.*, 1986). While virtually all cells express class I MHC antigens, class II MHC antigens are expressed on only a few cell types. Mature B-lymphocytes constitutively express class II MHC antigens and are capable of presenting foreign antigen to class II restricted T lymphocytes (Chestnut and Grey, 1981; Rock *et al.*, 1984).

It is well known that the functioning of the immune system declines during the process of aging. It has been suggested that this decline results in an increased susceptibility of the elderly to infections, autoimmune diseases and cancer (Haaijmans, 1987). Previous studies have suggested that the cell surface density of class I and class II antigens can influence the magnitude of immune response (Henry *et al.*, 1977; Bottomly *et al.*, 1983; Matis *et al.*, 1983 Bekkoucha *et al.*, 1984; Goldstein and Mescher, 1987). Therefore, an alteration in the level of expression of MHC antigens during aging could possibly contribute to age-related alterations in immune function.

Indeed, the studies presented in this paper demonstrate that there is an increase in the density of class I MHC antigens on both peripheral blood and spleen lymphocytes with age (Figure 1A and 2A). This increase was found to occur on both T and B lymphocyte populations in the spleen (data not shown). In contrast, the cell surface density of class II MHC antigens on C57BL/6 peripheral blood and spleen lymphocytes did not change significantly with age. Our results concerning class I density are in agreement with a similar study, however, our data regarding class II MHC density are not (Sidman *et al.*, 1987). Sidman and associates reported an increase in the expression of both class I and class II MHC antigens on lymphocytes of aged mice. A possible explanation for this discrepancy could be that different methods were used in these two studies to isolate lymphocytes. Thus, there may have been a selective loss of certain lymphocyte populations in either or both of these studies as a consequence of the method of lymphocyte preparation.

The increased class I MHC antigen density on lymphocytes was not accompanied by a change in the percentage of peripheral blood or spleen lymphocytes that were H-2K$^b$ or H-2D$^b$ positive (Figures 1B and 2B). The percentage of IA$^b$ positive peripheral blood lymphocytes also remained essentially unchanged (Figure 1B). In contrast, the percentage of spleen lymphocytes that expressed IA$^b$ decreased in older mice. These data indicate that the lymphocyte populations in these two tissue types may be affected differently during the aging process.

The age-related decrease in spleen lymphocytes expressing IA$^b$ was due to a decrease in the percentage of B lymphocytes and a concomitant increase in Thy 1.2$^+$ cells (Figure 3). This was reflected in a decreased level of class II mRNA present in the total spleen RNA of old mice (Figure 4). The percentage of null cells in the spleen did not change significantly with age. An age-related increase in the T lymphocyte population in the spleen has been reported previously using C57BL/6 mice (Utsuyama and Hirokawa, 1987). Although Utsuyama and Hirokawa demonstrated that the population of splenic T lymphocytes was increased in old mice, the mitogen reactivity and cell-mediated cytolytic activity of these cells was decreased relative to T lymphocytes obtained from spleens of young mice. Thus, although the T lymphocyte population may increase or stay the same in a given lymphoid compartment in old mice, T lymphocyte function is impaired (Kay *et al.*, 1979; Stutman, 1974; Utsuyama and Hirokawa, 1987). We have not yet tested T lymphocyte function in the older mice in our colony.

Although the increased density of class I MHC antigens on murine lymphocytes is statistically significant, it is not known whether it is, in fact, biologically significant. Sidman and coworkers (1987) demonstrated that the 1.5 fold increase in MHC antigen observed in their study resulted in a 3-4 fold increase in the ability of old lymphocytes to stimulate allogeneic lymphocytes. They suggested that the increased expression of MHC antigens in the old mice could result in more efficient foreign antigen presentation, perhaps by activating certain T lymphocytes (*e.g.*, autoreactive clones) in older mice that would be inactive in young mice. Indeed, this could contribute to the enhanced incidence of autoimmune disease in older individuals, who exhibit an immune system with otherwise compromised function.

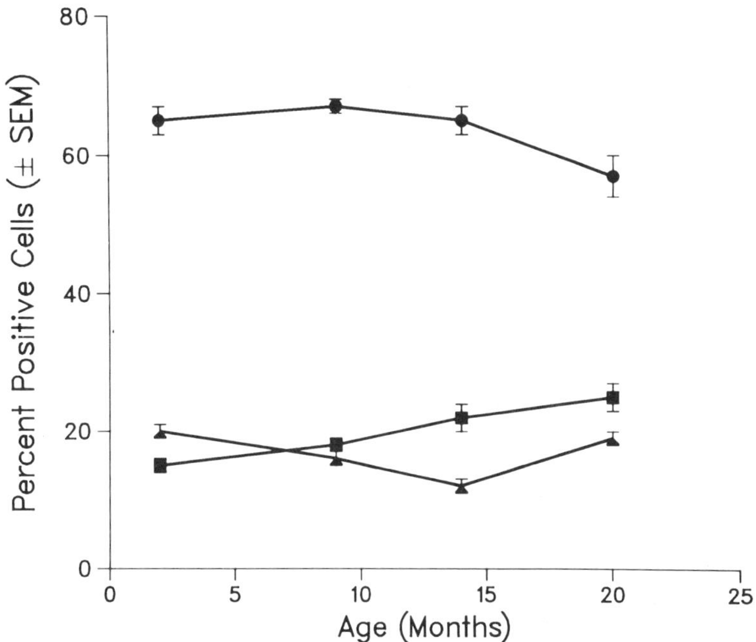

**Figure 3.** Percentages of B (●) and T ( ■) lymphocytes and null ( ▲) cells (sIgM⁻, Thy 1.2⁻) in the spleens of C57BL/6 mice at 2, 9, 14 and 20 months. Values represent the mean ± SEM of 3 female and 3 male mice.

It is not known at the present time what is responsible for these age-related changes in MHC antigen expression. MHC antigen expression is influenced by several endogenous factors including $\alpha$-, $\beta$- and $\gamma$-interferon, interleukin-4, as well as lymphotoxin and tumor necrosis factor (Fellous *et al.*, 1982; Koeffler *et al.*, 1984; Polla *et al.*, 1986, Lapierre *et al.*, 1988). It is of interest to determine whether lymphocytes from old mice respond in a similar or different manner following exposure to these compounds as compared to young mice. This may indicate whether there has been a change in the regulation of MHC antigen expression in old mice.

## ACKNOWLEDGEMENTS

The authors wish to thank Nancy Harvey for excellent technical assistance and Dr. David Cox for assistance with statistical analyses. Work supported by NIH grant AG02440.

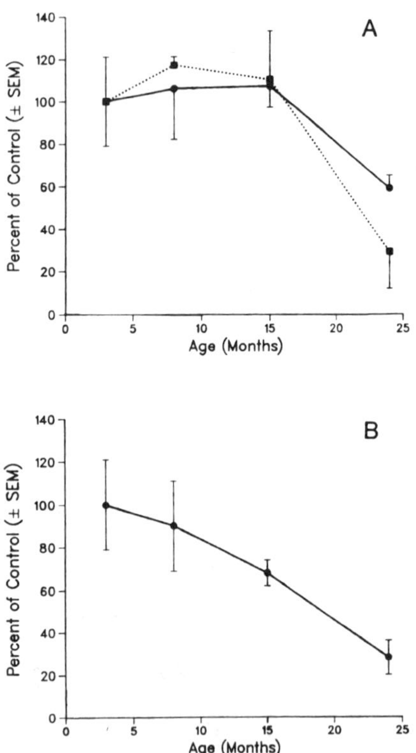

**Figure 4A.** Steady state levels of A$\alpha$ (■) and A$\beta$ (●) class II MHC mRNAs in the spleen, expressed relative to the amount of actin. Each point represents the mean ± SEM of 6 mice (3 female and 3 male).**Figure 4B.** Splenic levels of E$\beta$ class II MHC RNA. Data is expressed as percent of actin control. Each point represents the mean ± SEM from the same used in Figure 4A.

## REFERENCES

BEKKOUCHA, M. AND NAQUET, P., PIERRES, A., MARCHETTO, S., and PIERRES, M. (1984) Efficiency of antigen presentation to T cell clones by (B cell × B cell lymphoma) hybridomas correlated quantitatively with cell surface Ia antigen expression. *Eur. J. Immunol.* **14**: 807-814

BOTTOMLY, K., JONES, B., KAYE, J. and JONES, F. (1983) Subpopulations of B-cells distinguished by cell surface expression of Ia antigens. Correlation of Ia and idiotype during activation by cloned Ia-restricted T-cells. *J. Exp. Med.* **58**: 265-279

CHESTNUT, R. W. and GREY, H. M. (1981) Studies on the capacity of B cells to serve as antigen presenting cells. *J. Immunol.* **126**: 1075-1079

CHEUNG, H. T., REHWALDT, C. A., TWU, J. S., LIAO, N. S. and RICHARDSON, A. (1987) Aging and lymphocyte cytoskeleton: age-related decline in the state of actin polymerization in T lymphocytes from Fischer F344 rats. *J. Immunol.* **138**: 32-36

CHEUNG, H. T., TWU, J. S. and RICHARDSON, A. (1983) Mechanism of age related decline in lymphocyte proliferation: a role of IL-2 production and protein synthesis. *Exp. Gerontol.* **18**: 451-460

DAVIS, M. M., COHEN, D. I., NIELSEN, E. A., STEINMETZ, M., PAUL, W. E. and HOOD, L. (1984) Cell-type-specific cDNA probes and the murine I region: the localization and orientation of A-alpha$^d$. *Proc. Natl. Acad. Sci. USA* **82**: 2194-2198

DEMBIC, Z., AYANE, M., KLEIN, J., STEINMETZ, M., BENOIST, C. O. and MATHIS, D. J. (1985) Inbred and wild mice carry identical deletions in their E-alpha MHC genes. *EMBO J.* **4**: 127-131

DOWER, S. K. and SEGAL, D. M. (1985) Interaction of monoclonal antibodies with MHC class I antigens on mouse spleen cells. II. Levels of expression of H-2K, H-2D and H-2L in different mouse strains. *J. Immunol.* **134**: 431-435

ENNIST, D., JONES, K. H., ST. PIERRE, R. L. and WHISTLER, R. L. (1986) Functional analysis of the immunoscenescence of the human B cell system: dissociation of normal activation and proliferation from impaired terminal differentiation into IgM immunoglobulin-secreting cells. *J. Immunol.* **136**: 99-105

FELLOUS, M., NIR, U., WALLACH, D., MERLIN, G., RUBINSTEIN, M., and REVEL, M. 1982. Interferon-dependent induction of mRNA for the major histocompatibility antigens in human fibroblasts and lymphoblastoid cells. *Proc. Natl. Acad. Sci. USA* **79**: 3082-3086

FLAVELL, R. A., ALLEN, H., BURKLY, L. C., SHERMAN, D. H., WANECK, G. L. and WIDERA, G. (1986) Molecular biology of the H-2 histocompatibility complex. *Science* **233**: 437-443

GOLDSTEIN, S. A. N. and MESCHER, M. F. (1987) Cytotoxic T cell activation by class I protein on cell-size artificial membranes: antigen density and Lyt2/3 function. *J. Immunol.* **138**: 2034-2043

HAAIJMANS J. J. (1987) Perspectives in immunogerontology. In: *Immunoregulation in Aging.* (Ed. A. Facchini, J. J. Haaijman, G. Labo), pp. XI-XXX. Rijswijk: EURAGE.

HAMMERLING, U., CHIN, A. F. and ABBOTT, J. (1976) Ontgeny of murine B lymphocytes. Sequence of B cell differentiation from surface-immunoglobulin negative precursors to plasma cells. *Proc. Natl. Acad. Sci. USA* **73**: 2008-2012

HARA, H., NEGORO, S., MIYATA, S., SAIKO, O., YOSHIZAKI, K., TANAKA, T., IGARASHI, T. and KISHIMOTO, S. (1987) Age associated changes in the proliferation and differentiative response of human B cells and production of T cell derived functions regulating B cells functions. *Mech. Ageing and Dev.* **38**: 245-258

HENRY, C., CHAN, E. L. and KODLIN, D. (1977) Expression and function of I region products on immunocompetent cells. II. I region products in T-B interaction. *J. Immunol.* **119**: 744-748

JANEWAY, C. A., CONRAD, P. J., LERNER, E. A., BABICK, J., WETTSTEIN, P. and MURPHY, D. B. (1984) Monoclonal antibody specific for Ia glycoprotein raised by immunization with activated T-cells: possible role of T cells bound to Ia antigens as targets of immunoregulatory cells. *J. Immunol.* **132**: 662-667

JONES, P. P., MURPHY, D. B. and McDEVITT, H. O. (1981) Variable synthesis and expression of E-α and Aε (A-beta) Ia polypeptide chains in mice of different H-2 haplotypes. *Immunogenetics* **12**: 321-337

KAY, M. M. B., MENDOZA, J., DIVEN, J., DENTON, T., UNION, N. and LAJINESS, M. (1979) Age related changes in the immune system of mice of 8 medium and long lived stains and hybrids. I. Organ, cellular and activity changes. *Mech. Ageing Dev.* **11**: 295-346

KEARNEY, J. F., COOPER, M. D., KLEIN, J., ABNEY, E. R., PARKHOUSE, R. M. E. and
LAWTON, A. R. (1977) Ontogeny of Ia and IgD on IgM-bearing B lymphocytes in mice.
*J. Exp. Med.* **146**: 297-301

KOEFFLER, H. P., RANYARD, J., YELTON, L., BILLING, R. and BOHMAN, R. (1984)
γ-Interferon induces expression of the HLA-D antigens on normal and leukemic human
myeloid cells. *Proc. Natl. Acad. Sci. USA* **81**: 4080-4084

KOHLER, K. and LINDAHL, K. F. (1981) Characterization of a monoclonal anti-H-2K$^b$ antibody. In: *Immunological Systems* Vol. 2. (Ed. C. M. Steinberg and I. Lefkovits), pp.
202-208. Basel: S.Karger A.G.

KROGSRUD, T. L. and PERKINS, E. H. (1977) Age related changes in T-cell function. *J.
Immunol.* **118**: 1607-1611

LAPIERRE, L. A., FIERS, W. and POBER, J. S. (1988) Three distinct classes of regulatory
cytokines control endothelial cell MHC expression. Interaction with immune gamma-inter-
feron differentiate the effects of tumor necrosis factor and lymphotoxin from those of
leukocyte alpha and fibroblast beta interferons. *J. Exp. Med.* **167**: 794-804

MALISSEN, M., HUNKAPILLER, T. and HOOD, L. (1983) Nucleotide sequence of a light chain
gene of the mouse I-A subregion: A-β$^d$. *Science* **221**: 750-755

MANIATIS, T., FRITSCH, E. I. and SAMBROOK, J. (1982) *Molecular cloning. A laboratory
manual.* New York: Cold Spring Harbor Laboratory.

MANYAK, C., HARLEY, T., FISCHER, P., COKER, L., SIGAL, N. H. and KOO, G. C. (1988)
Regulation of class II MHC molecules on human endothelial cells. Effects of IFN and
dexamethasone. *J. Immunol.* **140**: 3827-3821

MATIS, L. A., GLIMCHER, L. H., PAUL, W. E. and SCHWARTZ, R. H. (1983) Magnitude of
response of histocompatibility-restricted T-cell clones is a function of the product of
concentration of antigen and Ia molecule. *Proc. Natl. Acad. Sci. USA* **80**: 6019-6023

McDEVITT H. O. (1981) The role of the H-2 I-region in the regulation of the immune response.
*J. Immunogenetics.* **8**: 287-295

MENGLE-GAW, L. and McDEVITT, H. O. (1983) Isolation and characterization of a cDNA
clone for the murine I-Eβ polypeptide chain. *Proc. Natl. Acad. Sci. USA* **80**: 7621-7625

MENGLE-GAW, L. and McDEVITT, H.O. (1985). Predicted protein sequence of the murine
IE-β$^s$ polypeptide chain from cDNA and genomic clones. *Proc. Natl. Acad. Sci. USA* **82**:
2910-2914

MILLER, R. A. (1986) Immunodeficiency and aging: restorative effects of phorbol esters combined with calcium ionophore. *J. Immunol.* **137**: 805-808

NEGORO, S., HARA, H., MIYATA, S., SAIKI, O., TANAKA, T., YOSHIZAKI, K.,
IGARASHI, T. and KISHIMOTO, S. (1986) Mechanism of age related decline in antigen
specific T cell proliferation response: IL-2 receptor expression and recombinant IL-2
induced proliferative response of purified Tac-positive T cells. *Mech. Ageing Dev.* **36**:
223-241

NEGORO, S., HARA, H., MIYATA, S., SAIKI, O., TANAKA, T., YOSHIZAKI, K.,
NISHIMOTO, I. and KISHIMOTO, S. (1987) Age related changes of the function of T cell
subsets: predominant defect of the proliferative response in CD8 positive T cell subsets in
aged persons. *Mech. Ageing Dev.* **39**: 263-274

NORDIN, A. A. and MAKINODAN, T. (1974) Humoral immunity in aging. *Fed. Proc.* **33**:
2033-2035

OZATO, K. and SACHS, D. H. (1981) Monoclonal antibodies to mouse MHC antigens. III.
Hybridoma antibodies reacting to antigens of the H-2$^b$ haplotype reveal genetic control of
isotype expression. *J. Immunol.* **126**: 317-321

PIKÓ, L., HAMMONS, M. D. and TAYLOR, K. D. (1984) Amount, synthesis, and some
properties of intracisternal A particle-related RNA in early mouse embryos. *Proc. Natl.
Acad. Sci. USA* **82**: 488-492

POLLAB, B. S., POLJAK, A., GEIER, S. G., NATHENSON, S. G., OHARA, J., PAUL, W. E. and GLIMCHER, L. H. (1986) Three distinct signal can induce class II gene expression in a murine pre-B-cell line. *Proc. Natl. Acad. Sci. USA* **83**: 4878-4882

PROUST, J. J., FILBURN, C. R., HARRISON, S. A., BUCHHOLZ, M. A. and NORDIN, A. A. (1987) Age related defect in signal transduction during lectin activation of murine T-lymphocytes. *J. Immunol.* **139**: 1472-1478

ROCK, K. L., BENACERRAF, B. and ABBAS, A. K. (1984) Antigen presentation by hapten specific B lymphocytes. I. Role of surface immunoglobulin receptors. *J. Exp. Med.* **160**: 1102-1113

SERGE, D. and SERGE, M. (1975) Humoral immunity in aged mice. II. Increased suppressor T cell activity in immunologically deficient old mice. *J. Immunol.* **116**: 735-746

SIDMAN, C. L., LUTHER, E. A., MARSHALL, J. D., NGUYEN, K-A., ROOPMAN, D. C., WORTHEN, S. W. (1987) Increased expression of major histocompatibility complex antigens on lymphocytes from aged mice. *Proc. Natl. Acad. Sci. USA* **84**: 7624-7628

SOLOMON, L. R. and RUBENSTEIN, P. A. (1987) Studies on the role of actin N-mehtylhistidine using oligodeoxynucleotide-directed site-specific mutagenesis. *J. Biol. Chem.* **262**: 11382-11388

STUTMAN, O. (1974) Cell mediated immunity and aging. *Fed. Proc.* **33**: 2028-2032

THOMAN, M. L. and WEIGLE, W. O. (1982) Cell mediated immunity in aged mice: an underlying lesion in IL-2 synthesis. *J. Immunol.* **128**: 2358-2361

UNANUE, E. R., BELLES, D. C., LU, C. Y. and ALLEN, P. M. (1984) Antigen presentation: comments on its regulation and mechanism. *J. Immunol.* **132**: 1-5

UTSUYAMA, M. and HIROKAWA, K. (1987) Age-related changes of splenic T cells in mice - a flow cytometric analysis. *Mech. Ageing Dev.* **40**: 89-102

WEKSLER, M. E. and HUTTEROTH, T. H. (1974) Impaired lymphocyte function in aged humans. *J. Clin. Invest.* **53**: 99-110

WHISTLER, R. L., NEWHOUSE, Y. G., ENNIST, D. and BLACHMAN, L. (1985) Human B-lymphocyte colony response: suboptimal colony responsiveness in aged humans associated with defective functions of B-cells and monocytes. *Cellular Immunol.* **94**: 133-146

# 23

# STUDIES ON THE EFFECTS OF AGE, OVARIAN STEROIDS AND GENOTYPE ON REPRODUCTIVE NEUROENDOCRINE CHANGES IN FEMALE MICE

Steven P. Lerner, Steven G. Kohama and Caleb E. Finch

## ABSTRACT

Long-term exposure of the hypothalamic-pituitary axis to ovarian factors has been demonstrated to play a key role in the reproductive senescence of female mice (Finch *et al.*, 1984). We now have support for the hypothesis that estradiol-17$\beta$ ($E_2$) is an essential component in this aging process. Intact and ovariectomized female mice experience irreversible damage to the mechanism controlling ovarian cyclicity after 12 weeks of treatment with $E_2$. This effect is manifested as an inability to support estrous cycles after grafting of young ovaries, and is viewed as a model of accelerated aging. Genotypic differences among closely-related strains of mice apparently influence the sensitivity of the cyclicity-controlling mechanism to disruption mediated by endogenous $E_2$. In a comparison of C57BL/6J, C57BL/10Sn, and mice of 2 strains congenic to the C57BL/10Sn (B10.BR and B10.RIII), an age-related lengthening of estrous cycles and early onset of acyclicity was observed only in C57BL/6J mice. This phenomenon was independent of modal cycle length, since C57BL/10Sn and B10.RIII mice had a 5-day mode and B10.BR mice had a 4-day mode in the absence of any difference in onset of acyclicity. We hypothesized that there are genetic loci, the product(s) of which influences the sensitivity of the neuroendocrine axis to $E_2$.

## INTRODUCTION

Neuroendocrine aging as it relates to female reproductive senescence has previously been established to be dependent upon the presence of the ovary (Finch *et al.*, 1984). That is to say, that some factor(s) of ovarian origin, produced as a consequence of normal ovarian function, significantly augments the age-dependent decrease in the animal's ability to support ovarian cycles. This phenomenon is manifested as an increase in the variability and length of estrous cycles (Nelson *et al.*, 1982). The mechanism through which the ovary contributes to this process is proposed to be long-term exposure of the hypothalamic-pituitary axis to ovarian hormones, resulting in dysfunction to the point where gonadotropic support of the ovaries for normal follicular development and/or ovulation cannot be maintained. By using two approaches, *i.e.* supplementation with exogenous hormone and ablation/replacement-type experiments, we have established that $E_2$ of ovarian origin is an essential factor.

Genetic polymorphisms within and outside the major histocompatibility complex (H-2 in mice) have been shown to affect the length of estrous cycles and the age of onset of acyclicity in closely-related and histocompatibility-congenic strains of mice (Lerner *et al.*, 1987). Since these strains show consistent differences in cycle lengths and onsets of acyclicity in the absence of ovarian morphological differences, we hypothesize that there are genetic differences in neuroendocrine sensitivity to $E_2$.

## MATERIALS AND METHODS

### Exogenous Administration of Estradiol-17β

#### *Animals*

Young, virgin female C57BL/6J mice were purchased from Jackson Laboratories (Bar Harbor) and were singly housed in controlled conditions of light (12:12 L:D) and temperature ($22 \pm 2°C$). Beginning at 3-4 months of age, estrous cycles were monitored by daily vaginal lavage. Only mice displaying repeated patterns of 4- and 5-day estrous cycles for a period of one month were used in the experiments.

#### *Experimental Groups*

At 4-5 months of age, normally-cycling mice were either bilaterally ovariectomized (OVX) or left intact. Four groups of intact mice were treated with 850 μg/kg body weight/day of $E_2$ or ethanol vehicle in drinking water for 6 or 12 weeks. Patterns of estrous cycles were observed by vaginal smear cytology in two groups of intact mice for a period of 4 months post-treatment. The remaining two groups of intact mice were observed for estrous cycle patterns for 1 month and were then bilaterally OVX, transplanted with 2 young ovaries, and observed for an additional 2 months. Four groups of OVX mice were treated with 850 μg/kg body weight/day of $E_2$ or ethanol vehicle in drinking water for 6 or 12 weeks. Following treatment, OVX mice were given two young ovaries and patterns of estrous cycles were observed in these groups of OVX mice for a period of 4 months post-treatment.

## Genetic Influences on Reproductive Parameters

### Animals

Young, virgin female mice and middle-aged, retired breeders of four stains (C57BL/B10Sn H-2$^b$, "B10"; B10.BR/Sg H-2$^k$, "B10.BR"; and B10.RIII H-2$^r$, "B10.RIII"; C57BL/6J H-2$^b$, "B6") were purchased from Jackson Laboratories. Mice were singly housed under controlled conditions of light (12:12 L:D) and temperature (22 ± 2°C).

### Experimental Groups

Beginning at 5 or 11 months of age (virgin and retired-breeder, respectively), estrous cycles were monitored by daily vaginal lavage for 10 months. For each mouse, normal estrous cycles, long cycles, putative pseudopregnancies and short periods of acyclicity (≥14 days) were sorted into four categories: those events lasting 4, 5, 6, or 7-14 days. For each 2 months period, the mean number of cycles per category for each strain were taken together as a measure of cyclicity for that period. Mice were considered to be acyclic after displaying two or more months of continuous acyclic vaginal smears (*i.e.*, persistent vaginal cornification or repetitive spontaneous pseudopregnant-like smears, > 14 days in length).

## RESULTS AND DISCUSSION

### Effect of E$_2$ on Estrous Cycles and Acyclicity

Oral treatment of intact mice with high physiologic levels of E$_2$ decreased ($p < 0.05$), in a duration-dependent manner ($p < 0.05$, 6 *vs.* 12 weeks), the number of estrous cycles observed in the post-treatment period as compared to control mice. The percent of mice able to sustain estrous cycles also decreased ($p < 0.05$), in a duration-dependent manner ($p < 0.05$, 6 *vs.* 12 weeks; Table 1) in E$_2$-treated as compared to control mice. Twelve weeks of E$_2$ treatment completely eliminated the ability of intact mice to support estrous cycles when transplanted with young ovaries. Among the OVX groups, 12 weeks of treatment with E$_2$ reduced the ability of OVX mice to support transplanted young ovaries as quantified by the number of estrous cycles and the percent of mice showing estrous cycles during the post-transplantation period ($p < 0.05$, control *vs.* E$_2$; Table 1). In contrast, 6 weeks of treatment with E$_2$ had no significant permanent affect on these neuroendocrine parameters.

**Table 1.** Effect of the presence of the ovary during treatment and duration of treatment on the ability of mice to sustain estrous cycles with endogenous ovaries (intact groups) or with grafted ovaries (ovariectomized groups)

| Groups | Number of estrous cycles | |
|---|---|---|
| | Control (ethanol) | Estradiol (850 µg/kg/day) |
| **Intact** | | |
| 6 weeks[a] | 21.8 ± 2.7 | 6.3 ± 3.4 |
| 12 weeks[a] | 10.2 ± 2.4 | 0 |
| 12 weeks followed by ovarian replacement with young ovaries[b] | 4.4 ± 1.7 | 0 |
| **Ovariectomized** | | |
| 6 weeks followed by ovarian replacement with young ovaries[a] | 20.2 ± 2.6 | 17.8 ± 2.2 |
| 12 weeks followed by ovarian replacement with young ovaries[b] | 10.4 ≥ 0.9 | 3.3 ± 0.8 |
| Groups | Percentage of mice showing estrous cycles | |
| | Control (ethanol) | Estradiol (850 µg/kg/day) |
| **Intact** | | |
| 6 weeks[a] | 80% | 25% |
| 12 weeks[a] | 80% | 0 |
| 12 weeks followed by ovarian replacement with young ovaries[b] | 60% | 0 |
| **Ovariectomized** | | |
| 6 weeks followed by ovarian replacement with young ovaries[b] | 100% | 82% |
| 12 weeks followed by ovarian replacement with young ovaries[b] | 95% | 50% |

[a] 4 months of post-transplantation observation
[b] 2 months of post-transplantation observation

These data clearly demonstrate that exogenously administered $E_2$ effects a change in the mechanism controlling ovarian function, presumably at the level of the neuroendocrine axis, in a treatment duration-dependent manner that advances the onset of acyclicity and impairs the animal's ability to regulate ovarian function. This change is clearly not related to direct $E_2$-mediated damage at the level of the ovary because treated, unlike control mice, were not able to sustain estrous cycles when transplanted with young ovaries. We contend that these adverse changes are the result of a direct or indirect action of $E_2$ at the level of the hypothalamus and/or pituitary and represent a temporally-accelerated version of what occurs during the normal aging process. While it is the direct action of exogenous $E_2$ and not the ovary

| Table 2. Effect of strain and age on numbers of 4-, 5- and 6-day estrous cycles in virgin mice | | | | |
|---|---|---|---|---|
| Strain[*] Cycle | Ages 5-6 | 7-8 | 9-10 | 11-12 | 13-14 |
| C57Bl/6J | | | | | |
| 4-day | 5.2 ± 1.5[a] | 1.9 ± 0.9[a] | 1.8 ± 1.1[-] | 1.6 ± 0.8[ab] | 0.2 ± 0.2[b] |
| 5-day | 2.9 ± 0.8[a,b] | 3.5 ± 1.0[ab] | 1.4 ± 0.5[a] | 3.6 ± 1.2[ab] | 3.2 ± 1.3[-] |
| 6-day | 1.9 ± 0.8[a] | 1.4 ± 0.5[a] | 2.8 ± 0.6[a] | 0.8 ± 0.5[-] | 1.0 ± 0.6[-] |
| % acyclic | 0.0 | 11.1 | 44.4 | 44.4 | 44.4 |
| C57BL/10Sn | | | | | |
| 4-day | 1.0 ± 0.2[b] | 1.3 ± 0.2[b] | 2.4 ± 0.3[-] | 1.7 ± 0.3[b] | - |
| 5-day | 4.3 ± 0.6[a] | 4.1 ± 0.7[a] | 4.8 ± 0.5[a] | 5.2 ± 0.6[a] | - |
| 6-day | 1.6 ± 0.3[a] | 1.5 ± 0.2[a] | 1.2 ± 0.2[b] | 1.0 ± 0.2[-] | - |
| % acyclic | 0.0 | 0.0 | 9.5 | 9.5 | - |
| B10.BR | | | | | |
| 4-day | 3.6 ± 0.6[a] | 3.2 ± 0.7[a] | 2.5 ± 0.7[-] | 3.2 ± 0.6[a] | 3.2 ± 0.8[a] |
| 5-day | 2.2 ± 0.5[b] | 1.7 ± 0.6[b] | 1.8 ± 0.4[b] | 2.7 ± 0.5[a] | 2.0 ± 0.4[-] |
| 6-day | 0.4 ± 0.2[b] | 0.5 ± 0.2[b] | 0.8 ± 0.3[b] | 0.4 ± 0.2[-] | 0.3 ± 0.3[-] |
| % acyclic | 0.0 | 0.0 | 7.7 | 15.4 | 23.1 |
| B10.RIII | | | | | |
| 4-day | 2.0 ± 0.5[b] | 1.3 ± 0.4[b] | 1.8 ± 0.4[-] | 1.4 ± 0.4[b] | 0.7 ± 0.2[b] |
| 5-day | 3.5 ± 0.7[a.b] | 3.8 ± 0.7[ab] | 2.4 ± 0.5[b] | 2.8 ± 0.4[b] | 2.4 ± 0.6[-] |
| 6-day | 1.5 ± 0.4[a] | 1.7 ± 0.4[a] | 1.1 ± 0.3[b] | 1.1 ± 0.3[-] | 1.0 ± 0.3[-] |
| % acyclic | 0.0 | 0.0 | 7.1 | 14.3 | 14.3 |
| * Strains with different superscripts for each individual cycle length within and age group differ (p < 0.05) | | | | | |

*per se* that is causing the changes we have observed, the presence of the ovary during the $E_2$ treatment results in a greater impact on subsequent cyclicity. OVX, as compared to intact mice, supported grafted ovaries significantly better after being treated for 6 or 12 weeks. Most likely, endogenous $E_2$ secreted from the ovaries of treated mice, induced into a polyfollicular state by the exogenous $E_2$, is responsible for this effect.

## Effect of Genotype on Estrous Cycles and Acyclicity

B10 and B10-congenic strains of mice showed age-independent strain specific patterns of estrous cycles (p < 0.001; Table 2; Lerner *et al.*, 1988). B10 mice and, to a lesser extent, B10.RIII mice had a preponderance of 5-day cycles, and B10.BR mice had a preponderance of 4-day cycles. The majority of virgin mice of these strains (54/57) did not become acyclic during this study. Furthermore, retired breeders displayed a similar incidence of acyclicity at all ages, except at 19-20 months of age when B10 mice had a greater incidence of acyclicity compared to the congenic strains (p < 0.05; Table 3). In contrast to B10 and B10-congenic mice, B6 mice showed marked age-dependent changes in patterns of estrous cycle, their initial

| Table 3. Effect of strain and age on numbers of 4-, 5- and 6-day estrous cycles in retired breeder mice | | | | | |
|---|---|---|---|---|---|
| Strain[*] Cycle | Ages 11-12 | 13-14 | 15-16 | 17-18 | 19-20 |
| C57Bl/6J | | | | | |
| 4-day | $2.9 \pm 0.3^a$ | $0.9 \pm 0.2^-$ | - | - | - |
| 5-day | $2.7 \pm 0.4^a$ | $2.2 \pm 0.5^{ab}$ | - | - | - |
| 6-day | $0.5 \pm 0.1^a$ | $0.9 \pm 0.3^-$ | - | - | - |
| % acyclic | 0.0 | 64.9 | 97.3 | 100.0 | 100.0 |
| C57BL/10Sn | | | | | |
| 4-day | $1.1 \pm 0.2^b$ | $1.0 \pm 0.2^-$ | $0.6 \pm 0.1^-$ | $0.5 \pm 0.1^-$ | $0.1 \pm 0.1^-$ |
| 5-day | $3.5 \pm 0.4^a$ | $2.7 \pm 0.3^a$ | $1.3 \pm 0.2^-$ | $0.6 \pm 0.2^-$ | $0.9 \pm 0.3^-$ |
| 6-day | $1.2 \pm 0.2^b$ | $1.2 \pm 0.2^-$ | $0.9 \pm 0.2^-$ | $0.2 \pm 0.1^b$ | $0.6 \pm 0.1^-$ |
| % acyclic | 0.0 | 2.2 | 26.1 | 50.0 | 76.1 |
| B10.BR | | | | | |
| 4-day | $2.0 \pm 0.5^a$ | $1.2 \pm 0.4^-$ | $0.9 \pm 0.4^-$ | $0.8 \pm 0.4^-$ | $0.5 Y 0.3^-$ |
| 5-day | $2.3 \pm 0.5^{ab}$ | $1.2 \pm 0.6^b$ | $2.1 \pm 0.6^-$ | $0.3 \pm 0.2^-$ | $0.7 \pm 0.2^-$ |
| 6-day | $1.3 \pm 0.4^b$ | $1.1 \pm 0.3^-$ | $1.3 \pm 0.3^-$ | $1.8 \pm 0.6^a$ | $0.3 \pm 0.3^-$ |
| % acyclic | 0.0 | 0.0 | 9.1 | 45.5 | 45.5 |
| B10.RIII | | | | | |
| 4-day | $0.0 \pm 0.0^b$ | $0.6 \pm 0.4^-$ | $0.8 \pm 0.3^-$ | $1.3 \pm 0.9^-$ | $0.0 \pm 0.0^-$ |
| 5-day | $0.6 \pm 0.4^b$ | $1.8 \pm 0.8^{ab}$ | $0.5 \pm 0.3^-$ | $0.7 \pm 0.3^-$ | $0.3 \pm 0.3^-$ |
| 6-day | $0.6 \pm 0.4^{ab}$ | $0.8 \pm 0.8^-$ | $0.0 \pm 0.0^-$ | $1.0 \pm 0.6^{ab}$ | $0.0 \pm 0.0^-$ |
| % acycli | 0.0 | 0.0 | 20.0 | 40.0 | 40.0 |

* Strains with different superscripts for each individual cycle length within and age group differ (p < 0.05).

preponderance of 4-day cycles before 6 months of age decreased sharply so that 4-day cycles were rare after 10 months of age. This rapid age-associated loss (p < 0.001) of 4-day cycles was unique to B6 mice since no age-related loss of 4-day cycles occurred in either the 4-day dominant B10.BR mice or the 5-day dominant B10 and B10.RIII mice. By 10 months of age, a greater percentage of virgin B6 mice had become acyclic (Table 2) compared to the other strains. Also, among retired breeders, the rate at which B6 mice became acyclic as a function of age was also significantly greater than that observed for B10 strains (Table 3).

The observation that B6 mice display both the greatest degree of age-related change in patterns of estrous cycles and the most rapid onset of acyclicity compared to B10-congenic strains has led us to postulate that there is a genetic difference in the sensitivity of the neuroendocrine axis to ovarian-hormone-mediated feedback and subsequent damage. "Cycle lengthening" seen in B6 mice as a function of age (Nelson et al., 1982), but not in B10-congenic mice, could be due to a delayed LH-surge-response to preovulatory rises in E2 because of cumulative damage to this surge-mechanism acquired during previous estrous cycles. In contrast, the lack of cycle lengthening among the B10-congenic mice could reflect a relative insensitivity to either $E_2$-mediated damage or the effects of such damage. The mechanism controlling frequency of estrous cycles is clearly independent from that which is effected by $E_2$ and mediates the onset of acyclicity; for neither 4-day nor 5-day cycling B10-congenic mice showed any difference in onset of acyclicity.

In conclusion, we have demonstrated that $E_2$ acts to limit the reproductive lifespan of mice, possibly through a mechanism that, in a time-dose manner, alters the responsiveness of the neuroendocrine axis to hormonal feedback. The apparent differential sensitivity of the various inbred strains of mice to this $E_2$-mediated change provides us with a tool to explore the interaction of genetic components and those factors controlling reproductive senescence.

## ACKNOWLEDGEMENTS

This research was supported by Grant AG-04419. The authors would like to thank Robert Mitchell for his diligent collection of daily vaginal smears.

## REFERENCES

ASCHEIM, P. (1965) Resultats fournis par le greffe heterochone des ovaries dans l'etude de la regulation hypothalamus-hypophyso-ovarienne de la ratte senile. *Gerontologie* **10** 65-75

BRAWER, J. R., SCHIPPER, H. and NAFTOLIN, F. (1980) Ovary-dependent degeneration in the hypothalamic arcuate nucleus. *Endocrinology* **107**: 274-279

FINCH, C.E., FELICIO, L.S., MOBBS, C.V. and NELSON, J.F. 1984. Ovarian and steroidal influences on neuroendocrine aging processes in female rodents. *Endo. Rev.* **5**: 467-497.

GORDON, M. N., OSTERBURG, H. H., MAY, P. C. and FINCH, G. E. (1986) Effective oral administration of 17β-estradiol to female C57BL/6J mice through the drinking water. *Biol. Reprod.* **35**: 1088-1095

KOHAMA, S. G., ANDERSON, C. P., OSTERBURG, H. H., MAY, P. G. and FINCH, G. E. (1989) Oral administration of estradiol to young C57BL/6J mice induces age-like neuroendocrine dysfunctions in the regulation of estrous cycles. *Biol. Reprod.* in press

LERNER, S.P., ANDERSON, C.P. and FINCH, C.E. 1987. Genotype and reproductive functions of inbred female mice: Effects of H-2 alleles. *Soc. Neurosci. Abstr.* **13**, 402.

LERNER, S.P., ANDERSON, C.P., WALFORD, R.L. and FINCH, C.E. 1988. Genotypic influences on reproductive aging of inbred female mice: effects of H-2 and non-H-2 alleles. *Biol. Reprod.* **38, 1035-1043.**

NELSON, J.F., FELICIO, L.S., RANDALL, P.K., SIMS, C. and FINCH, C.E. 1982. A longitudinal study of estrous cyclicity in aging C57BL/6J mice. I. Cycle frequency, length, and vaginal cytology. *Biol. Reprod.* **27**, 327-339.

## DISCUSSION

1. Differences in cycling patterns (or any other differences) between B6 and B10 mice are likely to be due to differences at a single locus, as these strains are very similar. Of course, backcrosses are needed to verify this.

2. Differences within the H-2 complex may not be in either the K or D regions but in the Q region; this can be mapped using congenic lines with cross-overs within H-2.

3. Cycling does not stop in all strains due to ovarian secretion. There are many possible responses to estrogen and many genes controlling them. Lerner agreed with this point, but commented that increased levels of gonadotropin may affect follicle cell populations and thus affect hormone levels.

# 24

## USE OF GENETIC MODELS TO INVESTIGATE THE HYPOPHYSEAL REGULATION OF SENESCENCE

K. Flurkey and D.E. Harrison

The hypothesis that patterns of aging are determined by genetic pleiotropisms (*i.e.*, post-maturational effects of genes that were fixed because of their benefit to reproductive fitness) predicts that rates of development will correlate positively with rates of aging (Williams, 1957; discussed in the chapters by Charlesworth, Kirkwood and Rose, this volume). Tests to determine if a direct causal relationship exists between rates of development and rates of aging generally have not been successful: induced delays of development through environmental manipulations did not prolong post-maturational survival in *C. elegans* (see chapter by Johnson, this volume) or in *Drosophila* (see chapter by Grigliatti, this volume); and lifespan was not markedly prolonged in rats that were food restricted from 6 weeks to 6 months compared to rats fed *ad libitum* (Yu *et al.*, 1985) Thus, if "rapid morphogenesis is associated with rapid senescence ", as Williams (1957) predicts, it may be because some genes which accelerate development subsequently have adverse consequences on survival only as they continue to act in the adult, not because a physiological link necessarily exists between rates of development and rates of aging. In order to examine the relationship between rates of development and rates of aging in mammals using genetic rather than environmental models, we investigated patterns of aging in mice with mutations that alter growth and development. We tested the hypothesis that mutations that retard or block developmental processes will also retard or prevent aging processes. We focused on the "dwarfing" mutations that affect the classical neuroendocrine developmental axes: the little mutation (growth hormone deficient, Eicher and Beamer, 1976), the hypothyroid mutation (thyroid hormone deficient, Beamer *et al.*, 1981) and a mutation that affects both of these axes, Snell's dwarf (growth hormone, thyrotrophin and prolactin deficient, Cheng *et al.*, 1983). These mutations are extreme experimental manipulations used to produce a maximum effect so that possible relationships between developmental hormones and aging might be identified. To examine patterns of aging in these mice, we determined the effects of these mutations on lifespan and on a set of biomarkers of aging, *i.e.* assays of biological age that are simple and relatively noninvasive (Harrison and Archer, 1988), which are specifically related to growth and cell proliferation (body weight, tail length and hematocrit). We also examined effects on aging in another system, the immune system, to determine if endocrinologically directed developmental impairments would retard aging in a system that does not contain classical growth hormone and thyroid hormone target tissues. Finally, by comparing effects of these mutations on endocrine-dependent biomarkers of aging to effects on immunologic aging, we illustrate how these mutations may be used to identify neuroendocrine influences on patterns of aging in any system.

## MICE

All mice used in these studies were maintained in a single research colony of The Jackson Laboratory. They received rodent chow (Emory Morse Co.) and tap water *ad libitum*. No endocrine supplements were given to any of the mice in these studies. Only male mice were used.

The *dw* mutation (Snell's dwarf) is a single locus autosomal recessive that is maintained on the DW/J background by mating known heterozygotes. The littermates used as controls included both heterozygotes and wild type homozygotes, which are phenotypically indistinguishable. Dwarf (*dw/dw*) mice were housed with at least one normal littermate to provide warmth; extra pine shavings were added to their cages to insure access to water bottles. Homozygosity for *dw* results in defective transcription of the genes for growth hormone (GH), prolactin (Cheng *et al.*, 1983) and probably thyroid stimulating hormone (TSH; Roti *et al.*, 1978). Thus, *dw/dw* mice lack GH, prolactin, TSH and are deficient in circulating thyroid hormones (TH). The potential for gonadotrophin secretion appears normal, although the dwarf mouse is infertile, with underdeveloped gonads (Bartke, 1964). There are conflicting reports on the function of the adrenocortical axis (Bartke, 1964; Shire and Hambly, 1973; Schneider, 1976).

The little (*lit*) and hypothyroid (*hyt*) mutations are also single locus autosomal recessives. *Lit/lit* mice are insensitive to growth hormone releasing hormone, causing a specific deficiency in circulating levels of GH (Jansson *et al.*, 1986). The *lit* mutation arose spontaneously and is maintained on the C57BL/6J background by mating male *lit/+* heterozygotes with female *lit/lit* homozygotes. Therefore, littermates are all heterozygous at the *lit* locus. *Hyt/hyt* mice are insensitive to thyrotrophin, resulting in severe hypothyroidism (Beamer *et al.*, 1981). The *hyt* mutation arose on the RF/J background and was transferred to the BALB/cBy background for breeding purposes. It is maintained by breeding heterozygotes; therefore, littermates are heterozygous or wild-type homozygous.

## LIFESPAN

Although *dw/dw* mice were once considered as models of accelerated aging because they typically exhibited characteristics of senescence preceding early death (at about 4-5 months, Fabris *et al.*,1972), later anecdotal reports indicated that they may live up to 16-20 months of age in apparently good health. Dwarf C3H/HeJ mice carrying a remutation at the *dw* locus called *dw^J/dw^J* were reported to live beyond 2 years (Eicher and Beamer, 1980). Therefore, we reassessed the effects of the original dwarf (*dw*) mutation on lifespan in DW/J mice (Figure 1). Both median (540 days) and maximum (the oldest 10th decile: 740 days) lifespans of male dwarf mice were 20-30% lower than for normal littermates under conditions described above (Figure 1). Although this indicates that the *dw* mutation does shorten lifespan slightly, the effect is much less than that observed by Fabris *et al.*, (1972). Furthermore, the survival curve of dwarf mice appeared to have two components, in contrast to the more "square" survival curve of the littermates. The earlier component (100-500 days) is typical of survival curves of populations that are subject to random effects on mortality that result in a constant mortality rate. It is possible that stresses related to their small size, such as dominance behavior of the normal male littermates and an occasional insufficiency of wood shavings to lift the dwarf to the water spout (due, for example, to random digging by littermates) may have caused this early mortality. If determinants of this early component continue to act throughout the lifespan in dwarf mice, they will affect the second portion of the curve (500-750 days) that is more typical of "aging" populations. We estimated the "senescence-specific" mortality by adjusting this second portion of the mortality curve for a constant rate of mortality assumed to be independent of aging (8% of the survivors per 100 days, the difference between control and dwarf mice in slope of the linear regression of survival on age from 100-500 days). Beginning with 88% survivorship at 500 days (the proportion of control mice alive at that age), subsequent survivorship was plotted based on the actual rate of death in the *dw/dw* mice plus the number that would have survived if there were no greater constant mortality in the dwarfs than in the controls. The resulting hypothetical curve suggested that median lifespan of dwarf mice would be about 625 days if all non-senescence related sources of mortality were removed (Figure 1). Predicted maximum lifespan would be about the same as without adjustment. Although the lifespan of these dwarf mice was less than that reported by Eicher and Beamer (1980), differences in back-

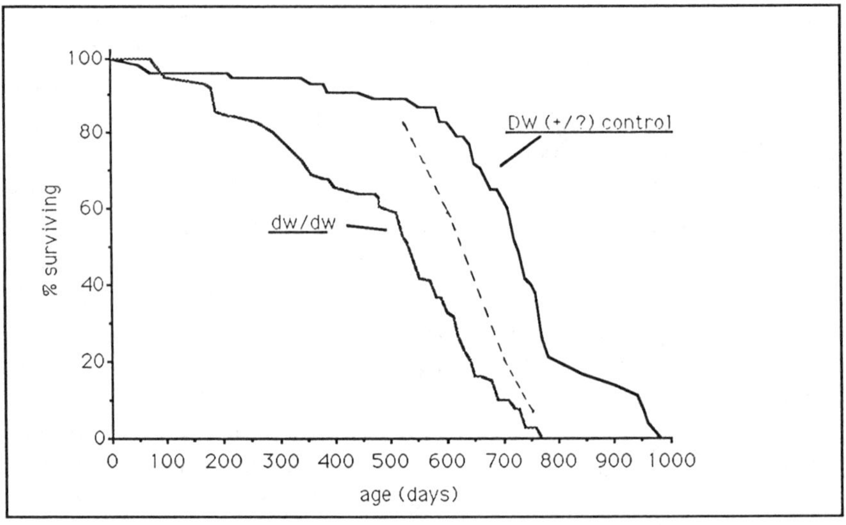



**Figure 1.** Survivorship in male DW/J Snell dwarf mice. Control mice are male littermates that may be either heterozygous or wild-type homozygous at the *dw* locus (+/?). See text for husbandry. Calculations were based on an initial population of 55-60 mice per group until 550 days. Afterward the calculation for percent surviving at each age was based on a progressively smaller population as mice were removed for studies. Whenever mice were removed, data from all their littermates (surviving and dead) were also eliminated from subsequent survival calculations to avoid any artificial selection bias. By 750 days, when almost all *dw/dw* mice were dead, survivorship calculations were based on an original population of 35-40 mice per group. The dashed line is the estimated senescence-specific survival curve for *dw/dw* mice (see text for details).

ground strain (C3H/HeJ *vs.* DW/J), specific mutation ($dw^J/dw^J$ *vs. dw/dw*) and husbandry (housing with normal BALB/cJ females rather than males and use of special drinking bottles) may have been involved.

The effect of the *lit* mutation on lifespan is unclear. In the present study mortality among *lit/lit* male mice was relatively greater than among heterozygote littermates from 350-650 days. This was not due to dominance behavior of the heterozygotes since early deaths occurred whether or not mutant mice were housed with heterozygotes. However, the rapid increase in

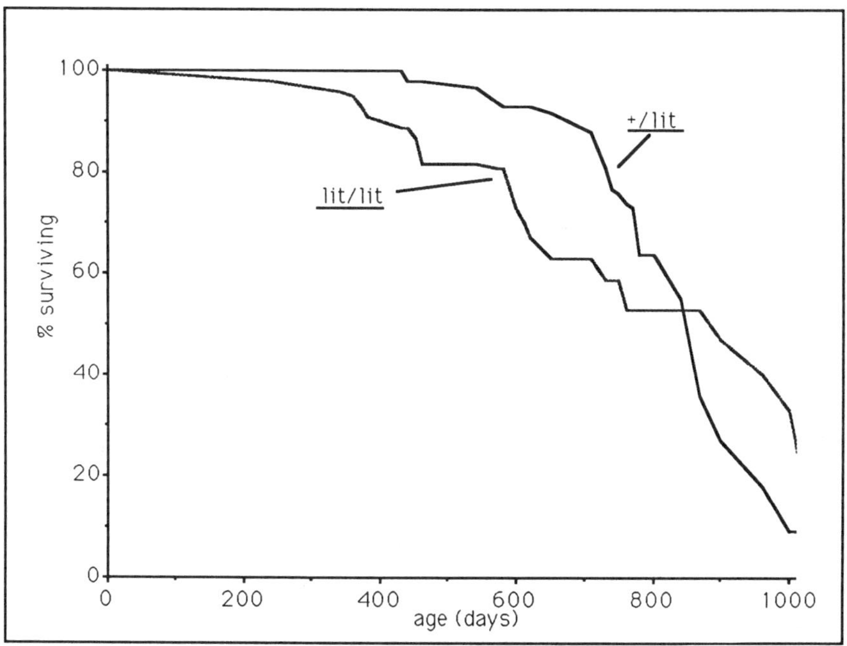


**Figure 2.** Survivorship in male C57BL/6J +/*lit* and *lit/lit* mice. Calculations were based on an initial population of 40-45 mice per group until 500 days, 20-45 mice until 750 days and 10- 15 mice afterward.

mortality that occurred among heterozygote littermates after 700 days did not appear among the *lit/lit* mice; survivorship among *lit/lit* mice was greater than among heterozygotes after 850 days (Figure 2). Earlier studies with 12-24 mice per group identified no effect of the *lit* mutation on lifespan in males and either no effect or a slight increase in lifespan of *lit/lit* females (Beamer, Archer and Harrison, Table 1). These results suggest that there may be subtle interactions of the *lit* mutation with unidentified environmental influences that may either delay or advance mortality for some individuals. We find no evidence that a chronic specific growth hormone deficiency will consistently accelerate or retard expression of determinants of mortality. Effects of

| Table 1. Effect of the *lit* mutation on lifespan in C57Bl/6J mice | | | | | |
|---|---|---|---|---|---|
| Investigator | genotype | n (mice) | X ± SEM (days) | Median | 2 oldest |
| Beamer | +/*lit* female | 18 | 955 ± 29 | 910 | 1199, 1220 |
|  | *lit/lit* female | 21 | 935 ± 56 | 1030 | 1125, 1193 |
| Beamer | +/*lit*, male | 13 | 969 ± 56 | 940 | 1268, 1477 |
|  | *lit/lit*, male | 21 | 1029 ± 38 | 970 | 1367, 1416 |
| Archer and | +/*lit* female | 9 | 742 ± 42 | 770 | 975, 1005 |
| Harrison | *lit/lit* female | 12 | 928 ± 60 | 950 | 1060, 1225 |
| Flurkey and | +/*lit*, male | 11 | 842 ± 41 | 850 | 1001, 1042 |
| Harrison | *lit/lit*, male | 15 | 739 ± 88 | 885 | 1160, 1171 |

heterozygosity at the *lit* locus were not directly tested, however, the lifespan of the +/*lit* C57BL/6J male mice of this study is comparable to that of normal C57BL/6J males in this laboratory.

Although the survivorship curve for hypothyroid (*hyt/hyt*) male mice is based on a small population, the effect of the mutation is quite apparent (Figure 3). There was no mortality until about 400 days; 80% of the population died within the next 170 days. In this study, *hyt/hyt* mice were housed separately from littermate controls. Lifespan was even shorter, with a similar precipitous increase in mortality, when males were caged with their normal littermates (not shown). Apparently there is some distinct interaction of the *hyt* mutation with age that severely limits survivorship in BALB/cBy.RFJ mice after 1 year. These data are consistent with the suggestion by Fabris *et al.*, (1982) that age-related hypothyroidism may be a part of the etiology of senescence, based on their studies of immune function in thyroid hormone-deficient or treated young and old BALB/C mice. However, we did not observe an accelerated "aging" in the T cell mitogen response of *hyt/hyt* mice (Table 4) that would have been predicted from Fabris's work. Furthermore, these mice appeared quite healthy, even at 400 days.

The somewhat shorter lifespan of the BALB/cBy +/? littermate controls, as well as the DW/J +/? littermates, compared to the C57BL/6J +/*lit* controls, probably results from strain differences since these mice were all maintained in the same colony.

In general, these data indicate that chronic deficiencies of developmentally important hormones can affect patterns of age-related mortality even in specific pathogen-free colonies such as those at The Jackson Laboratory. The present data suggest that a chronic growth hormone insufficiency has only a

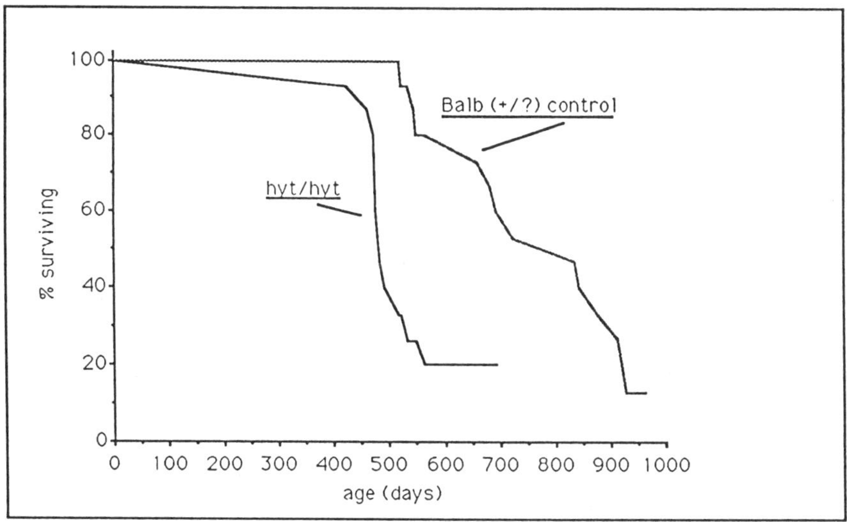



**Figure 3.** Survivorship in male BALB/cBy.RFJ *hyt/hyt* mice. Controls are heterozygous or wild-type homozygous at the *hyt* locus. There were 15 mice per group in the original population. The 3 remaining *hyt/hyt* mice were killed at 700 days and 2 remaining controls at 970 days for necropsy.

slight effect on mortality that may require unidentified environmental factors for expression, whereas a chronic hypothyroidism may severely limit maximum lifespan . A consistently greater mortality among young adults (2-12 months) was observed only for the *dw/dw* mice, which may be an indirect result of the severe dwarfism in these mice rather than a direct physiological effect of their endocrine deficiency. Clearly, our working hypothesis, that retardation of development would result in a delay in the onset of the age-related mortality, was not supported by our observations of population-mortality. However, complications due to interactions of the chronic hormone deficiencies with age-related impairments may have masked beneficial effects of the hormone deficiency on patterns of aging in specific systems. In order to address this issue, effects of aging on specific systems were determined in these mice.

## BIOMARKERS OF AGING

Biomarkers of aging are tests used to assay rates of aging that are specific for separate biological systems (Harrison and Archer, 1988). In these studies effects of age and mutation were determined for three biomarkers: body weight, tail length and hematocrit. The specific effects of each mutation are used to indicate which biomarkers may be developed as noninvasive "bioassays" of TH and GH in adults.

## BODY WEIGHT

Body mass, indicated by weight, progressively increased for adult littermate controls of all three strains until about 20 months (Figure 4). Body weight in young adult *dw/dw* mice was only 25% of normal, demonstrating the well-known effect of the *dw* mutation on development. Post-maturational changes in body weight occurred in two phases for dwarf mice; weight continued to increase up to 7 months of age, but it remained stable afterward. This indicates that at least some of the post-maturational increase in body mass is independent of hypophyseal hormones, although for growth to continue after 7 months, GH and/or TH are required. It is also at 7-8 months that the rate of weight gain became slower for the normal males in all three strains. These observations suggest that a shift in the regulation of growth occurs at this age. Thus, a useful parameter of body mass as a biomarker may be the increase in weight after 7-8 months of age. This measure may help identify specific post-maturational effects of GH and TH secretion, whereas total body weight reflects a summation of influences on growth over the animal's lifespan.

Although both young adult *lit/lit* and *hyt/hyt* mice were about 60% of the body weight of their respective controls, these mutants showed very different patterns of weight gain during aging. Normal patterns of post-maturational weight gain were observed among *lit/lit* mice, while *hyt/hyt* mice appeared to gain weight faster than normal, as also observed by Chubb and Henry (1988). Thus, although both GH and TH are necessary for normal development, neither is an absolute requirement for post-maturational weight gain; deficits of both, as in the *dw/dw* mice, appear to be necessary to prevent post-maturational increases in body mass.

Skeletal and connective tissue growth, indicated by increases in tail length, is slow but very consistent even after 7 months (Harrison and Archer, 1988). For example, even though tail length of heterozygote +/*lit* mice of this study increased only 0.3 cm from 8 to 16-19 months, the standard error was 0.08 cm, permitting detection of a significant effect of age (P < 0.05, T-test).

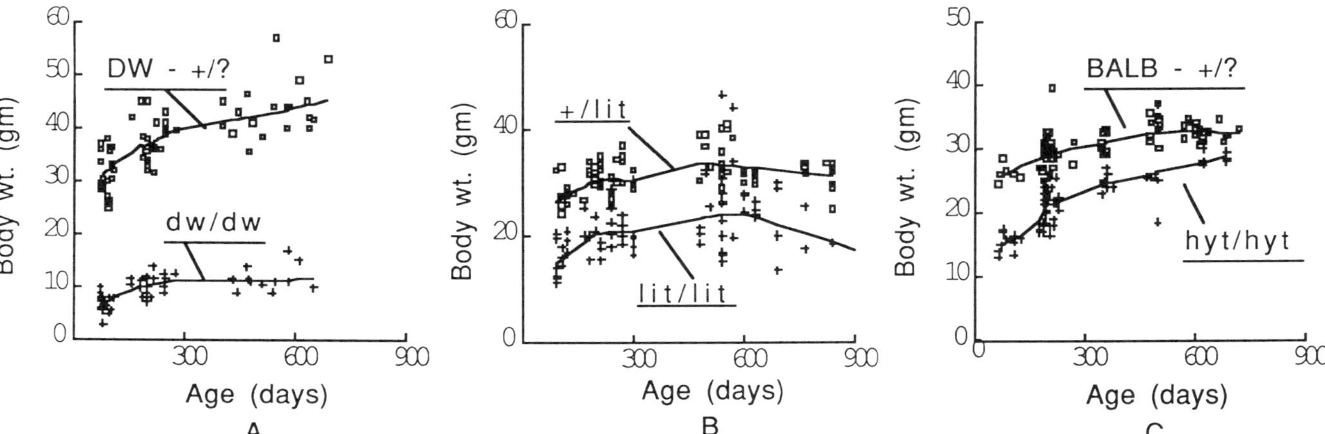



**Figure 4.** Effects of endocrine mutation on post-maturational changes in body weight (weight in gms, age in days). Panel A: Snell's dwarf mice and DW/J control littermates, 50-60 values per group (the scattergrams show fewer data points due to overlap); Panel B: little mice and C57BL/6J +/*lit* control littermates, 85-90 values per group; Panel C, hypothyroid mice and BALB/cBy.RF control littermates, 75-85 values per group (note change in Y axis scale) Age- profiles were estimated using a "running average" technique (Lowess: Cleveland, 1981) provided in the Systat graphics package for the MacIntosh (1987). In some cases, mice were weighed at more than one age. Body weight continued to increase during adulthood for all genotypes except *dw/dw*. (P < O.Ol for a positive linear regression of body weight on age from 150 to 650 days for all genotypes except *dw/dw*).

As with body mass, skeletal and connective tissue growth: 1) continued progressively throughout adulthood in most normal control mice; 2) were affected during maturation by all three mutations, and 3) for *dw/dw* mice, ceased after 7 months (Figure 5). However, unlike body mass, skeletal growth did not continue after 7-10 months in *lit/lit* mice (7-9 months, 6.8 ± 0.07 cm, n = 10; 16-19 months, 6.7 ± 0.1 cm, n = 10), indicating that there may be a specific requirement for normal levels of serum GH in order to continue skeletal and connective tissue growth after 7 months.

Although tail length is generally a good predictor of body weight during aging in mice (Harrison, unpublished), after 7-10 months in *lit/lit* mice tail growth ceased while body weight continued to increase. Thus, tail length appears to be a better parameter than body weight as an approximate "bioassay" for cumulative exposure to GH after 7-10 months. These genetic models may be useful to help determine whether age-related phenomena that correlate with body weight are associated primarily with increased adiposity, in which case they will appear in *lit/lit* but not in *dw/dw* mice, or if they are associated with true growth, exemplified by skeletal system growth, in which case they will not appear in either *lit/lit* or *dw/dw* mice. The distinction between consequences of continued growth *vs.* accumulation of body fat in post- maturational animals can be subtle, yet critical for studies of the determinants of age-related impairments and pathology (*e.g.* Harrison *et al.*, 1984). In contrast to the above two biomarkers, hematocrit progressively decreases during aging for the DW/J, C57BL/6J and BALB/cBy.RFJ strains used in these studies, as is commonly found for many strains of mice. Hematocrit is also low among young *dw/dw* (Fabris *et al.*, 1971) and *hyt/hyt* adults (Beamer *et al.*, 1981), but not among *lit/lit* mice (Figure 6). This suggests that the decrease in *dw/dw* mice may result primarily from their TH deficiency. TH replacement partially restores hematocrit in normal old mice as well as in *hyt/hyt* mice (data not shown) indicating that age-related decrements in hematocrit may be partially due to a reduction of or insensitivity to circulating TH. Therefore, hematocrit may be a useful marker for identification of other age-related impairments that are associated with the thyroid axis if that impairment shows the same distribution among these mutants as the deficiencies in hematocrit, and if it correlates with hematocrit in normal aging mice. The use of these biomarkers to identify neuroendocrine etiologies for age-related impairments is illustrated below with respect to immunologic aging.

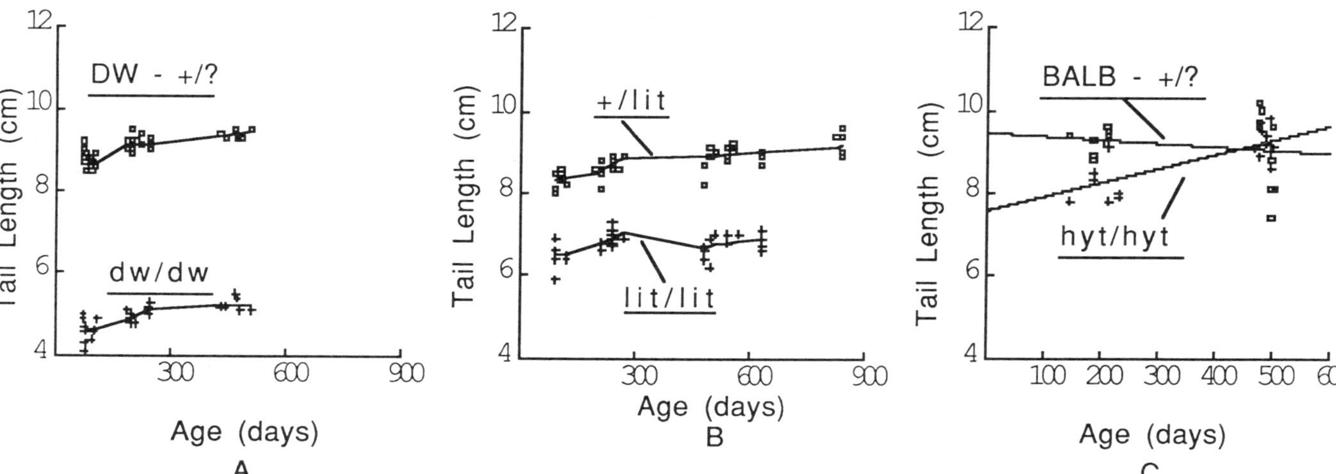



**Figure 5.** Effects of endocrine mutation on post-maturational skeletal growth indicated by tail length (cm).Panel A, Snell's dwarf mice, 35-40 mice per group; Panel B, little mice, 30-45 mice per group; Panel C hypothyroid mice, 17 mice per group (note change in scale of X axis). A running average procedure (Lowess) was used to calculate profiles for comparisons of *dw/dw* and *lit/lit* mice to controls, but a linear estimation is given for the comparison of *hyt/hyt* mice to controls since data were available at only 2 ages (150-230 days and 480-510 days). The change in tail length from 7 to 18 months was greater in control than in mutant mice for *dw/dw* and for *lit/lit* mice (interaction from 2-way ANOVA, P=0.04 for both comparisons).

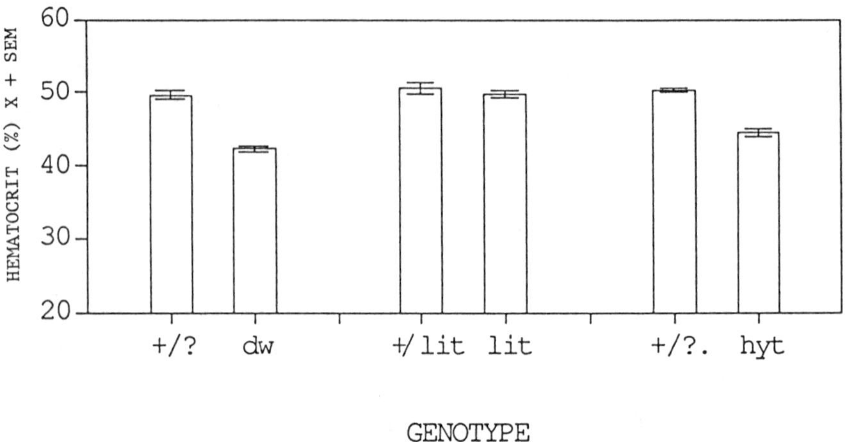


**Figure 6**. Effect of endocrine mutations on hematocrit (mean ± SEM) in 3-6 month-old mice (8-10 mice per group). Hematocrit was lower in *dw/dw* and *hyt/hyt* mice than in respective controls (P < 0.001, T-test).

## RELATIONSHIPS TO IMMUNOLOGIC AGING

### Thymic Involution

Progressive thymic involution is a universal characteristic of mammalian aging. Thymic weight of the *dw/dw* mouse, as a proportion of body weight, has been reported as lower (Fabris *et al.*, 1971; Duquesnoy *et al.*, 1970) or equivalent to (Shire, 1973; Dumont *et al.*, 1979) thymic weight in normal littermates. Thymic weight (adjusted for body weight) of young male *dw/dw* and *hyt/hyt* mice in our colony was about 25% lower than in controls (Table 2). This suggests that the decrease we observed in young *dw/dw* mice results from their TH deficiency rather than GH deficiency, because adjusted thymic weight was unaffected in young *lit/lit* mice. Since hematocrit was also affected in young *dw/dw* and *hyt/hyt*, but not in *lit/lit* mice, age-related decreases in hematocrit may be partially linked with thymic involution by a common dependence on thyroid hormone (Table 3). Based on this hypothesis we examined data from a separate study of hypophysectomized, old B6CBA

| Table 2. Thymus weight in mice with endocrine mutations | | | | | | |
|---|---|---|---|---|---|---|
|  | *DW* +/? | *dw/dw* | Balb +/? | *hyt/hyt* | +/lit | lit/*lit* |
| Weight (mg) | 26.6 ± 1.6 | 4.4 ± 0.4 | 31.6 ± 4.0 | 19.3 ± 4.0 | 42.8 ± 2.5 | 34.3 ± 2.5[*] |
| per gm. body weight | 0.82 ± 0.05 | 0.6 ± 0.06[**] | 0.92 ± 0.07 | 0.69 ± 0.04[*] | 1.47 ± 0.11 | 1.75 ± 0.08 |
| no. mice | 26 | 21 | 4 | 4 | 5 | 7 |

[*] P < 0.05, [**] P < 0.01, t-test. Values are mean ± SEM. Mice were 2.5-6 months old. (Data from Flurkey *et al.*, 1989b)

**Table 3.** Biomarkers of aging may be related to immunologic aging through common endocrine-dependencies: indications from patterns of aging in mice with endocrine mutations

| Physiology | Effect in mutant | Mutation | | |
|---|---|---|---|---|
|  |  | *dw/dw* | lit/*lit* | hyt/*hyt* |
| **Endocrine Deficiency** |  | GH, Prl, TH | GH | TH |
| body weight | gain prevented | Y | N | N |
| tail length | growth prevented | Y | Y | N |
| hematocrit | age effect mimicked | Y | N | Y |
|  |  |  |  |  |
| **Immunologic Change** |  |  |  |  |
| splenic hyperplasia | prevented | Y | Y | N |
| thymic involution | mimicked | Y | N | Y |
| impaired mitogenesis | prevented | Y | N | Y |

Y = effect observed, N = effect not observed. Under the hypothesis that aging patterns are not affected by hormones that regulate development, all the entries above should be N. Instead, age-related changes in both biomarkers of aging and in some immunologic markers are affected in similar ways, *e.g.*, a low hematocrit and evidence of early thymic involution are observed in both *dw/dw* and *hyt/hyt* mice but not in *lit/lit* mice, suggesting that these markers may be regulated by common endocrine determinants.

Fl hybrid mice that received TH supplements in their drinking water; the correlation coefficient for thymus weight and hematocrit was 0.52 (n =12) which was significant at P = 0.05 for the directional test. If similar correlations are found for a number of strains and conditions, more detailed etiologic studies involving modulation of circulating TH levels would be warranted.

## T Cell Mitogen Response

In Table 3 the spleen cell response to T cell mitogens is presented for aging mice as a percent of young controls. Mitogen response was unaffected in young *dw/dw*, *lit/lit* and *hyt/hyt* mice compared to their respective controls. Dumont *et al.*, (1979) also observed no effect of the *dw* mutation on spleen

**Table 4.** Effect of endocrine mutation on mitogen response in old mice (% of response of young littermate controls)

| mitogen | +/? | dw/dw | +/lit | lit/lit | +/? | hyt/hyt |
|---|---|---|---|---|---|---|
| ConA | 79 ± 12 | 151 ± 10[**] | 74 ± 13 | 92 ± 16 | 84 ± 6 | 126 ± 17[*] |
| PHA | 64 ± 11 | 148 ± 12[**] | 64 ± 11 | 61 ± 11 | 74 ± 7 | 114 ± 16[*] |

[*] $P < 0.05$, [**] $P < 0.01$ for comparison of spleen cell mitogen response for 6 old mutant *vs.* 6 old control (littermate heterozygote or wild-type homozygote) mice. Each value is the mean (± SEM) of the percent response of 3-6-month-old young control mice. Old mice were 14-16.5 mo (DW +/? and *dw/dw*), 15.5-16.5 mo (Balb/cBy +/? and *hyt/hyt*) or 22.5-23.5 mo (C57BL/6J +/*lit* and *lit/lit*). (Data are given for optimal mitogen doses; from Flurkey *et al.*, 1989)

cell mitogen response. Surprisingly, both the *dw* and the *hyt* mutations appear to have prevented the age-related decline in splenic mitogen response, a particularly striking effect for the aging *hyt/hyt* mice since they probably would have lived no more than 30-50 days beyond the age at which they were tested. This suggests the possibility that the age-related decline in T cell mitogen response, a classic marker for immunologic aging, may be a pleiotropic effect of exposure to normal levels of thyroid hormone during maturation and adulthood. This contrasts with conclusions based on the effects of thyroidectomy in young rats (Fabris, 1973) and thyroid hormone administration in old mice (Fabris *et al.*, 1982), which suggested that T cell mitogen responses are dependent on thyroid hormone and that the age-related loss of mitogen response may result from reduced levels of circulating thyroid hormone. Such studies are difficult to interpret since thyroidectomy also removes calcitonin and the parathyroid glands, which can alter calcium homeostasis, and since pharmacologic doses of TH may have been used in the replacement studies. Our present studies in *dw* and *hyt* mice clearly demonstrate that major decreases in circulating TH do not inevitably result in impaired T cell responses to mitogens, even in aging animals (Table 4). Our results may be reconciled with Fabris's (above) if exposure to physiological levels of thyroid hormone induces a subsequent thyroid hormone-dependency during aging. Long-term hormone replacement studies in *hyt/hyt* and *dw/dw* mice using physiological treatments will be necessary to characterize the relationship between TH and T cell mitogen response during aging.

Aspects of the relationship of thyroid hormone to age-related immunologic impairment may be indicated by correlational studies using biomarkers. For example, comparison of effects of the *dw*, *hyt* and *lit* mutations on T cell mitogen responses in aging mice to effects on hematocrit (Table 3) generates an interesting hypothesis: if the decline in hematocrit during aging does result from a functional hypothyroidism, as suggested above, then hematocrit may be <u>inversely</u> related to T cell mitogen response within aging individuals. This predicts an apparently paradoxical relationship: accelerated "aging" indicated by one marker could be associated with delayed aging in another. Initial tests of this hypothesis can be incorporated easily into almost any study of mitogen response and aging, including studies in humans, simply by determining if hematocrit correlates inversely with mitogen response. This illustrates one of the advantages of biomarkers of aging; they are easily incorporated into other studies since they are simple to perform and relatively non-invasive.

## Age-related Splenic Hyperplasia

Age-related increases in spleen weight are common in mice and result almost exclusively from increases in the number of cells of the immunohematopoietic lineage, since the spleen comprises primarily white and red blood cells which do not enlarge appreciably during aging. This splenic hyperplasia appeared in the DW/J and in C57BL/6J +/*lit* mice of these studies. Both the *dw* and *lit* mutations prevented this hyperplasia (Figure 7), suggesting that a GH deficiency alone is sufficient to prevent splenic hyperplasia. Since post-maturational skeletal and connective tissue growth was also prevented in *dw/dw* and *lit/lit* mice, the age-related splenic hyperplasia may be associated with a generalized continuation of post-maturational GH-dependent growth processes. One prediction from this hypothesis, that tail length will correlate with spleen weight in aging mice, was not supported when tested using data from 16-24-month-old +/*lit* mice of this study (P = 0.5, n = 16). If the more relevant parameter, the increment in tail length after 7 months of age, also does not correlate with spleen weight, then we would conclude that the degree of splenic hyperplasia is determined by some factor other than GH, even though GH may be necessary for age-related splenic hyperplasia to occur.

One potential difficulty with the use of biomarkers of aging as endocrine bioassays is that few, if any, of these biomarkers are regulated by a single endocrine axis. For example, the low hematocrit in hypophysectomized mice is improved by TH replacement, but not restored to normal (Flurkey, unpublished) suggesting that hematocrit is also affected by hormones of other hypophyseal axes. Therefore, a simple correlation between a biomarker of aging and another age-related change in normal mice does not imply that a particular neuroendocrine determinant is involved. However, when a relationship between a biomarker and another age-related phenomenon is indicated first by comparable effects of these endocrine mutations, then a shared

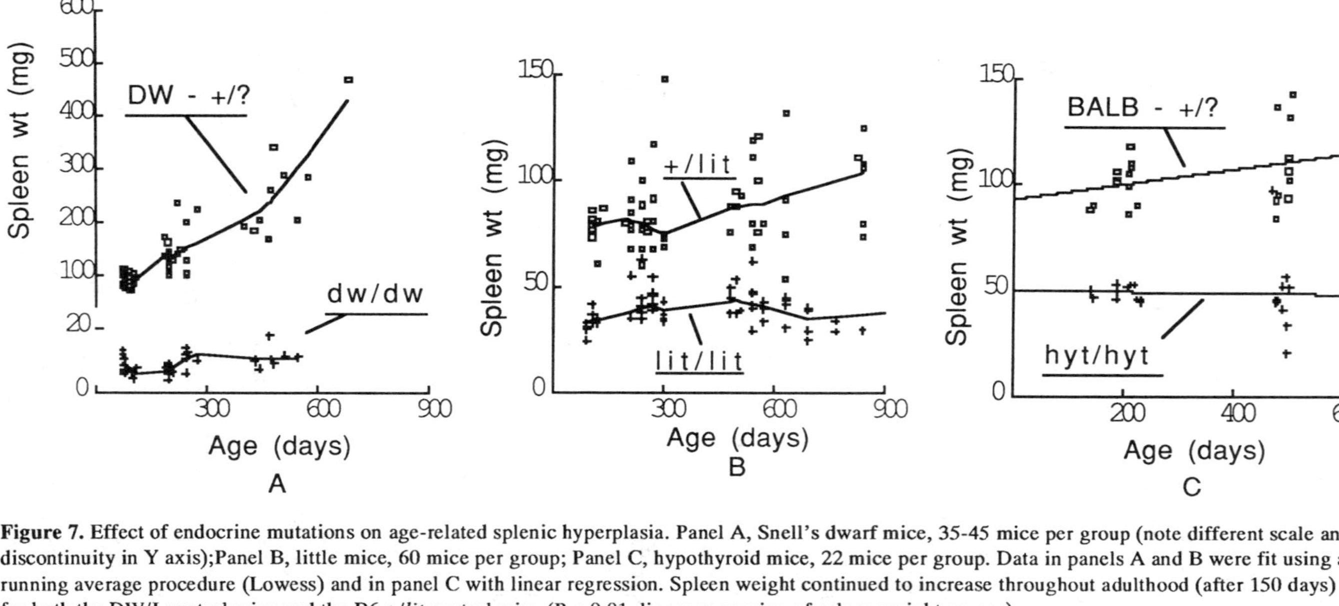


**Figure 7.** Effect of endocrine mutations on age-related splenic hyperplasia. Panel A, Snell's dwarf mice, 35-45 mice per group (note different scale and discontinuity in Y axis);Panel B, little mice, 60 mice per group; Panel C, hypothyroid mice, 22 mice per group. Data in panels A and B were fit using a running average procedure (Lowess) and in panel C with linear regression. Spleen weight continued to increase throughout adulthood (after 150 days) for both the DW/J control mice and the B6 +/*lit* control mice (P < 0.01, linear regression of spleen weight on age),

etiologic role for a single endocrine axis is more plausible. Once a hypothesis is suggested this way, then further correlational analyses in normal mice can help support or refine it.

## ROBUSTNESS OF HYPOTHESES

A potential problem with the use of a mutation on a single genetic background is that of background effects, *i.e.*, effects that result from an interaction of the mutation with the genetic background. This problem is diminished in these studies because of the overlapping physiological effects of the mutations used. Thus, the effect of chronic hypothyroidism is studied on two backgrounds (DW/J and BALB/cBy.RFJ) as is the effect of hyposomatotrophism (DW/J and C57BL/6J). When an effect appears in only one mutant strain, as with the effect of *dw* on postmaturational increases in body mass, a possible background effect becomes a greater consideration. A second potential pitfall is that even consistent effects of a chronic hormone deficiency may be an artifact of the deficiency that is unrelated to aging. This criticism is applicable to any study of chronic effects of endocrine deficiency. A particular advantage of the approach presented here, a consequence of the convenience of biomarkers, is that the hypotheses generated by these studies may be tested simply through correlational analysis in subsequent studies of normal aging mice of a variety of genotypes. Thus, a simple means of determining the generalizability of any of these hypotheses is built into these experiments.

## CONCLUSIONS

Genetic models in which development is altered by mutations that affect neuroendocrine axes were used to identify age-related changes that may be dependent on these developmental axes. Different endocrine determinants were suggested for age-related changes in each of three biomarkers of aging (summarized in Table 3). Similarly, aspects of immunologic aging were differentially affected by each mutation. The specific pattern of effects suggested that age- related changes in each immunologic function may be linked to changes in other axes by common dependencies on developmental hormones: age-related thymic involution may be associated with decrements in hematocrit by a dependency on TH; age-related splenic hyperplasia and post-maturational skeletal system growth may be pleiotropic effects of GH secretion, although correlational studies suggest that the mechanism may differ for each effect; impairments in spleen cell mitogen response may be a pleiotropic consequence of TH which could be inversely related to hematocrit. Easily performed correlational studies can help refine hypotheses concerning the endocrine determinants of immunologic aging so that replacement studies can be designed to test these hypotheses effectively. We suggest that this paradigm may be used to help identify the number, the extent of influence, and the mechanisms of hypothesized neuroendocrine "clocks" that may regulate aging in many systems (Everitt, 1973; Finch, 1987; Meites, 1987).

Although the hypothesis that genetic manipulations that delay or block development would also delay senescence was not supported by lifespan data in these studies, lifespan in laboratory reared inbred mice may reflect only a limited range of pathologies. Therefore, the exclusive use of lifespan as the dependent measure in such studies limits the construct of aging to the set of biological determinants that are associated with a characteristic limiting disease (see chapter by Bronsen, this volume). Age-related changes that may be important to survival under other conditions, such as the loss of lymphoid mitogenic capacity, were affected in a manner consistent with the proposal that negative pleiotropy may result from selection for rapid development or growth. A further consideration that may help clarify these results is the possibility that the *lit* mutation may be less valuable as a model for the study of antagonistic pleiotropisms than we originally assumed; the timing of sexual maturation has not been closely examined for this genotype; however, Chubb (1987) has proposed that its subfertility is a result of small size, not developmental impairment. On the other hand, fertility is delayed in *hyt/hyt* mice (Cubb and Henry, 1988) and *dw/dw* mice are completely infertile. These two genotypes may be more valuable for characterization of developmentally associated antagonistic pleiotropisms.

More generally, these observations indicate the multifactorial nature of mammalian aging; either an "endocrine-deficiency" model, in which aging is viewed as a result of progressive endocrine decrements (*e.g.* Meites, 1987), or a "developmental pleiotropy" model (*e.g.* Everitt, 1973) may apply depending on the specific system and endocrine axis studied. The best endocrine conditions for survivorship may lie somewhere between chronic severe deficiency and the endocrine levels observed in normal mice, which are a result of selection for optimal development and reproduction, not optimal aging. For example, chronic low-dose TH replacement beginning at 10 months of age in *hyt/hyt* mice may minimize detrimental effects of the TH deficiency while delaying the onset of TH-dependent aging. Such selective endocrine replacement studies may be necessary before we can effectively evaluate the extent to which neuroendocrine-associated developmental pleiotropisms determine the patterns of mammalian aging.

## ACKNOWLEDGMENTS

We are grateful to W. Beamer (DK-17947) for helpful discussions and for the mice used in these studies. This research was supported by grants to KF (AGO5429) and to DEH (AGO6232, and AGO0594) from the National Institute on Aging.

## REFERENCES

BARTKE, A. (1964) Histology of the anterior hypophysis, thyroid and gonads of two types of dwarf mice. *Anat. Rec.* **149**: 225-233.

BEAMER, W. G., EICHER, E. M., MALTAIS, L. M., and SOUTHARD, J. L. (1981) Inherited primary hypothyroidism in mice. *Science* **212**: 61-62.

CHENG, T. C., BEAMER, W. G., PHILLIP, J. A., BARTKE, A., MALLONEE, R. L. and DOWLING, C. (1983) Etiology of growth hormone deficiency in little, Ames and Snell dwarf mice. *Endocrinology* **113**: 1669-1 678.

CHUBB, C. (1987) Sexual behavior and fertility of little mice. *Biol. Reprod.* **37**: 564-569.

CHUBB, C. and HENRY, L. (1988) The fertility of hypothyroid male mice. *J. Reprod. Fert.* **83**: 819-823.

DUQUESNOY, R. J., KALPAKTSOGLOU, P. K. and GOOD, R. A. (1970) Immunological studies of the Snell-Bagg pituitary dwarf mouse. *Proc. Soc. Biol. Med.* **133**: 201-206.

DUMONT, F., ROBERT, F. and Bischoff, P. (1979) T and B lymphocytes in pituitary dwarf Snell-Bagg mice. *Immunology* **38**: 23-31.

EICHER, E. M. and BEAMER, W. G. (1976) Inherited ateliotic dwarfism in mice: characteristics of the mutation little (*lit*). *J. Heredity* **67**: 87-91.

EICHER E. M. and BEAMER, W. G. (1980) New mouse *dw* allele: genetic location and effects on lifespan and growth hormone levels. *J. Heredity* **71**: 187-190.

EVERITT, A. V. (1973) The hypothalamic-pituitary control of aging and age-related pathology. *Exp. Gerontol.* **8**: 265-277.

FABRIS, N. PIERPAOLI, W. and SORKIN, E. (1971) Hormones and the immunologic capacity 111. The immunodeficiency disease of the Snell-Bagg dwarf mouse. *Clin. Exp. Immunol.* **9**: 209-225.

FABRIS, N., PIERPAOLI, W. and SORKIN, E. (1972) Lymphocytes, hormones and ageing. *Nature* **240**: 557-559.

FABRIS, N. (1973) Immunodepression in thyroid deprived animals. *Clin. Exp. Immunol.* **15**: 601 -611.

FABRIS, N., MUZZOLI, M. and MOCCHEGIANI, E. (1982) Recovery of age-dependent immunological deterioration in BALB/C mice by short-term treatment with L-thyroxin. *Mech. Aging and Dev.* **18**: 327-338.

FINCH, C. E. (1987) Neural and endocrine determinants of senescence: investigation of causality and reversibility by laboratory and clinical interventions. In: *Modern Biological Theories of Aging* (Eds. H. R. Warner, R. N. Butler, R. L. Sprott and E. L. Schneider) pp. 261-308. N.Y. Raven Press.

FLURKEY, K., MILLER, R. and HARRISON, D. E. (1990) The Snell dwarf (*dw*) and hypothyroid (*hyt*) mutations, but not the little (*lit*) mutation, prevent age-related decrements in spleen cell mitogen response and diminish general lymphoid cellularity. In prep.

HARRISON, D. E. and ARCHER, J. R. (1988) Biomarkers of aging: Tissue markers. Future research needs, strategies, directions and priorities. *Exp. Geront.* **23**: 309-321.

HARRISON, D. E., INGRAM, D. K. and ARCHER, J. A. Longevity prediction by 13 physiological, behavioral and growth parameters in 6 mouse strains (submitted).

HARRISON, D. E., ARCHER, J. R. and ASTLE, C. M. (1984) Effects of food restriction on aging: separation of food intake and adiposity. *Proc. Nat. Acad. Sci. USA.* **81**: 1835-1838.

JANSSON, J.-O., DOWNS, T. R., BEAMER, W. G. and FROHMAN, L. A. (1986) Receptor-associated resistance to growth hormone-releasing factor in dwarf "little" mice. *Science* **232**: 511-512.

MEITES, J., GOYA, R. and TAKAHASHI, S. (1987) Why the neuroendocrine system is important in the aging process. *Exp. Gerontol.* **22**: 1-15.

ROTI, E., CHRISTIANSON, D., HARRIS, A. K. R., BRAVERMAN, L. E. and VAGINAKIS, A. G. (1978) Short loop feedback regulation of hypothalamic and brain thyrotrophin releasing hormone content in the rat and dwarf mouse. *Endocrinology* **103**: 1662-1667.

SCHNEIDER, G. B. (1976) Immunological competence in Snell-Bagg pituitary dwarf mice: response to the contact sensitizing agent oxazalone. *J. Anat.* **145**: 371-380.

SHIRE, J. G. M. (1973) Growth hormone and premature aging. *Nature* **245**: 215-216.

SHIRE, J. G. M. and HAMBLY, E. A. (1973) The adrenal glands of mice with hereditary pituitary dwarfism. *Acta Pathol. Microbiol. Scand.* **Sect.A 81**: 225-

WILLIAMS, G. C. (1957) Pleiotropy, natural selection and the evolution of senescence. *Evolution* **11**: 398-411.

YU, B. P., MASORO, E. J. and McMAHAN, C. A. (1985) Nutritional influences on aging of Fischer 344 rats: 1. Physical, metabolic and longevity characteristics. *J. Geront.* **40**: 657-670.

## DISCUSSION

1. Might *dw/dw* mice age more slowly than normal in some biological systems? Flurkey noted that this may be so in the immune system, although the extremely low spleen weights in *dw/dw* mice must be considered.

2. What is the pathology at death in these mutants? While complete pathological data were not collected in these preliminary studies, Flurkey suspects that there are a lot of nonaging "accidental" deaths in dwarf mice. Human dwarfs may have reduced longevities, but there are many different mechanisms, and some seem to have normal longevities.

3. The importance of the pituitary as the classical "master" gland for growth makes its role in aging interesting especially in relating growth and aging. However, further studies are needed to define mechanisms. Removing the pituitary proved difficult as a surgical technique in old mice, although it was possible. The mutations remove a repeatable portion of the pituitary functions. Of course, the animals may adapt to the losses more effectively in pituitary mutants than when the pituitary is removed in adults.

# 25

# *PEROMYSCUS* AS A GERONTOLOGIC ANIMAL: AGING AND THE MHC

George S. Smith, Mark D. Crew and Roy L. Walford

## ABSTRACT

The much longer lifespan of rodents of the genus *Peromyscus*, the white-footed mouse, and especially of *P. leucopus*, as compared to the common laboratory mouse, genus *Mus*, warrants the development of inbred lines of *Peromyscus* as a gerontologic model for comparison to *Mus* in aging studies. We are inbreeding 14 lines of *P. leucopus*, and have currently one line each at generations $F_{11}$, $F_{10}$, $F_9$ and four at $F_8$. Preliminary RFLP results toward definition of the *P. leucopus* MHC using human and mouse Class I and Class II DNA probes are presented. Studies of the effect on aging in *Mus* of transfection with *Peromyscus* MHC genes are in progress. We also here review the limited amount of gerontologic investigations which have used the comparative *Peromyscus/Mus* model (DNA repair, loss of 5′-methyl-deoxycytidine residues, *etc.*), as well as a variety of non-aging studies in *Peromyscus* which might contribute background material on this species relevant to aging studies.

## INTRODUCTION

The study of aging and the genetic and environmental factors which influence it has involved the pursuit of numerous theories using a broad range of animal species and methodologies. The role of genetics in determining life span in vertebrates has largely been inferred from data on the life spans of various species, as well as interspecies comparisons of physical and metabolic parameters such as body weight, brain weight and metabolic rates (Sacher and Hart, 1978). The evidence for genetic control of aging in invertebrates and vertebrates was recently reviewed by Lints (1978), Cutler (1982), and Johnson (1988).

Our demonstration of a significant influence of H-2 alleles on the life spans of various H-2 congenic lines of mice (Smith and Walford, 1977, 1978), subsequently confirmed by Williams *et al.* (1981), focused attention on the major histocompatibility complex (MHC) and its adjacent regions. Statistical analysis of Smith/Walford data demonstrating considerable differences in life spans between inbred strains of mice congenic at H-2 led Buckley (1982) to the conclusion that differences in the H-2 region could account for about 22 percent of the differences in longevity, whereas 57 percent of life span variation among the congenics was due to non-H-2 strain background effects. Ingram and Reynolds (1982) estimated that the strain background effect on aging accounts for 50% of the variances.

Sacher and Hart (1978) reported an 8 year maximum life span for *Peromyscus leucopus*, and found no other reports of long lived rodent species with comparable life span. Nor have any appeared since, to our knowledge. *Peromyscus*, and especially *Peromyscus leucopus*, seems to be a unique rodent in this regard, and presents an exceptional opportunity to develop a comparative research model companion for studying aging in the laboratory mouse *Mus*. The species are similar in size, structure, and behavior, but show a significant difference in life span. Other differences, for example in DNA-repair capacities or oxidative defense mechanisms, may be relevant gerontologically speaking.

## MATERIALS AND METHODS

Since 1981 we have maintained breeding groups of *Peromyscus*. Our colonies were started with 20 pairs of *P. leucopus* breeders from the colony at Argonne National Laboratories, developed there from wild, locally trapped, animals, randomly bred, with periodic addition of wild animals during its early period, and with 13 pairs of *P. maniculatis* breeders from the University of California, Irvine, which had been randomly bred for 18 months and originated from the colony of J. H. Bower at Weylin Baptist College, Plainsville, Texas (originally established from animals trapped in Chihuahua, Mexico). A small group of *P. maniculatus* derived from Canada were also obtained. These breed poorly. Some were retained for lifespan observation.

Animals were bred and maintained in 5 × 7 × 11 inch plastic mouse cages with metal covers, fed *ad libitum* water and Wayne Research Animal Diet Rodent Blox. They were bedded on wood shavings and provided cotton balls for nesting. The room was maintained at 22-24°C and on a 14 hour light 10 hour dark daily cycle.

We followed brother-sister matings to develop inbred lines, occasionally using half sib, cousin or father-daughter matings to maintain some lines. Pups were weaned between 21 and 30 days dependent on the condition of the dame and the litter. The father usually remained with the pregnant female and subsequent litters(s). Sibs were generally been mated at 8 to 10 weeks of age, usually as pairs but not infrequently as one male with two females.

Small groups of original deermice and $F_1$ animals (including some retired breeders) were set aside to observe for lifespan and diseases. They were housed as above, two to three per cage. Cages were regularly examined for dead mice. A portion of tail tissue was taken from representative animals of the various lines for preliminary DNA extraction and analysis. The detailed methods are described elsewhere (Crew *et al.*, 1988).

## RESULTS

Inbreeding is continuing in 14 lines (many with sublines), and it is likely that a sizeable proportion of the original gene pool continues. Diversity is evident in size, coat color and markings, behavior, and by RFLP patterns shown using human and *Mus* cDNA probes for MHC.

We presently have two original lines of *P. leucopus* (lines 10 and 13, Figure 1) with $F_{10}$ and $F_{11}$ litters respectively. Among "rejuvenated" lines established during 1985 and 1986, one (12) has $F_9$ litters, one (16) $F_8$ litters, two (7, 109) have $F_6$ litters, and four have $F_5$ litters; among 10 × 13 CR, two (752 and 754) have $F_8$ litters and one has $F_7$ litters (753). The rejuvenated lines represent a cross between a male from a failed original line and a 13 × 10 cross $F_{2-3}$ female, followed by a backcross to the original lines male, as well as sib-subline matings, in order to retain much of the original line genotype. Line 109 is a cross between a line 10 female and an original line 9 male. Cross lines 752, 753 and 754 were derived from a 13 × 10 mating. These relationships are shown in Figure 1.

While there is a great temptation to quickly institute compromises in the brother-sister inbreeding, we have limited this to father-daughter, half sib or cousin, similar to the choices exercised by Chai (1969) during inbreeding of rabbits. So far it appears that John King (personal communication) was correct in suggesting that past failures to inbreed *Peromyscus* were a result of too narrow a base and an inadequate breadth of resources, *i.e.*, too few sublines continued at each generation to break through the inbreeding barriers.

The life spans of original and early generation animals in our colony have been observed since November, 1981. The much longer life span of *P. leucopus* compared to *P. maniculatus* and to *Mus* is apparent from the survivorship curves shown in Figure 2 and the data in Table 1. We have three living *P. leucopus* males near 78 months (6 1/2 years). The much longer life span of *Peromyscus* as compared to *Mus*, is evident. It is important to note the difference between lifespans of *P. leucopus* and *P. maniculatus*. We are aware that two other laboratories have also found that *P. maniculatus* has the shorter lifespan, which would seem therefore a less optimal species for gerontologic comparisons to *Mus* than *P. leucopus*. Large differences in life span may

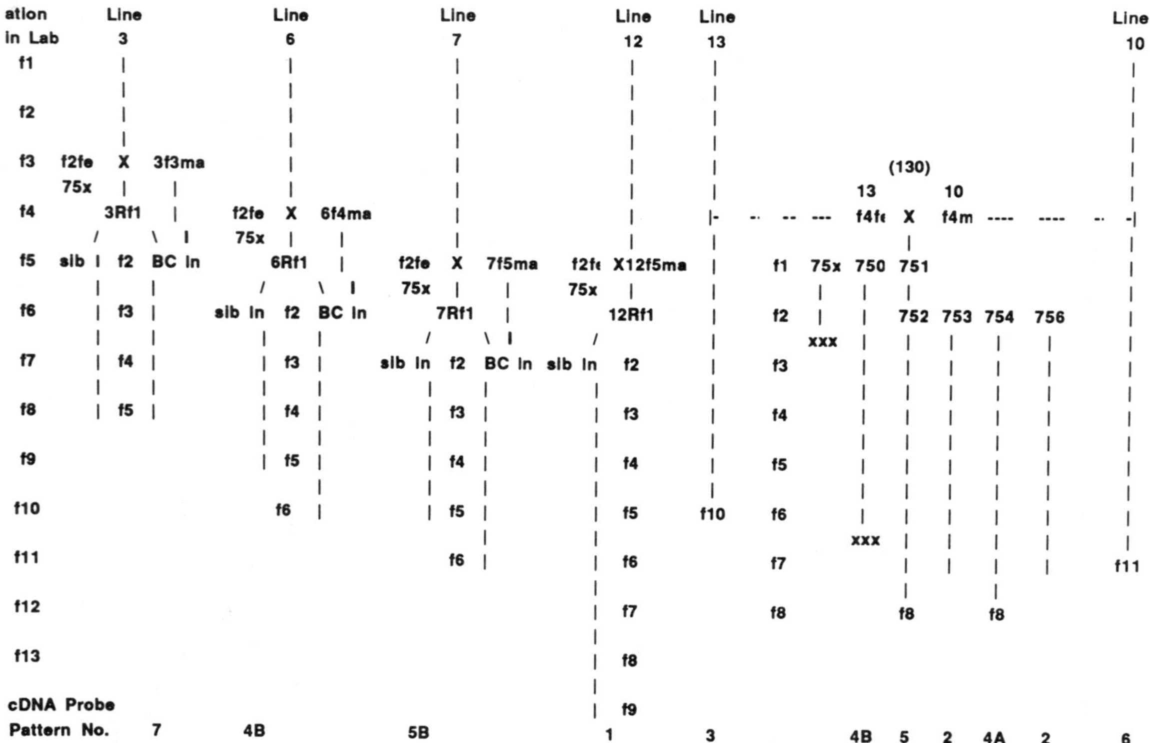

Generation in Lab
f1
f2
f3
f4
f5
f6
f7
f8
f9
f10
f11
f12
f13
cDNA Probe Pattern No.

Line 3
f2fe X 3f3ma
75x
3Rf1
sib f2 BC ln
f3
f4
f5
7

Line 6
f2fe X 6f4ma
75x
6Rf1
sib ln f2 BC ln
f3
f4
f5
f6
4B

Line 7
f2fe X 7f5ma
75x
7Rf1
sib ln f2 BC ln
f3
f4
f5
f6
5B

Line 12
f2fe X12f5ma
75x
12Rf1
sib ln f2
f3
f4
f5
f6
f7
f8
f9
1

Line 13
f10
3

(130)
13      10
f4fe X f4m
f1 75x 750 751
f2      752 753 754 756
xxx
f3
f4
f5
f6
xxx
f7
f8      f8      f8
4B  5   2  4A  2

Line 10
f11
6

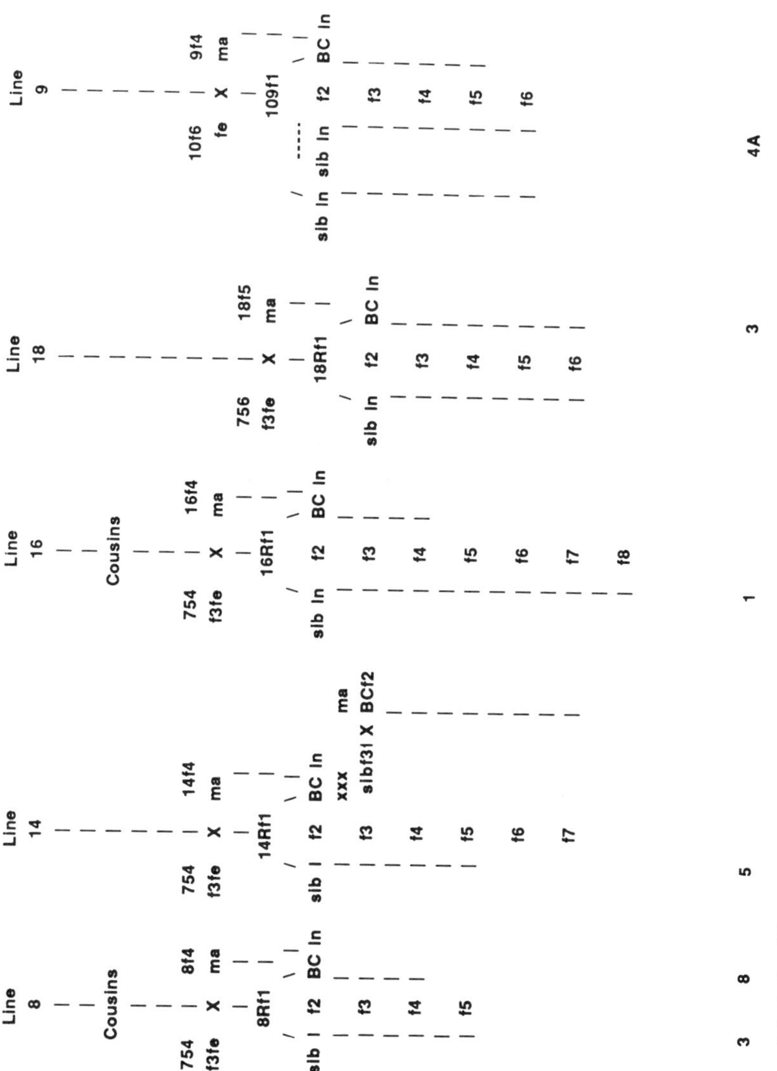


Figure 1. Relationships and status of inbred lines of *Peromyscus leucopus*

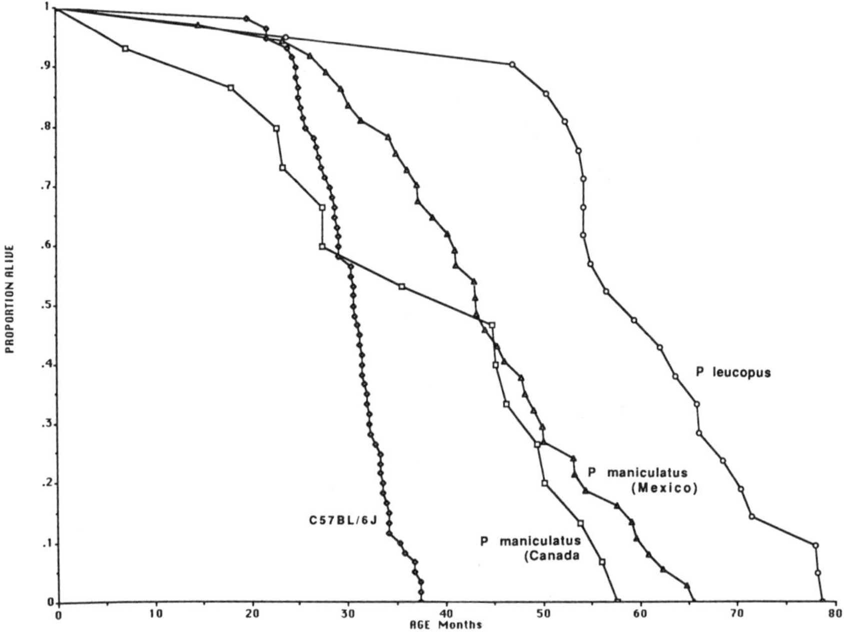


**Figure 2.** Survivorship curves of *P. leucopus* and two lines of *P. Maniculatus* (one derived from Canada; one derived from Mexico) as compared to C57BL/6 male mice (*Mus*).

correlate with large differences in physiologic parameters between species which are similar in other aspects.

In the relatively small population (21 animals) of *P. leucopus* set aside to determine survival, autopsies of all animals dying spontaneously have not revealed any diseases of substantial frequency corroborating the observations of Sacher and Hart (1978). We have not corroborated the disease patterns reported by Thomson *et al.* (1986). We have seen an occasional lymphoma, ovarian papillary carcinoma, adrenal cortical tumor, a liver hamartoma, usually at two or more years of age. Occasional chronic nephritis (end stage) has been noted. Subcutaneous or perianal abscesses are not uncommon. Among *P. maniculatus* we have noted an occasional lymphoma or lung tumor, and uterine sarcoma. Chronic glomerulonephritis is the most common lesion in animals dying beyond two years of age. Breeding mates fight, sometimes fatally. This has substantially declined with time and inbreeding.

| TABLE 1. LIFE SPANS of *PEROMYSCUS* species | | | | | | |
|---|---|---|---|---|---|---|
| Species Sex | No. Mice | Mean (Days) | Mean (Months) | Longest (Days) | Longest (Months) | |
| *P. leucopus* | | | | | | |
| Males | ?166 | 1451+626 | (47.6) | 3000 | (98.5) | Sacher 1978 |
| Females | ?159 | 1388+612 | (45.6) | 2850 | (93.6) | Thomson 1986 |
| Males | 409 | 1447+479 | (47.5) | 2180 | (71.6) | Smith 1989 |
| Males | 21 | | 57.1+3.8 | | 78.6 | |
| | | | | | | |
| *P. maniculatus* | | | | | | |
| **Canadian** | | | | | | |
| Males | 7 | | 39.4+17.5 | | 56 | Smith 1989 |
| Females | 8 | | 35.9+14.8 | | 57.6 | |
| | | | | | | |
| **Mexican** | | | | | | |
| Males | 23 | | 44.7+10.7 | | 62.1 | Smith 1989 |
| Females | 14 | | 41.9+14.5 | | 65.4 | |

An occasional mating (< 1%) results in pregnancy without fetal delivery. The fetuses (usually near term size) are retained and eventually the mother dies, sometimes after 2 or 3 months. Cultures of the resulting retained fetuses and often associated purulent uterine contents have shown no pathogenic organisms so far.

Efforts to characterize the *Peromyscus* MHC at the genomic (RFLP) level (Figure 3 and 4) are in progress, using human and mouse probes. A variety of human and mouse MHC Class I and Class II DNA probes applied to the several lines of *Peromyscus* demonstrate patterns consistent with known breeding relationships. Various lines can be grouped together as demonstrating essentially identical patterns with multiple probes, even though they may have had no breeding relationship since coming to our colony in 1981. The pattern number indicated for each line is also shown at the bottom in Figure 1. We have made a *Peromyscus* genomic library, and MHC genes are being cloned therefrom. We have to date obtained one Class I *Peromyscus* genomic clone and are planning additional efforts in the near future to define the MHC, including serologic methods to identify alleles among the lines and skin graft exchanges.

## DISCUSSION

Over the past 148 years, mammologists have extensively studied *Peromyscus* largely because of its wide geographic distribution and the variety of species in the genus. A considerable literature exists on the biology,

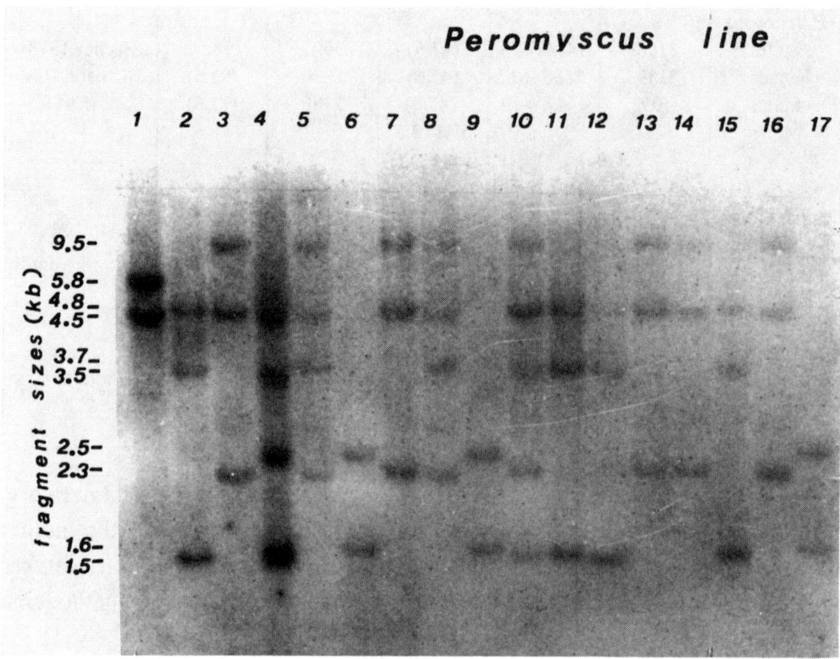


**Figure 3.** Restriction fragment length polymorphisms of DQ alpha-like genes in inbred lines of *P. leucopus*. Bg1 II digested DNA from animals of 17 lines were fractionated by agarose gel electrophoresis, blotted to nitrocellulose and probed with human DQ alpha cDNA at high stringency and washed at high stringency. Sizes of the resulting fragments (in kb) are given to the left of the autoradiogram.

habitats, reproduction and physiology of deermice, including breeding and fertility (Svihla, 1932; Terman, 1965; Rood, 1966; Whitsett and Miller, 1982) reproductive endocrinology, hypothalamic pituitary-gonadal axis, linkage groups of genetic loci, and brain and liver metabolism (Butler, 1988). Wild populations are readily available and adapt and breed well in the laboratory. A complete bibliography of the 1980's includes extensive references on physiology, biology, taxonomy and evolutionary genetics (Butler, 1988). A new book (Advances in the study of Peromyscus, edited by Kirkland and Layne, in press) provides an in depth review of these topics.

Both *Peromyscus* (deermouse) and the laboratory mouse *Mus musculus* belong to the superfamily Muroidea; *Peromyscus* in the family Cricetiae and *Mus* in the family Murinae. *Peromyscus* contains six subgenera (with as many

LINE →

| kb | 10 | 752 | 14 | 7 | 753 | 756 | 16 | 12 | 754 | 109 | 750 | 6 | 8.8 | 3 | 8 | 18 | 13 |
|---|---|---|---|---|---|---|---|---|---|---|---|---|---|---|---|---|---|
| DQ beta/ Bgl II | | | | | | | | | | | | | | | | | |
| 6600 | XXX | XXX | XXX | XXX | XXX | XXX | XXX | XXX | | | | | | | | | |
| 6100 | XXX | | | | | | | | XXX | XXX | XXX | XXX | XXX | | | | |
| 5800 | XXX | XXX | XXX | XXX | XXX | XXX | XXX | XXX | | | | | | XXX | | | |
| 5000 | | | | | | | | | | | | | | XXX | | | |
| 4800 | XXX | XXX | XXX | XXX | XXX | XXX | XXX | XXX | XXX | XXX | XXX | XXX | XXX | XXX | XXX | XXX | XXX |
| 4200 | | | | | | | | | | | | | | | XXX | XXX | XXX |
| 3900 | XXX | XXX | XXX | XXX | | | | | | | | | | XXX | | | |
| 3800 | | | | | | | | | | | | | | XXX | | | |
| 3600 | | | | | | | XXX | XXX | XXX | XXX | | | XXX | | | | |
| 3500 | XXX | XXX | XXX | XXX | XXX | XXX | XXX | XXX | | | | | XXX | | XXX | XXX | XXX |
| 3000 | XXX | XXX | XXX | XXX | XXX | XXX | XXX | XXX | | | | | | | | | |
| 2500 | XXX | XXX | XXX | XXX | XXX | XXX | XXX | XXX | | | | | | XXX | | | |
| 2100 | XXX | XXX | XXX | XXX | XXX | XXX | XXX | XXX | XXX | XXX | XXX | XXX | XXX | XXX | XXX | XXX | XXX |
| 2000 | XXX | | | | | | | | XXX | XXX | XXX | XXX | | | | | |
| 1800 | XXX | | | | | | | | XXX | XXX | XXX | XXX | XXX | | | | |
| 1600 | XXX | XXX | XXX | XXX | XXX | XXX | XXX | XXX | | | | | XXX | | XXX | XXX | XXX |
| 1300 | XXX | | | | | | | | XXX | XXX | XXX | XXX | | | | | |
| 900 | XXX | XXX | XXX | XXX | XXX | XXX | XXX | XXX | | | | | XXX | XXX | XXX | XXX | XXX |
| DQ alpha/ Bgl II | | | | | | | | | | | | | | | | | |
| 9500 | XXX | XXX | XXX | XXX | XXX | XXX | XXX | XXX | | | | | | | | | |
| 5800 | | | | | | | | | | | | | | XXX | | | |
| 4800 | XXX | XXX | XXX | XXX | XXX | XXX | XXX | XXX | XXX | XXX | XXX | XXX | XXX | | | | |
| 4500 | | | | | | | | | | | | | | XXX | | | |
| 3700 | XXX | | | | | | | | XXX | XXX | XXX | XXX | XXX | | | | |
| 3500 | | | | | | | | | | | | | | | | | |
| 2450 | | | | | | | | | | | | | XXX | | XXX | XXX | XXX |
| 2250 | XXX | XXX | XXX | XXX | XXX | XXX | XXX | XXX | | | | | | | | | |
| 1600 | | | | | | | | | | | | | XXX | | XXX | XXX | XXX |
| 1500 | XXX | | | | | | | | XXX | XXX | XXX | XXX | XXX | | | | |
| C4/ Eco RI | | | | | | | | | | | | | | | | | |
| 2350 | XXX | XXX | XXX | XXX | XXX | XXX | XXX | XXX | XXX | XXX | XXX | XXX | XXX | XXX | XXX | XXX | XXX |
| 1800 | XXX | XXX | XXX | XXX | XXX | XXX | XXX | XXX | | | | | | | | | |
| 1550 | XXX | | | | | | | | XXX | XXX | XXX | XXX | XXX | XXX | XXX | XXX | XXX |
| 1400 | XXX | | | | | | | | XXX | XXX | XXX | XXX | | | | | |
| E alpha (DR alpha)/BAM HI | | | | | | | | | | | | | | | | | |
| 2000 | XXX | XXX | XXX | XXX | XXX | XXX | XXX | XXX | XXX | XXX | XXX | XXX | XXX | | | | |
| 850 | XXX | XXX | XXX | XXX | XXX | XXX | XXX | XXX | XXX | XXX | XXX | XXX | XXX | XXX | XXX | XXX | XXX |
| DQ beta/ BAM | | | | | | | | | | | | | | | | | |
| 6400 | | XXX | XXX | | XXX | XXX | | | | | | | XXX | | XXX | XXX | XXX |
| 5500 | XXX | | XXX | | XXX | XXX | | | | | | | XXX | | | | |
| 4200 | | | | | XXX | XXX | | | | | | | | | | | |
| 3700 | | | | | | | | | | | | | XXX | | | | |
| 2800 | | | | XXX | | | | | XXX | XXX | XXX | XXX | XXX | XXX | XXX | XXX | XXX |
| 2600 | XXX | XXX | XXX | | XXX | XXX | XXX | XXX | | | | | | | | | |
| 2100 | XXX | XXX | XXX | XXX | XXX | XXX | XXX | XXX | | | | | | | | | |
| 0 | | | | | | | | | | | | | | | | | |
| Pattern No. | 6 | 5 | 5 | 5B | 2 | 2 | 1 | 1 | 4A | 4A | 4B | 4B | 8 | 7 | 3 | 3 | 3 |

**Figure 4.** Computer representation of Southern blot RFLP DNA banding patterns with several human MHC probes (Class II and III) is shown for 17 lines of inbred *P. leucopus*. Lines with similar patterns are shown adjacent to each other. Methods used were similar to those in Figure 3.

as 50 species), including the subgenus *Peromyscus*, which includes at least eighteen species. *P. leucopus* and *P. maniculatus* are widely distributed in virtually all geographic areas of America. Numerous outbred colonies are maintained in North America, including an NSF supported *Peromyscus* Stock Center at the University of South Carolina. Under the auspices of Wallace Dawson at the Stock Center, a Peromyscus Newsletter was begun in March 1986. *Peromyscus* is reasonably small and not overly expensive to maintain in large colonies, breeds reasonably well, and a number of species are available for inbreeding.

The reproductive portion of life-span of *Peromyscus* is long, with litters being produced at over four years of age (Peluso *et al.*, 1980). Giesel (1979) noted parallels between age specific mortality and age specific fertility in small mammals in general. *Peromyscus* has been used in several aging studies subsequent to the demonstration of its long life span, as reported by Sacher and Hart (1978), and herein confirmed (Figure 2). Harrison *et al.* (1978) studied tail collagen aging in rodents (including *Peromyscus*) and found that age-related changes occurred among females of *Peromyscus* at half the rate of *Mus*. Cohen *et al.* (1987) reported that aged *Peromyscus* had accelerated wound healing compared to young *Peromyscus* and *Mus*. Martin *et al.* (1983) reported that primary cloning efficiency of thoracic aorta smooth muscle cells was twice as much in *Peromyscus leucopus* as in *Mus*, and that a large linear decline occurred in both species. The rate of decline with age was significantly greater in *Peromyscus*. Hart *et al.* (1979) and Su *et al.* (1984) compared DNA repair between *Peromyscus* and *Mus* and reported that UV-induced unscheduled DNA synthesis was 2.5 times greater in the former. On the other hand, single strands produced by gamma rays and the rate of repair of such breaks were similar in the two species. According to Wilson *et al.* (1987), *Peromyscus leucopus* loses genomic DNA 5-methyldioxycytidine residues at a rate about half that of *Mus* over life span.

Significant changes with age in brain lipids in *Peromyscus* and *Mus* were described by Torello *et al.* (1986), and these also varied between the two species. Examining the ovaries and uterus histologically and hormonally as to changes with age, Peluso *et al.* (1980) found substantive differences between *Peromyscus leucopus* and *Mus*. Furthermore, they observed that the maintenance of fertility throughout most of the life span of *Peromyscus* stands "in marked contrast to most other rodents whose fertility and functional capacity of the hypothalamic-pituitary-ovarian axis decline well before the end of their life span." Such a situation may to some extent challenge a neuroendocrine interpretation of aging. Examining aging effects on the hypothalamic hypophyseal-testicular axis in *P. leucopus*, Steger *et al.* (1980) noted that changes in related hormone concentrations and testicular weights were relatively minor when compared to those occurring in comparably aged mice (*Mus*). King *et al.* (1982) observed age-associated pinealocyte changes, suggesting a decrease in neurosecretory-like secretory processes. Dapson *et al.* (1980) compared lipofuscin accumulation in Purkinje cells as a measure of the rates of aging of *Peromyscus* in natural populations. Age-related linear accumulation was noted up to 322 days. According to Rletweld *et al.* (1985), there is evidence for a shortening of the period of circadian rhythm during aging in *Peromyscus*.

Knowledge regarding the immunologic system of *Peromyscus* is quite limited. A multiallelic histocompatibility system can be inferred from the demonstration of skin graft rejection among members of random bred colonies between various species of *Peromyscus*, and from the delay in graft rejection following immunosuppressive treatment (Dawson *et al.*, 1982). Further support for this inference is provided by the immunosuppressive regimens used in pregnancy and placental fetal studies (Bell *et al.*, 1983 and En-Yu *et al.*, 1986). Olson and Hinsdill (1984) and Fairbrother *et al.* (1986) have studied the effects of various chemicals on the *Peromyscus* immune system including plaque forming cell assays, organ weights and marrow-hematologic parameters. Fairbrother *et al.* (1986) found a significant age related influence, causing older (3 years) animals to die more quickly than young animals following viral infection after being fed specific toxicants. Conjugated *Mus* antisera are apparently unable to recognize immunoglobulins of *Peromyscus* whereas rabbit antisera can do so (C. R. Bold, personal communication). The distribution of lymphoid tissue in the intestinal tract of *Peromyscus* is similar to that of most other small mammal species (Barry, 1986). A wide range of infectious diseases have been reported in wild *Peromyscus* including a considerable variety of pathogenic organisms, many similar to human pathogens.

Preliminary work in our laboratory to elucidate the MHC of *Peromyscus* using various human and mouse Class I, II and III DNA probes has shown restriction fragment length polymorphism (RFLP) patterns that are distinctly different among the seventeen lines and sublines examined (Figure 3). There appear to be several unique banding patterns on Southern blots with DQ alpha probes. This suggests multiple alleles among these lines. Similar results were obtained using multiple Class II and complement probes (Figure 4). Note that some lines show essentially identical patterns with all these probes although they have been separated for several generations since inbreeding was started.

We are the first to identify the MHC in *Peromyscus*, using molecular genetic techniques (Crew *et al.*, 1989) (Figs. 3, 4). The main thrust of our current work with *Peromyscus* aims at creating transgenic *Mus* containing MHC genes from the longer-lived species, as a test of the hypothesis that the MHC influences maximum life span and the rate of aging.

Motulsky *et al.* (1962) achieved successful bone marrow transplantation in newborn *Peromyscus* with hereditary spherocytosis and found skin graft rejection between random members of their colony. Prolonged skin graft survival accompanied further successful marrow engraftment.

Lasker (1986) examined microsomal cytochrome p-450 in rodents (including *Peromyscus*) and primates, and reported a protein immunochemically homologous to hamster liver p-450-4 which increased in ethanol treated animals. Mixed function oxidation has been studied by Gellert *et al.* (1986), comparing normal *Peromyscus* with a strain lacking alcohol dehydrogenase. Doyle and Sellinger (1980) found differences in cerebral methyltransferases and monoamine oxidase between audiogenic seizure susceptible and resistant mice and deermice. Lens proteins of *Peromyscus* were studied by Brenner and Atno (1983). Folk *et al.* (1984) noted unusual blood coagulation characteristic in *P. leucopus*.

Although food selection and short term food deprivation studies have been conducted, (Jaeger, 1982; Vickery, 1984; Gray, 1979; Nelson, 1987) we have found no information on chronic dietary restriction. However, *Peromyscus* is known to display increased periods of daily torpor when subjected to food restriction (Tannenbaum and Pivorum, 1987; Hill, 1983). Duffy *et al.* (1987) reported episodes of daily torpor in old animals fed *ad libitum*. This would greatly complicate experimental dietary restriction studies as well as studies of lifetime energy expenditure.

Extensive cytogenetic studies and standardization of *Peromyscus* karyotypes have been done for many of the 50 known species (The Committee for Standardization of Chromosomes of *Peromyscus*, 1977), utilizing trypsin G-Banding and C-banding. All species have a diploid number of 48; however, unlike other genera such as *Mus*, the genus displays considerable chromosomal variation (Robbins and Baker, 1981). A new committee, under the auspices of the *Peromyscus* Stock Center is currently re-evaluating data to achieve a set of current standards. Maps prepared under auspices of the NIH report six linkage groups (Dawson, 1987). A seventh linkage group has also been suggested. Efforts to establish linkage homologies with mouse genetic markers are also in progress.

The inbred lines of *P. maniculatus* at Jackson Laboratories, currently at $F_{18}$, are evidence that persistence can result in inbred lines. However, the gene pool of the JAX inbred lines is probably quite limited, judging from the history of that effort and the number of animals used to originate the lines, (personal communication, David Harrison). It seems most likely that the two groups of *Peromyscus* (JAX and UCLA) will be complimentary and quite different genetically (aside from the species differences).

The long lifespan of *Peromyscus* in the laboratory contrasts with the observation that relatively few animals in the wild survive beyond one or two years. The biological explanation for the long life span potential is unknown. The factors which determine the lifespan of one species as different from other species appear to be more important than the factors affecting life span among strains of a species. Once set, the determinants of maximum life span of a species might be less influenced by environmental influences that those modulating variation of potential life span among strains of a species.

Detailed biochemical and genetic research has been extended immeasurably by the use of inbred strains of animals (as well as more selective breeding systems such as the development of congenic and recombinant inbred lines). Although the long lived *Peromyscus* have been useful for research, the development of inbred strains is essential for more technically advanced biochemical and genetic investigation. Further, the development of such an interspecies gerontologic model may open additional avenues of investigation into genetic control of longevity.

## ACKNOWLEDGEMENTS

We gratefully acknowledge Betty Aalseth whose knowledge and skill in handling these animals has been invaluable. This investigation was supported by grants from the National Institutes of Health (AG-004419).

## REFERENCES

BARRY, R. E., JR. (1986) Distribution of lymphoid tissue in the intestinal tracts of eight species of small mammals. *J. Mamm.* **67**: 593-597

BELL, F. E., PALMER, J. S. and DAWSON, W. D. (1983) Medroxyprogesterone, immunosuppression and conceptus size in *Peromyscus. J. Exp. Zool.* **226**: 273-279

BRENNER, F. J. and ATNO, D. K. (1983) Morphological and eye lens protein characteristics of three species of small mammals. *Proc. Penn. Acad. Sci.* **57**: 173-176

BUTLER, B. (1988) Peromyscus *(Rodentia) 1980-1987 Bibliography* Biology Department, Canadian Union College.

BUTTLER, B. (1988) *Dispersal of* Peromyscus (Rodentia): A Bibliography. Biology Department, Canadian Union College.

CHAI, C. K. (1969) Effects of inbreeding in rabbits. *J. Heredity* **60**: 64-70

COHEN, B. J., CUTLER, R. G. and ROTH, G. S. (1987) Accelerated wound repair in old deer mice (*Peromyscus maniculatus*) and white-footed mice (*Peromyscus leucopus*). *J. Geron.* **42**: 302-307

COMMITTEE FOR STANDARDIZATION. 1977. Standardized karyotype of deer mice, *Peromyscus* (Rodentia). *Cytogenet. Cell Genet.* **19**: 38-43

CREW, M. D., SMITH, G. S., ZELLLER, E., WALFORD, R. L. (1989) Polymorphism in the major histocompatibility complex class II genes of the deermouse, *Peromyscus leucopus*, *Immunogenetics*, (in press).

CUTLER, R. G. (1982) Longevity is determined by specific genes: testing the hypothesis. **In:** *Testing the theories of aging.* CRC Press: Adelman, R.C. and Roth, G.S. (Eds.).

DAPSON, R. W., FELDMAN, A. T. and PANE, G. (1980) Differential rates of aging in natural populations of old-field mice (*Peromyscus polionotus*). *J. Geront.* **35**: 39-44

DAWSON, W. D., REUNING, S. C. and FINLAY, M. F. (1982) Immunological factors in *Peromyscus* speciation. *J. Exp. Zool.* **224**: 1-12

DAWSON, W. D. (1987) The genetic linkage map of the deer mouse (*Peromyscus maniculatus*). **In:** *Genetic Maps.* **4**: 470-473. Cold Spring Harbor Press:

DOYLE, R. L. and SELLINGER, O. Z. (1980) Differences in activity in cerebral methyltransferases and monoamine oxidases between audiogenic seizure susceptible and resistant mice and deermice. *Pharm. Biochem. Behav.* **13**: 589-591

DUFFY, P. H., FEUERS, R. J. and HART, R. W. Effect of age and torpor on the circadian rhythms of body temperature, activity, and body weight in the mouse (*Peromyscus leucopus*). Advances in Chronobiology, Part B. Alan R. Liss, Inc., pp. 111-120.

EN-YU, L. and DAWSON, W. D. (1986) Paternal antigen and progesterone effects on conceptus size in laboratory mice. *Biol. Rep.* **35**: 524-530

FAIRBROTHER, A., YUILL, T. M. and OLSON, L. J. (1986) Effects of three plant growth regulators on the immune response of young and aged deer mice *Peromyscus maniculatus*. *Arch. Environ. Contam. Toxicol.* **15**: 265-276

FOLK, G. E. JR., OWEN, W. and SMITH, D. (1984) Unusual blood coagulation in a hibernator, the deer mouse (*P. leucopus*). *Physiologist* **27**: 230

GELLERT, J., ALDERMAN, J. and LIEBER, C. S. (1986) Interaction between ethanol metabolism and mixed-function oxidation in alcohol dehydrogenase positive and negative deermice. *Biochemical Pharmacology* **35**: 1037-1041

GIESEL, J. T. (1979) Association between age specific mortality and fecundity rates in mammals. *Exp. Geront.* **14**: 189-192

GRAY, L. (1979) Feeding diversity in deer mice. *J. Comp. and Phys. Psych.* **93**: 1118-1126

HARRISON, D. E., ARCHER, J. R., SACHER, G. A. and BOYCE F. M. III. (1978) Tail Collagen aging in mice of thirteen different genotypes and two species: Relationship to biological age. *Exp. Gerontol.* **13**: 63-73

HART, R. W., SACHER, G. A. and HOSKINS, T. L. (1979) DNA repair in a short and long-lived rodent species. *J. Geront.* **34**: 808-817

HILL, R. W. (1983) Thermal Physiology and energetics of *Peromyscus*; ontogeny, body temperature, metabolism, insulation and microclimatology. *J. Mamm.* **64**: 19-37

INGRAM, D. K. and REYNOLDS, M. A. (1982) The relationship of genotype, sex, body weight, and growth parameters to lifespan in inbred and hybrid mice. *Mech. Aging Dev.* **20**: 253-266

JAEGER, M. M. (1982) Feeding Pattern in *Peromyscus maniculatus*: The response to periodic food deprivation. *Phys. Behav.* **28**: 83-88

JOHNSON, T. E. (1988) Genetic specification of life span: processes, problems and potentials. *J. Gerontol.* **43**: B87-93

KING, T. S., KARASEK, M., PETTERBORG, L. J., HANSEN, J. T. and REITER, R. J. (1982) Effects of advancing age on the ultrastructure of pinealocytes in the male white-footed mouse (*Peromyscus leucopus*). *J. Exp. Zool.* **224**: 127-134

LASKER, J. M., *et al.*. (1986) Immunochemical evidence for an ethanol-inducible form of liver microsomal cytochrome P-450 in rodents and primates. *Fed. Proc.* **45**: 1665

LINTS, F. A. (1978) Genetics and Aging, Interdisciplinary Topics in Gerontology 14.

MARTIN, G. M., OGBURN, C. E. and WIGHT, T. N. (1983) Comparative rates of decline in the primary cloning efficiencies of smooth muscle cell from the aging thoracic aorta of two murine species of contrasting maximum life span potentials. *Am. J. Path.* **110**: 236-245

MOTULSKY, A. G., ANDERSON, R., SPARKES, R. S. and HUESTIS, R. H. (1962) Marrow Transplantation In Newborn Mice with Hereditary Spherocytosis: A Model System. *Trans. Assoc. Amer. Phys.* **25**: 64-71

NELSON, R. J. (1987) Gonadal regression induced by caloric restriction is not mediated by the pineal gland in deer mice. *J. Pin. Res.* **4**: 339-345

OLSON, L. J. and HINSDILL, R. D. (1984) Influence of feeding chlorocholine chloride and glyphosine on selected immune parameters in deermice, *Peromyscus maniculatus. Toxicology* **30**: 103-114

PELUSO, J. J., MONTGOMERY, M. K., STEGER, R. W., MEITES, J. and SACHER G. (1980) Aging and ovarian function in the white-footed mouse (*Peromyscus leucopus*) with specific reference to the development of preovulatory follicles. *Exper. Aging Res.* **6**: 317-328

RIETVELD, W. J., BOON, M. E., KORVING, J. and VAN SCHRAVENDIJK, K. (1985) Circadian rhythms in elderly rats. *J. Interdiscipl. Cycle Res.* **16**: 154

ROBBINS, L. W. and BAKER, R. J. (1981) An assessment of the nature of chromosomal rearrangements in 18 species of *Peromyscus* (Rodentia: Cricetidae). *Cytogenet. Cell Genet.* **31**: 194-202

ROOD, J. P. (1966) Observations on the reproduction of *Peromyscus* in captivity. *The Am. Midland Naturalist* **76**: 496-503

SACHER, G. A. and HART, R. W. (1978) Longevity, aging and comparative cellular and molecular biology of the house mouse, *Mus musculus*, and the white-footed mouse, *Peromyscus leucopus. Birth Defects* Original Article Series **14** No. 1, 71-96.

SMITH, G. S. and WALFORD, R. L. (1977) Influence of the main histocompatibility complex on aging in mice. *Nature* **270**: 727-729

SMITH, G. S. and WALFORD, R. L. (1978) Influence of the H-2 and H-1 Histocompatibility Systems Upon Life Span and Spontaneous Cancer Incidences in Congenic Mice. *Birth Defects* Original Article Series. **14** No. 1, 281-312.

STEGER, R. W., HUANG, H. H., HODSON, C. A., LEUNG, F. C., MEITES, J. and SACHER G. A. (1980) Effects of Advancing Age on Hypothalamic-Hypophysial-Testicular Functions in the Male White-footed Mouse (*Peromyscus leucopus*). *Biol. Reprod.* **22**: 805-809

SU, C. M., BRASH, D. E., TURTURRO, A. and HART, R. W. (1984) Longevity-dependent organ-specific accumulation of DNA damage in two closely related murine species. *Mech of Ageing and Dev.* **27**: 239-247

SVIHLA, A. (1932) *A comparative life history study of the mice of the genus* Peromyscus. The University of Michigan Press: Misc. Publ. 24, July 8.

TANNENBAUM, M. G. and PIVORUN, E. (1987) Differential effect of food restriction on the induction of daily torpor in *Peromyscus maniculatus* and *P. leucopus. J. Therm. Biol.* **12**: 159-162

TERMAN, C. R. (1965) A study of population growth and control exhibited in the laboratory by Prairie Deermice. *Ecology* **46**: 890-895

THOMSON, J. F., WILLIAMSON, F. S. and GRAHN D. (1986) Life Shortening in mice exposed to fission neutrons and gamma rays. *Rad. Res.* **108**: 176-188

TORELLO, L. B., YATES, A. J., HART, R. and LEON, K. S. (1986) A comparative-evolutionary study of lipids in the aging brain of mice. *Neurobiol. Aging* **7**: 337-346

VICKERY, W. L. (1984) Optimal diet models and rodent food consumption. *Anim. Behav.* **32**: 340-348

WHITSETT, J. M. and MILLER, L. L. (1982) Photoperiod and reproduction in female deer mice. *Biol. Reprod.* **26**: 296-304

WILLIAMS, R. M., *et al.*. (1981) Genetics of Survival in Mice: Localization of Dominant Effects to Subregions of the Major Histocompatibility Complex. **In**: *Immunological Aspects of Aging.* Marcel Dekker, Inc., pp. 247-261.

WILSON, V. L., SMITH, R. A., MA, S. and CUTLER, R. G. (1987) Genomic 5-Methyl-deoxycytidine Decreases with Age. *J. Biol. Chem.* **262**: 9948-9951

## DISCUSSION

1. The subspecies *Peromyscus maniculatus* and *Peromyscus leucopus* will not breed to produce inter-species hybrids. The former are not nearly as long lived as the latter.

2. One of the major purposes in constructing the inbred *Peromyscus leucopus* strains was to provide gene donors for making transgenic laboratory mice using *Peromyscus leucopus* genes, especially the MHC. When it was noted that inbred strains are not required for this purpose, Smith agreed, but noted that it would be essential for studying such transgenic mice, for defining the MHC of *Peromyscus*, and for studying the gerontological comparative model of *Peromyscus* and *Mus*, to develop inbred lines. Currently, human MHC probes are best, although genes for MHCs of many species have been cloned. Why not use those for transgenic mice? Smith noted that the phylogenetic distance might be too great with human genes in laboratory mice. Possibly, laboratory mice have inverted MHC genes compared to human and rat. Also, transgenic mice would not be like MHC congenics for the *Peromyscus leucopus* genes, since the laboratory mouse genes will still be there. Using embryonal stem cells (ESC) homologous recombinations might occur replacing resident loci with those transferred. Are ESC lines from *Peromyscus leucopus* available?

3. How important is torpor in the longevity of *Peromyscus leucopus*? Tutarro suggested that the deep sleep of torpor in laboratory mice was sensitive to the amount of food and water, claiming that their body temperatures fall to ambient levels when food restricted. Others disagreed with this, based on oxygen consumption data over 24 hours, but those mice may not have behaved normally in the metabolic cages. Tutarro's group used surgically implanted temperature meters. Laboratory mice are so small that their temperature can change very rapidly in portions of the body due to their low "thermal mass". Possibly the surgically implanted temperature meters were not in a place representative of the most metabolically active tissues in sleeping mice, such as the brain or kidney.

# 26

# MURINE CHROMOSOMAL REGIONS INFLUENCING LIFE SPAN

Ada L. M. Watson, Rebecca S. Gelman, R. Michael Williams, and Edmond J. Yunis

## ABSTRACT

We have used three different experimental models to study chromosomal regions that influence life span in mice.

### *H-2* Congenic Mice

This study of B10 background congenic mice and their hybrids with DBA/2J mice showed there was a significant effect of birth date on survival, perhaps due to a Sendai virus infection which occurred when the mice were between 1 and 74 weeks old. The effect of birth date was about as strong as the genetic effect, but both were significant in models including both. The D-end of the *H-2* region is more significantly associated with life span than is the K-end. In the D subregion, hybrid mice which were $H\text{-}2^d$ had shorter life spans than $H\text{-}2^b$, $H\text{-}2^q$, or $H\text{-}2^k$. In this subregion, parental mice which were $H\text{-}2^d$, $H\text{-}2^k$, or $H\text{-}2^s$ had shorter life spans than $H\text{-}2^b$. Among strain-sex groups in which we studied parentals and hybrids with appropriate overlaps in date of birth, 2 of 6 comparisons showed significantly longer life span in the hybrids.

### Backcross Mice [(C57BL/6xDBA/2)$F_1$ × DBA/2].

Among these mice the females lived longer than males. Among the male mice the $H\text{-}2^{b/d}$ mice lived longer than the $H\text{-}2^{b/b}$ mice. The Chromosome 4 marker (brown locus) was seen to have a significant effect on life span among the female mice (+/*b* mice lived longer than *b*/*b* mice). In general, the longest survival was observed in the most heterozygous mice. The more heterozygous the longer the survival. We also observed a significant interaction between Chromosome 4, Chromosome 17 and birth date.

## Recombinant Inbred (RI) Mice of (C57BL/6xDBA/2)F₁.

In twenty strains studied, 101 of the 141 typed chromosomal regions were distinguishable.Two strains had significantly shorter survival and 5 had longer survival than the remaining 13.Despite the fact that C57BL/6 (B) mice live longer than DBA/2 (D) mice, strains with the most B markers didn't live the longest.Statistical models identified 7 chromosomal regions which together account for most of the variation of survival. These regions are determined by the following markers: *Coh B* type on Chromosome 7, *Ly-24* B type and *H-3* D type on Chromosome 2, *Lamb-2* D type and *Ltw-4* B type on Chromosome 1, *Igh* region D type and *D12Nyu1* D type on Chromosome 12.

## INTRODUCTION

Our research has been focussed on identifying possible genes that interact with environmental factors to affect murine life span. We aim to characterize mouse strains that have a short or a long life span and to correlate them with chromosomal regions and causes of death. We have used three different experimental models: congenic strains to associate life span to different *H-2* (MHC - the major histocompatibility complex); backcross mice to test the influence of *H-2* on life span in relation to other genetic factors; and the effect of many chromosomal regions in life span using recombinant inbred strains of mice. In studying mice that differ in more genetic regions than the *H-2* region, we have found that *H-2* is not the major genetic influence on longevity.

## Genetic Influences on Longevity

Genes affecting life span have been identified in nematodes and fruit flies (Klass, 1983; Johnson and Wood, 1982; Clark and Gould, 1970; Gould and Clark, 1983), but it has not been possible to determine a single gene that can predict long life in outbred populations. The different life spans observed in various inbred strains of mice also suggest a genetic influence on longevity. Some of the life span differences in inbred mouse strains have been associated with specific diseases; *e.g.*, leukemia in AKR mice and mammary tumors in C3H female mice. The gross pathology at death and mean survival times of many inbred mouse strains have been documented to differ by strain (Storer, 1966; Festing and Blackmore, 1971; Russell, 1972; Goodrich, 1975; Smith, *et al.*, 1973; Myers, 1978; Storer, 1978). In other strains and hybrids the differences in life span could not be accounted for by specific diseases (Russell, 1975).

It has been possible to show that heterosis prolongs life span in some mouse strains (Russell, 1975). In some $F_1$ hybrid mice the mean life spans are longer than those of their parents (Myers, 1978; Smith and Walford, 1977), however, some long lived inbred strains have longer life spans than do some types of $F_1$ hybrid mice (Myers, 1978). This suggests that heterozygosity, per se, does not universally increase longevity in mice. In fruit flies a similar effect has been seen (Baird and Linzczynsyj, 1985), however, in nematodes no survival benefit of heterosis has been found (Johnson, 1984; Johnson, *et al.*, 1984).

The studies of different life spans in *H-2* congenic mice (differing only in *H-2* haplotypes) led to the hope that a genetic effect on longevity would be relatively simple and based on one or a few selected genes. Since genes of the MHC control the immune system, it was anticipated that longevity may be associated with the expression of certain *H-2* phenotypes (Benacerraf, 1981; Greenberg and Yunis, 1975; Greenberg and Yunis, 1978; Katz, *et al.*, 1976; Meredith and Walford, 1977; Popp, 1978; Williams, *et al.*, 1981). There was a correlation between *H-2*, life span and maintenance of immune vigor (Meredith and Walford, 1977; Popp, 1978). In some congenic strains non-chromosomal effects have been shown, *e.g.*, the reciprocally bred $F_1$ hybrids between $H\text{-}2^n$ and $H\text{-}2^b$ showed differences in life span (Popp, 1978). Although congenic experiments are important, they do not examine the role of other genetic factors alone or the effect of combined genes on life span. Association of immune functions with genotypes and life span has not been done but it would be possible now to use strains differing at genotypes to monitor immune function without sacrificing the experimental animals. The development of limiting dilution assays using peripheral blood lymphocytes makes it possible to study these relationships. For example, retardation of the rate at which precursor cell frequencies decline in long lived strains or long lived individuals (Miller and Harrison, 1985) would suggest that this cell type plays an important role in life span and that such decline is the result of genetic influences. Furthermore, dietary restriction may change these functions in relation to life span and incidence of tumors.

Tumors and infections are some of the common factors responsible for the mortality of aged mice and man. NK cells form an important arm of the surveillance mechanism against tumor development, and viral and bacterial infections (Herberman and Ortaldo, 1981). Low NK activity is correlated with high incidence of tumors. When NK cells were injected into NK deficient histocompatible mice, these mice developed a capability, comparable to that of normal counterparts, to reject syngeneic tumors and inhibited the development of radiation induced thymic leukemia (Warner and Dennert, 1981). Also, when mice with a propensity to reject tumors were injected with anti-AGMI antibody (which is know to bind primarily mouse NK cells) and challenged with tumor cells, a significant increase in tumor take and growth was observed (Kasai, *et al.*, 1979). Such studies would provide evidence that NK cells in vivo are involved in the control of tumor growth.

The regulation of immune response is predominantly under genetic control, but non-lymphoid factors, such as nutrition, hormone levels and drugs are also influential. Yunis and collaborators (Fernandes, *et al.*, 1981; Fernandes, *et al.*, 1983; Lane and Yunis, 1981) demonstrated that, in the autoimmune-prone NZB mouse strain, diets low in fat and high in protein and fiber content lead to delayed development of auto-immunity and are associated with prolonged life span in both males and females.

Since we, as well as others, have shown that genetic profiles may predict association of cause of death by tumors it would be helpful to analyze immune functions during life in order to find out if genetic factors can be identified which are associated to immune vigor and cause of death.

## EXPERIMENTAL DESIGNS AND RESULTS

### *H-2* Congenic Studies

In a study of *H-2* congenic mice, F$_1$ hybrids between DBA/2J (D2) females and C57BL/10 (B10) background *H-2* congenic male mice were bred (11 strains). Also followed for survival were F$_1$ hybrids between B10 female mice and three strains of B10 congenic male mice. In addition, ten of the parental *H-2* congenic strains were followed for survival. The mice were bred over a period of two years. Towards the end of the breeding period, there was documentation of sendai infection in the mouse rooms. One-third of the mice followed for survival were male and two-thirds were female. Eighteen percent of the mice were censored at various times because they were removed from the colony for use in other experiments. Table 1 shows the *H-2* haplotypes and subregion markers for the strains in this study.

There were some differences in survival by sex, with females of the B10.A5R strain surviving significantly longer than males. All analyses were done separately for the two sexes. Although it did not appear that an unusually high number of mice died during the time the colony was infected with Sendai, there was a highly significant tendency for mice who were younger at the time of the Sendai infection to have shorter survival than mice who were older at that time point. This was true for male parental, male hybrid and female hybrid mice, but not for the female parental mice, see Table 2. The effect of birth date on survival was about as significant as the effect of strain

**Table 1.** *H-2* and Closely Linked Loci of Parental Strains

| Parental Strain | I | | | | | | | |
|---|---|---|---|---|---|---|---|---|
| | *H-2* Haplotype | K/Aα/Aβ/Eβ | Eα | S | D/L | Qa-2 | Qa-1 | Tla |
| DBA/2 | d | d | d | d | d | a | b | c |
| B10 | b | b | b | b | b | a | b | b |
| B10.A | a | k | k | d | d | a | a | a |
| B10.A2R | h2 | k | k | d | b | a | b | b |
| B10.A4R | h4 | k | b | b | b | a | b | b |
| B10.A5R | i5 | b | k | d | d | a | a | a |
| B10.BR | k | k | k | k | k | b | b | b |
| B10.HTT | t3 | s | k | k | d | a | b | c |
| B10.T6R[a] | y2 | q | q | q | d | a | a | a |
| B10.AKM | m | k | k | k | q | a | a | a |
| B10.D2N[b] | d | d | d | d | d | a | b | c |
| B10.S[c] | s | s | s | s | s | a | b | b |

[a] Only one parental mouse followed for survival.
[b] No parental mice followed for survival.
[c] No hybrids were made from this parental.

**Table 2.** Effect of Birth Date on Life Span

| | Median Survival (in months) | | | | | | | | |
|---|---|---|---|---|---|---|---|---|---|
| | | | | | | | Period of Sendai Infection | | |
| Year | 76 | 76 | 76 | 77 | 77 | 77 | 77 | 78 | 78 |
| Quarter | 2nd | 3rd | 4th | 1st | 2nd | 3rd | 4th | 1st | 2nd |
| Male parental | 30 | - | - | 28 | 26 | 21 | 24 | - | 22 |
| Female parental | - | - | 26 | 26 | 27 | 25 | 28 | 24 | 25 |
| Male D2 hybrid | - | 29 | - | 28 | 27 | - | 27 | - | - |
| Female D2 hybrid | - | 31 | 33 | 26 | 24 | - | 22 | - | - |

on survival (Table 3). Hence all analyses of genetic effects on survival were either done within subsets of mice born in the same quarter of a particular year or else included date of birth variables in survival models.

Among parental strains (within specific birth dates), strain was a more significant factor for females than for males. However, among DBA/2 hybrids (within specific birth dates), strain was a more significant factor in males than females (Table 4). The same relative relationship based on sex was found in survival models adjusting for date of birth. Of the 18 possible comparisons of pairs of strains which overlapped in birth dates and differed only in the D-end of *H-2*, 5 were associated with highly significant survival differences. Of the 10 pairs of strains which overlapped in birth date and differed only in the K end of *H-2*, none were associated with significant survival differences (Table 5). In models of survival based on birth date and alleles for one of the four

**Table 3**. The Effect of Strain on Survival After Birth Date Taken Into Account (and vice versa)

| | Male P-value[a] | Female P-value[a] |
|---|---|---|
| **D2 Hybrids** | | |
| all strains | $<10^{-10}$ | 0.00005 |
| all quarters | 0.0007 | 0.04 |
| **Parentals** | | |
| all strains | $1\times10^{-8}$ | $2\times10^{-7}$ |
| all quarters | 0.0002 | $1\times10^{-7}$ |

[a] The P-values represent the overall significance of strains (or birth date) in proportional hazards models after the effect of birth date (or strains) is removed.

**Table 4.** Comparisons of Strains Within Common Birth Dates

| | Male P-value | Direction[a] | Female P-value | Direction[a] |
|---|---|---|---|---|
| **Quarter** | | | | |
| **D2 Hybrids** | | | | |
| 3rd of 1976 | .002 | D2×B10 < D2×B10.BR | - | — |
| 1st of 1977 | .005 | D2×B10.A2R, D2×B10 < D2×B10.A | .10 | — |
| 2nd of 1977 | .004 | D2×B10.A5R < D2×B10.A < D2×B10 | .01 | — |
| 4th of 1977 | .03 | — | .96 | — |
| **Parentals** | | | | |
| 1st of 1977 | .03 | — | .000001 | B10.A < B10.A2R < B10.HTT |
| 2nd of 1977 | .08 | — | .03 | |
| 3rd of 1977 | .003 | — | .0002 | B10.A5R, B10.A < B10, B10.A4R |
| 4th of 1977 | .05 | — | .47 | — |
| 2nd of 1978 | .04 | — | — | — |

[a] C, A < B Survival on strains C and A significantly less than survival on strain B.

subregions (KAEβ, Eα, S, DL), the KAEβ alleles were seldom (2/8 models) associated with significant survival differences but the other regions usually were associated with significant survival differences (Eα in 6/8, S in 8/8, DL in 7/8). The most consistent results in comparing alleles in these models among hybrid strains were: *d* was associated with shorter survival than *b*, *q*, or *k*. Among parentals, *d* or *k* or s was associated with shorter survival than b.

**Table 5.** Strains Which Differ on Only Parts of *H-2* Region; Analysis Within Common Birth Quarter

| *H-2* Differences | Parental Male | Parental Female | D2 Hybrid Male | D2 Hybrid Female |
|---|---|---|---|---|
| K End | | | | |
|    KAE$_\beta$[a] | | | | |
|       B10 *vs.* B10.A4R | -[b] | .08 | - | - |
|       B10.A *vs.* B10.A5R | .82, .05 | .77 | .24 | .17 |
|    KAE$_\beta$E$_\alpha$ | | | | |
|       B10.A5R *vs.* B10.D2 | .07 | - | - | - |
|    KAE$_\beta$E$_\alpha$S | | | | |
|       B10 *vs.* B10. A2R | - | - | .19 | .28 |
|       B10.HTT *vs.* B10.T6R | - | - | .03 | .54 |
| | | | | |
| D End | | | | |
|    DL | | | | |
|       B10.A *vs.* B10.A2R | .98 | <.0001 | .003 | .02 |
|    SDL | | | | |
|       B10.A *vs.* B10.BR | .73 | - | - | .0002, .76 |
|       B10.A2R *vs.* B10.AKM | - | - | - | .07 |
|       B10.A2R *vs.* B10.BR | - | - | - | .19 |
|    E$_\alpha$SDL | | | | |
|       B10 *vs.* B10.A5R | .001, .65 | .02 | .007 | .53 |
|       B10.A *vs.* B10.A4R | - | .003, .52 | - | - |
|       B10.A4R *vs.* B10. AKM | - | - | .40 | .93 |

[a] Strains which differ at K, A, E$\beta$, loci but have same alleles for E$\alpha$, S, D, L loci.
[b] - = Too few dead mice or no overlap in birth seasons

We conclude that it is very important for survival studies to be based on animals bred at approximately the same time, since age differences at the time of an environmental stress may result in significant differences in longevity, even among mice who survive the acute health threat. We also conclude that mice differing genetically only at the *H-2* (and perhaps closely linked) loci differ significantly in survival. These data also suggest that the D end of *H-2* may have more of an effect on survival than the K end; future experiments in these strains, their hybrids, and other congenic strains will be needed to verify this.

## Backcross Study

Our work on backcross mice [(C57BL/6 × DBA/2)F$_1$ × DBA/2] suggested that several chromosomal regions and the environment act together to influence longevity in mice (Yunis, *et al.*, 1984). The Cox model, used to test for interactions between the different variables, revealed two significant three-way interactions. *H-2*$^b$/*H-2*$^d$ mice differed significantly in life span from the *H-2*/*H-2*$^d$, both in animals born 5/29/79 and heterozygous for *b* (*B/b*)

**Table 6.** Median Survival of Backcross Mice

| | All Mice | | Females | | Males | |
|---|---|---|---|---|---|---|
| | Median Survival | P-value | Median Survival | P-Value | Median Survival | P-value |
| Sex | | | | | | |
| females | 27 | | | | | |
| | | .0006 | | | | |
| males | 26 | | | | | |
| *Chromosome 17* | | | | | | |
| $H\text{-}2^d/H\text{-}2^d$ 25 | | 26 | | 25 | | |
| | | .02 | | .38 | | .01 |
| $H\text{-}2^b/H\text{-}2^d$ 27 | | 28 | | 26 | | |
| *Chromosome 4* | | | | | | |
| *b/b* | 25 | | 25 | | 25 | |
| | | .006 | | .008 | | .30 |
| *B/b* | 28 | | 29 | | 29 | |
| *Chromosome 9* | | | | | | |
| *d/d* | 26 | | 28 | | 25 | |
| | | .38 | | .23 | | .08 |
| *D/d* | 27 | | 27 | | 27 | |

Modified from Yunis, *et al.*, 1984.

(median survival in months: 29.3 *vs.* 27.9) and in mice born on 8/8/79 and homozygous for *b* (*b/b*) (median survival in months: 27.7 *vs.* 23.8). There was also an interaction between sex, *H-2* and the *b* locus of chromosome 4. The $H\text{-}2^b/H\text{-}2^d$ mice differed significantly in life span from the $H\text{-}2^d/H\text{-}2^d$ in males homozygous for (*b/b*) at the brown locus (median survival in months: 26.2 *vs.* 24.1) and in females heterozygous for (*B/b*) of the brown locus (median survival in months: 30.5 *vs.* 28.1). Ignoring interactions there was a significant effect of sex on survival, but not the D locus on chromosome 9. In males, there was a significant effect of chromosome 17, but the effect in females was not significant. In females, there was a significant effect of chromosome 4, but in males the effect was not significant (Table 6).

Longevity was also analyzed by ranking the mice according to the number of heterozygotes at each locus studied. The median survival was ranked in the same order as the number of heterozygous markers studied. Using the log rank test, there was a significant difference (P = 0.0004) between the five groups but the survival rates were not equally spread. Increased heterozygosity directly correlates with longer life span. The longest lived mice were females (in which one or the other of the two X chromosomes was activated), heterozygous at the *H-2* and brown (b) loci. The shortest lived group were males (with only one X chromosome), homozygous at the *H-2* and brown (b) loci. This may represent a case of hybrid vigor (heterosis), associated either with the dominance of favorable alleles not held in common by the parental strains (Roderick and Schlager, 1975) or with avoidance of the deleterious effects of recessive genes which limit life span (Russell, 1975).

## Recombinant (RI) Study

We studied twenty strains of BxD recombinant inbred mice (Gelman, *et al.*, 1988). We obtained 395 female BxD mice from the Jackson Laboratory: on 11/9/82, 12/1/82, 1/17/83, 2/1/83, 2/8/83 and on 3/22/83. At the time of receipt at the Michael Redstone Animal Facility of the Dana-Farber Cancer Institute, the mice were between 5 and 10 weeks old. The mice were born between September, 1982 and February, 1983, with the majority born in 1982. These female mice were representative of the 23 BxD recombinant inbred strains available in 1982. Fifteen of the strains analyzed included 19 to 21 mice and five included 9 or 10 mice.

Beginning in March, 1983, dead mice that were not severely autolysed nor destroyed by cannibalism were necropsied. Tissues were fixed in 10% neutral buffered formalin and examined histopathologically for significant lesions. Gross lesions were described at necropsy and representative sections of lesions and major organs were sampled for histopathological evaluation. The organs usually included were brain, heart, lung, liver, kidney, intestines, and reproductive organs; often the intestines and brain were too autolysed for evaluation. The last mouse died on 1/21/86.

Published strain distribution patterns (Taylor, 1981) were available for up to 141 genes (actually, markers of an area of a chromosome) which were identified as being from the B or D parent. Most of the strains were missing data on between one and six genes (mostly *Ly-22* on chromosome 4, *Saac* on chromosome 9, *Igh*-Bgl, *Igh*-Npa on chromosome 12, and *Lyb-7* on an unknown chromosome). In this study two strains were associated with significantly shorter life spans and one strain was definitely associated with significantly longer life span while four other strains were possibly associated with longer life span than the other 13 strains in a proportional hazards model of survival. Mean survival of the shortest lived strain was 479 days; the mean survival of the longest lived strain was almost double (904 days). Ranges of survival within strains were very large (averaging 642 days), and strain accounted for only 29% of the variation of survival, showing that there were important environmental effects on longevity, even in this colony housed in a single room. Each strain had been typed for markers of 141 regions on 15 chromosomes; 101 of these markers had distinguishable distributions on the 20 strains. The two shortest lived strains had the same alleles for 63% of the markers. The single region most significantly correlated with survival (marked by *Coh, Xmmv-35* on chromosome 7) divided the mice into two groups with survival medians which differed by 153 days (755 days for mice with a B genotype; 602 days for mice with a D genotype). Evaluated individually, 44% of the genetic markers (including some markers on 11 of 15 chromosomes with any markers typed) were found to be significantly correlated with survival ($p < 0.05$). While this does not adjust for multiple comparisons, any experiment with only one of these markers typed might have concluded that the marker was a significant predictor of survival. Two types of multiple regression models were used to examine the correlation with survival of groups of chromosomal regions. When a proportional hazards model for survival was done in terms of genotype regions, a six genetic region model correlated best with survival: that marked by *P450, Coh, Xmmv-35* on chromosome 7 (B allele lives longer), *Ly-24* on chromosome 2 (B allele lives longer), β2M and *H-3* on chromosome 2 (D allele lives longer), *Lamb-2* on chromosome 1 (D allele lives longer), *Ltw-4* on chromosome 1 (B allele lives longer), and the *Igh* area of chromosome 12 (*Igh*-Sa4, *Igh*-Sa2, *Igh*-Bgl, *Igh*-Nbp, *Igh*-Npid, *Igh*-Gte, Odc-8, and *Ox-1*; D allele lives longer). A linear model that regressed mean survival (per strain) on genetic markers found a similar six region model to be best, but replaced *Coh* by *D12Nyu-1* on chromosome 12 (Table 7). It should be noted that in both types of regression, there were many other models almost as good as the best one. The total number of chromosomal regions marked by the genotype of the longer lived B parent (out of a possible 141) was not, in general, correlated with survival, although the two shortest lived strains had the most B genes.

## DISCUSSION

Age-associated loss of immune function has been well documented in mice in investigations of the antibody response (Makinodan and Kay, 1980; Callard and Basten, 1978), the generation of cytotoxic T cell (Bach, 1977; Zharhary and Gershon, 1981) and natural killer cells (Weindruch, *et al.*, 1983), anti-tumor immunity (Flood, *et al.*, 1981), and the role of regulatory cells in preventing autoimmunity (Ben-Nun, *et al.*, 1980). Advances in our understanding of T cell collaboration in the initiation of immune reactions have led to the analysis of immune deficiencies, including aging, in terms of the roles played by lymphokine-reacting cytotoxic T lymphocytes (CTL) and B cells. Several laboratories (Gillis, *et al.*, 1981; Thoman and Weigle, 1981; Gilman, *et al.*, 1982), including ours (Miller and Stutman, 1982), have reported age-associated declines in the ability to produce interleukin-2 (IL-2), a T cell growth factor now thought to be of critical importance in the amplification of CTL responses. In addition, age-associated loss of CTL

**Table 7.** Proportional Hazards Regression Models and Linear Regression Models on Genetic Markers

| Chromosome | Statistically indistinguishable[a] markers | Allele associated with longer survival[b] | Significance level in final proportional hazards model | Significance level in final linear model |
|---|---|---|---|---|
| 7 | P450 | | | |
| | Coh | B | 0.0011 | N/A[c] |
| | Xmmv-35 | | | |
| 2 | Ly24 | B | <0.0001 | 0.0006 |
| 2 | b2m | | | |
| | H-3 | D | 0.0006 | 0.0012 |
| 1 | Lamb-2 | D | <0.0001 | 0.0006 |
| 1 | Ltw-4 | B | <0.0001 | <0.0001 |
| 12 | Igh-Sa4 | | | |
| | Igh-Sa2 | | | |
| | Igh-Bgl | | | |
| | Igh-Nbp | D | 0.0018 | <0.0001 |
| | Igh-Npa | | | |
| | Igh-Gte | | | |
| | Odc-8 | | | |
| | Ox-1 | | | |
| | Npid | | | |
| 12 | D12Nyu1 | D | N/A | 0.0011 |

[a] Markers are indistinguishable if their genotypes were not known to differ in any of the twenty strains in the model.
[b] B means means allele the same as that for C57BL/6 and D means allele the same as that for DBA/2.
[c] Not applicable (marker is not in final model)Modified Gelman, *et al.*, 1988.

function, even in the presence of excess IL-2, has been reported under some (Gillis, *et al.*, 1981; Thoman and Weigle, 1981; Gilman, *et al.*, 1982; Thoman and Weigle, 1982), though not all (Thoman and Weigle, 1981; Gilman, *et al.*, 1982; Thoman and Weigle, 1982; Miller and Stutman, 1982; Chang, *et al.*, 1982) circumstances.

Since genes of the MHC (*H-2*) govern immune function it was anticipated that the *H-2* haplotype influenced longevity (Benacerraf, 1981; Greenberg and Yunis, 1975; Greenberg and Yunis, 1978; Katz, *et al.*, 1976). Such studies were significant because not only the *H-2* haplotype was correlated with life span but that there was an association between immune vigor and life span (Meredith and Walford, 1977; Popp, 1978). We have corroborated these findings using parental and hybrid congenic strains, as well as congenic strains hybrid to DBA/2. It was found that the heterozygotes lived longer than the parental strains in only 2 out of 5 combinations studied and that $H\text{-}2^b$ congenics live longer than $H\text{-}2^a$ and $H\text{-}2^k$.

We found a highly significant correlation of date of birth and survival in the congenic experiment. The birth date had approximately as significant an effect on survival as the *H-2* haplotypes. Our analyses was complicated because we demonstrated a significant correlation between survival and date of birth on 6 of the 16 strains which had birth dates ranging over more than three months. Hence all analyses of genetic effects on survival were either done with subsets of mice from the same season of a particular year or else included date of birth variables in survival models.

Of the 18 possible comparisons of pairs of strains which overlapped in birth dates and differed only in the D-end of *H-2*, 5 were associated with highly significant survival differences. Of the 10 pairs of strains which overlapped in birth date and differed only in the K-end of *H-2* none were associated with significant survival differences. In models of survival based on birth date and alleles for one of the four regions (KAE$\beta$, E$\alpha$, S, DL), the KAE$\beta$ alleles were seldom (2/8 models) associated with significant survival differences (E$\alpha$ in 6/8, S in 8/8, DL in 7/8). The most consistent results in comparing alleles in these models were; *b* associated with longer survival than *s* or *d* or *k*, *q* was associated with longer survival than *d*, and *k* with longer survival than *d*. In models of survival based on birth dates and alleles for one of three regions closely linked with *H-2* (Qa and Tla), these alleles were never significant.

We conclude that it is very important for survival studies to be based on animals bred at approximately the same time and that mice differing genetically only at the *H-2* (and perhaps closely linked) loci differ significantly in survival. Our data also suggested that the D-end of *H-2* may have more of an effect on survival than the K-end.

Our findings regarding heterozygosity may represent hybrid vigor associated either with codominance of favorable alleles not held in common by the parental strains (Roderick and Schlager, 1975), or with the avoidance of deleterious effects of recessive genes which limit life span. In general, genetic interactions or additive effects of several genes and the environment are more important in conferring longer life span than the presence of specific individual alleles (Yunis, *et al.*, 1984).

Histopathological findings on mice that died at or after 28 months of age were comparable for all genetic combinations except that there was an increased frequency of lymphoma in females and an increased frequency of amyloidosis in males. Our analysis emphasizes the need for comprehensive studies of aging and life span that would simultaneously determine the effects of several genetic regions and their interactions with the environment with respect to possible causes of death.

It appears that BxD recombinant strains can vary widely in survival, that no single genetic marker which has yet been identified can account for much of this variance, (although groups of 6 or more markers may do so), and that it is not always those strains which inherit the most genes from the long-lived parent B which live longest. The large number of genetic markers found to be significantly correlated with survival raises questions of the reliability of conclusions based on survival studies of only one or two genetic regions (Gelman, *et al.*, 1988, Figure 4).

Taken together our studies suggest that life span results from environmental factors interacting with several genes. Our studies represent an attempt to identify some of the genes that are involved. They emphasize the need to use several genetic models. The congenic mice are useful only to study one genetic region but in other models other genes may be more important. For example, *H-2* is believed to influence life span but differences at *H-2* using backcross animals suggested that they are less important in females. In recombinant strains the *H-2* region is not as important as at least 16 out of 101 informative chromosomal regions studied. The use of recombinant inbred strains have the disadvantage that genetic studies based on mapping of genes depend on the map as it exists today. There could be other, as yet unmapped, genes which more strongly influence survival than the genes we have identified so far. It is remarkable that even after minimizing the genetic and environmental variations we found complex patterns of disease and survival, which raise doubts as to the feasibility of studying genetic effects of life span in outbred populations. It is obvious that it would be necessary to study life span in other recombinant inbred strains in order to find out if some of the results for chromosomal regions described in our studies are generalizable.

## REFERENCES


BACH, M. A. (1977) Lymphocyte-mediated cytotoxicity: Effects of aging, adult thymectomy and thymic factor. *J. Immunol.* **119**: 641-647

BAIRD, M. B., and J. LINZCZYNSYJ (1985) Genetic control of adult life span in Drosophila melanogaster. *Exp. Gerontol.* **20**: 171-177

BEN-NUN, A., Y. RON AND I. R. COHEN (1980) Spontaneous Remission Of Autoimmune Encephalomyelitis Is Inhibited By Splenectomy, Thymectomy Or Aging. *Nature* **288**: 389-390

BENACERRAF, B. (1981) A hypothesis to relate the specificity of T lymphocytes and the activity of I-region-specific Ir genes in macrophages and B lymphocytes. *J. Immunol.* **120**: 1809

CALLARD, R. E. and A. BASTEN (1978) T cell and B cell function in antibody production by old mice. *Eur. J. Immunol.* **8**: 552-558

CHANG, M.-P., T. MAKINODAN, W. J. PETERSON and B. L. STREHLER (1982) Role of T-cell in adherent cells in age-related decline in murine interleukin-2 production. *J. Immunol.* **129**: 2426-2430

CLARK, A. M. and A. B. GOULD (1970) Genetic control of adult life span in *Drosophila melanogaster. Exp. Gerontol.* **5**: 157

FERNANDES, G., D. R. ALONSO, T. TANAKA, H. T. THALER, E. J. YUNIS and R. A. GOOD (1983) Influence of diet on vascular lesions in autoimmune-prone B/W mice. *Proc. Natl. Acad. Sci. USA* **80**: 874

FERNANDES, G., R. A. GOOD and E. J. YUNIS (1981) Responses of autoimmune diseases and diseases of aging to dietary restriction, **In:** *Immunological Aspects of Aging*, p. 207 (D. Segre and L. Smith, Eds.) Marcel Dekker, Inc., New York.

FESTING, M. F. W. and D. R. BLACKMORE (1971) Life span of specific pathogen free (MRC Category 4) mice and rats. *Lab. Animal* **5**: 179-197

FLOOD, P. M., J. L. URBAN, M. L. KRIPKE and H. SCHREIBER (1981) Loss of tumor-specific and ideotype-specific immunity with age. *J. Exp. Med.* **154**: 275-290

GELMAN, R., A. WATSON, R. BRONSON, and E. YUNIS (1988) Murine chromosomal regions correlated with longevity. *Genetics* **118**: 693-704

GILLIS, S., R. KOZAK, M. DURANTE and M. E. WEKSLER (1981) Immunological studies of aging. Decreased production of and response to T cell growth factor by lymphocytes from aged humans. *J. Clin. Inv.* **67**: 937-942

GILMAN, S. C., J. S. ROSENBERG and J. D. FELDMAN (1982) T-lymphocytes of young and aged rats. *J. Immunol.* **128**: 644-650

GOODRICH, C. L. (1975) Life span and inheritance of longevity of inbred mice. *J. Gerontol.* **30**: 257-263

GOULD, A. B. and A. M. CLARK (1983) Behavior of life shortening genes in genetic mosaics of *Drosophila melanogaster. Mech. Aging Develop.* **23**: 1-10

GREENBERG, L. J. And E. J. YUNIS (1975) Immunopathology Of Aging. *Hum. Pathol.* **5**: 122

GREENBERG, L. J. and E. J. YUNIS (1978) Genetic control of autoimmune disease and immune responsiveness and the relationship to aging, **In:** *Genetic Effects of Aging*, **Vol. XIV** (D. Gergsma and D. Harrison, Eds.). Alan R. Liss, New York p. 249.

HERBERMAN, H. B. and J. ORTALDO (1981) Natural killer cells: Their role in defense against disease. *Science* **214**: 24.

JOHNSON, T. E. (1984) Analysis of the biological basis of aging in the nematode, with special emphasis on *Caenorhabidites elegans.* **In:** *Invertebrate Models in Aging Research*, CRC Press. (D. H. Mitchell and T. E. Johnson, Eds). CRC Press p. 59-93.

JOHNSON, T. E., and WOOD, W. B. (1982) Genetic analysis of life span in *Caenorhabidites elegans. Proc. Natl. Acad. Sci. USA* **79**: 6603

JOHNSON, T. E., D. H. MITCHELL, S. KLINE, R. KEMAL and J. FOY (1984) Arresting development arrests aging in the nematode *Caenorhabditis elegans. Mech. Ageing Develop.* **28**: 23-40

KASAI, J., J. C. LECLERC, L. McVAY-BOURDEAU, F. W. SHEN and H. CANTOR (1979) Direct evidence that natural killer cells in non-immune spleen cell populations prevent tumor growth *in vivo. J. Exp. Med.* **149**: 12

KATZ, D. H. and B. BENACERRAF (Eds.) (1976) *The Role of the Products of the Histocompatibility Gene Complex in Immune Responses*, Academic Press, New York.

KLASS, M. R. (1983) A method for the isolation of longevity mutants in the nematode *Caenorhabditis elegans* and initial results. *Mech. Aging Develop.* **22**: 279-280

LANE, M. A. and E. J. YUNIS (1981) Nutritional alteration in aging and immune reactivity: Application of the rate-limit concept. **In:** *Integrated Medicine: Volume II of A Companion to the Life Sciences*, p. 238 (S. B. Day, Ed.) Van Nostrand Reinhold Company, New York.

MAKINODAN, T. and M. M. KAY (1980) Age influence on the immune system. *Adv. Immunol.* **29**: 287-330

MEREDITH, P. J. and R. L. WALFORD (1977) Effect of age on response to T- and B-cell mitogens in mice congenic at the *H-2* locus. *Immunogenetics* **5**: 109

MILLER, R. A. and D. E. HARRISON (1985) Delayed reduction in T-cell precursor frequencies accompanies diet-induced life span extension. *J. Immunol.* **134**: 1426-1429

MILLER, R. A. and O. STUTMAN (1982) Decline, in aging mice, of the anti-2,4,6-trinitrophenyl (TNP) cytotoxic T cell response attributable to loss of *Lyt-2-*, interleukin 2-producing helper cell function. *Eur. J. Immunol.* **11**: 751-756

MYERS, D. D. (1978) Disease patterns in aging inbred mouse strains. Interaction of genetics and environment. In: *Genetic Effects of Aging* **Vol. XIV** (D. Gergsma and D. Harrison, Eds.) Alan R. Liss, New York. pp. 41-53.

POPP, D. M. (1978) Use of congenic mice to study the genetic basis of degenerative disease. In: *Genetic Effects of Aging,* **Vol. XIV** (D. Gergsma and D. Harrison, Eds.) Alan R. Liss, New York. pp 261-279.

RODERICK, T. H. and G. SCHLAGER (1975) Multiple factor inheritance, In: *Biology of the Laboratory Mouse,* 2nd Revised Edition (The Staff of the Jackson Laboratory, Eds.) Dover Publ., Inc., New York, p.151.

RUSSELL, E. S. (1975) Life span and aging patterns. In: *Biology of the Laboratory Mouse,* Dover Publications, Inc. New York, pp 511-519.

RUSSELL, E. S. (1972) Genetic considerations in the selection of rodent species and strains for research in aging. In: *Development of the Rodent as a Model System of Aging* (D. Gibson, Ed.) DHEW publication *(NIH) G2-121, Bethesda, MD, pp. 33-35.*

SMITH, G. W., and R. L. WALFORD (1977) Influence of the main histocompatiblity complex on aging in mice. *Nature* **270**: 727-729

SMITH, G. W., R. L. WALFORD and M. R. MICKEY (1973) Life span and incidence of cancer and other diseases in selected long lived inbred mice and their $F_1$ hybrids. *J. Natl. Cancer Inst.* **50**: 1195-1213

STORER, J.B. (1966) LONGEVITY AND GROSS PATHOLOGY AT DEATH IN 22 INBRED MOUSE STRAINS. *J. GERONTOL.* **21**: 404-409.

STORER, J. B. (1978) Effect of aging and radiation in mice of different genotypes. In: *Genetic Effects of Aging,* **Vol. XIV** (D. Gergsma and D. Harrison, Eds.) Alan R. Liss, New York. pp.55-70.

TAYLOR, B. A. (1981) *Genetic Variants and Strains of the Laboratory Mouse* 2nd Edition. Oxford University Press, Oxford.

THOMAN, M. L. and W. O. WEIGLE (1981) Lymphokines and aging: interleukin-2 production and activity. *J. Immunol.* **127**: 2101-2106

THOMAN, M. L. and W. O. WEIGLE (1982) Cell-mediated immunity in aged mice: an underlying lesion in IL-2 synthesis. *J. Immunol.* **128**: 2358-2361

WARNER, J. F. and G. DENNERT (1981) Effect of a cloned cell line with NK activity on bone marrow transplants, tumor development and metastasis *in vivo. Nature* **300**: 31

WEINDRUCH, R., B. H. DEVENS, H. V. RAFF and R. L. WALFORD (1983) Influence of dietary restriction and aging on natural killer cell activity in mice. *J. Immunol.* **130**: 993-996

WILLIAMS, R. M., L. J. KRAUS, P. T. LAVIN, L. L. STEELE, and E. J. YUNIS (1981) Genetics of survival in mice: Localization of dominant effects to subregions of the major histocompatibility complex. In: *Immunological Aspects of Aging,* (D. Segre and L. Smith, Eds.) Marcel Dekker, Inc., New York, p 247.

YUNIS, E. J., A. L. M. WATSON, R. S. GELMAN, S. J. SYLVIA, R. BRONSON, M. E. DORF (1984) Traits that influence longevity in mice. *Genetics* **108**: 999-1011

ZHARHARY, D. and H. GERSHON (1981) Allogeneic T-cytotoxic reactivity of senescent mice: affinity for target cells and determination of cell number. *Cellular Immunology* **60**: 470-479

## DISCUSSION

1. Yunis noted that he did not find the $F_1$ hybrids to always outlive the parental strains. Similar findings have been reported by Smith and by Harrison. Asked to compare the longest-lived RI lines between B6 and D2 with B6, Yunis noted that strain 19 had more D2 type genes of the 101 loci tested. The H-2 locus did not come out as one of the 7 that defined regions affecting longevities significantly.

2. Asked whether the longest-lived congenic strains outlived the B6 parent, Yunis noted that this could not be determined due to seasonal variations in longevity.

3. About 44% of the loci tested in recombinant mice had some effect on longevities. This suggests that a large proportion of the genome is important. Yunis noted that if he had typed all genotypes, some effects might disappear. Charlesworth cautioned that this may result from the genes altering components of fitness that all slightly affect viability. When testing mutants, many genes had small effects, and he expects similar results in any pair of inbred strains. The genome is already saturated with loci affecting fitness. Of course if there was a really important gene differing between B6 and D2 that greatly affected aging rates, it should have been found. None were. It was unfortunate that populations were so small, as these may have masked important effects.

# Section 6

## EXAMPLES OF MODERN MAMMALIAN GENETICS

# 27

# BIBLIOGRAPHIES

## GENE MAPPING AND GENOME ORGANIZATION

J.H. Nadeau

CHENG, S. V., G. R. MARTIN, J. H. NADEAU, J. L. HAINES, M. BUCAN, C. A KOZAK, M. E. MACDONALD, J. L. LOCKYER, F. D. LEDLEY, S. L. C. WOO, H. LEHRACH, T. C. GILLIAM, and J. F. GUSCFLA. (1989) Synteny on mouse Chromosome 5 of human DNA loci linked to the Huntington's disease gene. *Genomics* **4**: 419-426.

CHENG, S. V., J. H. NADEAU, R. E. TANZI, P. C. WATKINS, J. JAGADESH, B. A. TAYLOR, N. SACCHI, and J. F. GUSELLA (1988) Comparative mapping of DNA markers from the familial Alzheimer disease and Down syndrome regions of human chromosomes 21 to mouse chromosomes 16 and 17. *Proc. Natl. Acad. Sci. USA* **85**: 6032-6036.

LUNDIN, L.-G. (1979) Evolutionary conservation of large chromosomal segments reflected in mammalian gene maps. *Clin. Genet.* **16**: 72-8 1.

NADEAU, J. H. (1989) Maps of linkage and synteny homologies between mouse and man. *Trends in Genetics* **5**: 82-86

NADEAU, J. H. (1989) Genome duplication and comparative gene mapping. **In:** *Advanced Techniques in Chromosome Research.* (K. Adolph, Ed.) Marcel Dekker. (in press)

NADEAU, J. H. and A. H. REINER (1989) Linkage and synteny homologies in mouse and man. **In:** *Genetic Variants and Strains of the Laboratory Mouse.*(M. F. Lyon and A. G. Searle, Eds.) Oxford University Press, Oxford. pp. 506-536

NADEAU, J. H. and B. A. TAYLOR (1984) Lengths of chromosomal segments conserved since divergence of man and mouse. *Proc. Natl. Acad. Sci. USA* **81**: 814-818.

O'BRIEN, S. J., H. N. SEUANEZ, and J. E. WOMACK (1985) On the evolution of genome organization in mammals. **In:** *Molecular Evolutionary Genetics* (R. J. McIntyre, Ed.) Plenum Publ. Corp.

O'BRIEN, S. J., H. N. SEUANEZ, and J. E. WOMACK (1988) Mammalian genome organization: An evolutionary view. *Ann. Rev. Genet.* **22**: 323-35 1.

SEARLE, A. G., J. PETERS, M. F. LYON, E. P. EVANS, J. H. EDWARDS, and V. J. BUCKLE (1987) Chromosome maps of man and mouse. *Genomics* **1**: 3-18.

WOMACK, J. E. (1982) Linkage of mammalian isozyme loci: A comparative approach. Isozymes *Curr. Top. Biol. Med. Res.* **6**: 207-246.

## MURINE POLYSACCHARIDOSIS

Edward H. Birkenmeier

PAIGEN, K. (1979) Acid hydrolases as models of genetic control. Ann. Rev. Genet. 13, 417-466.

LUSIS, A. J., TOMINO, S., and PAIGEN, K. (1976). Isolation, characterization and radioimmunoassay of murine egasyn, a protein stabilizing glucuronidase membrane binding. *J. Biol. Chem.* **251**: 7753-7760.

LEVVY, G. A. (1953). β-Glucuronidase and related enzymes. *Br. Med. Bull.* **9**: 126-130.

TOMINO, S., PAIGEN, K., TULSIANI, D. R. P., and TOUSTER, O. (1975) Purification and chemical properties of mouse liver lysosomal (L-form) (β-glucuronidase. *J. Biol. Chem.* **250**: 8503-8509.

DORFMAN, A., and MATALON, R. (1976) The mucopolysaccharidoses (A Review). *Proc. Natl. Acad. Sci. USA* **73**: 630-637.

SLY, W. S., QUINTON, B. A., McALISTER, W. H., and RIMOIN, D. L. (1973) Beta glucuronidase deficiency: report of clinical, radiologic, and biochemical features of a new mucopolysaccharidosis. *J. Ped.* **82**: 249-257.

SLY, W. S., BROT, F. E., GLASER, J. H., STAHL, P. D., OUINTON, B. A., RIMOIN, D. L., and McALISTER, W. H. (1974) β-Glucuronidase deficiency mucopolysaccharidosis. *Birth Defects* **10**: 239-245.

HASKINS, M. E., DESNICK, R. J., DIFERRANTE, N., JEZYK, P. F., and PATTERSON, D. F. (1984) β-Glucuronidase deficiency in a dog: a model of human mucopolysaccharidosis VII. *Ped. Res.* **18**: 980-984.

PAIGEN, K. (1961) The effect of mutation on the intracellular location of β-glucuronidase. *Exp. Cell Res.* **25**: 286-301.

SWANK, R. T., PAIGEN, K., and GANSCHOW, R. E. (1973) Genetic control of glucuronidase induction in mice. *J. Mol. Biol.* **81**: 225-243.

LALLEY, P. A., and SHOWS, T. B. (1974) Lysosomal and microsomal gb glucuronidase: genetic variant alters electrophoretic mobility of both hydrolases. *Science* **185**: 442-444.

PALMER, R., GALLAGHER, P. M., BOYKO, W. L., and GANSCHOV, R. E. (1983) Genetic control of levels of murine kidney glucuronidase mRNA in response to androgen. *Proc. Natl. Acad. Sci. USA* **80**: 7596-7600.

MEREDITH, S. A., and GANSCHOV, R. E. (1978) Apparent *trans* control of murine β-glucuronidase synthesis by a temporal genetic element. *Genetics* **90**: 725-734.

LUSIS, A. J., CHAPMAN, V. M., WANGENSTEIN, R. W., and PAIGEN, K. (1983) *Trans*-acting temporal locus within the β-glucuronidase gene complex. *Proc. Natl. Acad. Sci. USA* **80**: 4398-4402.

GANSCHOV, R., and PAIGEN, K. (1968) Glucuronidase phenotypes of inbred mouse strains. *Genetics* **59**: 335-349.

GALLAGHER, P. M., D'AMORE, M. A., LUND, S. D., ELLIOTT, R. W., PAZIK, J., BOHMAN, C., KORFHAGEN, T. R., and GANSCHOV, R. E. (1987) DNA sequence variation within the β-glucuronidase gene complex among inbred strains of mice. *Genomics* **1**: 145-152.

HOOGERBRUGGE, P. M., POORTHUIS, B. J. H. M., MULDER, A. H., WAGEMAKER, G., DOOREN, L. J., VOSSEN, J. M. J. J., and VAN BEKKEN, D. V. (1987) Correction of lysosomal enzyme deficiency in various organs of β-glucuronidase-deficient mice by allogeneic bone marrow transplantation. *Transplantation* **43**: 609-614.

BEAMER, W. G., and COLEMAN, D. L. (1982) Adipose storage deficiency (asd). *Mouse News Lett.* **67**: 21.

SHOWS, T. B., RUDDLE, F. H., and RODERICK, T. H. (1969) Phosphoglucomutase electrophoretic variants in the mouse. *Biochem. Genet.* **3**: 25-35.

SHOWS, T. B., CHAPMAN, V. M., and RUDDLE, F. H. (1970) Mitochondrial malate dehydrogenase and malic enzyme: Mendelian inherited electrophoretic variants in the mouse. *Biochem. Genet.* **4**: 707-718.

GLASER, J. H., and SLY, W. S. (1973) β-Glucuronidase deficiency mucopolysaccharidosis: Methods for enzymatic diagnosis. *J. Lab. Clin. Med.* **82**: 969-977.

GEHLER, J., CANTZ, M., TOLKSDORF, M., and SPRANGER, J. (1974) Mucopolysaccharidosis VII: β-Glucuronidase deficiency. *Humangenetik* **23**: 149- 158.

LOWRY, O. H., ROSEBROUGH, N. J., FARR, A. L., and RANDALL, R. J. (1951) Protein measurement with the Folin phenol reagent. *J. Biol. Chem.* **193**: 265-275.

CHIRGWIN, J. M., PRZYBYLA, A. E., MACDONALD, R. J., and RUTTER, W. J. (1979) Isolation of biologically active ribonucleic acid from sources enriched in ribonuclease. *Biochemistry* **18**: 5294-5299.

MANIATIS, T., FRITSCH, E. F., and SAMBROOK, J. (1982) Molecular *Cloning, A Laboratory Manual*. Cold Spring Harbor Laboratory, Cold Spring Harbor, NY.

HEUCKEROTH, R. O., BIRKENMEIER, E. H., LEVIN, M. S., and GORDON, J. I. (1987) Analysis of the tissue-specific expression, developmental regulation, and linkage relationships of a rodent gene encoding heart fatty acid binding protein. *J. Biol. Chem.* **262**: 9709-9717.

FEINBERG, A. P., and VOGELSTEIN, B. (1983) A technique for radiolabeling DNA restriction endonuclease fragments to high specific activity. *Anal. Biochem.* **132**: 6-13.

SOUTHERN, E. M. (1975) Detection of specific sequences among DNA fragments sep%rated by gel electrophoresis. *J. Mol. Biol.* **98**: 5031-517.

LEITER, E. H., BEAMER, W. G., COLEMAN, D. L., and LONGCOPE, C. (1987) Androgenic and estrogenic metabolites in serum of mice fed dehydroepiandrosterone: relationship to antihyperglycemic effects. *Metabolism* **36**: 863-869.

MOORE, K. J., and PAIGEN, K. (1988) Genome organization and polymorphism of the murine β-glucuronidase region. *Genomics* **2**: 25-31.

BAILEY, D. V., and KOHN, B. I. (1965) Inherited histocompatibility changes in progeny of irradiated and unirradiated inbred mice. *Genet. Res.* **6**: 330-340.

WATSON, C. S., and CATTERALL, J. F. (1986) Genetic regulation of androgen-induced accumulation of mouse renal β-glucuronidase messenger ribonucleic acid. *Endocrinology* **118**: 1081-1086.

BERNSEN, P. L. J. A., WEVERS, R. A., GABREELS, F. J. M., LAMERS, K. J. B., SONNEN, A. E. H., and SCHUURMANS STEKHOVEN, J. H. (1987) Phenotypic expression in mucopolysaccharidosis VII. *J. Neurol. Neurosur. Psych.* **50**: 699-703.

KORNFELD, S. (1987) Trafficking of lysosomal enzymes. *FASEB J.* **1**: 462-468.

LEE, J. E. S., FALK, R. E., NG, W. G., and DONNELL, G. N. (1985) β-Glucuronidase deficiency. A heterogeneous mucopolysaccharidosis. *Am. J. Dis. Child.* **139**: 57-59.

SHULL, R. M., HASTINGS, N. E., SELCER, R. R., JONES, J. B., SMITH, J. R., CULLEN, W. C., and CONSTANTOPOULOS, G. (1987) Bone marrow transplantation in canine mucopolysaccharidosis I. Effects within the central nervous system. *J. Clin. Invest.* **79**: 435-443.


# UNRAVELING THE MECHANISM OF SEX DETERMINATION: MOLECULAR APPROACHES TO STUDIES ON SEX DETERMINATION


Eva M. Eicher


EICHER E. M. (1988) Autosomal genes involved in mammalian primary sex determination. *Phil. Trans. Roy. Soc. Lond. B* **322**: 109-118. (This issue of the *Phil. Trans. Roy. Soc. Lond. B* is dedicated to the subject of sex determination).

EICHER E. M and WASHBURN L. L. (1986) Genetic control of primary sex determination in mice. *Ann. Rev. Genet.* **20**: 327-360.

GERMAN, J. (1988) Gonadal dimorphism explained as a dosage effect of a locus on the sex chromosomes the gonad-differentiation locus (GDL). *Am. J. Hum. Genet.* 414-421.

PAGE, D. C. *et al.* (1987) The sex determining region of the human Y chromosome encodes a finger protein. *Cell* **51**: 1091-1104.

# Section 7

## PROGERIOD MUTANTS AND ALZHEIMER'S DISEASE

# 28

# SEGMENTAL AND UNIMODAL PROGEROID SYNDROMES OF MAN

George M. Martin

## ABSTRACT

Evolutionary arguments would suggest that at least a proportion of the pathophysiological details of senescence in man may be unique to that species. Moreover, the enormous degree of genetic heterogeneity in man permits a number of "private" patterns of senescence. Thus, in order to develop rational strategies for the prevention and treatment of geriatric disabilities, it is essential to investigate the biochemical genetic basis of *specific* aspects of senescence in our own species. One such approach is the investigation of segmental and unimodal progeroid syndromes. Segmental progeroid syndromes involve a number of different aspects of the senescent phenotype. The prototype is Werner's syndrome, an autosomal recessive characterized by limitation of growth, premature arteriosclerosis, osteoporosis, cataracts, diabetes, skin and gonadal atrophy, and benign and malignant neoplasms, with onset at adolescence. Somatic cells of these patients are prone to chromosomal and intragenic deletions and rearrangements. Localization of the gene should be feasible *via* homozygosity mapping. Unimodal progeroid syndromes affect a single major aspect of the senescent phenotype. The prototype is familial Alzheimer's disease, an autosomal dominant. A number of abnormalities have been reported in peripheral cells, but none have yet received wide confirmation. Linkage analysis indicates genetic heterogeneity. A previously reported linkage to 21q21 markers could not be confirmed with a set of ethnically homogeneous pedigrees (Volga Germans).

Strong arguments have been made by evolutionary biologists in favor of non-adaptive theories of the evolution of various maximum life-span potentials (Rose, 1984; see contributions by Charlesworth, Kirkwood, Rose, this volume ). The two favored non- adaptive evolutionary mechanisms are: 1) the accumulation, in the absence of selection, of deleterious mutations acting post-reproductively, and 2) antagonistic pleiotropy (selection for alleles conferring enhanced reproductive fitness, with the expression of paradoxical deleterious effects during the post-reproductive life span). There is no reason, *a priori*, to expect that the subset of relevant genes and, consequently, the detailed pathophysiological events that play out during senescence, would be identical among all species (Rose, 1984), or even among all mammalian species. It may be the case, however, that a proportion of genetic loci are indeed of universal importance (operative in *all* species), or of importance to how senescence develops in a large group of species ("public" genetic markers of aging) (Martin, 1988).

Given these considerations, a case might be made that the conduct of basic biogerontologic research should be guided, at least to a degree, by the famous dictum of Alexander Pope: "The proper study of mankind is man" (Essay on Man, 1733-1734, *Oxford Dictionary of Quotations*, 1953). [Pope was also a developmental gerontologist of sorts, as he noted that man was "Created half to rise, and half to fall" (Essay on Man, 1733-1734).]

## Some Definitions

Botanical gerontologists generally use the term aging to refer to all changes in structure and function from birth to death, while reserving the term senescence for those deteriorative changes in structure and function of an organism that develop post- maturationally and that lead to organ and organismal death (Leopold, 1975). Perusal of the animal gerontological literature reveals much less rigor in the use of these terms, but it is generally the case that the terms aging and senescence (or, more properly, "senescing") are both used to refer to post-maturational alterations. Most of these changes are presumed to be non-adaptive, *i.e.*, they are thought to contribute to the exponential increase, as a function of chronological age, in the probability of organismal death among populations of post-reproductive individuals (Gompertz, 1825).

Although the term progeria ("premature aging") is well entrenched in the medical literature and is a synonym for the Hutchinson-Gilford syndrome (McKusick, 1988), the term should probably be abandoned. Many aspects of the phenotype of that syndrome differ from what is observed in ordinary aging (Martin, 1978; Brown, this volume). Moreover, no other syndrome has been discovered, either genetic or environmental, that can bring forward in time all of the features associated with aging, either symmetrically or asymmetrically. The regimen that comes closest to doing this is *ad libidum* feeding of rodents (Masoro, 1988), if we were to take the view that the dietarily restricted cohorts of animals represent the normal controls! But even here, there are several features of aging that seem not to be altered significantly by food intake (Weindruch and Walford, 1988). Finally, on theoretical grounds, given the evolutionary considerations discussed above, it would seem highly improbable that mutation at a single genetic locus could result in a true progeria. Given the limited state of our knowledge, "progeroid syndrome" is suggested as a more conservative term for genetically or environmentally induced syndromes suggestive of premature aging. The suffix "-oid" means "-like;" it does not indicate identity.

The term "segmental progeroid syndrome" was introduced to describe a set of genetic disorders of man that mimicked, to some degree, a *number* of features of the senescent phenotype of man (see below) (Martin, 1978). Subsequently, the term "unimodal progeroid syndrome" was used to refer to genetic syndromes of man that appeared to accelerate, predominately, only a *single* aspect of the senescent phenotype (Martin, 1982).

## An Alternative to the "Casarett Rules": Particularization of the Senescent Phenotype

Radiation biologists have recognized for many decades that the long-term consequences of ionizing radiation could include a shortening of the life span, an acceleration of the development of a number of cancers and other diseases, and the premature greying of hair. It was generally believed, however, that ionizing radiation could not be regarded as an agent capable of accelerating the aging "process." This view was epitomized in an influential review by George W. Casarett (1964) in which he spelled out the criteria for concluding that an agent can be "regarded as causing premature aging." To briefly paraphrase, the agent should: 1) accelerate the force of mortality in a population without alteration of the shape of the entire mortality curve; 2) accelerate proportionately the times of onset and rates of development of all age-associated diseases or causes of death found in control groups, "without alteration of degree, sequence, or absolute incidence of the disease and causes of death, and without induction of disease" (presumably, of qualitatively unique types of disease); and 3) accelerate, proportionately, all morphological and physiological manifestations of aging.

These rigorous criteria were subsequently applied by geneticists to the consideration of genetic mutations in man that might accelerate aging (Epstein *et al.*, 1966); the disorder of special interest in that study, to be discussed below in more detail, was the Werner syndrome (Salk *et al.*, 1985a). Not surprisingly, it was concluded that the mutation could not be considered as accelerating aging, but might be viewed as resulting in a "caricature of aging" (Epstein *et al.*, 1966). This view was reiterated in 1985 (Epstein, 1985).

It is probably the case, however, that no single agent, either genetic or environmental, could possibly satisfy the Casarett rules. Such an outcome could only be expected if aging were the result of a single process or mechanism. Aging is likely to be multifactorial in origin, however (Martin, 1978; Rose, 1984); one should speak of aging processes, not *the* aging process (Warner *et al.*, 1987). Given this view, it becomes essential to *particularize the phenotype* when considering agents that might influence aging. The question should not be :"Does this gene affect aging?"; it should be:"Does this gene affect the development of varieties of ocular cataracts associated with aging?", or "Does this gene affect the times of onset and rates of development of specific age-associated post-translational modifications of particular proteins?", or "Does this gene influence the deposition of A4 (beta) amyloid in the cerebral vasculature?", or "Does this gene influence the probability of the emergence of adenocarcinoma of the prostate in a human male?", *etc., etc.*

## Synopsis of 1978 Review

The above views on the importance of particularizing the senescent phenotype were the basis of a review presented at the first conference in this series (Martin, 1978). At that time I noted the paucity of physiologic (and biochemical) markers of aging that had been investigated by human geneticists; this is still the case. Thus, I had to be largely concerned with constitutional genetic factors that may modulate the times of onset and/or the rates of progression of specific components of the "senescent phenotype" of man as it is generally recognized by physicians, pathologists, gerontologists and, to some degree, laymen. Included in the analysis were such parameters as premature greying and loss of hair, ocular cataracts, dementias and certain types of relevant degenerative neuropathology, various types of arteriosclerosis, depositions of amyloid and lipofuscins, various neoplasms characteristic of the elderly population, alterations in the amounts and distributions of adipose tissue, and diabetes mellitus (see Martin, 1978 for a complete tabulation). In retrospect, one parameter (which involved a search for loci of potential relevance to the intrinsic mutagenesis hypothesis of aging) (Burnet, 1974) was inappropriate, as it dealt with a potential mechanism of aging rather than with a phenotype and produced "hits" that, by definition, had to overlap with certain other parameters, such as chromosomal instability and susceptibility to age-related neoplasms.

What emerged from that investigation was an estimate that up to 6.9% of the human genome could play a role in modulating specific aspects of the senescent phenotype of man. Given estimates of about 100,000 human genes (the minimum figure is currently cited as 50,000) (McKusick, 1986), mutation and allelic variation at up to almost 7,000 loci might have the potential of making some impact on the patterns of aging in individual subjects. It was apparent, however, that there were some genetic loci that might prove to be of particular significance because they had the potential to influence many important aspects of the senescent phenotype. These were classified as segmental progeroid syndromes. The prototype example, to be discussed below, is the Werner syndrome.

Of equal significance, however, are certain progeroid syndromes that, while individually impacting upon only a single aspect of the senescent phenotype, can potentially lead to an understanding of the pathogenesis of geriatric disabilities that are of compelling medical and social importance. These are included among a group of heritable conditions that were classified as unimodal progeroid syndromes (Martin, 1982). Because of its great medical significance, and its contrast with the mode of inheritance and phenotype of Werner's syndrome, the prototype example I have chosen to discuss is familial Alzheimer's Disease.

My current research efforts and those of a number of my close colleagues are presently largely focussed upon attempts to understand the genetic basis and pathogenesis of each of these disorders.

## THE WERNER SYNDROME

### Mendelian Pattern of Inheritance

Werner's syndrome is clearly inherited as an autosomal recessive. Pedigrees often reveal two or more affected siblings in a single generation without evidence of affected individuals in other generations. Using two different methods of correction for ascertainment bias, the proportion of affected sibs in a review of 53 sibships was found to range from $17.9 \pm 2.5\%$ to $26.5 \pm 3.2\%$, close to the theoretical value of 25% on the hypothesis of autosomal recessive inheritance (Epstein *et al.*, 1966). The sex ratio of affected homozygotes is approximately 1:1.

As in all rare autosomal recessive disorders, there is a striking increase in the prevalence of consanguinity among the parents of affected homozygotes. Among the 196 patients studied by Goto *et al.* (1985), there was parental consanguinity in 70%.

### Geographical Distribution

The following nationalities/ethnic groups were represented among the 92 sibships investigated by Epstein *et al.* (1966): Hungarian, Hungarian (Jewish), Polish, Russian, Russian (Jewish), Yugoslavian, Bulgarian, Persian (Jewish),

Iraqi (Jewish), Turkish, Italian, German, Dutch, Africaans, Swiss, French, Belgian, Danish, Norwegian, Swedish, English, Irish, New Zealander, Australian, American, American (Jewish), Puerto Rican, Argentinean, Negro, Japanese. Thus, the mutation (or mutations, if genetic heterogeneity can be established), appears to be distributed around the world. The lack of any case reports from certain parts of the world (for example, I have been unable to discover a case report in the Chinese literature) may be attributable to less efficient ascertainment and/or publication.

## Estimates of Prevalence

Estimates of gene frequencies and prevalence rates of the homozygotes have usually been derived from formulas that are based upon estimates of consanguinity. Using such methods, Epstein *et al.* (1966) reported a world-wide prevalence of homozygotes ranging from 1-22.1/million, and Fraccaro *et al.* (1985) gave estimates, for the population of Sardinia, ranging from 2.2-10.8/million. Goto and his colleagues (reviewed in Goto *et al.*, 1985), using such methods as well as large scale population surveys of relatively closed Japanese communities, reported homozygote frequencies ranging from 2.5-3.3/million. Thus, while Werner's syndrome is a rare disease, it is probably being under-diagnosed. Experience among interested investigators in the United States, Europe and Japan would suggest that comparatively few patients are being ascertained. In Japan, for example, with a population of some 110,000,000 people and a relatively high level of awareness of the problem, only 162 living cases were reported between 1961 and 1985 (Goto *et al.*, 1985). The fact that, in Japan, the average age at diagnosis is 36.7 yrs. (Goto *et al.*, 1985), whereas an array of signs and symptoms usually become apparent during the twenties, would support that conclusion.

## Phenotype: Clinical and Pathological Features

The phenotypic features of the disorder have been well described in a number of reviews (see Salk *et al.*, 1985a, for a collection of these). Homozygotes show no detectable abnormalities at birth. It is possible, but not yet documented, that there is somewhat less growth during childhood when compared to siblings. The first sign of any unusual problem, however, is the failure to undergo the usual adolescent growth spurt. There then ensues premature greying of the hair, atrophic, hyperkeratotic and pigmentary changes of skin, hair loss, a weak, high-pitched and squeaky voice, visual difficulties associated with bilateral ocular cataracts, ulcers of the skin of the distal extremities, diabetes mellitus, several forms of arteriosclerosis (Monckeberg's medial calcinosis, calcification of heart ring valves,

| Table 1. Principal Features of the Werner Syndrome (Percentages of Cases). Modified from Tollefsbol and Cohen (1984), from Data of Murata and Nakashima, 1982. | | | |
|---|---|---|---|
| Bilateral cataracts | 95 | ↓ II$^{\mathrm{o}}$ sexual development | 47 |
| Cutaneous atrophy | 86 | Osteoporosis | 41 |
| Short stature | 86 | Cutaneous leg ulcers | 39 |
| Graying or loss of hair | 80 | Nail deformity | 38 |
| Thin limbs, stocky trunk | 77 | Soft tissue calcification | 25 |
| High-pitched or hoarse voice | 70 | Mental disorders | 21 |
| Hyperkeratosis | 68 | Atherosclerosis | 18 |
| Parental consanguinity | 68 | Telangiectasia | 13 |
| Skin pigmentation | 64 | Malignant neoplasms | 8 |
| Diabetic tendency | 61 | Flat feet | ? |
| Hypogonadism | 61 | Irregular tooth arrangement | ? |
| Tight skin | 59 | Hyperreflexia | ? |
| Bird-like facies | 56 | | |

atherosclerosis, arteriosclerosis), osteoporosis, hypogonadism (atrophic changes of testes and ovaries), diminutions of secondary sexual development and a variety of benign and malignant neoplasms. The short stature of the adult patient is striking and is typically associated with very thin limbs but a relatively stocky trunk. Flat feet appear to be very common among Japanese subjects but have not been properly evaluated in Caucasian subjects. Telangiectasia, irregular tooth arrangements, hyperreflexia and "mental disorders" have also been reported, although there is no evidence of an increased susceptibility to any of the histopathological hallmarks of dementia of the Alzheimer's type. A "bird-like," pinched facies is typical, due to facial subcutaneous atrophy and skin alterations.

Quantitative assessments of these various features are given in Table 1.

The median age of death is 47 yrs. The major cause of death is coronary artery atherosclerosis with myocardial infarction. Atherosclerosis appears to be relatively more severe in Caucasian subjects, however. The second most common cause of death is cancer. Of twenty necropsies of Werner syndrome subjects in Japan, five had malignant neoplasms (Ishii *et al.*, 1985).

Salk (1982) has reviewed the literature as regards neoplasia. A relative preponderance of mesenchymal types of neoplasms, such as meningiomas, appears to be well established, but a number of types of benign and malignant epithelial neoplasms have been reported. Of great theoretical and practical interest is the report of Goto *et al.* (1981) suggesting that heterozygotic carriers might be more susceptible to neoplasms; 4.2% of siblings of patients with Werner's syndrome had neoplasms, as compared to 0.11% of controls in the general population. It is essential that additional systematic investigations be carried out, since the frequency of heterozygotes in the general population may range from about 1-5/thousand.

The fact that the phenotype of the Werner's syndrome differs from ordinary aging in a number of ways has been discussed elsewhere (Epstein *et al.*, 1966; Martin, 1978; Salk, 1982); these references should be consulted for a fuller discussion of this issue. We have already noted that mesenchymal tumors appear to be more prevalent than epithelial tumors, the opposite of the situation in ordinary aging. Also, as noted above, is the lack of histopathological evidence of premature aging in the CNS. (Certain of these features will be reviewed in the section on Familial Alzheimer's Disease.) The osteoporosis appears to be more severe in the long bones than in the vertebral bones, contrary to what geriatricians typically observe.

### Phenotype: Cultured Somatic Cells

Martin *et al.* (1970) demonstrated a marked reduction in the replicative potential of fibroblast-like cells taken from the skin, vertebral bone marrow and prostate of patients with the Werner syndrome. Statistical studies of fibroblasts from the dermis of the mesial aspect of the mid-upper arm showed that cultures from these patients gave cumulative population doublings that were two to three standard deviations below the means of age-matched controls. Control cultures gave highly significant negative regressions of replicative potentials as functions of donor age (Martin, 1970; Martin *et al.*, 1981; Nikaido *et al.*, 1985; see also Schneider and Mitsui, 1976 for evidence of decreased growth potential as a function of donor age). A number of other investigators have confirmed the diminished growth potential of cultured cells from subjects with the Werner syndrome (Goldstein, 1979; Aso *et al.*, 1980; Salk *et al.*, 1981a; Schonberg *et al.*, 1984; Thompson and Holliday, 1983; Nikaido *et al.*, 1985; Gawkrodger *et al.*, 1985).

Since Werner's syndrome is recessive, one might expect some degree of complementation of the limited life-span potential in hybrid synkaryons between homozygous affected and wild type. The limited research to date on this question has failed to show such complementation, but since only two hybrid clones have so far been evaluated, no definitive conclusions can be made (Salk *et al.*, 1981a). The interpretation of heterokaryon experiments is also uncertain (Norwood *et al.*, 1979; Pendergrass *et al.*, 1985; Tanaka *et al.*, 1979, 1980 and 1985). The extent of initiation of semi-conservative DNA synthesis in such constructs can depend upon a number of variables, perhaps including the extent of dilution of DNA polymerases and their associated factors by the abundant cytoplasmic mass of senescent or senescing cells (Pendergrass *et al.*, 1982). Given the use of very early passage Werner syndrome cells, it does appear that heterokaryotic fusion with normal young cells or with HeLa cells can increase the proportion of nuclei capable of commencing DNA synthesis (Tanaka *et al.*, 1985).

In a single experiment, co-cultivation of normal cells (foreskin fibroblasts from a newborn male) with skin fibroblasts from a female with Werner's syndrome showed no evidence of either inhibition or complementation of the growth rates or population doublings of the respective cultures (Salk *et al.*, 1981a). Variable (strain dependent) growth enhancement effects were detected, however, in experiments with feeder layers, particularly with SV 40 transformed fibroblasts (Ohno and Yamaguchi, 1984).

Hoehn *et al.* (1975) coined the term "variegated translocation mosaicism" to describe their observations of the propensity of cultured cells from Werner's syndrome patients to exhibit a variety of clonally propagated reciprocal translocations. McKusick (1988), incorrectly attributed the origin of this term to Nichols. The first intimation of a chromosomal abnormality in such cultured cells was based upon the finding, by R. Miller and W. W. Nichols of the Institute for Medical Research, of a deletion in a strain submitted by our laboratory. They raised the question of a constitutional deletion. This led to the discovery, by Hoehn *et al.* (1975), that mosaicism for chromosomal mutations was commonly observed in such cultures. In addition to reciprocal translocations, these included deletions and inversions.

This aspect of the phenotype was more extensively investigated by Salk *et al.* (1981b). Apparent "hot spots" of chromosomal breakage were described, involving sites differing from those associated with such chromosomal instability syndromes as Bloom's syndrome, Fanconi's anemia, ataxia telangiectasia and ionizing radiation. Salk *et al.* (1985b) also presented evidence that chromosomal lesions could arise *in vivo*.

Nordenson (1977), Scappaticci *et al.* (1982) (see also Fraccaro *et al.*, 1985), Schonberg *et al.* (1984) and Gebhart *et al.* (1985) have also demonstrated evidence of chromosomal instability in somatic cells from affected patients. Neither Darlington *et al.* (1981) nor Gebhart *et al.* (1985) could demonstrate increased frequencies of sister chromatid exchanges, however.

In a thoughtful commentary on the paper by Schonberg *et al.* (1984), Benn (1985) has given persuasive arguments supporting his view that the observations of multiple clonal chromosomal abnormalities seen in cultures from Werner syndrome subjects also occur *in vivo* and that they may be extreme examples of a normal phenomenon associated with aging, made particularly apparent by the comparatively limited competitive replication of normal diploid sister clones within the slowly growing and rapidly senescing Werner cultures. There is indeed a great deal of evidence that a number of different types of chromosomal aberrations increase in the tissues of aging mammals (see Martin *et al.*, 1985, for a relatively recent experimental study).

Somatic cells from patients with Werner's syndrome have also been shown to exhibit a mutator phenotype at the single gene level. The forward mutation rates to 6-thioguanine resistance (reflecting mutation at the X-linked locus, HPRT) were measured in cells that had been transformed by the simian vacuolating virus (SV 40) in the laboratories of T. Matsumura and R. Holiday; this conferred apparently unlimited growth potential, permitting an analysis of the rates of mutation with two different methods (Luria and Delbruck, 1943; Newcombe, 1948). The results demonstrated 10-100 fold increases in mutation rates in comparison to SV 40 transformed control cell lines (Fukuchi *et al.*, 1985; Fukuchi *et al.*, 1989a). The great majority (76%) of the forward mutations found in Werner cells proved to be partial or complete deletions (Fukuchi *et al.*, 1989a). These interesting results have obvious implications for the pathogenesis of certain age-related aspects of the senescent phenotype, especially neoplasia. Perhaps of equal significance, however, is the fact that they indicate an expression, in transformed and, hence, experimentally tractable cultures, of an underlying basic biochemical genetic defect. That the observations are not mere artifacts of cell culture is supported by recent studies by Fukuchi *et al.* (1989b) establishing an eight fold increase in the frequencies of spontaneous 6-thioguanine resistant peripheral blood lymphocytes of five patients with well documented Werner's syndrome as compared to age-matched controls. Observations by Scappaticci *et al.* (1982), Gahan and Middleton (1984) and Salk *et al.* (1985b) are also consistent with chromosomal instability *in vivo*.

The chromosomal instability and propensity for deletion mutagenesis has so far not been shown to be related to an abnormality in DNA repair (Fujiwara *et al.*, 1977). Studies with a single strain of Werner syndrome cells (Barenfeld *et al.*, 1986) indicated that, like the well documented results with cells from subjects with ataxia telangiectasia (see Lavin and Schroeder, 1988, for review), the progress of DNA synthesis is relatively resistant to gamma irradiation. This could be due to a deficiency in the recognition of, or response to, DNA damage unrelated to deficiencies in DNA repair (Painter and Young, 1980). Thus, the basic lesion in Werner's syndrome could be some defect in the synthesis of DNA. Schimke *et al.* (1986) have made compelling arguments in favor of the proposition that a variety of perturbations in the S phase of the mitotic cell cycle that lead to the interruption and subsequent reinitiation of DNA synthesis can result in a number of chromosomal rearrangements and deletions. The S phase of the cell cycle and the cell division time are increased in Werner syndrome cells. The rate of DNA elongation appears to be normal (at least up to 2-3 replicons) but the frequency of replicon initiation is decreased (Fujiwara *et al.*, 1977; Takeuchi *et al.*, 1982a; Takeuchi *et al.*, 1982b; Hanaoka *et al.*, 1983 and 1985). Fujiwara *et al.* (1985) have proposed a misfiring and/or delay of initiation due to a "sticky" attachment of replicating DNA to the nuclear matrix of Werner cells.

It is also possible, of course, that any perturbation in DNA synthesis may only be peripherally related to some inborn error of metabolism - for example, some defect in energy metabolism. There have been reports of abnormalities in glucose-6-phosphate dehydrogenase activity (Shindo *et al.*, 1986), proteoglycan metabolism (Tajima *et al.*, 1981; Fujiwara and Ichihashi, 1985; Murata *et al.*, 1985; Bryant *et al.*, 1985; Kieras *et al.*, 1986; Cowles *et al.*, 1987); diminished response to growth factors (Bauer *et al.*, 1986); and reduced sensitivity to catecholamine (Bannai *et al.*, 1987), but these studies require additional controls and further confirmations, and have not been collectively reconciled into some kind of rational pathogenetic perspective.

Although some type of regulatory abnormality is not yet ruled out, and a multi-locus deletion remains a possibility, the most likely explanation for Werner's syndrome is an enzyme deficiency. Those who are enamored of the free radical theory of aging will be disappointed to learn that the specific activities of CuZn and Mn superoxide dismutases, glutathione peroxidase and catalase appear to be normal in the few cell types so far examined (Marklund *et al.*, 1981; Marklund, 1981).

## Future Directions

The rate of progress of the discovery of highly polymorphic genetic markers and their application to the construction of a comparatively high resolution genetic map of man has been such that it is now quite feasible to map (and, ultimately, to clone) the gene for Werner's syndrome using the method of homozygosity mapping (Lander and Botstein, 1987). This method requires DNA from a relatively small number of affected homozygotes who are the progeny of consanguineous matings. Our group in Seattle (John McKay, Gerard Schellenberg, Ellen Wijsman and myself) have embarked upon such a project with the collaboration of colleagues in Japan (Y. Fujiwara and others), Europe (M. Fraccaro, H. Hoehn) and the United States (W.T. Brown). We would be most grateful if additional such patients could be brought to our attention.

An alternative approach to isolating the gene is *via* complementation of the phenotype of limited growth potential *via* transfection with normal DNA. This approach was first suggested by L.E. Orgel in 1982 at the United

States-Japan Cooperative Seminar on Werner's Syndrome and Human Aging (Salk *et al.*, 1985a) and is now being pursued by G.C. Burmer and L.A. Loeb at our institution and by at least two other laboratories.

## FAMILIAL ALZHEIMER'S DISEASE

### Mendelian Pattern of Inheritance

By 1963, a Yale University neurologist and his colleagues were able to collect 19 pedigrees from the world literature in which there were from 2-13 demented individuals in 2-5 generations, with at least one autopsy confirmation of Alzheimer's disease (Feldman *et al.*, 1963). Included in that report was original research on a 6-generation pedigree with 13 affected individuals. The authors acknowledged the assistance of a state official in Catanzaro, the capital city of the Calambria region of southern Italy. It is highly probable that subsequent publications in both the French and American literature have included members of this same kindred (see, for example, David *et al.*, 1987; St. George- Hyslop *et al.*, 1987a).

Although not yet systematically compiled, it is probably the case that there are at least 100 pedigrees now being investigated around the world on the hypothesis that they represent familial forms of Alzheimer's disease in which there is segregating a single major autosomal dominant gene determining susceptibility, with nearly complete penetrance, provided the individual lives long enough to express the disorder. In many of these presumptive autosomal dominant forms, time of onset is generally comparatively early—in the thirties, forties, or fifties (St. George-Hyslop *et al.*, 1987a; Sadovnick *et al.*, 1988; Bird *et al.*, 1989). Some investigators, however, believe there is a separate subset of autosomal dominantly inherited disease of later onset (Pericak-Vance *et al.*, 1988).

Feldman *et al.* (1963) also included in his tabulation 6 families with 2 affected sibs in a single generation. Such familial aggregations are not unusual in routine clinical practice and are usually interpreted as apparently independent instances of sporadic Alzheimer's disease, although, particularly in the case of early onset disease, one should be alert to the possibility of autosomal recessive inheritance, or, in the case of affected males, X-linked inheritance. There is at present, however, no evidence for such Mendelian modes of inheritance.

## Geographical Distribution

Pedigrees consistent with autosomal dominant modes of inheritance have been ascertained in many different regions of the world, but rarely have efforts been undertaken to determine evidence of genetic founder effects (Goudsmit *et al.*, 1981). A particularly striking example was recently uncovered by members of the Alzheimer's Disease Research Center at the University of Washington and their colleagues. A subset of 9 pedigrees, ascertained from various parts of the U.S. west, mid-west and south- west, and originally assumed to be independent, were all discovered to be ethnic "Volga Germans," all of whom were descended from ancestors who migrated from the Hesse area of what is now West Germany to one of two small villages on the west side of the Volga River, now part of the U.S.S.R. (Bird *et al.*, 1988, 1989) (Figure 1). In the 1760's, these farmers were given land by Catherine the Great, who was herself a German. They maintained their native customs and prospered until, with changing political and economic conditions, large numbers of them emigrated to the United States and elsewhere (including Argentina), beginning in the latter half of the nineteenth century. During World War II, a number of remaining families were relocated to other regions of the Soviet Union. Our colleague Holger Hoehn, Chairman of the Department of Human Genetics at the University of Würtzburg, is currently attempting to trace the origins of these kindreds back to the Frankfort-Hesse region of West Germany.

## Estimates of Prevalence

A recent review of the literature on prevalence estimates of dementias (the majority of which are attributable to Alzheimer's disease) indicates a general agreement that prevalence rates double every 5.1 years after the age of 65 (Jorm *et al.*, 1987). This exponential increase in vulnerability as a function of chronological age is consistent with the hypothesis that the disorder is somehow coupled to an intrinsic biological aging process or processes (see also the discussion of the phenotype below). In a longitudinal study of normative aging, the prevalence was estimated to exceed 50% among subjects aged 95 and over (Sayetta, 1986). The proportion of such cases which might be associated with dominant alleles at a single genetic locus is unknown. Mohs *et al.* (1987) found that the cumulative frequency of probable Alzheimer's disease among first-degree relatives of 50 index cases was 46% by age 86, about four times that of values for a control population. They concluded that the data are suggestive of a relatively common autosomal dominant gene for susceptibility to Alzheimer's disease, the expression of which may be delayed

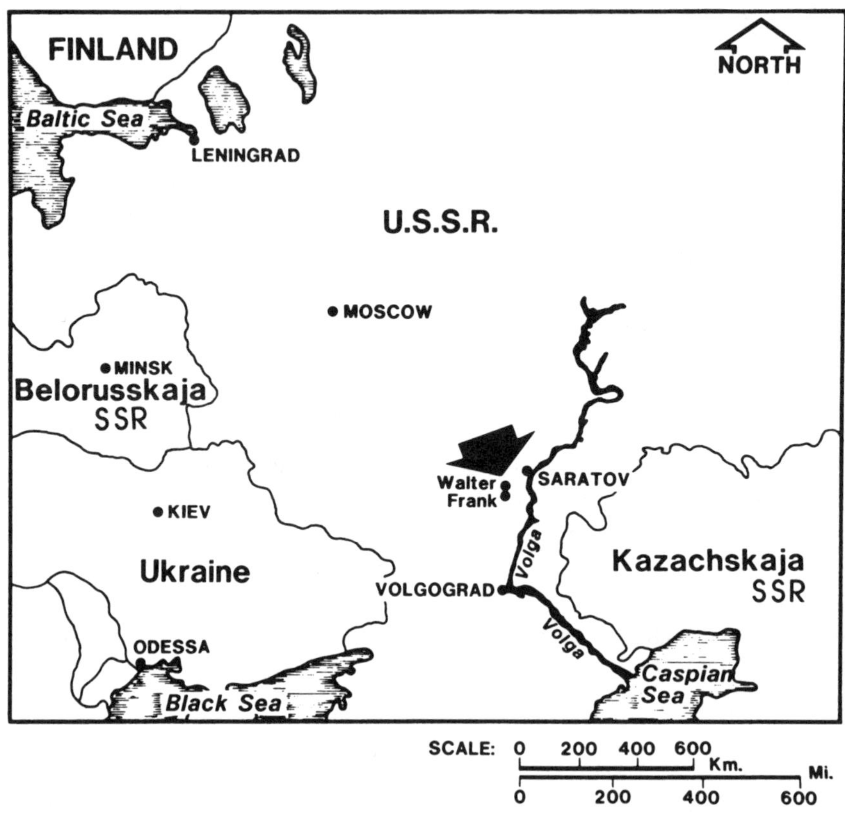



**Figure 1.** The Volga German villages of Walter and Frank, west of the Volga River and near the city of Saratov, are indicated by the arrow (After Bird *et al.*, 1988, with permission.)

until late old age, but is essentially completely penetrant by about age 90. These conclusions have been challenged (Heston, 1988) and rebutted (Mohs *et al.*, 1988).

## Phenotype: Clinical and Pathological Features

No definitive distinctions have yet been made between the clinical and pathological features of familial *vs.* sporadic (*i.e.*, no known family history) Alzheimer's disease, except for the comparatively early onset and disease severity of at least subsets of the former. Patients show the insidious onset and gradual progression of cognitive deterioration, including deficits in judgment, problem solving, orientation, personal care, interest in community and family affairs. There is no loss in alertness, however, as might be observed in various other neuropsychiatric illnesses. Differential diagnosis involves the exclusion of a large number of other neurological and psychiatric conditions capable of causing dementia, including certain reversible dementias (Morris *et al.*, 1988). There are no specific laboratory tests. The monoclonal antibody, Alz 50, recognizes abnormal filaments associated with Alzheimer's disease and its utility for diagnosis using cerebral spinal fluid is currently being evaluated, but it is not likely to be specific (Tabaton *et al.*, 1988).

The "gold standard" for diagnosis is the histopathological examination, in which a set of very characteristic lesions are noted, including neuritic plaques, neurofibrillary tangles, granulovacuolar degeneration, and a specific type of amyloid deposition in the walls of blood vessels and within plaques (Khachaturian, 1985). These lesions also have characteristic distributions, the hippocampal cortex being particularly vulnerable (Hyman *et al.*, 1984), although lesions appear to be quite widespread, perhaps particularly in advanced familial cases (McDuff and Sumi, 1985). Unfortunately, however, none of the lesions are pathognomonic. Moreover, rarely are quantitative methods utilized to establish a diagnosis. There is evidence, of variable quality, that each of the histopathological parameters may be detected, albeit in much lesser abundance, in the brains of elderly individuals who did not display obvious cognitive impairments (Morimatsu *et al.*, 1975). This is another argument in favor of the hypothesis that dementia of the Alzheimer type may reflect an exaggerated form of intrinsic biological aging in our species. For one parameter, beta (or A4) amyloid deposition, the notion of a coupling to intrinsic aging is strongly supported by the observations that this protein accumulates in the aging brains of a number of mammalian species with very different maximum life-span potentials, thus arguing against a simple relationship to chronological aging (Selkoe *et al.*, 1987).

Quite recently, heparan sulfate proteoglycans have been documented to co-localize with the amyloid deposits of Alzheimer's disease, both within the plaques and blood vessels (Snow *et al.*, 1988; Snow and Wight, 1989). It remains to be seen to what extent such materials accumulate as a function of chronological and/or intrinsic biological aging.

## Phenotype: Non-neuronal Somatic Cells

A bewildering array of observations are being reported using fresh peripheral blood lymphocytes, red blood cells, platelets, cultured skin fibroblast-like cells, or lymphoblastoid cell lines from subjects with Alzheimer's disease. The situation is somewhat reminiscent of the flurry of papers, some years ago, concerning putative markers in non-neuronal somatic cells from subjects with Huntington's disease; while some of those claims may yet be substantiated, none have reached the status of proven fact. Those who, for example, utilize cultured skin fibroblast-like cells, could profit from the experience of Goetz *et al.* (1981), who learned, the hard way, about the importance of controlling such variables as the methodologies utilized in establishing the cultures, such as biopsy site and innoculum size. Moreover, it would seem prudent to assume that many aspects of the phenotype of serially cultivated human diploid cells of finite growth potential change as a function of percent of life span achieved; this parameter should therefore be rigorously controlled. While there is no evidence of a systematic difference in the replicative life spans of strains of fibroblasts from patients with Alzheimer's disease and age-matched controls (Balin *et al.*, 1988), there is a great deal of variance within these groups, so that comparison of 2 or 3 pairs of strains could be misleading. Moreover, the use of small inocula of replicating cells for the establishment of cultures could result in large variances of levels of *in vitro* senescence even among multiple biopsies from the same individual, as there is a great deal of clonal heterogeneity in growth potential (Martin *et al.*, 1974; Smith *et al.*, 1978).

As with Huntington's disease, there is not yet any fully confirmed and widely accepted phenotype of this kind for Alzheimer's disease, either familial or sporadic, although there are some promising possibilities. It would, of course, be of great diagnostic and pathogenetic significance if expressions of an autosomal dominant gene could in fact be detected in non-neuronal somatic cells. This approach proved to be the key to the sudden explosion of information concerning the pathogenesis of familial hypercholesterolemia and of atherogenesis in general (Brown and Goldstein, 1984).

Zubenko *et al.* (1987a) have measured the fluorescence anisotropy of 1,6-diphenyl-1,3,5-hexatriene in labeled platelet membranes as an index of "membrane fluidity" and have observed patterns within families consistent with autosomal dominant inheritance of a trait associated with an increase in this index. A possible anatomical substrate for this result is the presence of unusually abundant internal systems of smooth membranes within the platelets of subjects with Alzheimer's disease, suggestive of a dysregulation of platelet membrane biosynthesis (Zubenko *et al.*, 1987b). These interesting observations need to be confirmed by other laboratories and extended to an analysis within a number of well- defined pedigrees.

In another promising line of research, also mainly attributable to the work of one investigator and her colleagues (Christine Peterson), there is evidence of altered calcium homeostasis in cultivated fibroblasts from subjects with Alzheimer's disease; these alterations, including differences in the response to agents that elevate cytosolic calcium, and effects upon the cytoskeleton (cell spreading) appear to be exaggerations of qualitatively similar alterations related to age of donor (Peterson and Goldman, 1986; Peterson *et al.*, 1986; Peterson *et al.*, 1988). Small decreases (10-15%) have also been noted in the mitogen-induced uptake of calcium by lymphocytes in Alzheimer's subjects compared to age-matched controls (Gibson *et al.*, 1987). More work is needed to determine the extent to which these various findings may be characteristic of particular familial types of Alzheimer's disease.

The literature on putative chromosomal instability and hypersensitivity to ionizing radiation and radiomimetic chemicals is inconclusive (Sulkava *et al.*, 1979; Buckton *et al.*, 1983; Moorhead and Heyman, 1983; Fischman *et al.*, 1984; Smith *et al.*, 1984; Morimoto *et al.*, 1984; Matsuyama and Fu, 1988; Robbins *et al.*, 1983; Otsuka *et al.*, 1985; Das, 1986; Scudiero *et al.*, 1986; Kidson and Chen, 1986; Kinsella *et al.*, 1987; Bradley *et al.*, 1987; Smith *et al.*, 1987). With my associate, Eileen M. Bryant, we have tested the hypothesis of radiation hypersensitivity using lymphoblastoid cell lines from members of individual pedigrees, using comparable cultures from a known radiosensitivity disorder (ataxia telangiectasia) as positive controls in each experiment. Although there are important caveats relative to methodological limitations, the results have so far failed to provide support for the hypothesis.

Numerous other observations have been reported with cells from Alzheimer's subjects, the significance of which await clarification: increased $CO_2$ production from glucose and increased lactate, but decreased $CO_2$ production from glutamine and decreased $O_2$ uptake in skin fibroblasts (Sims *et al.*, 1987); reduced activity of transketolase in red cells and fibroblasts (Gibson *et al.*, 1988); increased prostaglandin E1 receptor activity in lymphocytes (Ebstein *et al.*, 1984); increased prostaglandin E1-stimulated cyclic AMP accumulation in lymphocytes (Ebstein *et al.*, 1986); reduction in cholinergic muscarinic binding capacity in lymphocytes (Rabey *et al.*, 1986); reduction of number of both muscarinic and nicotinic binding sites in lymphocytes (Adem *et al.*, 1986); decreased binding of corticotropin releasing factor in monocytes and T cells (Singh and Fudenberg, 1988); decreased production of IL-1 by monocytes, decreased number of autologous rosette forming cells, increased glucose metabolism of B cells (Khansari *et al.*, 1985); attenuated delayed type hypersensitivity response and decreased mitogenesis (with Con A stimulation) of T lymphocytes (Torack, 1986); decreased mitogenic response of lymphocytes to phytohemagglutinin, pokeweed mitogen and OKT3 monoclonal antibody to T3 antigen (Singh *et al.*, 1986-87); deficiency of fibroblasts in synthesizing or excreting a factor that induces the activity of choline acetyl transferase in cultured sympathetic neurons (Kessler, 1987).

## Linkage Analysis

It should be apparent that it will take some time to sort out the many leads to pathogenesis suggested by the research that we have briefly summarized above. A number of the findings may turn out not to be reproducible. Some could have comparatively trivial explanations, such as shifts in population heterogeneity (for the case of studies with unfractionated lymphocytes) or lack of appropriate controls (as discussed above for the case of skin fibroblasts). It should also be apparent that, while an epidemiological approach to pathogenesis is potentially very powerful, it too is fraught with difficulties in the development of rigorous controls and the statistical interpretation of results (Feinstein, 1988).

Meanwhile, however, there is a much more robust approach to pathogenesis—the mapping, cloning and characterization of specific autosomal dominant genes and their gene products. This is made possible by the existence of a number of multiplex pedigrees with such forms of inheritance and the great progress in the development of polymorphic markers for linkage analysis (White and Lalouel, 1987). Considering the complexity of the pathology, however, it would seem likely, *a priori*, that mutation or allelic variation at a number of different loci might be playing a role. If this indeed proves to be the case, as is suggested by the evidence to be discussed below, it is both a strength and a weakness. On the one hand, genetic heterogeneity greatly complicates the task of linkage analysis, since the pooling of pedigrees is typically required to obtain the requisite number of subjects for the statistical rejection or acceptance of the hypothesis of linkage with a given marker. On the other hand, given the approach of pooling of specific subsets of pedigrees for which there is evidence of a genetic founder effect, as in the case of the Volga Germans discussed above, one has the possibility of mapping several genes, each of which could provide invaluable clues to the pathogenesis. The eventual identification of a family of critical gene products could lead to conclusions concerning pathogenetic mechanisms based upon a single integral biochemical pathway *vs.* independent pathways.

The first evidence of genetic linkage was provided by St. George-Hyslop *et al.* (1987a). Four apparently unrelated pedigrees were investigated: 1) a Nova Scotian kindred of British origin; 2) a pedigree of German, but apparently not of Volga German origin; 3) a kindred of Russian origin; and 4) the Southern Italian kindred mentioned above. A multipoint linkage analysis revealed linkage with markers in the proximal portion of the long arm of chromosome 21 (21q21); 2-point linkage analysis, however, did not achieve the requisite level of statistical significance (a LOD score equal to or greater than +3) for the 21q21 markers.

It should be noted that these investigators focussed upon chromosome 21 markers because of the well-established relationship between trisomy 21 and the early development of Alzheimer's disease (reviewed by Cooper and Hall, 1988). The region thought to be essential for the principal components of the Down syndrome, however, maps distally to Alzheimer assignment (St. George-Hyslop *et al.*, 1987a; Cooper and Hall, 1988). Moreover, the great majority of patients with Alzheimer's disease do not show evidence of a submicroscopic duplication of chromosome 21 (St. George-Hyslop *et al.*, 1987b).

Using a 21q21 marker identical to the one employed by St. George-Hyslop *et al.* (1987a), Schellenberg *et al.* (1988) ruled out linkage, for the case of their Alzheimer's disease pedigrees, in the 21q21 region, thus arguing strongly for genetic heterogeneity, although there remains the formal possibility that the initial assignment of St. George- Hyslop *et al.* (1987a) may have resulted from chance. There were two notable features of the experimental design of Schellenberg *et al.* (1988). Firstly, autopsy confirmation was required for the diagnosis for at least one affected member of each pedigree; secondly, a homogeneous subset of their pedigrees (the Volga Germans) could be segregated for the linkage analysis; this analysis also led to a rejection of the hypothesis of linkage to 21q21 markers.

Pericak-Vance *et al.* (1988) have also failed to support the hypothesis of linkage to 21q21 markers in a group of pedigrees that were predominately of the late onset type.

It should be emphasized, however, that it is still the case that there could exist a linkage with a marker elsewhere on chromosome 21. One pathogenetically promising candidate gene on chromosome 21, the locus coding for the amyloidogenic protein of Alzheimer's disease and the aging brain, has been ruled out, since a number of recombinations have been noted between a polymorphism at that locus and the Alzheimer gene (Tanzi *et al.*, 1987; Van Broeckhoven *et al.*, 1987; Schellenberg *et al.*, 1988).

## CONCLUSIONS

It is my belief that progress in gerontology and geriatric medicine will require a biochemical genetic analysis of each of a number of specific components of aging, *i.e.*, we must particularize the phenotype. In view of the enormous fund of knowledge of the biology and pathobiology of man and the striking recent advances in the formal genetic analysis of our species, human genetics offers vast opportunities for such an approach. While the lack of emphasis on the Mendelian inheritance of unusually well-preserved structure and function is regrettable, the identification of genetic loci that lead to the premature onset and/or the accelerated rate of development of a particular senescent process or age-related disorder opens the door for the discovery of potential allelic variants that may in fact enhance structure and function over the life span, given a certain range of environmental conditions.

## REFERENCES

ADEM, A., NORDBERG, A., BUCHT, G., and WINBLAD, B. (1986) Extraneural cholinergic markers in Alzheimer's and Parkinson's disease. *Prog. Neuropsychopharmacol. Biol. Psychiatry* **10**: 247-257.

ASO, K, KENDO, S., and AMANO, M. 1980. A case of Werner's syndrome in which lowered activity of a platelet-dependent serum factor for cell growth and reduced growth potential of fibroblasts and epidermal cells were demonstrated. *Nippon Hifuka Gakkai Zasshi* **90**: 929-934.

BAUER, E. A., SILVERMAN, N., BUSIEK, D. F., KRONBERGER, A., and DEUEL, T. F. (1986) Diminished response of Werner's syndrome fibroblasts to growth factors PDGF and FGF. *Science* **234**: 1240-1243.

BALIN, A. K., BAKER, A. C., LEONG, I. C., and BLASS, J. P. 1988. Normative replicative lifespan of Alzheimer skin fibroblasts. *Neurobiol. Aging* **9**: 195-198.

BANNAI, S., OKAMURA, N.,ISHII, T., SUGITA, Y., BANNAI, C., and YAMASHITA, K. (1987) Reduced sensitivity to catecholamine in Werner's syndrome fibroblasts. *Biochem. Biophys. Res. Commun.* **145**: 183-189.

BARENFELD, L. S., PLESKACH, N. M., BILDIN, V. N., PROKOFJEVA, V. V., and MIKHEL-SON, V. M. (1986) Radioresistant DNA synthesis in cells of patients showing increased chromosomal sensitivity to ionizing radiation. *Mutat. Res.* **165**: 159-164.

BENN, P. A. (1985) Chromosome translocations in fibroblast cultures derived from patients with Werner's syndrome. *Am. J. Hum. Genet.* **37**: 221-223.

BIRD, T. D., LAMPE, T. H., NEMENS, E. J., MINER, G. W., SUMI, S. M., and SCHELLEN-BERG, G. D. (1988) Familial Alzheimer's disease in American descendants of the Volga Germans: Probable genetic founder effect. *Ann. Neurol.* **23**: 25-31.

BIRD, T. D., LAMPE, T., NEMENS, E. J., SUMI, S. M., NOCHLIN, D., SCHELLENBERG, G., WIJSMAN, E., and MINER, G. (1989) Characteristics of familial Alzheimer's disease in nine kindreds of Volga German ancestry. *Alzheimer's Dis. Assoc. Disorders* **2** in press.

BRADLEY, W. G., ROBISON, S. H., and TANDAN, R. (1987) Deficient repair of alkylation damage of DNA in Alzheimer's disease and amyotrophic lateral sclerosis cells. *Adv. Exp. Med Biol.* **209**: 3-6.

BROWN, M. S. and GOIDSTEIN, J. L (1984) How LDL receptors influence cholesterol and atherosclerosis. *Sci. Am.* **251**: 58-66.

BRYANT, E., SALK D., and WIGHT, T. (1985) Proteoglycans in the Werner syndrome and aging: A review and perspective. *Adv. Exp. Med. Biol.* **190**: 553-565.

BUCKTON, K. E., WHALLEY, L. J., LEE, M., and CHRISTIE, J.E. (1983) Chromosome changes in Alzheimer's presenile dementia. *J. Med. Genet.* **20**: 46-51.

BURNET, M. (1974) *Intrinsic Mutagenesis.* New York: John Wiley and Sons.

CASARET, G. W. (1964). Similarities and contrasts between radiation and time pathology. *Adv. Gerontol. Res.* **1**: 109-163.

COOPER, D. N. and HALL, C. (1988) Down's syndrome and the molecular biology of chromosome 21. *Prog. Neurobiol.* **30**: 507-530.

COWLES, E. A., BRAUKER, J. H., and ANDERSON, R. L. (1987) Turnover of sulfated glycosaminoglycans in fibroblasts derived from patients with Werner's syndrome. *Exp. Cell Res.* **168**: 347-357.

DARLINGTON, G. J., DUTKOWSKI, R., and BROWN, W. T. (1981) Sister chromatid exchange frequencies in progeria and Werner syndrome patients. *Am. J. Hum. Genet.* **33**: 762-766.

DAS, R. K. (1986) Mitomycin C and ethyl methanesulphonate-induced sister-chromatid exchanges in lymphocytes from individuals with Alzheimer's pre-senile dementia. *Mutat. Res.* **173**: 127-130.

DAVID, F., HALLE, L, and LUCOTTE, G. (1987) Absence de liaison entre la maladie d'-Alzheimer et une sonde polymorphe du bras long du chromosome 21. *CR Acad. Sci. Paris* **305**: 21-24.

EBSTEIN, R. P., OPPENHEIM, G., and STESSMAN, J. (1984) Alzheimer's disease: Isoproterenol and prostaglandin E l-stimulated cyclic AMP accumulation in lymphocytes. *Life Sci.* **34**: 2239-2243.

EBSTEIN, R. P., OPPENHEIM, G., EBSTEIN, B.S., AMIRI, Z., and STESSMAN, J. (1986) The cyclic AMP second messenger system in man: The effects of heredity, hormones, drugs, aluminum, age and disease on signal amplification. *Prog. Neuropsychopharmacol. Biol. Psychiatry* **10**: 323-353.

EPSTEIN, C. J., MARTIN, G. M., SCHULTZ, A. L., and MOTULSKY, A. G. (1966) Werner's syndrome: A review of its symptomatology, natural history, pathologic features, genetics and relationship to the natural aging process. *Medicine* **45**: 177-221.

EPSTEIN, C. J. (1985) Werner's syndrome and aging: A reappraisal. *Adv. Exp. Med Biol.* **190**: 219-228.

FELDMAN, R. G., CHANDLER, K. A., LEVY, L. L., and GLASER, G. H. (1963) Familial Alzheimer's disease. *Neurology* **13**: 811-824.

FEINSTEIN, A. R. (1988) Scientific standards in epidemiologic studies of the menace of daily life. *Science* **242**: 1257-1263.

FISCHMAN, H. K., REISBERG, B., ALBU, P., FERRIS, S. H., and RAINER, J. D. (1984) Sister chromatid exchanges and cell cycle kinetics in Alzheimer's disease. *Biol. Psychiatry* **19**: 319-327.

FRACCARO, M., SCAPPATICCI, S., and CERIMELE, D. (1985) A population and cytogenetic study of the Werner syndrome in Sardinia. *Adv. Exp. Med. Biol.* **190**: 547-552.

FUJIWARA, Y., and ICHIHASHI, M. (1985) Glycosaminoglycan synthesis in untransformed and transformed Werner syndrome fibroblasts: A preliminary report. *Adv. Exp. Med. Biol.* **190**: 613 -625.

FUJIWARA, Y., KANO, Y.,ICHIHASHI, M., NAKAO, Y., and MATSUMURA, T. 1985. Abnormal fibroblast aging and DNA replication in the Werner syndrome. *Adv. Exp. Med. Biol.* **190**: 459-477.

FUJIWARA, Y., HIGASHIKAWA, T., and TATSUMI, M. (1977) A retarded rate of DNA replication and normal level of DNA repair in Werner's syndrome fibroblasts in culture. *J. Cell Physiol.* **92**: 365-374.

FUKUCHI, K-1., TANAKA, K., NAKURA, J., KUMAHARA, Y., UCHIDA, T., and OKADA, Y. (1985) Elevated spontaneous mutation rate in SV40-transformed Werner syndrome fibroblast cell lines. *Somat. Cell Mol. Genet.* **11**: 303-308.

FUKUCHI, K-I., MARTIN, G. M., and MONNAT, R. J. JR. (1989a) The mutator phenotype of Werner syndrome is characterized by extensive deletions. *Proc. Natl. Acad. Sci. USA* **86**: 5893-5897

FUKUCHI, K-I., TANAKA, K., KUMAHARA, Y., MARUMO, K., PRIDE, M., MARTIN, G. M., and MONNAT, R.J. JR. (1989b) Increased frequency of 6-thioguanine-resistant peripheral blood lymphocytes in Werner syndrome patients. *Hum. Genet.* in press

GAHAN, P. B., and MIDDLEToN, J. (1984) Euploidization of human hepatocytes from donors of different ages and both sexes compared with those from cases of Werner's syndrome and progeria. *Exp. Gerontol.* **19**: 355-358.

GAWKRODGER, D. J., PRIESTLEY, G. C., VIJAYALAXMI, ROSS, J. A., NARCISI, P., and HUNTER, J. A. A. (1985) Werner's syndrome: Biochemical and cytogenetic studies. *Arch. Dermatol.* **121**: 636-641.

GEBHART, E., SCHINZEI, M., and RUPRECHT, K. W. (1985) Cytogenetic studies using various clastogens in two patients with Werner syndrome and control individuals. *Hum. Genet.* **70**: 324-327.

GIBSON, G. E., NIELSEN, P., SHERMAN, K. A., and BLASS, J. P. (1987) Diminished mitogen-induced calcium uptake by lymphocytes from Alzheimer patients. *Biol. Psychiatry* **22**: 1079-1086.

GIBSON, G. E., SHEU, K. F., BIASS, J. P., BAKER, A., CARLSON, K. C., HARDING, B., and PERRINO, P. (1988) Reduced activities of thiamine-dependent enzymes in the brains and peripheral tissues of patients with Alzheimer's disease. *Arch. Neurol.* **45**: 836-840.

GOETZ, I. E., ROBERTS, E., and WARREN, J. (1981) Skin fibroblasts in Huntington disease. *Am. J. Hum. Genet.* **33**: 187-196.

GOLDSTEIN, S. (1979) Studies on age-related diseases in cultured skin fibroblasts. *J. Invest. Dermatol.* **73**: 19-23.

GOMPERTZ, B. (1825) On the nature of the function expressive of the law of human mortality and on a new mode of determining life contingencies. *Phil. Trans. R Soc. London* **II**: 513-585.

GOTO, M., TANIMOTO, K., HORIUCHI, Y., and SASAZUKI, T. (1981) Family analysis of Werner's syndrome: A survey of 42 Japanese families with a review of literature. *Clin. Genet.* **19**: 8-15.

GOTO, M., TAKEUCHI, F., TANIMOTO, K., and MIYAMOTO, T. 1985. Clinical, demographic, and genetic aspects of the Werner syndrome in Japan. *Adv. Exp. Med. Biol.* **190**: 245-261.

GOUDSMIT, J., WHITE, B. J., WEITKAMP, L. R., YEATS, B. J., MORROW, C. H., and GAJDUSEK, D. C. (1981) Familial Alzheimer's disease in two kindreds of the same geographic and ethnic origin. A clinical and genetic study. *J. Neurol. Sci.* **49**: 79-89.

HANAOKA, F., TAKEUCHI, F., MATSUMURA, T., GOTO, M., MIYAMOTO, T., and YAMADA, M. (1983) Decrease in the average size of replicons in a Werner syndrome cell line by Simian Virus 40 infection. *Exp. Cell Res.* **144**: 463-467.

HANAOKA, F., YAMADA, M-A., TAKEUCHI, F., GOTO, M., MIYAMOTO, T., and HORI, T-A. (1985) Autoradiographic studies of DNA replication in Werner's syndrome cells. *Adv. Exp. Med. Biol.* **190**: 439-457.

HESTON, L. L (1988) Morbid risk in first-degree relatives of persons with Alzheimer's disease. *Arch. Genl. Psychiatry* **45**: 97-98.

HOEHN, H., BRYANT, E. M., AU, K, NORWOOD, T. H., BOMAN, H., and MARTIN, G. M. (1975) Variegated translocation mosaicism in human skin fibroblast cultures. *Cytogenet. Cell Genet.* **15**: 282-298.

HYMAN, B. T., VAN HORSEN, G. W., DAMASIO, A. R., and BARNES, C. L. (1984) Alzheimer's disease: Cell-specific pathology isolates the hippocampal formation. *Science* **225**: 947-949.

ISHII, T., HOSODA, Y., HAMADA, Y., NAKAGAWA, S., ASANO, G., and HORIBE, Y. (1985) Pathology of the Werner Syndrome. Pathology of the Werner syndrome. *Adv. Exp. Med. Biol.* **190**: 187-214.

JORM, A. F., KORTEN, A. E., and HENDERSON, A. S. (1987) The prevalence of dementia: A quantitative integration of the literature. *Acta Psychiatr. Scand.* **76**: 465-479.

KESSLER, J. A. (1987) Deficiency of a cholinergic differentiating factor in fibroblasts of patients with Alzheimer's disease. *Ann. Neurol.* **21**: 95-98.

KHACHATURIAN, Z. S. (1985) Diagnosis of Alzheimer's disease. *Arch. Neurol.* **42**: 1097-1105.

KHANSARI, N., WHITTEN, H. D., CHOU, Y. K., and FUDENBERG, H. H. (1985) Immunological dysfunction in Alzheimer's disease. *J. Neuroimmunol.* **7**: 279-285.

KIDSON, C. and CHEN, P. (1986) DNA damage, DNA repair and the genetic basis of Alzheimer's disease. *Prog. Brain Res.* **70**: 291 -301.

KIERAS, F. J., BROWN, W. T., HOUCK, G. E., JR., and ZEBROWER, M. (1986) Elevation of urinary hyaluronic acid in Werner's syndrome and progeria. *Biochem. Med. Metab. Biol.* **36**: 276-282.

KINSELLA T. J., DOBSON, P. P., FORNACE, A. J. JR., BARRETT, S. F., GANGES, M. B., and ROBBINS, J. H. (1987) Alzheimer's disease fibroblasts have normal repair of N-methyl-N-nitro-N-nitrosoguanidine-induced DNA damage determined by the alkaline elution technique. *Biochem. Biophys. Res. Commun.* **149**: 355-361.

LANDER, E. S. and BOTSTEIN, D. (1987) Homozygosity mapping: A way to map human recessive traits with the DNA of inbred children. *Science* **236**: 1567-1570.

LAVIN, M. F., and SCHROEDER, A. L. (1988) Damage-resistant DNA synthesis in eukaryotes. *Mutat. Res.* **193**: 193-206.

LEOPOLD, A. C. (1975) Aging, senescence, and turnover in plants. *Bioscience* **25**: 659-662.

LURIA, S. E. and DELBRUCK, M. (1943) Mutations of bacteria from virus sensitivity to virus resistance. *Genetics* **28**: 491-511.

MARKLUND, S. L (1981) Superoxide dismutase, catalase and glutathione peroxidase in degenerative diseases. *Bull. Europ. Physiopath. Resp.* **17**:(suppl.) 259-263.

MARKLUND, S. L., NORDENSSON, I., and BÄCK, 0. 1981. Normal CuZn superoxide dismutase, Mn superoxide dismutase, catalase and glutathione peroxidase in Werner's syndrome. *J. Gerontol.* **36**: 405-409.

MARTIN, G. M. (1978) Genetic syndromes in man with potential relevance to the pathobiology of aging. *Birth Defects - Original Article Series* **14**: 5-39.

MARTIN, G. M. (1982) Syndromes of accelerated aging. *Natl. Cancer Inst. Monogr.* **60**: 241-247.

MARTIN, G. M. (1988) Constitutional genetic markers of aging. *Exp. Gerontol.* **23**: 257-267.

MARTIN, G. M., SPRAGUE, C. A. and EPSTEIN, C. J. (1970) Replicative life-span of cultivated human cells: Effects of donor's age, tissue, and genotype. *Lab. Invest.* **23**: 86-92.

MARTIN, G. M., SPRAGUE, C. A., NORWOOD, T. H., and PENDERGRASS, W. R. (1974) Clonal selection, attenuation and differentiation in an *in vitro* model of hyperplasia. *Am. J. Path.* **74**: 137-154.

MARTIN, G. M., OGBURN, C. E., and SPRAGUE, C. A. (1981) Effects of age on cell division capacity. **In**: *Aging, A Challenge to Science and Society, Vol. I Biology* (Eds. D. Danon, N. W. Shock, and M. Marvis), pp. 124-135. Oxford: Oxford University Press.

MARTIN, G. M., SMITH, A. C., KETTERER, D. J., OGBURN, C. E., and DISTECHE, C. M. (1985) Increased chromosomal aberrations in first metaphases of cells isolated from the kidneys of aged mice. *Israel J. Med. Sci.* **21**: 296-301.

MASORO, E. J. (1988) Food restriction in rodents: An evaluation of its role in the study of aging. *J. Gerontol. Biol. Sci.* **43**: B59-B64.

MATSUYAMA, S. S. and FU, T-K. (1988) Sister chromatid exchanges and dementia of the Alzheimer type. *Neurobiol. Aging* **9**: 405-408.

McDUFF, T. and SUMI, S. M. (1985) Subcortical degeneration in Alzheimer's disease. *Neurology* **35**: 123-126.

McKUSICK, V. A. (1986) The genetic map of *Homo sapiens*: Status and prospectus. **In**: *Molecular Biology of Homo Sapiens. Symposium on Quantitative Biology,* **51**: pp. 15 - 27. New York: Cold Spring Harbor Laboratory.

McKUSICK, V. A. (1988) *Mendelian Inheritance in Man 8th Edition.* Baltimore: The Johns Hopkins University Press.

MOHS, R. C., BREITNER, J. C. S., SILVERMAN, J. M., and DAVIS, K. L. (1987) Alzheimer's disease: Morbid risk among first-degree relatives approximates 50% by 90 years of age. *Arch. Genl. Psychiatry* **44**: 405-408.

MOHS, R. C., BREITNER, J. C. S., SILVERMAN, J. M., and DAVIS, K. L. (1988) In reply. *Arch. Genl. Psychiatry* **45**: 98.

MOORHEAD, P. S. and HEYMAN, A. (1983) Chromosome studies of patients with Alzheimer disease. *Am. J. Med. Genet.* **14**: 545-556.

MORIMATSU, M., HIRAI, S., MORAMATSU, A., and YOSHIWAKA, M. (1975) Senile degenerative brain lesions and dementia. *J. Am. Geriatr. Soc.* **23**: 390-406.

MORIMOTO, K., MIURA, K., KANEKO, T., IIJIMA, K., SATO, M., and KOIZUMI, A. (1984) Human health situation and chromosome alterations: Sister chromatid exchange frequency in lymphocytes from passive smokers and patients with hereditary diseases. *Basic Life Sci.* **29** (Pt B), 801-811.

MORRIS, J. C., McKEEL, D. W., FULLING, K., TORACK, R. M., and BERG, L. (1988) Validation of clinical diagnostic criteria for Alzheimer's disease. *Ann. Neurol.* **24**: 17-22.

MURATA, K. and NAKASHIMA, H. (1982) Werner's syndrome: 24 cases of Werner's synrome: With a clinical review of the Japanese medical literature. *Am. Geriatr. Soc.* **30**: 303-308.

MURATA, K., HIWATARI, R., and MATSUMURA, T. (1985) Acidic glycosaminoglycans in Werner's syndrome: Studies on levels in tissue, organ, cell, and fluid. *Adv. Exp. Med. Biol.* **190**: 587-606.

NEWCOMBE, H. B. (1948) Delayed phenotypic expression of spontaneous mutations in *Escherichia coli*. *Genetics* **33**: 447-476.

NIKAIDO, O., NISHIDA, T., and SHIMA, A. (1985). Cellular mechanisms of aging the Werner syndrome. *Adv. Exp. Med. Biol.* **190**: 421-438.

NORDENSON, 1. (1977) Chromosome breaks in Werner's syndrome and their prevention *in vitro* by radical-scavenging enzymes. *Hereditas* **87**: 151-154.

NORWOOD, T. H., HOEHN, H., SALK, D., and MARTIN, G. M. (1979) Cellular aging in Werner's syndrome: A unique phenotype? *J. Invest Dermatol.* **73**: 92-96.

OHNO, T. and YAMAGUCHI, N. (1984) Life span elongation of Werner's syndrome fibroblasts by co-culture with origin-defective SV-40 DNA transformed cells. *Hum. Genet.* **68**: 209-210.

OTSUKA, F., TARONE, R. E., SEGUIN, L. R., and ROBBINS, J. H. (1985) Hypersensitivity to ionizing radiation in cultured cells from Down syndrome patients. *J. Neurol. Sci.* **69**: 103-112.

Oxford Dictionary of Quotations 2nd Edition. 1953. London: Oxford University Press.

PAINTER, R. B. and YOUNG, B. R. (1980) Radiosensitivity in ataxia telangiectasia: A new explanation. *Proc. Natl. Acad. Sci. USA* **77**: 7315-7317.

PENDERGRASS, W. R., SAULEWICZ, A. C., BURMER, G. C., RABINOVITCH, P. S., NORWOOD, T. H., and MARTIN, G. M. (1982) Evidence that a critical threshold of DNA polymerase-alpha activity may be required for the initiation of DNA synthesis in mammalian cell heterokaryons. *J. Cell Physiol.* **113**: 141-151.

PENDERGRASS, W., SALK, D., and NORWOOD, T. (1985) Cell fusion studies and biochemical analysis of DNA synthesis in Werner and non-Werner cultured cells. *Adv. Exp. Med. Biol.* **190**: 353-372.

PERICAK-VANCE, M. A., YAMAOKA, L. H., HAYNES, C. S., SPEER, M. C., HAINES, J. L., GASKELL, P. C., HUNG, W.-Y., CLARK, C. M., HEYMAN, A. L., TROFATTER, J. A., EISENMENGER, J. P., GILBERT, J. R., LEE, J. E., ALBERTS, M. J., DAWSON, D. V., BARTLETT, R.J., EARL, N. L., SIDDIQUE, T., VANCE, J. M., CONNEALLY P. M., and ROSES, A. D. (1988) Genetic linkage studies in Alzheimer's disease families. *Exp. Neurol.* **102**: 271-279

PETERSON, C. and GOLDMAN, J. E. (1986) Alterations in calcium content and biochemical processes in cultured skin fibroblasts from aged and Alzheimer donors. *Proc. Nat. Acad. Sci. USA* **83**: 2758-2762.

PETERSON, C., RATAN, R. R., SHELANSKI, M. L, and GOLDMAN, J. E. (1986) Cytosolic free calcium and cell spreading decrease in fibroblasts from aged and Alzheimer donors. *Proc. Nat. Acad. Sci. USA* **83**: 7999-8001.

PETERSON, C., RATAN, R. R., SHELANSKI, M. L. and GOLDMAN, J. E. (1988) Altered response of fibroblasts from aged and Alzheimer donors to drugs that elevate cytosolic free calcium. *Neurobiol. Aging* **9**: 261-266.

RABEY, J. M., SHENKMAN, L., and GILAD, G. M. (1986) Cholinergic muscarinic binding by human lymphocytes: Changes with aging, antagonist treatment, and senile dementia of the Alzheimer type. *Ann. NeuroL* **20**: 628-631.

ROBBINS, J. H., OTSUKA, F., TARONE, R. E., POLINSKY, R. J., BRUMBACK, R. A., MOSHELL, A. N., NEE, L. E., GANGES, M. B., and CAYEUX, S. J. (1983) Radiosensitivity in Alzheimer disease and Parkinson disease. *Lancet* **1**: 468-469.

ROSE, M. R. (1984) The evolution of animal senescence. *Can. J. Zool.* **62**: 1661-1667.

SADOVNICK, A. D., TUOKKO, H., HORTON, A., BAIRD, P. A., and BEATTIE, B. L (1988) Familial Alzheimer's disease. *Can. J. Neurol. Sci.* **15**: 142-146.

SALK, D. (1982) Werner's syndrome: A review of recent research with an analysis of connective tissue metabolism, growth control of cultured cells, and chromosomal aberrations. *Hum. Genet.* **62**: 1-15.

SALK,, D., BRYANT, E., AU, K., HOEHN, H., and MARTIN, G. M. (1981a) Systematic growth studies, cocultivation, and cell hybridization studies of Werner syndrome cultured skin fibroblasts. *Hum. Genet.* **58**: 310-316.

SALK,, D., AU, K., HOEHN, H., and MARTIN, G. M. (1981b) Cytogenetics of Werner's syndrome cultured skin fibroblasts: variegated translocation mosaicism. *Cytogenet. Cell Genet.* **30**: 92-107.

SALK, D., FUJIWARA, Y., and MARTIN, G. M. (Eds.) (1985a) Werner's Syndrome and Human Aging. *Advances in Experimental Medicine and Biology* **Vol. 190.** New York: Plenum Press.

SALK, D., AU, K., HOEHN, H., and MARTIN, G. M. (1985b) Cytogenetic aspects of Werner syndrome. *Adv. Exp. Med. Biol.* **190**: 541-546.

SAYETTA, R. B. (1986) Rates of senile dementia—Alzheimer's type in the Baltimore longitudinal study. *J. Chron. Dis.* **39**: 271 -286.

SCAPPATICCI, S., CERIMELE, D., and FRACCARO, M. (1982) Clonal structural chromosomal rearrangements in primary fibroblast cultures and in lymphocytes of patients with Werner's syndrome. *Hum. Genet.* **62**: 16-24.

SCHELLENBERG, G. D., BIRD, T. D., WIJSMAN, E. M., MOORE, D. K., BOEHNKE, M., BRYANT, E. M., LAMPE, T. H., NOCHLIN, D., SUMI, S. M., DEEB, S. S., BEYREUTHER, K., and MARTIN, G. M. (1988) Absence of linkage of chromosome 21q21 markers to familial Alzheimer's disease. *Science* **241**: 1507-1510.

SCHIMKE, R. T., SHERWOOD, S. W., HILL, A. B., and JOHNSTON, R. N. (1986) Overreplication and recombination of DNA in higher eukaryotes: Potential consequences and biological implications. *Proc. Nat. Acad. Sci. USA* **83**: 2157-2161.

SCHNEIDER, E. L. and MITSUI, Y. (1976) The relationship between *in vitro* cellular aging and *in vivo* human age. *Proc. Nat. Acad. Sci. USA* **73**: 3584-3588.

SCHONBERG, S., NIERMEIUER, M. F., BOOTSMA, D., HENDERSON, E., and GERMAN, J. (1984) Werner's syndrome: Proliferation *in vitro* of clones of cells bearing chromosome translocations. *Am. J. Hum. Genet.* **36**: 387-397.

SCUDIERO, D. A., POLINSKY, R. J., BRUMBACK, R. A., TARONE, R. E., NEE, L. E., and ROBBINS, J. H. (1986) Alzheimer disease fibroblasts are hypersensitive to the lethal effects of a DNA damaging chemical. *Mutat. Res.* **159**: 125-131.

SELKOE, D. J., BELL, D. S., PODLISNY, M. B., PRICE, D. L., and CORK L. C. (1987) Conservation of brain amyloid proteins in aged mammals and humans with Alzheimer's disease. *Science* **235**: 873-877.

SHINDO, Y., AKIYAMA, J., MATSUMOTO, K., TAKASE, Y., and HASHIMOTO, T. (1986) Low glucose-6-phosphate dehydrogenase activity in cultured skin fibroblasts from Werner's syndrome. *J. Dermatol.* **13**: 396-398.

SIMS, N. R., FINEGAN, J. M., and BLASS, J. P. (1987) Altered metabolic properties of cultured skin fibroblasts in Alzheimer's disease. *Ann. Neurol.* **21**: 451-457.

SINGH, V. K. and FUDENBERG, H. H. (1988) Binding of [$^{125}$I]-corticotropin releasing factor to blood immunocytes and its reduction in Alzheimer's disease. *Immunol. Lett.* **18**: 5-8.

SINGH, V. K., FUDENBERG, H. H., and BROWN, F. R. 3d. (1986-87) Immunologic dysfunction: Simultaneous study of Alzheimer's and older Down's patients. *Mech. Ageing Dev.* **37**: 257-264.

SMITH, A., BROE, G. A., and WILLIAMSON, M. (1984) Chromosome fragility in Alzheimer's disease. *Clin. Genet.* **25**: 416-421.

SMITH, J. R., PEREIRA-SMITH, O., and SCHNEIDER, E. L. (1978) Colony size distributions as a measure of *in vivo* and *in vitro* aging. *Proc. Nat. Acad. Sci. USA* **75**: 1353-1356.

SMITH, T. A., NEARY, D., and ITZHAKI, R. F. (1987) DNA repair in lymphocytes from young and old individuals and from patients with Alzheimer's disease. *Mutat. Res.* **184**: 107-112.

SNOW, A. D., MAR, H., NOCHLIN, D., KIMATA, K., KATO, M., SUZUKI, S., HASSELI, J., and WIGHT, T. N. (1988) The presence of heparan sulfate proteoglycans in the neuritic plaques and congophilic angiopathy in Alzheimer's disease. *Am. J. Pathol.* **133**: 456-463.

SNOW, A. D. and WIGHT, T. N. (1989) The involvement of proteoglycans in the pathogenesis of Alzheimer's disease and other amyloidoses. *Neurobiol. Aging*, in press.

ST. GEORGE-HYSLOP, P. H., TANZI, R. E., POLINSKY, R. J., HAINES, J. L, NEE, L., WATKINS, P. C., MYERS, R. H., FELDMAN, R. G., POLLEN, D., DRACHMAN, D. *et al.* (1987a) The genetic defect causing familial Alzheimer's disease maps on chromosome 21. *Science* **235**: 885-890.

ST. GEORGE-HYSLOP, P. H., TANZI, R. E., POLINSKY, R. J., NEVE, R. L., POLLEN, D., DRACHMAN, D., GROWDON, J., CUPPLES, L. A., NEE, L., MYERS, R. H., *et al.* (1987b) Absence of duplication of chromosome 21 genes in familial and sporadic Alzheimer's disease. *Science* **238**: 664-666.

SULKAVA, R., ROSSI, L., and KNUUTILA S. (1979) No elevated sister chromatid exchange in Alzheimer's disease. *Acta Neurol. Scand.* **59**: 156-159.

TABATON, M., WHITEHOUSE, P. J., PERRY, G., DAVIES, P., AUTILIO-GAMBETTI, L., and GAMBETTI, P. (1988) Alz 50 recognizes abnormal filaments in Alzheimer's disease and progressive supranuclear palsy. *Ann. Neurol.* **24**: 407-413.

TAJIMA, T., WATANABE, T., IIJIMA, K., OHSHIKA, Y., and YAMAGUCHI, H. (1981) The increase of glycosaminoglycans synthesis and accumulation on the cell surface of cultured skin fibroblasts in Werner's syndrome. *Exp. Path.* **20**: 221-229.

TAKEUCHI, F., HANAOKA, F., GOTO, M., AKAOKA,I., HORI, T-A., YAMADA, M-A., and MIYAMOTO, T. (1982a) Altered frequency of initiation sites of DNA replication in Werner's syndrome cells. *Hum. Genet.* **60**: 365-368.

TAKEUCHI, F., HANAOKA, F., GOTO, M., YAMADA, M-A., and MIYAMOTO, T. (1982b) Prolongation of S phase and whole cell cycle in Werner's syndrome fibroblasts. *Exp. Gerontol.* **17**: 473-480.

TANAKA, K., NAKAZAWA, T., OKADA, Y., and KUMAHARA, Y. (1979) Increase in DNA synthesis in Werner's syndrome cells by hybridization with normal human diploid and HeLa cells. *Exp. Cell. Res.* **123**: 261 -267.

TANAKA, K, NAKAZAWA, T., OKADA, Y., and KUMAHARA, Y. (1980) Roles of nuclear and cytoplasmic environments in the retarded DNA synthesis in Werner syndrome cells. *Exp. Cell Res.* **127**: 185 -190.

TANAKA, K, YAMAMURA, K-I., FUKUCHI, F., KAWAI, K., and KUMAHARA, Y. (1985) Cell fusion studies in the Werner syndrome. *Adv. Exp. Med. Biol.* **190**: 341 -351.

TANZI, R. E., ST. GEORGE-HYSLOP, P. H., HAINES, J. L., POLINSKY, R. J., NEE, L., FONCIN, J. F., NEVE, R. L., McCLATCHEY, A. I., CONNEALLY, P. M., and GUSELLA, J. F. (1987) The genetic defect in familial Alzheimer's disease is not tightly linked to the amyloid beta-protein gene. *Nature* **329**: 156-157.

THOMPSON, K. V. A., and HOLLIDAY, R. (1983) Genetic effects on the longevity of cultured human fibroblasts. I. Werner's syndrome. *Gerontology* **29**: 73-82.

TOLLEFSBOL, T. O. and COHEN, H. J. (1984) Werner's syndrome: An underdiagnosed disorder resembling aging. *Age* **7**: 75-88.

TORACK, R. M. (1986) T-lymphocyte function in Alzheimer's disease. *Neurosci. Lett.* **71**: 365-369.

VAN BROECKHOVEN, C., GENTHE, A. M., VANDENBERGHE, A., HORSTHEMKE, B., BACKHOVENS, H., RAEYMAEKERS, P., VAN HUL, W., WEHNERT, A., GHEUENS, J., CRAS, P., BRUYLAND, M., MARTIN, J. J., SALBAUM, M., MULTHAUP, G., MASTERS, C. L, BEYREUTHER, K., GURLING, H. M. D., MULLAN, M. J., HOLLAND, A., BARTON, A., IRVING, N., WILLIAMSON, R., RICHARDS, S. J., and HARDY, J. A. (1987) Failure of familial Alzheimer's disease to segregate with the A4-amyloid gene in several European families. *Nature* **329**: 153-155.

WARNER, H. R., BUTLER, R. N., SPROTT, R. L., and SCHNEIDER, E. L. (Eds.) (1987) *Modern Biological Theories of Aging.* New York, Raven Press.

WEINDRUCH, R. and WALFORD, R. L (1988) *The Retardation of Aging and Disease by Dietary Restriction.* Springfield, Illinois: C. C. Thomas.

WHITE, R. and LALOUEL, J. M. (1987) Investigation of genetic linkage in human families. *Adv. Hum. Genet.* **16**: 121-128.

ZUBENKO, G. S., WUSYLKO, M., COHEN, B. M., BOLLER, F., and TEPLY, 1. (1987a) Family study of platelet membrane fluidity in Alzheimer's disease. *Science* **238**: 539-542.

ZUBENKO, G. S., MALINAKOVA, I., and CHOJNACKI, B. (1987b) Proliferation of internal membranes in platelets from patients with Alzheimer's disease. *J. Neuropathol. Exp. Neurol.* **46**: 407-418.

## DISCUSSION

1. Clinical and pathological manifestations of familial Alzheimer's disease can arise from at least 2 different loci independently, *i.e.* one or the other must be present, and one is not located on chromosome 21 (not for at least 17 cM on either side of the D2151 locus), but there still may be only a single pathogenetic pathway in developing the disease. Aging plays a large role in Alzheimer's disease generally, but we don't understand it. The evolutionary hypothesis may predict that Alzheimer's is the price that mankind pays for large brains. Although neuronal loss has not been found in normal aging mice, Bronson and Harrison (unpublished) found evidence of neuronal loss in 48-57 month old mice that were so long- lived because they were dietarily restricted. Controls are not yet available, but must be done, comparing fully fed and restricted mice at the same ages (this is possible up to about the 36 month maximum longevity of the fed mice) to test whether amounts fed affect neuronal loss.

2. Asked whether the abnormality in hyaluronic acid may be the same as that for the Hutchinson-Gilford Syndrome, Martin replied that it was not known, but alterations of synthesis or turnover might be important. The H-G syndrome is dominant, but there are differences in times of onset and phenotype; Brown discusses it in detail in the next paper.

3. The effects of apparently accelerated aging syndromes on immune status are varied. Werner's syndrome patients may have depressed T-cell functions.

4. Why is the growth spurt during puberty lost in people with Werner's syndrome? This is hard to answer, as the disease is not recognized until middle age, while measurements would have to be made at puberty. Possibly there are inadequate responses to growth factors.

# 29

# PROGERIA : A GENETIC DISEASE MODEL OF PREMATURE AGING

W. Ted Brown, Michael Zebrower and Fred J. Kieras

## ABSTRACT

Progeria is a rare genetic disease with striking features that resemble accelerated aging. The inheritance pattern, paternal age effect, and lack of consanguinity argue that it is due to a sporadic dominant mutation. We have observed elevated levels of HA excretion in progeria and in WS patients. Their cultured cells also accumulate excessive HA. We hypothesize that the failure of patients with progeria and WS to thrive may be due to a lack of vasculogenesis caused by excess HA. Clinical features which support this hypothesis include the sclerodermatous appearance of the skin, the decreased number of blood vessels and the increased incidence of death due to cardiovascular problems found in patients with these disorders. The nature of such a genetic mutation leading to an increase in HA needs to be elucidated to understand the cause of progeria. Insight into the nature of this mutation may help in understanding a gene with a major effect on aging.

## INTRODUCTION

Aging appears to have a strong genetic component. This is reflected in the wide variation (approximately 50,000 fold) seen in the maximal lifespans of various animal species (Brown, 1979). Among mammals, an approximately 100-fold variation in maximal lifespan is observed. The smokey shrew appears to have a lifespan of only about one year (Hamilton, 1940), while the oldest documented human died at the age of 120 (Russell, 1988).

Analyses of the degree of genetic complexity underlying longevity have suggested it may be encoded by a limited number of genes, perhaps 20-50, which have a major gene effect on aging (Martin, 1977; Cutler, 1980; Sacher, 1980). Therefore, a useful approach to understanding the genetic basis of aging may be to study appropriate genetic mutants which appear to affect that process.

Although no mutations are known to extend the maximal human lifespan, there are a number which shorten the lifespan. Several genetic diseases have mutations which appear to accelerate many features of the aging process.

Since they do not appear to accelerate all segments of the aging process, they have been described as "segmental progeroid" syndromes by Martin (1977). Such diseases can serve as useful models for the study of aging. Insight into the nature of the basic mutations in these syndromes may identify the genes which play a major role in aging.

Two genetic diseases which appear to many to show the most striking clinical features suggestive of accelerated aging are the Hutchinson-Gilford Progeria Syndrome (progeria) and the Werner Syndrome (WS, also called progeria of the adult). The basic mutations underlying these two diseases are not known. However, recent findings in several laboratories, including our own, indicate that patients with these two diseases may excrete an excessive amount of the glycosaminoglycan, hyaluronic acid (HA) (Takunaga *et al.*, 1975, 1978; Goto *et al.*, 1978; Brown *et al.*, 1985a,b; Kieras *et al.*, 1986; Zebrower *et al.*, 1986a). Cultured cells from patients with these diseases show an excessive amount of HA accumulation (Tajima *et al.*, 1981; Brown *et al.*, 1986b). Experimentally, excess HA has also been shown to inhibit vascular development, and may act as an anti-angiogenesis factor (Feinberg and Beebe, 1983). These findings raise the possibility that one or several major genes affecting aging may relate to HA metabolism. Understanding the basis of these genetic abnormalities may help to further elucidate the molecular basis of normal aging. In the following, we review clinical aspects, genetic features and laboratory investigations of progeria as a model of accelerated aging.

## THE HUTCHINSON-GILFORD PROGERIA SYNDROME

Progeria, illustrated in Figure 1, is a rare genetic disease with a reported birth incidence of about 1 in 8 million and with striking clinical features that resemble premature aging (Debusk, 1972; Brown *et al.*, 1985b). Patients with this condition generally appear normal at birth but by about one year of age, severe growth retardation is usually seen. Balding occurs, and loss of eyebrows and eyelashes is common in the first few years of life. Widespread loss of subcutaneous tissue occurs. As a result, the veins over the scalp become prominent. The skin appears old, and pigmented age spots appear. The patients are very short and thin. They average about 40 inches in height, but they usually weigh no more than 25 or 30 pounds even as teenagers. The weight-to-height ratio is thus very low. The voice is thin and high pitched. Sexual maturation usually does not occur. They have a characteristic facial appearance with prominent eyes, a beaked nose, a "plucked-bird" appearance, and facial disproportion resulting from a small jaw and large cranium. The large balding head and small face give them an extremely aged appearance. The bones show distinctive changes, with frequent resorption of the clavicles

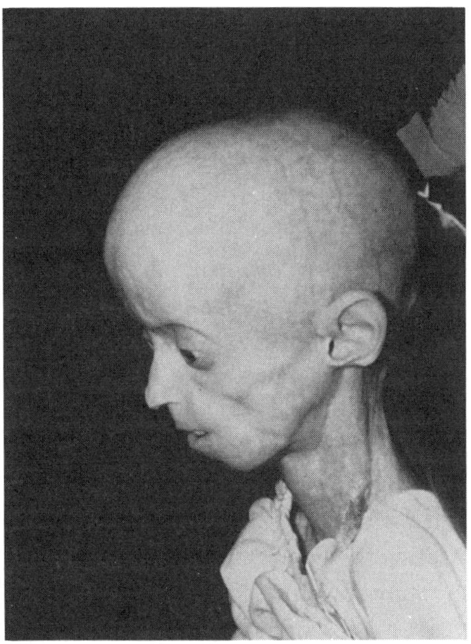

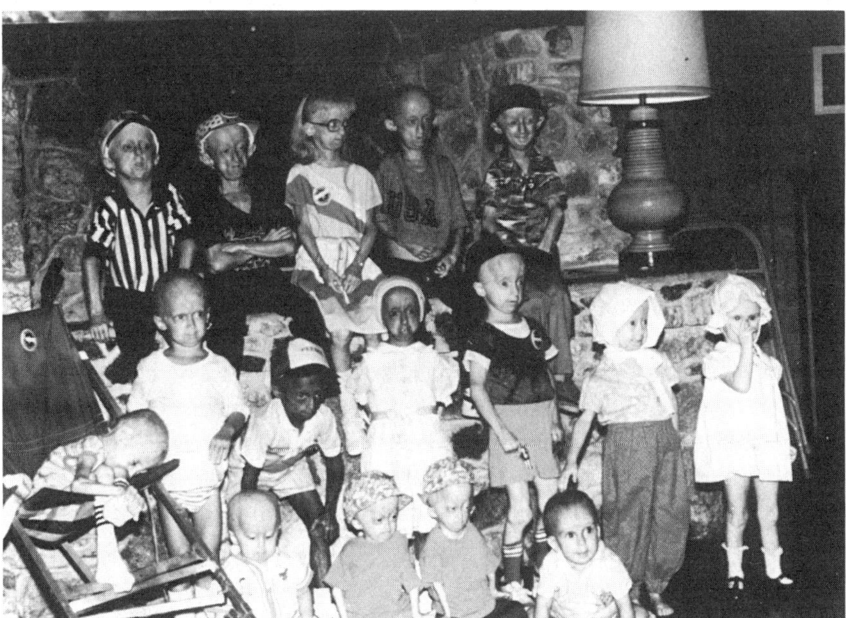

**Figure 1.** Progeria subjects. A. A 10 yr-old girl (TS) with progeria, who had suffered a stroke and had bilateral hip dislocations. She died of cardiac arrest at age 13. B. Fourteen children with progeria and 3 with progeroid conditions attending annual progeria family reunion.

and replacement by fibrous tissue. Resorption of the terminal finger bones (acroosteolysis), stiffening of finger joints, elbow and knee joint enlargement, coxa valga, and a resulting "horse-riding" stance are all seen. Asceptic necrosis of the head of the femur and hip dislocation are common (Moen, 1982; Gamble, 1984).

Progeria subjects have a normal to above-average intelligence. The median age of death is 12 years. Over 80% of deaths are due to heart attacks or congestive heart failure. Widespread atherosclerosis, with interstitial fibrosis of the heart, is usually seen at postmortem examination (Baker *et al.*, 1981). Occasionally marked enlargement of the thymus gland is noted. However, some features often associated with normal aging such as tumors, cataracts, diabetes, and hyperlipidemia although occasionally reported (King *et al.*, 1978, Villee and Powers, 1978, Rosenbloom *et al.*, 1983) are not usually present.

Over the past 15 years, we have had the opportunity to examine over 30 cases of progeria. Information on 25 cases is summarized in Table 1. We have established an International Progeria Registry. As of 1989, the Registry included 20 living cases: 16 living in the United States, 1 in Canada, 1 in Holland, 1 in Argentina and 1 in South Africa. We have had correspondence regarding other cases from Russia, China, Egypt and Iran, but confirmation that they have true progeria is lacking. We have helped to organize an annual progeria family conference. Beginning in the summer of 1981 all interested progeria families have been brought together for one week. At each meeting there have been 8 to 15 progeria children and their families present. This has allowed the children and families to meet each other, and to share common experiences. Several interested physicians have been present. Genetic counseling has been given to the families regarding this rare condition. This has been a unique and valuable experience for all concerned.

Consideration of the mode of inheritance in progeria is important for genetic counseling and may help us to understand the nature of the underlying mutation. Recessive diseases often appear to be due to enzymatic deficiencies which lead to metabolic abnormalities. Dominant diseases often involve structural proteins. However, they may be due to partial deficiencies of rate-limiting enzymes (*i.e.*, Porphyria) or cell-surface receptors (*i.e.*, familial hypercholesterolemia) where half the normal level of the gene product can lead to a disease.

Several genetic considerations suggest progeria is most likely a sporadic dominant mutation. First, high rates of consanguinity, *i.e.* first cousin marriages, are expected in rare recessive diseases. High consanguinity is not seen in progeria. Debusk (1972) noted that consanguinity was present in only 3 out of 19 families in which it was specifically discussed. Some of these cases had come from areas of the world with high background population levels of consanguinity. In addition, it was not reported in 41 other families. Thus, 3 of 60 or 5% was the reported frequency as of 1972. A family history of consanguinity was not present in any of the 24 progeria cases that we have reviewed since then. Thus, we estimate the frequency of progeria cases born to consanguinious marriages to be less than 3/84, (3.6%). For rare recessive diseases, an estimate of the expected frequency of consanguinity can be derived using the Dahlberg formula (Epstein *et al.*, 1966). Assuming a birth incidence of progeria to be 1 per 8 million, and a background population consanguinity frequency of 1% leads to an estimate of expected consanguinity of 64% in progeria families. Thus, the 3.6% observed consanguinity frequency in progeria is much lower than the high level that would be expected for such a rare recessive disease.

Although the reported incidence of progeria in the United States is about 1 in 8 million births (Debusk, 1972), the true population incidence may be somewhat higher, as not all cases are reported. Based on our experience, we estimate that about 50% of all cases in the United States are reported, which leads to an estimate of incidence of 1 in 4 million, this would still lead to a much higher expected consanguinity frequency, 45%, than the low frequency that is seen in progeria families. This lack of consanguinity suggests progeria is unlikely to be a rare recessive.

Secondly, a paternal age effect is seen in progeria which is also observed in some other sporadic dominant type mutations. Jones *et al.* (1975) reported that among 18 progeria cases the fathers were older than expected by an average of 2.56 years when controlled for maternal age, a difference which was highly significant (p = 0.005). In addition to progeria, they reported a paternal age effect in seven other disorders (Basal Cell Nevus Syndrome, Waardenburg Syndrome, Crouzon Syndrome, Cleido-cranial dysostosis, Oculo-dental-digital Syndrome, Treatcher-Collins Syndrome, and multiple exostoses) involving new mutations for which autosomal dominant inheritance had been clearly established and in four disorders (Achondroplasia, Apert Syndrome, Fibrodysplasia ossiicans progressiva, and Marfan Syndrome) in which older paternal age in the setting of new mutation has been previously shown.

We have also observed a paternal age effect in the 24 cases of progeria we have examined (Table 1). The fathers were older than the mothers by an average of 4.5 years which is higher than the expected control value of 2.8 years (Jones *et al.*, 1975). The paternal age effect observed in these 24 cases confirms the previously reported paternal age effect in the 18 earlier cases.

| Case | ID | Sex | Age At Exam | Birthdate | Died | Mother | Father | Diff | Sibs |
|---|---|---|---|---|---|---|---|---|---|
| | | | | **Table 1.** Summary of 24 cases of progeria. | | | | | |
| 1 | MC | F | 27 | 10/01/55 | 05/25/85 | 40.0 | 45.8 | 5.8 | 6 |
| 2 | RM | F | 15 | 08/06/66 | 04/24/83 | 27 | 27 | 0 | 1 |
| 3 | FM | M | 13 | 1966 | 1981 | 28 | 25 | -3 | 2 |
| 4 | KC | M | 10 | 1968 | —— | 24 | 24 | 0 | 2 |
| 5 | TS | F | 10 | 02/01/68 | 09/11/82 | 25.8 | 26 | 0.8 | 3 |
| 6 | AF | F | 12 | 09/12/69 | 12/19/85 | 27.4 | 35.6 | 8.2 | 3 |
| 7 | AG | F | 13 | 04/01/85 | 04/01/85 | 24.5 | 49.11 | 25.6 | 6 |
| 8 | BS | F | 10 | 12/15/71 | 01/30/88 | 26 | 38 | 12 | 2 |
| 9 | MH | M | 11 | 06/30/72 | —— | 19 | 26 | 7 | 1 |
| 10 | FG | M | 11 | 12/31/72 | —— | 21.0 | 27.0 | 6 | 1 |
| 11 | DP | M | 12 | 1973 | —— | 38 | 44 | 6 | 13 |
| 12 | RP | M | 9 | 11/26/73 | 06/20/73 | 20.0 | 27.4 | 7.4 | 1 |
| 13 | JE | M | 9 | 08/16/74 | —— | 17 | 17 | 0 | 1 |
| 14 | SK | F | 2 | 06/09/76 | 1982 | 33 | 47 | 14 | 1 |
| 15 | PS | M | 6 | 05/10/77 | —— | 24.0 | 23.9 | -0.3 | 2 |
| 16 | AK | F | 5 | 06/28/78 | 10/3/86 | 29.11 | 34.10 | 4.11 | 1 |
| 17 | AB | F | 6 | 09/10/78 | —— | 16.11 | 16.9 | -0.2 | 1 |
| 18 | LC | M | 4 | 08/20/79 | —— | 33.0 | 41.4 | 8.4 | 3 |
| 19 | AF | F | 3 | 04/18/80 | —— | 23.0 | 23.0 | 0 | 1 |
| 20 | BS | M | 3 | 07/26/80 | —— | 28.8 | 28.8 | 0 | 1 |
| 21 | C | M | 2 | 01/26/81 | 4/17/89 | 25.6 | 26.2 | 0.8 | 1 |
| 22 | *( CR | M | 2 | 01/26/81 | —— | 25.6 | 26.2 | 0.8 | 1) |
| 23 | KS | F | 1 | 06/22/82 | —— | 26.4 | 28.3 | 1.11 | 1 |
| 24 | MS | F | 1 | 07/11/82 | —— | 28.6 | 25.3 | -3.3 | 1 |
| Averages | | | | | | 26.4 | 31.0 | 4.6 | |
| Total | | | | | | | | | 55 |
| (21 & 22 Identical Twins) | | | | | | | | | |

(Jones *et al.*, 1975) and also suggests dominant inheritance. The paternal age effect appears to be due to an excess of a few older fathers which produces a secondary age peak, as is illustrated in Figure2. A similar secondary paternal age peak has been reported in new cases of neurofibromatosis, another dominant disease (Riccardi, 1983).

Third, for a recessive condition, the proportion of affected sibs is expected to be 25%. In progeria it is clearly much less than 25%. Almost all cases are sporadic and the is no evidence of increased miscarriage rates to suggest selection against the homozygote in utero. A case of identical progeria twins with 14 normal sibs was reported (Viegas *et al.*, 1974). Here, 3 or 4 affected sibs would be expected if it was a recessive disease. It is recognized that for new dominant mutations, occasionally the mutation can occur in a germ line leading to somatic mosaicism within the ovary or testes (McKusick, 1988).

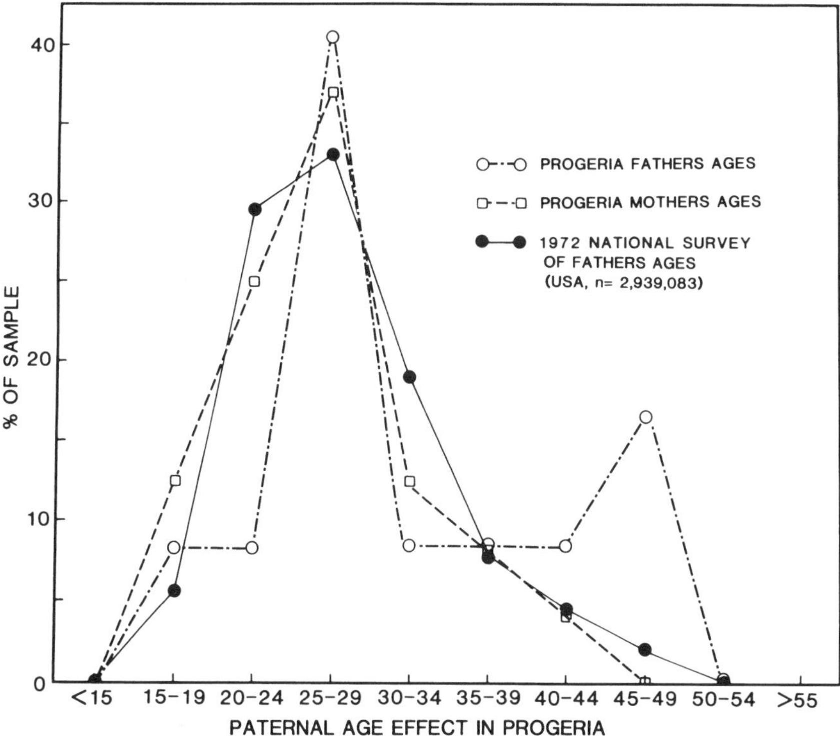


**Figure 2**. Paternal age effect in 24 families with cases of progeria. A secondary age peak (age 40-49) for 15-20% of the fathers is shown. This secondary age peak is not seen in a normal age distribution of fathers as compared to a national survey of fathers ages nor in the mothers of the progeria children.

Several cases could then occur within one family. Probable cases of familial progeria have been reported in only a few instances among more than 100 families (Mostafa and Gabr, 1954; Gabr *et al.*, 1960; Rautenstrauch and Snigula, 1977; Franklyn, 1976). We believe that these reports of progeria cases most likely represent misidentified cases of other progeroid syndromes. Among the 24 cases we have examined (Table 1), no family had more than one affected child except for one set of identified twins. There were 55 unaffected sibs. One would expect there to be 13 or 14 of the 55 sibs affected (25%) if a recessive mode of inheritance were to apply to these 24 progeria families.

In general, the lack of consanguinity, the paternal age effect, and the lack of affected sibs, argues that progeria is not a rare recessive, but most probably is a sporadic dominant mutation. Progeria was formerly considered to be a recessive disease and was so classified in early editions of McKusick's "Catalog of Mendelian Inheritance in Man." Because of a lack of consanguinity, a lack of affected sibs, and a paternal age effect, we suggested progeria should be classified as a sporadic autosomal dominant mutation (Brown and Darlington, 1980). Subsequently, it was moved from the recessive to the dominant section of the catalogue (McKusick, 1988). The possibility of genetic heterogeneity in progeria in which some cases have a similar clinical presentation but with a recessive mode of inheritance seems possible but unlikely because of the rarity of the condition. The majority of cases appear to represent isolated sporadic dominant mutations, although a few may be the result of a germ line mutation. For genetic counseling of families with a progeria child, the recurrence risk can be stated to be very low, but may be on the order of 1 in 500 with each pregnancy in order to allow for the possibility of somatic mosaicism such as has been occasionally seen in other new dominant mutations (See McKusick, 1988).

## WERNER SYNDROME

Werner Syndrome (WS), also called progeria of the adult, has a number of features which resemble premature aging but, in contrast to progeria, has an adult age of onset (Epstein *et al.*, 1966; Salk, 1982; Brown, 1984). WS subjects generally appear normal during childhood but cease growth during teenage years. Premature graying and whitening of hair occur at an early age. Striking features include early cataract formation, skin which appears aged, with a sclerodermatous appearance, a high-pitched voice, peripheral musculature atrophy, poor wound-healing, chronic leg and ankle ulcers, hypogonadism, widespread atherosclerosis, soft tissue calcification, osteoporosis, and a high prevalence of diabetes mellitus. About 10% of patients develop neoplasms with a particularly high frequency of sarcomas and meningiomas (German, 1984). The diagnosis of WS is usually made when patients are in their 30's. They commonly die of complications from atherosclerosis in their 40's. The mode of inheritance of WS is clearly autosomal recessive. Thus WS and progeria subjects show many similarities but have many differences as well (Brown *et al.*, 1985a).

## BASIC RESEARCH ON PROGERIA

Laboratory investigations of progeria have involved a search for a genetic marker in an attempt to help define the underlying defect. The cultured lifespan of progeric fibroblasts was initially reported to be greatly reduced (Goldstein, 1969). Subsequent studies have shown that although difficulties may sometimes occur in the initial establishment of a culture, once established, a normal or only a modest reduction in lifespan is seen (Martin *et al.*, 1970; Goldstein and Moerman, 1975). We have examined the *in vitro* lifespans of 11 progeria cell cultures, 4 WS cultures, 4 parents of progeria subjects, and 3 control cultures (Figure 3). The WS cell lines showed extremely rapid senescence with a range of 9-15 maximal population doubling levels. The progeria cell lines had a range from about 20 to 60 population doubling levels (Brown *et al.*, 1985b). This was reduced by about 1/3 compared to the parent lines and the normal controls. The WS line population doubling levels were greatly reduced. Thus, a markedly reduced *in vitro* lifespan of progeria cells such as was seen in WS was not present. The modest and variable reduction in lifespan in culture is unlikely to represent a useful marker for the disease.

Goldstein and Moerman (1975) reported finding an increased fraction of abnormally thermolabile enzymes, including glucose-6-phosphate dehydrogenase (G6PD), 6-phosphogluconate dehydrogenase (6PGD), and hypoxanthine phosphoribosyltransferase (HPRT) in progeria fibroblasts. Based in part on the Orgel error-catastrophe hypothesis of aging (1963), it was suggested that diseases resembling premature aging may be the result of widespread errors in protein synthesis (Goldstein and Moerman, 1976). Abnormally high thermolabile enzyme levels in circulating erythrocytes from one progeria patient with intermediate levels in the parents was also reported (Goldstein and Moerman, 1978a,b). It was suggested that this would support autosomal recessive inheritance. Our studies of three progeria patients and their families did not confirm these elevations as no increased erythrocyte thermolabile enzyme elevations were seen (Brown and Darlington, 1980). In our opinion, this lack of confirmation indicates that a defect in protein synthetic fidelity is unlikely to be the basic defect in progeria, and does not support the suggestion of autosomal recessive inheritance. Subsequent work by Wojityk and Goldstein (1980) on cell-free protein synthesis using progeria fibroblast extracts also found no decreased translation ability, which also argues against a generalized defect in progeria protein synthesis.

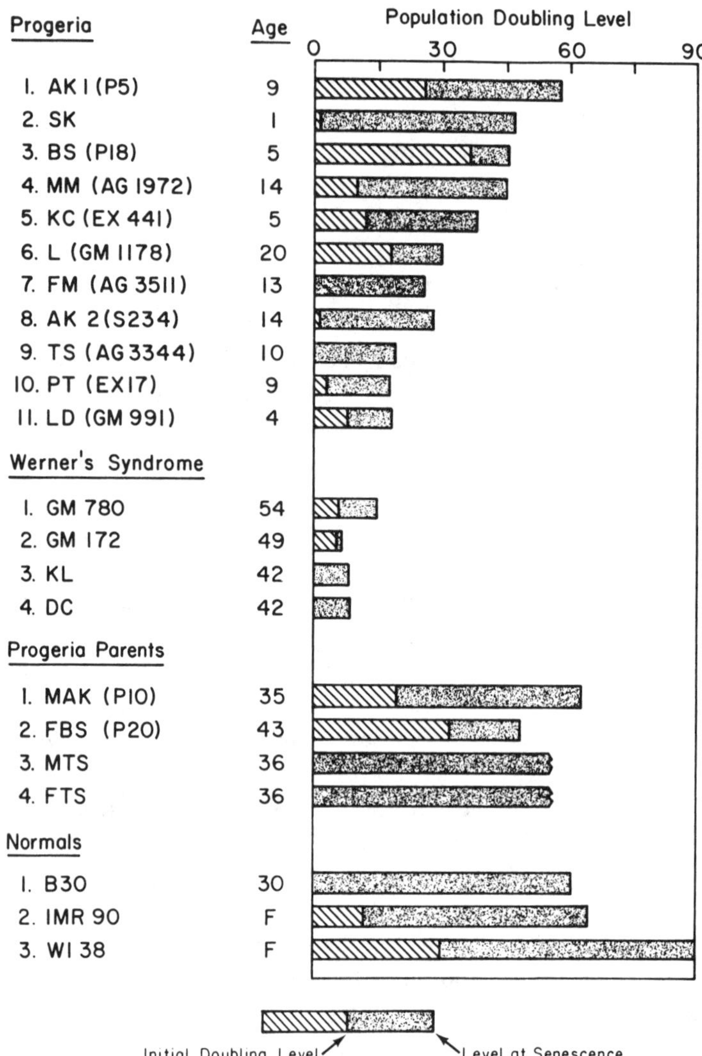


**Figure 3.** *In vitro* cell lifespans of progeria and Werner Syndrome fibroblasts. Cell cultures were initiated from skin biopsies(SK, FM, TS, KL, DFC, MTS, FTS, B30) or obtained from other investigators (AK1, BS, MM, KC, AK2, PT, MAK, FBS) or were obtained from the Camden Cell Repository (GM1178, GM991, GM780, GM712, IMR90, Wl38). Ages of subjects are indicated. F is fetal lung. Cultures were split 4:1 or 2:1 once a week which added 2 and 1 population doubling levels, respectively. Where cells became too sparse to be subcultured in one month, they were judged senescent. Progeria cells showed a variably modest reduction. WS cells showed a marked reduction in comparison to parents and normals.

Abnormal immune function has been postulated as a defect in progeria. Walford suggested that progeria could reflect an abnormality of immune function because of the similarity to experimental graft-versus-host reaction and to runting disease (1970). In support of this concept, Singal and Goldstein (1973) reported that HLA expression on two cultured progeria fibroblast strains was absent. They later reported that there was not an absence, but a greatly reduced concentration of HLA cell-surface molecules (Goldstein *et al.*, 1975; Goldstein and Moerman, 1976). In studies of ten progeria fibroblast strains, we were unable to confirm this reported abnormality. We found no evidence for either qualitative or quantitative abnormalities in HLA expression and no association with HLA type was detected (Brown *et al.*, 1980a). Thymic hormone levels have been reported as normal for the range of patient ages tested (Iwata *et al.*, 1981). Thus, no immune abnormalities have been established for progeria.

An abnormality in X-ray DNA-repair capacity in progeria fibroblasts was suggested by Epstein *et al.*, (1973, 1974) who detected decreased single-strand rejoining of gamma-irradiated DNA using alkaline sucrose gradients. The presence of altered DNA-repair capability was found in another study. Using a somewhat modified method for the assay of single-strand rejoining, no differences between one progeric strain and two atypical progeric strains were seen as compared to normals (Regan and Setlow, 1974). Brown *et al.* (1976, 1977) showed that co-cultivation of two progeric cell strains with normal strains or with each other reversed the single-strand DNA-rejoining defect and suggested that complementation groups for DNA repair might exist in progeria. Weichselbaum *et al.* (1980) assayed the X-ray sensitivity of various types of human fibroblasts by measuring their ability to form colonies following irradiation. They found two progeric strains with increased sensitivity and three strains with normal sensitivity. These studies suggested some increase in radiosensitivity but left open the possibility that damage to cellular components other than DNA might be responsible. Rainbow and Howes (1977) using a sensitive host-cell-reactivation (HCR) assay of X-irradiated adenovirus reported that two progeric strains showed a deficiency of DNA-repair capacity. Brown *et al.* (1980b) studied HCR in two other strains and found one strain showed decreased HCR while another showed normal HCR under a variety of cell growth conditions. These results suggest that heterogenicity of DNA-repair capacity exists among progeria fibroblasts. Defective DNA-repair capacity therefore does not appear to be a consistent marker for progeria and it seems unlikely to represent a basic genetic defect.

A few other isolated reports have suggested abnormalities in progeria. Elevated levels of the blood coagulant tissue factor were reported in both progeria and WS fibroblast cells (Goldstein and Niewiarowski, 1976). This could reflect variations in culture conditions or growth state of cells unrelated to genotype, such as has been reported for other cell types (Magniord *et al.*, 1977). A normal insulin-binding receptor response, but decreased binding of insulin to non-specific receptors in progeria cells has been reported (Rosenbloom and Goldstein, 1976). The significance of nonspecific receptor binding is unclear. An increased level of elastin mRNA and increased *in vitro* levels of elastin have been reported recently for cultured progeria fibroblasts (Sephel *et al.*, 1988). The reasons for this increase are unclear but may be due to loss of normal regulatory mechanisms *in vitro* or increased sensitivity to regulation *in vitro* by serum growth factors or some unusual cellular selection *in vitro*. No evidence of increased elastin production in patients has yet been seen.

## HYALURONIC ACID (HA) URINARY LEVELS IN PROGERIA AND WS

A potentially unique marker for both progeria and WS appears to be urinary HA excretion. HA excretion has been found to be elevated in these two syndromes and has not been reported to be elevated for any other genetic disease. HA levels in controls are normally considered to represent less than 1% of total GAGs. Elevated HA levels have been reported to vary from 2 to 22% of total GAGs in a series of Japanese WS subjects (Tokunaga *et al.*, 1975; Goto and Murata, 1978; Maekawa and Hayashibara, 1981; Murata, 1982). Urinary HA as a percent of total GAGs present was also reported to be elevated to 4.4% in one Japanese Progeria subject compared to controls of 0.2 and 0.3% (Tokunaga *et al.*, 1978).

In order to test the generality of this observation, we determined the total urinary excretion of GAGs and HA in three progeria patients, one patient with an atypical progeroid syndrome, one WS patient and a control subject using standard methods for GAG analysis using CPC precipitation, pronase digestion, TCA treatment, ethanol precipitation and uronic acid determination before and after hyaluronidase digestion (Kieras *et al.*, 1985). Normal levels of total urinary GAGs were observed in all affected individuals and the control. HA analyses for the patients and for the control showed that the WS patient and 3 progeria patients had increased levels of urinary HA which ranged from a high of 16% to a low of about 5%. The normal individual and the atypical progeroid subject showed no significant elevation of HA excretion. Although it has generally been accepted that urinary HA levels are

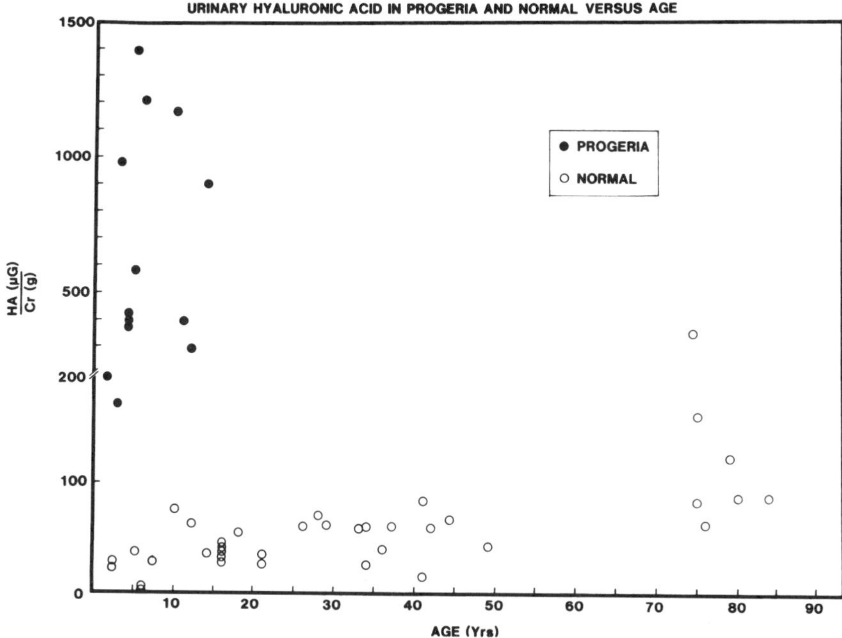


**Figure 4.** Urinary hyaluronic acid excretion by progeria and normal subjects versus age. A 10 to 20 fold elevation is seen in comparison to age matched controls and a modest increase with normal aging is observed. Figure plotted from data presented in Zebrower *et al.* (1985a) and additional unpublished data on older apparently normal subjects.

normally less than about 1% of GAGs, there was no systematic study available.

To determine HA levels in progeria and normal subjects as a function of age we developed an HPLC method of assay of HA and GAGs (Zebrower *et al.*, 1985b). Using this method, we studied 30 normal individuals to determine HA excretion as a function of age (Zebrower *et al.*, 1986a). These results are presented in Figure 4.

Our studies verified that HA content in young children and adolescents was low but with age there was found to be an elevation to 5-6%. These results suggest that elevated excretion of urinary HA may be a normal characteristic or biomarker of aging which occurs at an accelerated rate in progeria and WS patients.

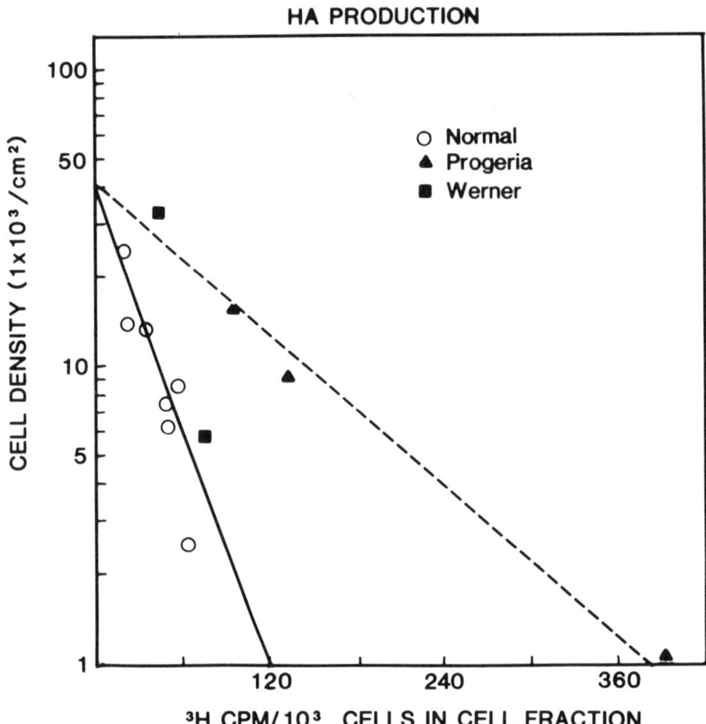



**Figure 5.** HA steady-state levels of progeria and Werner syndrome fibroblasts as a function of cell density in three day cultures. HA assayed by measurement of levels of $^3$H-glucosamine incorporation. Progeria and Werner syndrome fibroblasts were obtained from NIA Aging Cell Repository (AG 1972, AG 3513, AG 4110, AG 5230) or were established from primary biopsies of progeria subjects (SK). Control fibroblast lines were established from age-matched subjects without accelerated aging phenotypes. Approximately, a three-fold excess of HA level was observed in progeria and Werner fibroblasts at all cell densities studied.

## HA AND GAG PRODUCTION IN CULTURED CELLS

To determine if the elevated HA excretion seen in progeria was also reflected in cell culture, we analyzed steady-state HA and GAG levels in normal, progeria, and WS fibroblasts. HA and GAG levels in 3 day cultures of progeria, WS, and control cells were assayed by measuring both total glucosamine and sulfate incorporation into cells and media. HA levels were found to be elevated in progeria and WS compared to normal cultures at all cell densities measured, as shown in Figure 5. A pronounced difference in total GAG levels was also observed when normal fibroblasts were compared with WS and progeria fibroblasts as a function of cell density, as shown in

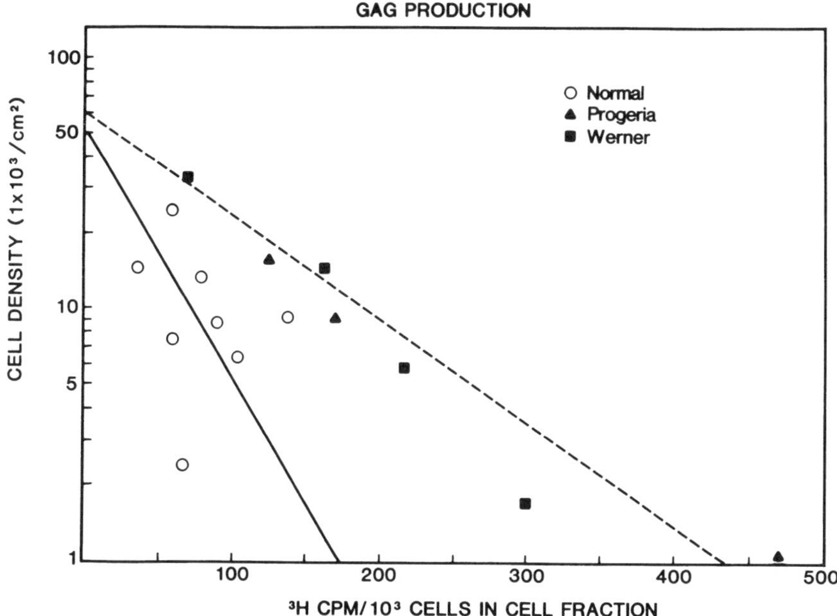


**Figure 6.** GAG levels in progeria and Werner syndrome fibroblasts. GAG was assayed following three-day culture of the same cultures in Figure 5. Approximately a three-fold elevation of levels was seen at all cell densities examined.

Figure 6. A similar difference in GAG and HA excretion into the media was seen in comparing WS and progeria to normals as a function of cell density. Non-HA containing GAGs, as assayed by sulfur incorporation, were also found to decrease as a function of cell density, and were found to be present in excess in WS and progeria fibroblasts.

In order to determine whether the elevated levels of GAGs, in general and HA, in particular, were related to increased synthesis or to faulty degradation, cultures from normal, WS, and progeria lines were labelled for 4, 8, and 24 hours and then assayed. There was little comparative difference in either total GAG or HA levels at these earlier times, unlike the marked difference that was seen at 72 hours of cultivation. This suggested a degradative pathway abnormality may be present since initial synthesis was relatively unimpaired.

## FACTORS GOVERNING HA AND GAG PRODUCTION LEVELS

The regulation of GAG production levels in fibroblasts appears to vary in a complex fashion as a function of age of the culture, age of the donor from which it was taken, the density of the culture, and possibly the disease afflicting the donor. The total production of GAGs and HA in fibroblast cultures has been found to vary inversely as a function of cell density (Hronowski and Anastassiades, 1980) regardless of the source of the fibroblasts. The composition of GAGs though has been found to change as a function of the population doubling level (PDL) of the cultures. Schachtschabel and Wever (1981) examined the synthesis and distribution of GAGs as a function of PDL in human embryonic fibroblasts. It was observed that GAG synthesis declined only during the last 5 divisions before phaseout. This decline was accompanied by a decline in HA production in both absolute and relative terms in cellular and media fractions. Production of another GAG, heparan sulfate, was found to increase continually during the very last population doublings. Vogel *et al.*, (1981) reported that HA production was found to increase in the medium fraction of an old donor relative to a young donor. Total GAG production appeared greater in the older than the young donor.

One complication in the interpretation of all these studies is that the data were normalized in terms of cell protein content as measured at the beginning of the labelling period rather than cell density at the end of the labelling period. As the growth rates of the lines may be significantly different, vastly different incorporation rates may be present because of the relationship between cell density and GAG production. The underlying biochemical reasons for these changes in GAG production have not been explained.

Excess HA and GAG production has been reported by Tajima *et al.* (1981) for one line of WS fibroblasts; however, these workers did not normalize their data to constant cell densities. Fibroblasts from another genetic disease affecting connective tissue, Marfan Syndrome, have been observed to accumulate significantly greater amounts of HA than normal lines (Malaton and Dofman, 1968). This HA production rate was elevated due to an overactive synthetase rather than the degradation defect that appears to be present in our experiments. In a cell-free system, increased rates of synthesis were observed even though the physical properties of the particular enzymes involved did not seem to change (Appel *et al.*, 1979). Production of HA in fibroblasts has been found to be elevated in Osteogenesis Imperfecta (Turakainen *et al.*, 1980). This elevation has also been found to be due to an overactive synthetase as measured in a cell-free system.

HA and GAG production during embryogenesis is believed to play a very important role in morphogenesis. HA production in particular is associated with the formation of the primary mesenchyme and the first cell-free spaces in the rat embryo (Solursh and Moriss, 1977). In chick embryos, a striking correlation between hyaluronate synthesis and cell movement and proliferation is observed as well as between HA degradation and differentiation. For example, in the check embryo cornea, a close correlation exists between the presence of HA and the period during which corneal mesenchyme migration and proliferation in the hydrated primary stroma occur. Both corneal mesenchyme migration and HA production occur during days 3-9 of development. The removal of HA by hyaluronidase begins on day 10 and corresponds with the cessation of migration and proliferation of the mesenchymal cells as well as their differentiation into corneal keratocytes (Hay, 1980; Toole and Trelstad, 1971; Trelstad *et al.*, 1974; Toole, 1981).

HA appears to act as an anti-angiogenesis factor. During development tissue regions that are high in HA concentration are invariably avascular zones. HA containing implants were shown to cause avascularity when implanted into normal vascular wing mesoderm (Feinberg and Beebe, 1983). HA thus appears to be crucial in the morphogenesis of blood vessels in the embryo and may be expected to play an equally important role as an anti-angiogenesis factor during maturation and aging. West *et al.* (1985) have reported that partial degradation products of HA (oligosaccharides between 4 and 25 residues in length) have the opposite effect. They stimulated angiogenesis on the chick chorioallantoic membrane when these partial degradation products were applied.

Our results in progeria and WS suggest abnormalities of excess HA excretion or abnormal degradation may provide a consistent marker. Mutations of HA metabolism may underlie these diseases, perhaps due to their pervasive effects on angiogenesis. This might explain the profound failure to thrive seen in progeria patients. Elucidation of the nature of a genetic mutation that may lead to an increase in HA production or accumulation may help to understand the cause of progeria. We believe that insight into the nature of the mutation which underlies progeria, this most remarkable experiment of nature, may help in understanding a gene or genes with a major effect on aging.

## REFERENCES

APPEL, A., HORWITZ, A., AND DORFMAN, A. (1979) Cell free synthesis of hyaluronic acid in Marfan syndrome. *J. Biol. Chem.* **254**: 12199-12203

BAKER, P. B., BABA, N., AND BOESEL, C. P. (1981) Cardiovascular abnormalities in progeria. *Arch. Pathol. Lab. Med.* **105**: 384-386

BROWN, W. T., LITTLE, J. B., EPSTEIN, J., AND WILLIAMS, J. R. (1977) DNA repair defect in progeria cells, In: *Genetic Effects on Aging.* (D. Bergsma, and D. E. Harrison, Eds.) Alan R. Liss, Inc., New York, p.417-430.

BROWN, W. T. (1979) Human mutations affecting aging: A review. *Mech. Ageing Dev.* 9: 325-326

BROWN, W. T., AND DARLINGTON, G. (1980a) Thermolabile enzymes in progeria and Werner syndrome: Evidence contrary to the protein error hypothesis. *Am. J. Hum. Genet..* 32: 614-619

BROWN, W. T., DARLINGTON, G. J., FOTINO, M., and ARNOLD A. (1980b) Detection of HLA antigens in progeria syndrome fibroblasts. *Clin. Genet.* 17: 213-219

BROWN, W. T., FORD, J., AND GERSHEY, E. (1980c) Variation of DNA repair capacity in progeria cells unrelated to growth conditions. *Biochem. Biophys. Res. Commun.* 97: 347-353

BROWN, W. T. (1983) Werner's syndrome In: *Chromosome Mutation and Neoplasia* (German, J., Ed.) Alan R. Liss, Inc., New York, pp 85-93.

BROWN, W. T., KIERAS, F. J., HOUCK, G. E., DUTKOWSKI, R., AND JENKINS, E. C. (1985a) A comparison of adult and childhood progerias: Werner syndrome and Hutchinson-Gilford progeria syndrome. **In:** *Werner's Syndrome and Human Aging.* (D. Salk, Y. Fujiwara, G. M. Martin, Eds.) Plenum Press, New York

BROWN, W. T., ZEBROWER, M. KIERAS, F. (1985b) Progeria, a Model Disease for the Study of Accelerated Aging. **In:** *Molecular Biology of Aging.* (Woodhead, A., Blackett, A. D., Hollaender, A., Eds.) Plenum Press, New York. 375-396.

CUTLER, R. (1980) Evolution of human longevity. *Adv. Pathobiol.* 7: 43-49

DEBUSK, F. (1972) The Hutchinson-Gilford progeria syndrome. *J. Pediat.* 80: 697-724

EPSTEIN, C., MARTIN, G., SCHULTZ, A., AND MOTULSKY, A. (1966) Werner's syndrome: A review of its symptomatology, natural history, pathologic features, genetics and relationship to the natural aging process *Medicine* 45: 177-221

EPSTEIN, J., WILLIAMS, J. R., AND LITTLE, J. B. (1973) Deficient DNA repair in human progeroid cells. *Proc. Natl. Acad. Sci. USA* 70: 977-981

EPSTEIN, J., WILLIAMS, J. R., AND LITTLE, J. B. (1974) Rate of DNA repair in progeria and normal fibroblasts. *Biochem. Biophys. Res. Commun.* 59: 850-857

FEINBERG, R., AND BEEBE, D. (1983) Hyaluronate in vasculogenesis. *Science* 220: 1177-1179

FRANKLIN, P. P. (1976) Progeria in siblings *Clin. Radiol.* 27: 327-333

FUJIWARA, Y., HIGASHIKAWA, T., AND TATSUMI, M. (1977) A retarded rate of DNA replication and normal level of DNA repair in Werner's syndrome fibroblasts in culture. *J. Cell. Physiol.* 92: 365-374

GABR, M., HASHEM, N., HASHEM, M., FAHNI, A., AND SATOUH, M. (1960) Progeria, a pathologic study. *J. Pediat.* 57: 70-77

GAMBLE, J. G. (1984) Hip Disease in Hutchinson-Gilford Progeria Syndrome. *J. Pediatric Orthopedics* 4: 585-589

GERMAN, J. (1983) Patterns of neoplasia associated with the chromosome-breakage syndromes. **In:** *Chromosome Mutation and Neoplasia.* p.97-119. (German, J. Ed.) Alan R. Liss, Inc., New York.

GOLDSTEIN, S. (1969) Lifespan of cultured cells in progeria. *Lancet* 1969(i):424.

GOLDSTEIN, S., AND MOERMAN, E. (1975) Heat-labile enzymes in skin fibroblasts from subjects with progeria. *New Engl. J. Med.* 292: 1305-1309

GOLDSTEIN, S., NIEWIAROWSKI, S., AND SINEGAL, D. P. (1975) Pathological implications of cell aging *in vitro. Fed. Proc. Am. Soc. Exp. Biol.* 34: 55-63

GOLDSTEIN, S., AND NIEWIAROWSKI, S. (1976) Increased procoagulant activity in cultured fibroblasts from progeria and Werner's syndrome of premature aging. *Nature (London)* 260: 711-713

GOLDSTEIN, S., AND MOERMAN, E. (1976) Defective protein in normal and abnormal fibroblasts during aging *in vitro. Interdiscip. Top. Gerontol.* 10: 24-43

GOLDSTEIN, S., AND MOERMAN, E. J. (1978a) Heat-labile enzymes in circulating erythrocytes of a progeria family. *Am. J. Hum. Genet.* **30**: 167-173

GOLDSTEIN, S., AND MOERMAN, E. J. (1978b) Unstable enzymes in erythrocytes of a family with the Hutchinson-Gilford progeria syndrome. **In**: *The Red Cell* (Brewer, G. J. Ed.) Alan R. Liss, Inc., New York, p.217-228.

GOTO, M., AND MURATA, K. (1978) Urinary excretion of macromolecular acidic glycosaminoglycans in Werner's syndrome. *Clin. Chim. Acta* **85**: 101-106

HAMILTON, W. J. (1940) The biology of the smokey shrew (*Sorex fumeus fumeus* Miller). *Zoologica (New York)* **23**: 473-491

HAY, E. D. (1980) Development of the vertebrate cornea *Int. Rev. Cytol.* **63**: 263-322

HRONOWSKI L., AND ANASTASSIADES, T. (1980) The effect of cell density on net rates of glycosaminoglycan synthesis and secretion by cultured rat fibroblasts *J. Biol. Chem.* **255**: 10091-10099

IWATA, T., INCEFY, G. S., CUNNINGHAM-RUNDLES, S., SMITHWICK, E., GELLER, N., O'REILLY, R., AND GOOD, R. A. (1981) Circulating thymic hormone activity in patients with primary and secondary immunodeficiency diseases. *Am. J. Med.* **71**: 385-394

JONES, K., SMITH, P., HARVEY M., HALL, B., AND QUAN, L. (1975) Older paternal age and fresh gene mutation: Data on additional disorders. *J. Pediatr.* **86**: 84-88

KIERAS, F. J., BROWN, W. T., HOUCK, G. E., AND ZEBROWER, M. (1985) Elevation of urinary hyaluronic acid in Werner syndrome and progeria. *Biochem. Med. and Metab. Biol.* **36**: 276-282

KING, C. R., LEMMER, J., CAMPBELL, J. R., AND ATKINS, A. R. (1978) Osteosarcoma in a patient with Hutchinson-Gilford progeria. *J. Med. Genet.* **15**: 481-482

MAEKAWA, Y., AND HAYASHIBAR, T. (1981) Determination of hyaluronic acid in the urine of a patient with Werner's syndrome. *J. Dermatol.* **8**: 467-472

MAGNIORD, J. R., DREYER, B. E., STEMERMAN, M. B., AND PITLICK, F. A. (1977) Tissue factor coagulant activity of cultured human endothelial and smooth muscle cells and fibroblasts. *Blood* **50**: 387-396

MARTIN, G. M., SPRAGUE, C. A., AND EPSTEIN, C. J. (1970) Replicative life-span of cultivated human cells: Effects of donor's age, tissue, and genotype. *Lab. Invest.* **23**: 86-92

MARTIN, G. M. (1977) Genetic syndromes in man with potential relevance to the pathobiology of aging. *Birth Defects Orig. Artic. Ser.* **14**: 5-39

MATALON, R., AND DORMAN, A. (1968) The accumulation of hyaluronic acid in cultured fibroblasts of the Marfan syndrome. *Biochem. Biophys. Res. Commun.* **32**: 150-154

McKUSICK, V. A. (1988) *Mendelian Inheritance in Man, Catalogues of Autosomal Dominant, Autosomal Recessive, and X-Linked Phenotypes* 8th ed., Johns Hopkins University Press, Baltimore.

MOEN, C. (1982) Orthopaedic aspects of progeria. *J. Bone Joint Surg.* **64A**: 542-546

MOSTAFA, A. H., AND GABR, M. (1954) Hereditary progeria with follow-up of two affected sisters. *Arch. Pediat.* **71**: 163-172

MURATA, K. (1982) Urinary acidic glycosaminoglycans in Werner's syndrome. *Experientia* **38**: 313-314

ORGEL, L. E. (1963) The maintenance of the accuracy of protein synthesis and its relevance to aging. *Proc.Natl. Acad. Sci. USA* **49**: 517-521

ORKIN, R., AND TOOLE, B. (1980) Isolation and characterization of hyaluronidase from cultures of chick embryo and muscle-derived fibroblasts. *J. Biol. Chem.* **255**: 1036-1042

RAINBOW, A. AND HOWES, M. (1977) Decreased repair of gamma ray damaged DNA in progeria. *Biochem. Biophys. Res. Commun.* **74**: 714-719

RAUTENSTRAUCH, T., SNIGULA, F., KREIG, T., GAY, AND MULLER, P. (1977) Progeria: A cell culture study and clinical report of familial incidence. *Eur. J. Pediat.* **124**: 101-111

REGAN, J. D., AND SETLOW, R. B. (1974) DNA repair in human progeroid cells, Biochem. *Biophys. Res. Commun.* **59**: 858-864

RICCARDI, V. M. (1983) Neurofibromatosis. **In:** *Principles and Practice of Medical Genetics* p.314, (A. Emery, and D. Rimoin, Eds.) Churchill Livingstone, New York.

ROSENBLOOM, A. L., AND GOLDSTEIN, S. (1976) Insulin binding to cultured human fibroblasts increases with normal and precocious aging. *Science* 19: 412-415

ROSENBLOOM, A. L., KAPPY, M. S., DEBUSK, F. L., FRANCIS, G. L., PHILPOT, T. J., AND MACLAREN, M. K. (1983) Progeria: Insulin resistance and hyperglycemia. *J. Pediat.* 102: 400-403

RUSSELL, A. (1988) Authenticated national longevity records, **In:** *Guinness 1988 Book of World Records*, p.15, Sterling Publishing Co., Inc., New York.

SACHER, G. (1980) Mammalian life histories: Their evolution and molecular-genetic mechanism. *Adv. Pathobiol.* 7: 21-42

SALK, D. (1982) Werner's syndrome: A review of recent research with an analysis of connective tissue metabolism, growth control of cultured cells, and chromosomal aberrations. *Hum. Genet.* 62: 1-20

SCHACHTSCHABEL, D., AND WEVER J. (1978) Age-related decline in the synthesis of glycosaminoglycans by cultured human fibroblasts. *Mech. Ageing Dev.* 8: 257-264

SEPHEL, G. C., STURROCK, A., GIRO, M. G., and DAVIDSON, J. M. (1988) Increased elastin production by progeria skin fibroblasts is controlled by the steady-state levels of elastin mRNA. *J. Investigative Dermatology* 90: 643-647

SINGAL, D. P., AND GOLDSTEIN, S. (1973) Absence of detectable HL-A antigens on cultured fibroblasts in progeria. *J. Clin. Invest.* 52: 2259-2263

SOLURSH, M., AND MORISS, G. (1977) Glycosaminoglycan synthesis in rat embryos during the formulation of the primary mesenchyme and neural folds. *Dev. Biol.* 57: 75-86

TAJIMA, T., WATANABE, T., IIJIMA, K., OPHSHIKA, Y. AND YAMAGUCHI, H. (1981) The increase of glycosaminoglycans synthesis and accumulation on the cell surface of cultured skin fibroblasts in Werner's syndrome. *Exper. Pathol.* 20: 221-229

TAKAEUCHI, F., HANAOKA, F., GOTO M., AKAOKA, I., HORI, T., YAMADA M., AND MIYAMOTO , T. (1982) Altered frequency of initiation sites of DNA replication in Werner's syndrome cells. *Human Genet.* 60: 365-368

TOKUNAGA, M., WAKAMATSU, E., SOTO, K., SATAKE, S., AOYAMA, K., SAITO, K., SUGAWARA, M., AND YOSIZAWA, Z. (1978) Hyaluronuria in a case of progeria (Hutchinson-Gilford syndrome). *J. Am. Geriat. Soc.* 26: 296-302

TOOLE, B., AND THRELSTAD, R. (1971) Hyalruonate production and removal during corneal development in the chick. *Dev. Biol.* 26: 28-35

TOOLE, B. (1981) Glycosaminoglycans in Morphogenesis. **In:** *Cell Biology of Extracellular Matrix*, p. 259-288 (E. Hay, Ed.) Plenum Press, New York.

TRELSTAD, R., HAYASHI, K., AND TOOLE, B. (1974) Epithelial collagens and glycosaminoglycans in the embryonic cornea. *J. Cell Biol.* 62: 815-830

TURAKAINEN, H., LARJAVA, H., SAARNI, H., AND PENTTINEN, R. (1980) Synthesis of hyaluronic acid and collagen in skin fibroblasts cultured from patients with Osteogenesis Imperfecta. *Biochim. Biophys. Acta* 628: 388-397

VIEGUS, J., SOUZA, P. L. R., AND SALZANIO, F. M. Progeria in twins. *J. Med. Genet.* 11: 384-376

VILLEE, D. B., AND POWERS, M. L. (1978) Progeria: A model for the study of aging. **In:** *Senile Dementia: A Biomedical Approach*, (K. Nandy, Ed.) Elsevier Biomedical Press, New York, p. 259-270.

VOGEL, K., KENDALL, V., AND SAPIEN, R. (1981) Glycosaminoglycan synthesis and composition in human fibroblasts during *in vitro* cellular aging (IMR-90). *J. Cell. Physiol.* 107: 271-281

WALFORD, R. L. (1970) Antibody diversity, histocompatibility systems, disease states, and aging. *Lancet* 1970(ii):1226.

WEICHSELBAUM, R. R., NOVE, J., AND LITTLE, J. B. (1980) X-ray sensitivity of fifty-three human fibroblast cell strains from patients with characterized genetic disorders. *Cancer Res.* **40**: 920-925

WEST, D. C., HAMPSON, I. N., ARNOLD, F., KUMAR, S. (1985) Angiogenesis Induced by Degradation Products of Hyaluronic Acid. *Science* **228**: 1324-1326

WOJTYK, R., AND GOLDSTEIN, S. (1980) Fidelity of protein synthesis does not decline during aging of cultured human fibroblasts. *J. Cell. Physiol.* **103**: 299-303

ZEBROWER, M., KIERAS, F. J., AND BROWN, W. T. (1986a) Urinary hyaluronic acid elevation in Hutchinson-Gilford Progeria Syndrome. *Mech. Ageing and Develop.* **35**: 39-46

ZEBROWER, M., KIERAS, F. J., AND BROWN, W. T. (1986b) Analysis by high-performance liquid chromatography of hyaluronic acid and chondroitin sulfates. *Analytical Biochem.* **157**: 93-99

## DISCUSSION

1. Dr. Brown's talk was a unique combination of hard science and humane concern for his patients. He gave the only scientific presentation that brought tears to our eyes. The relationships with the children that have this hopeless disease, and their families, has resulted in Dr. Brown's large and varied collection of Progeria patients for scientific research. But perhaps equally important, through the marvelous collection of pictures shown during Dr. Brown's talk shines a respect and love for those little people: they are always smiling!

2. Might changes with age in urinary HA (Hyaluronic Acid) excretion result from secondary changes; for example, it is normalized against creatinine excretion, and this changes with age due to changes in muscle mass. Amounts of HA throughout the body are very large as it is a GAG (glycosaminoglycan) and repeated subunits with molecular weights more than a million form "backbones" to which many proteins are attached. An implant of HA inhibits blood vessel development, yet this is enhanced by implanted HA cleaved into subunits of 20 - 40 sugar molecules. In Progeria only HA is elevated, not GAGs generally.

3. Asked whether progeria may be an accelerated model for primary circulation problems with aging, Brown answered that HA metabolism may be affected with age, indicated by increased time for wound healing due to slower blood vessel development. There are no animal models for Progeria; even if one was found, it is a dominant mutation and sterile, so the mutant could not reproduce. The "accelerated aging" in the "SAM" mouse does not seem related to Progeria or to Werner's syndrome. Would injections of HA into mice or rats cause Progeria-like symptoms to develop? HA may not be the primary cause of the syndrome; for example defects of connective tissue may cause the high HA excretion. Still HA injections would be useful in testing whether this alone caused Progeria, although developmental effects

might be required; perhaps this could be tested in transgenic mice with genes causing excess HA production.

# 30

# MODIFICATION OF HOST PRECURSOR PROTEINS TO AMYLOID FIBRILS IN ALZHEIMER'S DISEASE

D.C. Guiroy and D.C. Gajdusek

## ABSTRACT

The gene encoding the amyloid β-protein precursor is expressed in various human and animal tissues and is highly conserved in evolution. As a complex transcriptional unit, it utilizes alternative splicing and polyadenylation sites. This amyloid β-protein precursor protein without inserts contains 695 amino acids; mRNAs for the alternatively spliced forms contain inserts homologous to the Kunitz family of serine protease inhibitors. Aberrant proteolytic processing of the precursor may result from inhibition or the lack of inhibition of proteases and subsequent conformational change to β-pleated sheets of amyloid.

We suggest that such modified forms of the brain amyloid β-protein could act as amyloid-enhancing factors, nucleating and enhancing amyloid fibril formation and its fibril polymerization and copolymerization with other molecules. This would be analogous to the fibril amyloid-enhancing factors in AA amyloidosis. In Alzheimer's disease, the 42-amino acid subunit of the amyloid of the neurofibrillary tangles, amyloid plaque core, and congophilic angiopathy, could itself serve, in the form of oligomers or fibril microfragments, as nuclei patterning the configurational change to amyloid and its polymerization and deposition as amyloid fibrils.

## INTRODUCTION

Amyloid is a generic name for insoluble proteinaceous deposits exhibiting characteristic congophilia and birefringence under polarized light. Ultrastructurally, amyloid consists of 10 nm diameter fibrils, having a twisted β-pleated sheet configuration on X-ray diffraction. Such insoluble deposits of amyloid fibrils occur in the aging brain and, more extensively, in Alzheimer's disease as senile plaques and vascular amyloid deposits extracellularly and as neurofibrillary tangles intracellularly. These cerebral amyloid deposits which are composed of a 4.2 kilodalton (kDa) protein (Glenner and Wong 1984a,

**Table 1.** Diseases with amyloid-beta protein and congophilic lesions of the central nervous system

| Disease | Neurofibril-lary tangles (NFT) | Neuritic pla-ques | Cerebro-vascular amyloid | Amyloid-beta protein |
|---|---|---|---|---|
| Alzheimer's disease | +++ | +++ | +++ | + |
| Down's syndrome | +++ | +++ | +++ | + |
| Guamanian parkinsonism-dementia (PD) | +++ | - | - | + |
| Guamanian amyotrophic lateral sclerosis (ALS) | +++ | - | - | ? |
| Non-ALS, non-PD Guamanian Chamorro with NFT | ++ | - | - | + |
| Hereditary cerebral hemorrhage with amyloidosis (Dutch type) | - | ++ | +++ | + |
| Sporadic cerebral amyloid angiopathy | +/- | ++ | +++ | + |
| Asymptomatic age-related amyloidosis | ++ | ++ | + | + |

1984b; Masters *et al.*, 1985a; Prelli *et al.*, 1988), designated amyloid β-protein or A4 protein, are found also in Down's syndrome (Masters *et al.*, 1985a; Beyreuther *et al.*, 1986), Guamanian parkinsonism-dementia (Guiroy *et al.*, 1987), neurologically normal Guamanians (Guiroy *et al.*, 1989b), sporadic cerebral amyloid angiopathy, asymptomatic age-related amyloidosis and hereditary cerebral hemorrhage with amyloidosis (Dutch type) (Castaño and Frangione, 1988) (Table 1).

Oligonucleotide probes corresponding to the N-terminal amino acid sequence of amyloid β-protein (also called A4 protein) were used to screen normal human cDNA libraries to identify and characterize the gene coding for the amyloid β-protein, (Goldgaber *et al.*, 1987, 1988; Kang *et al.*, 1987; Tanzi *et al.*, 1987; Robakis *et al.*, 1987; Zain *et al.*, 1988). The gene, located on the long arm of human chromosome 21, contains an open reading frame coding for amyloid precursor protein (APP) of 695 amino acids, referred to as $APP_{695}$, with an internal sequence (positions 597-638) identical with that of the amyloid β-protein. Recent studies indicate that this single copy gene produces two other mRNAs: $APP_{751}$ with a 168 base pair insert (56 amino acids) (Ponte *et al.*, 1988; Tanzi *et al.*, 1988; Goldgaber *et al.*, 1988) and $APP_{770}$ with an insert of 225 base pairs (75 amino acids) (Kitaguchi *et al.*, 1988; Goldgaber *et al.*, 1988). The amino acid sequence of the 56-amino acid insert is highly homologous to the Kunitz family of protease inhibitors (KPI), a family of small, basic inhibitors with a highly conserved region consisting of six cysteines spaced in a minikringle structure (Kitaguchi *et al.*, 1988), which are specific for serine proteases such as trypsin, chymotrypsin, elastase, plasmin and cathepsin G (Palmert *et al.*, 1988). Examples of these KPI include bovine basic protease inhibitor precursor, human inter-alpha-trypsin inhibitor (domain 1 and 11), bovine inter-alpha-trypsin inhibitor (domain 1 and 11), viper venom basic protease inhibitor 11, snail isoinhibitor K, bovine colostrum inhibitor and bovine pancreatic inhibitor (Tanzi *et al.*, 1988; Ponte *et al.*, 1988).

The promoter of the gene for the human precursor of amyloid β-protein resembles promoters of housekeeping genes characterized by a lack of typical TATA box. It has been suggested that there are at least four mechanisms by which this promoter could be regulated: the stress-related heat shock response; the "oncogene related" AP-l/Fos binding site; the potential protein binding at the GC-rich element; and the possible methylation of the CpG region (Salbaum *et al.*, 1988). Goldgaber *et al.*, 1989 (personal communication) have shown that Homeobox gene 1.3 is not expressed in Alzheimer's disease as studied by immunocytochemistry.

The mechanism by which amyloid is formed and deposited in the brain is not understood. We propose that amyloidogenic fibril fragments or microfragments derived from modified forms of the amyloid precursor protein, act as amyloid enhancing factors similar to those in AA amyloidosis (Niewold *et al.*, 1987), which serve as nucleants promoting their own conformational change and polymerization, or copolymerization with other molecules, culminating in their deposition as insoluble amyloid fibrils.

## MECHANISMS OF AMYLOID FORMATION AND DEPOSITION

Amyloid formation and deposition involve a dynamic cascade of events with an interplay of several factors. The following sections offer a possible sequence of events that may be necessary for cerebral amyloidogenesis.

## AMYLOID PRECURSOR PROTEIN GENE EXPRESSION

Amyloid is produced and deposited locally, as demonstrated in experimental secondary amyloidosis (Teilum, 1965). Thus all cells in the body have the potential to produce amyloid; in so far as they express the necessary amyloid precursor protein.

The amyloid precursor protein gene is differentially expressed in human tissues. In fetal human tissues, amyloid β-protein mRNA is abundant in brain, kidney, heart and spleen. In human brain, $APP_{695}$ mRNA is highest in the frontal cortex and the anterior perisylvian cortex-opercular gyri (Tanzi *et al.*, 1987). An alternate form of the messenger RNA with the Kunitz protease inhibitor domain (APP$_{751}$) detected by Northern blot analysis is greatest in the kidney, while uniform levels are found in other human fetal tissues. APP$_{751}$ mRNA is more abundant in fetal than in adult human brain (Tanzi *et al.*, 1988). The other alternate form, APP$_{770}$, is expressed equally in adult and fetal human hippocampus (Kitaguchi *et al.*, 1988).

As determined by in-situ hybridization, mRNA encoding amyloid β-protein precursor has been found in neurons of layers III and V in the frontal cortex, in hippocampal neurons, in neurons of the visual cortex and in Purkinje cells of the cerebellum. Oligodendrocytes, fascicular astrocytes, endothelial cells, fibroblasts and meningeal cells also express amyloid β-protein mRNA (Bahmanyar *et al.*, 1987; Schmechel *et al.*, 1988).

## APP GENE AND ITS DIFFERENTIAL OVEREXPRESSION

The APP gene is overexpressed in Alzheimer's disease (Higgins *et al.*, 1988; Schmechel *et al.*, 1988; Cohen *et al.*, 1988). The distribution of the APP$_{695}$ mRNA in neurons parallels the pathological changes in Alzheimer's disease. Thus, neurons which are lost and develop NFTs in Alzheimer's disease are the very neurons that contain high levels of APP$_{695}$ mRNA (Bahmanyar *et al.*, 1988; Schmechel *et al.*, 1988; Higgins *et al.*, 1988). Moreover, the APP mRNA, principally the APP without the KPI domain, is increased twofold in neurons of the locus ceruleus and the nucleus basalis of Meynert in Alzheimer's disease (Palmert *et al.*, 1988).

In Down's syndrome, the increased expression of APP is related to an extra dose of the APP gene. In sporadic and familial cases of Alzheimer's disease, the mechanism by which APP gene expression is increased is still unknown. Amyloid precursor protein may be produced as a reaction to an environmental stimulus or stress. In Guamanian parkinsonism-dementia and amyotrophic lateral sclerosis, two diseases characterized by widespread intraneuronal amyloid formations, intracellular deposition of elements, such as calcium, aluminum and silicon, has been demonstrated in affected neurons (Garruto *et al.*, 1984, 1985, 1986). Manganese chloride, colloidal sulfur and selenium (Cohen, 1965), silver nitrate and silicon (Kisilevsky et al, 1977) can act as inflammatory stimuli in experimental amyloidosis in mice. These responses could constitute a heat shock response, which Lindquist *et al.* (1985) defined as a reaction to exposure to stressful conditions which are not limited to heat but may include hypoxia and a variety of toxic organic chemicals such as ethanol or cadmium chloride.

Other factors like cytokines and growth factors could modulate the expression of APP mRNA. For example, APP$_{695}$ mRNA expression in human vascular endothelial cells is augmented considerably by interleukin 1, phorbol myristate acetate and heparin-binding growth factor-1 (Goldgaber *et al.*, 1988).

## ROLE OF ENZYMES IN THE PROCESSING OF THE AMYLOID PRECURSOR PROTEIN

Enzymatic cleavage of a larger precursor to its smaller, biologically active molecule is a common step in many living systems. In Alzheimer's disease, the expression of the alternate forms of the APP mRNA with the KPI domain, with subsequent decrease or inhibition of specific protease activity, could cause defective processing of the APP. The degree of conservation of the KPI domain, together with the sequence of their reactive centers (Carrel, 1988) and the increased protease inhibitory activity in extracts of cells transfected with $APP_{770}$ cDNA containing the KPI domain (Kitaguchi *et al.*, 1988) indicate that the KPI domain is functional.

As products accumulate, other enzymes and enzyme systems not specific for processing of the APP could take over, leading to its abnormal cleavage. These abnormal cleavage products present as short polypeptides/microfibrils or oligomers, may undergo tertiary and quaternary configurational changes to form β-pleated sheets which polymerize into microfibrils of amyloid.

## MODIFIED FORMS OF THE AMYLOID PRECURSOR PROTEIN AS NUCLEATING AGENTS

AA amyloidosis, the most common type of amyloidosis, is characterized by extracellular deposition of proteinaceous fibrils composed principally of an 8 to 10 kDa peptide (protein AA), which is formed by proteolytic cleavage of its precursor, serum amyloid A (Niewold *et al.*, 1988). Similar to the fibril amyloid-enhancing factors (FAEF) in AA amyloidosis (Niewold *et al.*, 1987), short polypeptides, oligomers/microfibrils in Alzheimer's disease, formed through aberrant enzymatic processing of the APP, could act as nucleating agents for further amyloid fibril formation.

## AMYLOID-ENHANCING FACTORS (AEF)

AEF is a low-molecular weight glycoprotein found in systemic amyloidosis (Axelrad *et al.*, 1980). It is non-immunoglobulin in origin and distinct from the acute phase reactant amyloid protein (amyloid AA) and its precursor, and amyloid P, which is induced in mice and hamsters by non-specific activation of an inflammatory response following injections of casein, silver nitrate or lipopolysaccharide. The administration of AEF shortens the lag time for experimentally induced amyloidosis in mice and hamsters from two weeks to four days (Axelrad *et al.*, 1980, 1982). Because of its ability to complex with itself or other molecules in an indiscriminate fashion (Axelrad *et al.*, 1980, 1982), AEF can serve as a nucleus for fibril polymerization. Fibril AEF (Niewold *et al.*, 1987) is only a microfibril of amyloid AA and acts as a nucleant in accelerating its own production and the formation of amyloid. This fibril-derived AEF lacks typical birefringence after Congo red staining and appears amorphous by electron microscopy. It has beta-pleated sheet conformation by infrared spectroscopy, similar to that of the original fibrils. Active fractions contain proteins of three different sizes, with $M_r$ of 8-9, 16-17 and 27 kDa, respectively. Therefore, amyloid fibril fragments of various sizes appear to enhance amyloid formation in hamsters.

## ROLE OF GLYCOSAMINOGLYCANS AND POLYMERIZATION

The intimate relationship between amyloid fibrils and sulfated glycosaminoglycans has been demonstrated ultrastructurally and histochemically in experimental amyloidosis (Snow *et al.*, 1985, 1987a, 1987b), histochemically in Alzheimer's disease (Snow *et al.*, 1987c; Guiroy *et al.*, 1989a), in parkinsonism-dementia and. amyotrophic lateral sclerosis of Guam, Down's syndrome and Creutzfeldt-Jakob disease (Guiroy et. al., 1989a). Recent *in vitro* data suggest that the amyloid β-protein in Alzheimer's disease is possibly a heparan sulfate proteoglycan core protein (Schubert *et al.*, 1988) or is co-purified with such a protein (Beyreuther, personal communication). Heparan sulfate proteoglycan has been demonstrated in neuritic plaques and vascular amyloid deposits in Alzheimer's disease by immunocytochemistry and immunoelectronmicroscopy (Snow *et al.*, 1988).

A general biological theme of the laying down of extracellular matrix has been the extrusion of a transmembrane portion of a precursor molecule with subsequent copolymerization of the extracellular matrix polypeptide with glycosaminoglycans. These glycosaminoglycans are intimately involved in collagen polymerization from tropocollagen monomers. Like AEF, their oligomeric assemblies stimulate the nucleation phase of collagen fibril growth (Öbrink, 1972). In general, these oligomers inhibit the second phase of fibril growth by steric interference with the building pattern set by the nuclei. For this phase, fibril growth is stimulated by monomers. In the case of systemic amyloid fibril deposition, glycosaminoglycans seem to play a similar role of fibril nucleation and fibril growth acceleration. We can only speculate about a possible similar activity of fibril-derived AEFs in Alzheimer's disease. Hypothetically, fibril-derived AEF may serve as nucleating agent in Alzheimer's disease and other neurodegenerative disorders.

## SELF POLYMERIZATION OF AMYLOID β-PROTEIN/A4

Masters *et al.* (1985b) and Beyreuther *et al.* (1986) isolated several low molecular weight species (4, 8, 16, 32, 64 kDa and species above 64 kDa) in formic acid-treated extracts of amyloid isolated from amyloid plaque cores, neurofibrillary tangles and vascular amyloid deposits in Alzheimer's disease and Down's syndrome. They postulated that the 4.2-kDa protein, designated A4, could polymerize into multimeric aggregates to produce the amyloid fibril.

Synthetic homologs of the amyloid β-protein, specifically of the first 28 amino acids or fragments thereof, form fibrils *in vitro* resembling amyloid fibrils (Castaño *et al.*, 1986; Gorevic *et al.*, 1987; Kirschner *et al.*, 1987). The synthetic homolog of the complete 42-amino acid amyloid β-protein can also form fibrils (Beyreuther and Masters, personal communication). Computer predictions of the secondary structure of the amyloid β-protein indicate that the first 28 amino acids are hydrophilic, and the last 14 amino acids are hydrophobic with a β-pleated configuration (Goldgaber *et al.*, 1987; Gorevic *et al.*, 1987; Guiroy, unpublished data). Congo red staining of the non-polymerized, synthetic 42-amino acid homolog, whether treated with formic acid or not, reveals congophilia but no birefringence under polarized light. By electron microscopy, the synthetic homolog appears as amorphous structures (Guiroy and Miyazaki, unpublished data).

Birefringence of the amyloid fibrils under polarized light is attributed to the cross β-pleated configuration of its subfilaments which measures 42 Å in diameter and 76 Å in length with four β-pleated sheets constituting its thickness, where a β strand is estimated to comprise about 10 to 15 amino acid residues (Kirschner *et al.*, 1987). The conversion of the amyloid precursor protein into a cross β-pleated configuration is a process involving alteration of the quaternary configuration.

It has been shown immunologically and biochemically that the microtubule-associated protein tau is a component of the cerebral amyloid deposits in Alzheimer's disease (Grundke-Iqbal *et al.*, 1986; Kosik *et al.*, 1986; Nukina *et al.*, 1986). The core of the paired helical filaments in Alzheimer's disease has a molecular weight of about 100 kDa, 9.5 kDa of which is formed by the microtubule associated protein tau (Wischik *et al.*, 1988a, 1988b). Sequencing of cDNA clones encoding this 9.5 kDa fragment revealed homology to the sequence of mouse microtubule-associated protein tau (Goedert *et al.*, 1988). The presence of the microtubule-associated protein tau and other proteins can be attributed to the process of copolymerization with the core amyloid β-protein.

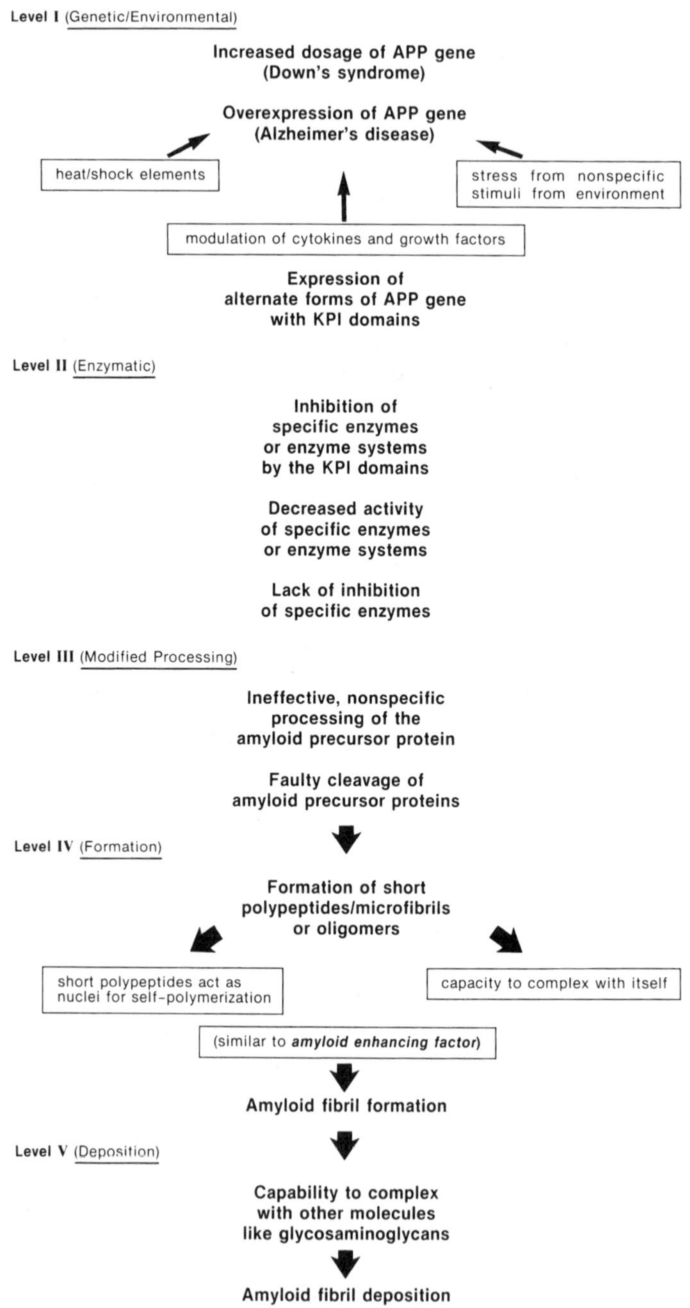


**Figure 1.** Hypothetical schema of amyloid formation and deposition.

## CONCLUSION

The increased production of the amyloid precursor protein is related to the overexpression of the APP gene in Alzheimer's disease, the mechanism of which is still unknown. Changes in expression of APP mRNA with KPI domains could contribute to the increased production of the precursor protein as a result of defective enzymatic processing. Aberrant and/or nonspecific processing of the APP through other enzymes or enzyme systems could inhibit or lead to abnormal catabolism, resulting in faulty protein cleavage, leading to the formation of modified β-pleated forms of the protein. This short β-pleated polypeptides polymerizes easily into oligomers or microfibrils, which may act as nucleating agents that enhance their own formation by polymerization and copolymerization with other molecules, culminating in amyloid fibril deposition (Figure 1).

## REFERENCES


AXELRAD, M. A. and KISILEVSKY, R. (1980) Biological characterizations of amyloid enhancing factor. In: *Amyloid and Amyloidosis* (Eds. Glenner, G. G., Costa, P. P. and de Freitas, A. F.), pp.527-533. Excerpta Medica, Amsterdam.

AXELRAD, M. A., KISILEVSKY, R., WILLMER, J., CHEN, S. J. and SKINNER, M. (1982) Further characterization of amyloid-enhancing factor. *Lab. Invest.* **47**: 139-146.

BAHMANYAR, S., HIGGINS, G. A., GOLDGABER, D., LEWIS, D. A., MORRISON, J. H., WILSON, M. C., SHANKAR, S. K. and GAJDUSEK, D. C. (1987) Localization of amyloid β-protein messenger RNA in brains from patients with Alzheimer's disease. *Science* **237**: 77-80

BEYREUTHER, K., MULTHAUP, G., SIMMS, G., POTTGIESSER, J., SCHROEDER, W., MARTINS, R. N. and MASTERS, C. L. (1986) Neurofibrillary tangles of. Alzheimer's disease and "aged" Down's syndrome contain the same protein as the amyloid of plaque cores and blood vessels. *Disc. Neurosci.* **3**: 68-79.

CASTAÑO, E. M. and FRANGIONE, B. (1988) Human amyloidosis, Alzheimer disease and related disorders. *Lab. Invest.* **58**: 122-132.

CASTAÑO, E. M., GHISO, J., PRELLI, F., GOREVIC, P.D., MIGHELI, A. and FRANGIONE, B. (1986) *In vitro* formation of amyloid fibrils from two synthetic peptides of different lengths homologous to Alzheimer's disease beta protein. *Biochem. Biophys. Res. Commun.* **141**: 782-789.

COHEN, M. L., GOLDE, T. E., USIAK, M. F., YOUNKIN, L. H., and YOUNKIN, S. G. (1988) *In situ* hybridization of nucleus basalis neurons shows increased beta-amyloid mRNA in Alzheimer's disease. *Proc. Natl. Acad. Sci. USA* **85**: 1227-1231.

COHEN, A. S. (1965) The constitution and genesis of amyloid. *Int. Rev. Exp. Pathol.* **4**: 159-243.

DeSAUVAGE, F., and OCTAVE, J. N. (1989) A novel mRNA of the amyloid precursor gene encoding for a possibly secreted protein. *Science* **245**: 651-653

GARRUTO, R. M., FUKATZU, R., YANAGIHARA, R., GAJDUSEK, D. C., HOOK, G. and FIORI, C.E. (1984) Imaging of calcium and magnesium in neurofibrillary tangle-bearing neurons in parkinsonism-dementia of Guam. *Proc. Natl. Acad Sci. USA* **81**: 875-879.

GARRUTO, R. M., SWYT, C., FIORI, C. E., YANAGIHARA, R., and GAJDUSEK, D. C. (1985) Intraneuronal deposition of calcium and aluminum in amyotrophic lateral sclerosis of Guam. *Lancet* **2**: 1353.

GARRUTO, R. M., SWYT, C., YANAGIHARA, R., FIORI, C. E., and GAJDUSEK, D. C. (1986) Intraneuronal co-localization of silicon with calcium.and aluminum. amyotrophic lateral sclerosis and parkinsonism-dementia of Guam. *N. Engl. J. Med.* **315**: 711-712.

GHISO, J., TAGLIAVINI, F., TIMMERS, W. F. and FRANGIONE, B. (1989) Alzheimer's disease amyloid presursor protein is present in senile plaques and cerebrospinal fluid : immunohistochemical and biochemical characterization. *Biochem. Biophys. Res. Commun.* **163**: 430-437

GLENNER, G. G., and WONG, C. W. (1984a) Alzheimer's disease: initial report of the purification and characterization of a novel cerebrovascular amyloid protein. *Biochem. Biophys. Res. Commun.* **120**: 885-890.

GLENNER, G. G. and WONG, C. W. (1984b) Alzheimer's disease and Down's syndrome: sharing of a unique cerebrovascular amyloid fibril protein. *Biochem. Biophys. Res. Commun.* **122**: 1131-1135.

GOEDERT, M., WISCHIK, C. M., CROWTHER, R. A., WALKER, J. E. and KLUG, A. (1988) Cloning and sequencing of the cDNA encoding a core protein of the paired helical filament of Alzheimer disease: identification as the microtubule-associated protein tau. *Proc. Natl. Acad. Sci. USA* **85**: 4051-4055.

GOLDGABER., D., LERMAN, M. I., McBRIDE O. W., SAFFIOTTI, U., and GAJDUSEK, D. C. (1987) Characterization and chromosomal localization of a cDNA encoding brain amyloid of Alzheimer's disease. *Science* **235**: 877-880.

GOLDGABER, D., TEENER, J. W., and GAJDUSEK, D. C. (1988) Multiple forms of amyloid β-protein precursor mRNAS. *Disc. Neurosci.* **5**: 40-46.

GOLDGABER, D., HARRIS, H. W., HLA, T., MACIAG, T., DONNELLY, R. J., JACOBSEN, J. S., VITEK, M. P. AND GAJDUSEK, D. C. (1989) Interleukin I regulates synthesis of amyloid β-protein precursor mRNA in human endothelial cells. *Proc. Natl. Acad. Sci. USA* **86**: 7606-7610

GOREVIC, P. D., CASTAÑO, E. M., SARMA, R. and FRANGIONE, B. 1987. Ten to fourteen residue peptides of Alzheimer's disease beta protein are sufficient for amyloid fibril formation and its characteristic X-ray diffraction pattern. *Biochem. Biophys. Res. Commun.* **147**: 854-862.

GRUNDKE-IQBAL, I., IQBAL, K., TURG, Y. C., QUINLAN, M., WISNIEWSKI, H. M. and BINDER, L. I. (1986) Abnormal phosphorylation of the microtubule-associated protein tau in Alzheimer cytoskeletal pathology. *Proc. Natl. Acad. Sci. USA* **83**: 4913-4917.

GUIROY, D. C., MIYAZAKI, M., MULTHAUP, G., FISCHER, P., GARRUTO, R. M., BEYREUTHER, K., MASTERS, C. L., SIMMS, G., GIBBS, C. J., Jr. and GAJDUSEK, D. C. (1987) Amyloid of the neurofibrillary tangles of Guamanian parkinsonism-dementia and Alzheimer disease share identical amino acid sequence. *Proc. Natl. Acad. Sci. USA* **84**: 2073-2077.

GUIROY, D. C., SNOW, A. D., GAJDUSEK, D. C. YANAGIHARA, R., and GARRUTO, R. M. (1989a) Sulfated glycosaminoglycans in amyotrophic lateral sclerosis and parkinsonism-dementia of Guam, Alzheimer's disease, Down's syndrome and Creutzfeldt-Jakob disease. *J. Cell. Biochem.* **Suppl 13C**: 157.

GUIROY, D. C., MIYAZAKI, M., HIRANO, A., GARRUTO, R. M., YANAGIHARA, R., and GAJDUSEK, D. C. (1989b) Isolation of low molecular weight amyloid proteins from neurofibrillary tangles of neurologically normal Guamanian Chamorros. *Alz. Dis. Assoc. Dis.* **3**: Suppl. 1, 1-36.

HIGGINS, G. A., LEWIS, D. A., BAHMANYAR, S., GOLDGABER, D., GAJDUSEK, D. C., YOUNG, W. G., MORRISON, J. H. and WILSON, M. C. (1988) Differential regulation of amyloid β-protein mRNA expression within hippocampal neuronal subpopulations in Alzheimer's disease. *Proc. Natl. Acad. Sci. USA* **85**: 1297-1301.

JOHNSTONE, E. M., CHANEY, M. G., MOORE, R. E., WARD, K. E., NORRIS, F. H. and LITTLE, S. P. (1989) Alzheimer's disease amyloid peptide is encoded by two exons and shows similarity to soybean trypsin inhibitor. *Biochem Biophys. Res. Commun.* **163**: 1248-1255

KANG, J., LEMAIRE, H. G., UNTERBECK, A., SALBAUM, J. M. MASTERS, C. L. GRZES-CHIK, K. H., MULTHAUP, G., BEYREUTHER, K., and MÜLLER-HILL, B. (1987) The precursor of Alzheimer's disease amyloid A4 protein resembles a cell surface receptor. *Nature* **325**: 733-736.

KIRSCHNER, D. A., INOUYE, H., DUFFY, L. K., SINCLAIR, A., LIND, M. and SELKOE, D. J. (1987) Synthetic peptide homologous to β-protein from Alzheimer disease forms amyloid-like fibrils *in vitro. Proc. Natl. Acad. Sci. USA* **84**: 6953-6957.

KITAGUCHI, N., TAKAHASHI, Y., TOKUSHIMA, Y., SHIOJIRI, S., and ITO, H. (1988) Novel precursor of Alzheimer's disease amyloid protein shows protease inhibitory activity. *Nature* **331**: 530-532.

KOSIK, K. S., JOACHIM C. L., and SELKOE D. S. (1986) The microtubule-associated protein, tau, is a major antigen component of paired helical filaments in Alzheimer's disease. *Proc. Natl. Acad. Sci. USA* **83**: 4044-4048.

LINDQUIST, S. (1986) The heat-shock response. *Ann. Rev. Biochem.* **55**: 1151-91.

MASTERS, C. L., SIMMS, G., WEINMAN, N. A., MULTHAUP, G., McDONALD, B. L. and BEYREUTHER, K. (1985a) Amyloid plaque core protein in Alzheimer disease and Down's syndrome. *Proc. Natl. Acad. Sci. USA* **82**: 4245-4249.

MASTERS, C. L., MULTHAUP, G., SIMMS, G., POTTGIESSER, J., MARTINS, R. N. and BEYREUTHER, K. (1985b) Neuronal origin of a cerebral amyloid: neurofibrillary tangles of Alzheimer's disease contain the same protein as the amyloid of plaque cores and blood vessels. *EMBO J.* **4**: 2757-2763.

NIEWOLD, Th.A., HOL, P. R., van ANDEL, A. C. J., LUTZ, E. T. G. and GRUYS, E. (1987) Enhancement of amyloid induction by amyloid fibril fragments in hamster. *Lab. Invest.* **56**: 544-549.

NUKINA, N. and IHARA, Y. (1986) One of the antigenic determinants of paired helical filaments is related to tau protein. *J. Biochem.* **99**: 1541-1544.

ÖBRINK, B. (1972) The influence of glycosaminoglycans on the formation of fibers from monomeric tropopcollagen *in vitro. Eur. J. Biochem.* **84**: 129-137.

OLTERSDORF, T., FRITZ, L. C., SCHENK, D. B, LIEBERSBURG, I., JOHNSON-WOOD, K. L., BEATTIE, E. C., WARD, P. J., BLCAHER, R. W., DOVEY, H. F. and SUKANTO, S. (1989) The secreted form of the Alzheimer's amyloid precursor protein with the Kunitz domain is protease nexin-II. *Nature* **341**: 144-147

PALMERT, M-R., GOLDE, T. E., COHEN, M. L., KOVACS, D. M., TANZI, R. E., GUSELLA, J. F., USIAK, M. F. YOUNKIN, L. H. and YOUNKIN, S. G. (1988) Amyloid protein precursor messenger RNAs: differential expression in Alzheimer's disease. *Science* **241**: 1080-1084.

PALMERT, N. R., PODLISNY, M. B., WITTKER, D. S., OLTERSDORF, T., YOUNKIN, L. H., SELKOE, D .J. and YOUNKIN, S. G. (1989) The β-amyloid protein precursor of Alzheimer disease has soluble derivatives found in human brain and cerebrospinal fluid. *Proc. Natl. Acad. Sci. USA* **86**: 6338-6342

PONTE, P., GONZALES-DeWHITT, P., SCHILLING, J., MILLER, J., HSU, D., GREENBERG, B., DAVIS, K., WALLACE, W., LIBERBURG, I., FULLER, F., and CORDELL, B. (1988) A new A4 amyloid mRNA contains a domain homologous to serine protease inhibitors. *Nature* **331**: 525-527.

ROBAKIS, N.K., RAMAKRISHNA, N., WOLFE, G., and WISNIEWSKI, H.M. (1987) Molecular cloning and characterization of a cDNA encoding the cerebrovascular and the neuritic plaque amyloid peptides. *Proc. Natl. Acad. Sci. USA* **84**: 4190-4194.

SAITOH, T., SUNDSMO, M., ROCH, J. M., KIMURA, N., COLE, G., SCHUBERT, D., OLTERSDORF, T. and SCHENK, D. B. (1989) Secreted form of amyloid beta precursor protein is involved in the growth regulation of fibroblasts. *Cell* **58**: 615-622.

SALBAUM, J. M.., WEIDEMANN, A., LEMAIRE, H. G., MASTERS, C. L. and BEYREUTHER, K. (1988) The promoter of Alzheimer's disease amyloid A4 precursor gene. *EMBO J.* **7**: 2807-2813.

SCHUBERT, D., SCHROEDER, R., LaCORBIERE, M., SAITOH, T. and COLE, G. (1988) Amyloid β-protein precursor is possibly a heparan sulfate proteoglycan core protein. *Science* **241**: 223-226.

SCHMECHEL, D. E., GOLDGABER, D., BURKHART, D. S., GILBERT, J. R., GAJDUSEK, D. C. and ROSES, A. D. (1988) Cellular localization of messenger RNA encoding amyloid β-protein in normal tissue and in Alzheimer disease. *Alz. Dis. Assoc. Dis.* **2**: 96-14.

SNOW, A. D. and KISILEVSKY, R., (1985) Temporal relationship between glycosaminoglycan accumulation and amyloid deposition during experimental amyloidosis. A. histochemical study. *Lab. Invest.* **53**: 3744.

SNOW, A. D., WILLMER, J., and KISILEVSKY, R. (1987a) Sulfated glycosaminoglycans: a common constituents of all amyloids. *Lab. Invest.* **56**: 120-123.

SNOW, A.D., WILLMER, J., and KISILEVSKY, R. (1987b) A close ultrastructural relationship between sulfated proteoglycans and AA amyloid fibrils? *Lab. Invest.* **57**: 687-698.

SNOW, A. D., WILLMER, J. P., and KISILEVSKY, R. (1987c) Sulfated glycosaminoglycans in Alzheimer's disease. *Hum. Pathol.* **18**: 506-510.

SNOW, A. D., MAR, H., NOCHLIN, D., KIMATA, K., KATO, M., SUZUKI, S., HASSELL, J. and WIGHT, T. N. (1988) The presence of heparin sulfate proteoglycans in the neuritic plaques and congophilic angiopathy in Alzheimer's disease. *Am. J. Pathol.* **133**: 456-463.

TANZI, R. E., GUSELLA, J. F., WATKINS, P. C., BRUNS, G. A., ST GEORGE-HYSLOP, G. A. P., van KEUREN, M-L., PATTERSON, D., PAGAN, S., KURNIT, D. M., and NEVE, R-L. (1987) Amyloid β-protein gene: cDNA, mRNA distribution, and genetic linkage near the Alzheimer locus. *Science* **235**: 880-884.

TANZI, R. E., McCLATCHEY, A. I., LAMPERTI, E. D., VILLA-KOMAROFF, L., GUSELLA, J. F., and NEVE, R. L. (1988) Protease inhibitor domain encoded by an amyloid precursor mRNA associated with Alzheimer's disease. *Nature* **331**: 528-530.

TEILUM, G. (1964) Pathogenesis of amyloidosis. The two-phase cellular theory of local secretion. *Acta Path. Microbiol. Scand.* **61**: 21-45.

van DUINEN, S. G., CASTAÑO, E. M., PRELLI, F., BOTS, G. T. A. B., LUYENDIJK, W. and FRANGIONE, B. (1987) Hereditary cerebral hemorrhage with amyloidosis in patients of Dutch origin is related to Alzheimer disease. *Proc. Natl. Acad. Sci. USA* **84**: 5991-5994

Van NOSTRAND, W. E., WAGNER, S. L., SUZUKI, M., CHOI, B. H., FARROW, J. S., GEDDES, J. W., COTMAN, C. W. and CUNNINGHAM, D. D. (1989) Protease nexin-II, a potent antichymotrysin, shows identity to amyloid β-protein precursor. *Nature* **341**: 546-549.

WHITSON, J. S., SELKOE, D. J. AND COTMAN, C. W. (1989) Amyloid beta-protein enhances the survival of hippocampal neurons *in vitro*. *Science* **243**: 1488-1490.

WISCHIK, C. M., NOVAK, M., THOGERSEN, H. C. EDWARDS, P. C., RUNSWICK, M. J., JAKES, R., WALKER, J. E., MILSTEIN, C., ROTH, M., and KLUG, A. (1988a) Isolation of a fragment of tau derived from. the core of the paired helical filament of Alzheimer disease. *Proc. Natl. Acad. Sci. USA* **85**: 4506-4510.

WISCHIK, C. M., NOVAK, M., EDWARDS, P. C., KLUG, A., TICHELAAR, W., and CROWTHER R. A. (1988b) Structural characterization of the core of the paired helical filament in Alzheimer disease. *Proc. Natl. Acad. Sci. USA* **85**: 4884-4888.

YANKER, B. A., DAWES, L. R., FISHER, S., VILLA-KOMAROFF, L., OSTER-GRANITE, M. L. and NEVE, R. L. (1989) Neurotoxicity of a fragment of the amyloid precursor associated with Alzheimer's disease. *Science* **245**: 417-420.

## DISCUSSION

1. There is a report from another group that Alzheimer's disease is transmissible in hamsters. Possibly, this was from contamination in the laboratory by hamster-adapted Creutzfeldt-Jakob disease virus. Gajdusek's group was not able to repeat this transmission.

2. Expression of the amyloid protein precursor has been found in various human tissues. What role do glycosaminoglycans play in the formation of amyloid fibrils? Amyloid fibril formation is dependent mainly on the formation of amyloidogenic fragments probably from modified host precursor protein, while glycosaminoglycans may facilitate amyloid fibril deposition.

3. Since the amyloid gene is expressed in all tissues, could the problems causing Alzheimer's disease be detected in tissues other than brain, perhaps as altered ratios of the different forms? Amyloid precursor protein is present in other tissues, such as muscles, but amyloid deposition has not been shown in muscles. More studies are necessary to determine amyloid deposition in tissues other than the brain.

4. Could Alzheimer's disease result from the action of genes that are useful early in life, but cause harm late? Or could a mutation produce the disease from a protein essential early in development? There are many genes implicated in Alzheimer's disease, like Hox 1.3. expression, which diminishes or may become absent in Alzheimer's disease. But the most likely candidate in amyloid fibril formation is the amyloid $\beta$-protein.

There is evidence to refute the suggestion that amyloid deposition is secondary to cell injury. Amyloid deposits could cause cell injury. If cell injury is not the primary cause, the amyloid protein may increase the damage. Amyloidogenesis is a cascade of events, so it is difficult to identify the primary cause. The cascade could include membrane injury, faulty proteolysis possibly through prolonged inhibition of enzymes or enzyme complexes thereby modifying the host precursor protein leading to formation of amyloidogenic fragments that could act as nucleants for amyloid fibril formation.

## ADDENDUM

In addition to the membrane-bound form of the amyloid precursor protein (APP$_{695}$), a secreted form, APP$_{751}$, which lacks the transmembrane domain (de Sauvage *et al.*, 1989; Oltersdorf *et al.*, 1989; Palmert *et al.*, 1989; Ghiso *et al.*, 1989), is now known to be homologous to protease nexin-II (Oltersdorf *et al.*, 1989; Van Nostrand *et al.*, 1989), a protease inhibitor, a potent antichymotrypsin, that forms SDS-resistant inhibitory complexes with epidermal growth factor-binding protein, the $\gamma$-subunit of nerve growth factor, and trypsin (Van Nostrand *et al.*, 1989). Furthermore, amyloid $\beta$-protein, specifically amino acid residues 4-36, shows 68% homology to residues 120-153 of soybean trypsin inhibitor (Kunitz) (Johnstone *et al.*, 1989).

Amyloid precursor protein and amyloid $\beta$-protein have trophic (Whitson *et al.*, 1989; Saitoh *et al.*, 1989).

Amyloid precursor protein and amyloid $\beta$-protein have trophic (Whitson et al., 1989; Saitoh *et al.*, 1989), as well as toxic effects (Yanker *et al.*, 1989; Guiroy, unpublished data). These contradictory effects could be explained by differences in the kinetics of enzyme inhibition.

Currently available data indicate that one aspect of cerebral amyloidogenesis can be explained by altered proteolysis. The mechanism by which these proteinase inhibitors accumulate in Alzheimer's disease and their conversion into cross $\beta$-pleated sheets remains unknown.

# 31

# LINKAGE ANALYSIS IN ALZHEIMER DISEASE


Jonathan L. Haines, Peter St George-Hyslop, Ronald Polinksy,
John Hardy, Leonard Heston, Sandra Sorbi,
Christine van Broeckhoven, and James F. Gusella


## ABSTRACT


Alzheimer disease (AD) is one of the most common neurodegenerative
disorders of man. Onset is quite variable, usually occurring after the third
decade of life, most commonly in the sixth to eighth decades of life. Familial
aggregation of AD has been observed, suggesting a genetic etiology for at
least some forms of AD. A subset of families with AD show clear evidence of
autosomal dominant transmission. In such families, linkage analysis can be
used to detect a marker cosegregating with the putative disease gene, thus
allowing the approximate location of the AD gene to be identified. Two
markers on chromosome 21, D21S1/D21S11 and D21S16 have shown such a
linkage, providing strong evidence that a gene for familial AD resides on the
proximal long arm of chromosome 21. A large set of 35 pedigrees with AD
have now been examined for linkage to D21s1/D21s11. The peak lod score is
3.28 at $\theta = 0.22$ However, linkage analysis is complicated by many factors,
including the distance between the markers and the AD gene, the variable
age-at-onset of AD, the poor quality of many of the pedigrees, and diagnostic
uncertainty. These factors will make it difficult to tease out any genetic
heterogeneity, and make identifying more closely linked (or flanking)
markers a long and involved process.


## INTRODUCTION

Much work has been expended to classify the clinical and pathological
aspects of Alzheimer disease. The disease affects upwards of two million
individuals in the United States alone, and millions more worldwide. Although Alzheimer disease (AD) is usually believed to occur only in the aged
(indeed, for a long time senility was considered part of the normal course in
human aging), individuals in their early forties have been known to suffer
symptoms completely concordant with AD (Nee *et al.*, 1983), including the
classical pathological findings in the brain upon autopsy. During the past 20
years, much effort and money has been focused on AD, partially in response

to the aging of the U.S. population and the ever increasing lifespan of its citizens. Major advances in defining the functional deficits and clinical course of the disease have been made. Unfortunately, there has been little progress toward understanding the basic underlying etiology of AD. This results from the lack of appropriate animal models, from the inability to obtain living tissue of the affected organ (brain) from patients with AD, and from a continued lack of understanding of the biochemical and physiological defects. The past few years have seen an explosion of methodologies for exploring human biology with the advent of the new and powerful techniques of molecular genetics. These techniques, in concert with more traditional yet powerful classical genetic techniques have opened many new avenues for understanding the underlying etiologies involved in Alzheimer disease.

## CLINICAL ASPECTS OF ALZHEIMER DISEASE

Alzheimer disease is a neurodegenerative disorder displaying chronic loss of mental and physical ability. It is characterized by progressive dementia together with deterioration of most cognitive functions (Terry and Davies, 1980). The classical brain pathology consists of a large number of amyloid plaques and neurofibrillary tangles. The age-at-onset of AD is quite variable, with a few individuals displaying clinical symptoms as early as their forties, while the vast majority do not display symptoms until their seventies or eighties. It has been estimated that as many as 10% of individuals will develop AD if they live into their eighties (Nee *et al.*, 1983; Breitner *et al.*, 1986). However, the problem with any estimates of incidence, prevalence, and risk of AD is that the study sample sizes have generally been small, the diagnostic criteria for inclusion have been vague, and appropriate life table analyses have not been employed. Before accurate epidemiology of AD can be obtained, these problems must be addressed.

## GENETICS OF ALZHEIMER DISEASE

It has long been noted that AD occasionally "runs in families". Unfortunately, a disease may "run in families" for several reasons. First, it may simply be a coincidence, and need not invoke a genetic etiology. If one accepts a population lifetime risk of 10%, then each relative of an AD proband (a proband is the person through which a family, and any other affected relative, is originally identified) has a 10% chance of also developing AD given a long enough life span, and thus many family constellations (multiplex families) will be identified. Second, there may be many genes, each with small effect, giving rise to AD. This would produce multiplex families, but with more relatives being affected than predicted by population incidence rates alone. However, simple mendelian modes of inheritance would not be followed, and the risks of AD as one moves from first to second to third degree relatives would drop dramatically. Finally, simple Mendelian inheritance (autosomal dominant, recessive, or X-linked) may be involved if there are one or a few major genes giving rise to AD. Of course, there may be environmental influences in all of these models, complicating the picture still further. Recent advances in the techniques of segregation analysis may help to distinguish between these possibilities. Unfortunately, these techniques are quite sensitive to methods of ascertainment, and require large population based studies to be used with any accuracy.

With such a possible mix of etiologies, teasing out the gene(s) involved is a complex task. Fortunately, there may be a certain subset of families that fit one or other of the models so well that formal segregation analysis is not necessary. Such a subset has been identified for AD showing a clear pattern of autosomal dominant inheritance (Nee *et al.*, 1983; Heston *et al.* 1978; St George-Hyslop *et al.*, 1987). These pedigrees are a natural choice for attempts to identify a putative familial Alzheimer disease (FAD) gene by the use of linkage analysis.

## APPROACHES TO FINDING AN ALZHEIMER GENE

There are several possible approaches in trying to uncover a gene or genes involved in the etiology of FAD. First, physiological and biochemical changes in the brain or other tissues may be studied to identify abnormalities in FAD patients. Unfortunately, this is akin to a fishing expedition, and may not produce significant results. Second, clues from animal models, either in suggesting which biochemical pathways to study or by comparative mapping of interesting neurological mutants, may be used to determine important mammalian systems in the FAD degenerative process. Unfortunately, no adequate animal models of Alzheimer disease have yet been identified. Finally, genetic analysis, primarily linkage analysis, can be used to identify the approximate location of the putative disease gene. This method has the advantage that no knowledge about the structure or function of the FAD gene is necessary, only the segregation of the disease need be observed.

The paradigm of "reverse" genetics is a useful one in this instance. Once the approximate location of the disease gene is identified, molecular techniques such as jumping, walking or sequencing can be employed to localize the disease gene, isolate it, and clone it. Given its sequence, the protein it codes for may be determined, and its localization and function within the body can be examined. Thus, instead of starting with biochemistry and ending with the gene, we start with the gene, and end with the biochemistry. The application of linkage analysis as a starting point for this "reverse" genetics is a recent event as discussed below.

## LINKAGE ANALYSIS

Linkage analysis is a powerful tool for identifying the approximate location of a gene relative to previously localized genes, but its application to humans was delayed until the late 1950's for several reasons. First, there was a lack of identifiable loci for which segregation could be observed. Until the early 1980's, marker loci were restricted to red cell antigen and serum protein polymorphisms which at best covered about 15% of the genome (Conneally and Rivas, 1980). Second, families segregating diseases were not large, and obtaining phase known mating information (generally requiring 3 generations of living individuals, a difficult finding especially since most diseases result in reduced fertility and/or early mortality) was virtually impossible. Third, methods for capturing all possible segregation information had not yet been developed, making even more essential the above family structures.

In 1955 Morton described a method of capturing the linkage information in a family through the use of a statistic he called the Lod score. The Lod score is simply the Logarithm (base 10) of the ODds of linkage versus random segregation. The lod score is generally calculated by dividing the likelihood that the observed segregation pattern arose in a pedigree (or set of pedigrees) given that two loci are linked at a certain recombination fraction by the likelihood of that segregation pattern given the two loci are completely unlinked. Thus there is a separate lod score for each possible recombination fraction. Morton suggested that a lod score of +3 was sufficient to indicate linkage, while -2 was sufficient to refute linkage at any given recombination fraction (for an excellent review of the history and methods of linkage analysis, see Ott, (1985)).

With the advent of restriction fragment length polymorphisms (RFLPs) (Botstein *et al.*, 1980) and variable number of tandem repeats (VNTRs) (Nakamura *et al.*, 1987), linkage analysis now can examine the entire genome for evidence of disease gene location. The plethora of new markers has allowed testing of multiple loci simultaneously using the technique of multi-point linkage analysis.

## COMPLICATIONS IN LINKAGE ANALYSIS

One must be careful when applying linkage analysis, as misleading results may be obtained if certain assumptions are not valid. Linkage analysis presumes that the genetic model (consisting of disease and marker allele frequencies, mutation rates, mode of inheritance, and penetrance functions) is known. For many diseases the mode of inheritance, be it autosomal dominant, autosomal recessive, or X-linked, is clear-cut, and mutation rates are generally so small that they may be ignored. Allele frequencies for markers can be satisfactorily estimated by examining approximately 50 unrelated individuals, but can be subject to variation in different populations or ethnic groups. Allele frequencies for disease genes are more difficult to estimate, but unless the disease is very common, its frequency will be so small as not to be a problem. Accurate penetrance functions may also be difficult to obtain. Fortunately, any reasonable estimate will usually suffice, as long as some estimate is used (Hodge, 1979). One must avoid gross errors in any of the above or they are likely to produce poor and perhaps unintelligible results.

Underlying genetic heterogeneity may also confound linkage analysis. If any disease is caused by abnormalities in a single gene, then all tested families of sufficient size should produce positive lod scores for closely linked markers. However, if some families have disease caused by another gene at a second locus, they will produce negative lod scores with markers linked to the first locus. Thus the overall lod score will be a result of both positive and negative scores, and may not reach significant values. Testing for heterogeneity may be done, but the tests are sensitive to the recombination fraction; it is difficult to prove heterogeneity when the linked marker is ten or more centiMorgans from the disease locus.

## LINKAGE ANALYSIS IN ALZHEIMER DISEASE

Initially, we identified four large pedigrees each with clear demonstration of autosomal dominant inheritance, and classical clinical and pathological findings of AD. Lymphoblastoid cell lines were created for all available living members of each pedigree to act as an inexhaustible source of DNA for the linkage studies (St George-Hyslop *et al.*, 1987).

Initial studies focused on markers residing on chromosome 21 because of the association of AD with Down syndrome (trisomy 21) (Heston, 1977). Virtually all adult Down syndrome patients will develop the classical Alzheimer brain pathology if they live into their 30's or 40's. Because the individuals have three copies of chromosome 21, it has been suggested that overexpression of a gene or genes on chromosome 21 might result in this pathology. In the case of families segregating autosomal dominant FAD, the argument is that a single genetic mutation resulting in overexpression might be the underlying cause.

Markers on the lower portion of chromosome 21 provided primarily negative lod scores, and reasonably large portions of the distal long arm have been excluded (St George-Hyslop *et al.*, 1987). However two markers,

D21S1/D21S11 and D21S16, provided positive lod scores in all four families. Unfortunately, neither marker by itself could provide a lod score greater than 3. When multipoint analysis was used, however, a lod score of over 4 was obtained, providing strong evidence for linkage of an FAD gene to these markers on the proximal long arm of chromosome 21.

A total of 35 families with multiple cases of AD have now been identified (Haines *et al.*, 1988, van Broeckhoven *et al.*, 1988, Goate *et al.*, 1989). Full descriptions of the pedigrees, along with clinical information, are presented elsewhere (St george-Hyslop *et al.*, in press, St George-Hyslop *et al.*, in preparation). Unfortunately, many of these families are small, can provide only limited amounts of segregation information, and may not show truly convincing evidence of autosomal dominant inheritance. If these families are not segregating the chromosome-21 linked AD gene, the individuals who are seen as recombinants, and who usually provide crucial information on gene location, will randomly point in either direction, totally confusing the analysis. In order to examine the possibility that such families might provide misleading results, we instituted selection criteria to identify and study the most useful families for continued linkage studies.

## SELECTION CRITERIA

Our first and most important selection criterion was to insist on using only families with clear autosomal dominant transmission. This was primarily done by demanding apparent transmission through at least three generations. This may be fulfilled in several ways, including direct transmission from grandparent to parent to child, or presumed transmission by observing an uncle/aunt, parent, and child constellation of affected individuals. Although documentation for the parent and child was almost always excellent (including pathological confirmation and medical/hospital records), documentation for the third generation was often less clear, usually consisting of multiple reports from other family members that the person in question had dementia consistent with AD. Of the 35 families, approximately 15 were excluded because no information on a third generation was available.

The second criterion required at least one case in each family to be diagnosed by a physician as having AD. The diagnosis must have fit the NINCDS-NIA diagnostic criteria, and must not have had any unusual clinical or pathological features. Other family members were considered to be affected if they met the same criteria, or were reported to have the same disease as the medically diagnosed individual. They were considered as unknown if any unusual features were reported. The remaining families all fulfilled this criterion. Pathological confirmation of AD was obtained on at least one patient from 20 of the families. Unfortunately, it is not yet available on any member of the remaining families.

The third criterion required a family structure that would allow observation of transmission of markers not only between at least two affected individuals but also from an affected parent to an affected child. This was introduced to remove some of the effects of genetic model parameters on the ensuing linkage analysis. In order to fulfill this criterion, the families must have at least two living first or second degree relatives, and at least one other affected relative who is either living, or potentially reconstructable (by having the spouse and at least two children). Additionally, this must also include an affected parent/child pair. This requirement provides that all families can potentially provide a lod score greater than +0.3 for any linked marker, or be substantially negative for any unlinked marker. It makes spurious positive or negative results less likely by reducing the number of untyped individuals in a pedigree. Spurious results are often obtained when most of the linkage information is being provided from the starting parameters of the genetic model (introduced primarily through untyped individuals), such as marker and disease allele frequencies, and disease gene penetrance. Additionally, families fulfilling these criteria will be useful when testing for genetic heterogeneity as they are more likely to provide substantial positive or negative lod scores. Three of the remaining families did not fulfill these criteria, leaving a total of 17 families for study.

## RESULTS

Because D21S16 has remained a relatively uninformative marker, efforts have been concentrated on the D21S1/D21S11 marker locus. Table 1 presents the lod scores between FAD and D21S1/D21S11 for all 35 families. As can be seen, numerous families provide positive lod scores, and the overall peak lod score is 3.28 at $\theta = 0.22$. Thus, even when all families are considered, a lod score above three is obtained. Table 2 presents the lod scores for the 17 families fulfilling our selection criteria. The peak lod score is 3.86 at $\theta = 0.13$. Absolute recombinants (those observed between affected individuals) between D21S1/D21S11 and FAD have been observed in six families, all but one providing an overall positive lod score. Five families had no positive lod scores. No single family had lod scores even approaching 3, leaving open the question of heterogeneity. There is always the possibility that a family may be segregating something other than AD if no pathological confirmation of AD in the family has been documented. If one considers only the 13 (of 17) families with pathologically confirmed FAD in our sample, then the peak lod score is 3.48 at $\theta = 0.15$.

| Pedigree | Lod Score | | | | | | |
|---|---|---|---|---|---|---|---|
| | 0.00 | 0.05 | 0.10 | 0.15 | 0.20 | 0.30 | 0.40 |
| Bel A | $-\infty$ | 0.01 | 0.18 | 0.23 | 0.24 | 0.20 | 0.11 |
| Bel B | $-\infty$ | -1.08 | -0.52 | -0.24 | -0.09 | -0.00 | -0.00 |
| Lon 46 | 0.01 | 0.01 | 0.00 | 0.00 | 0.00 | 0.00 | 0.00 |
| Lon 45 | -2.91 | -1.43 | -0.89 | -0.59 | -0.39 | -0.15 | -0.04 |
| Lon 44 | -3.81 | -0.84 | -0.54 | -0.36 | -0.24 | -0.10 | -0.02 |
| Lon 23 | 1.17 | 1.04 | 0.91 | 0.77 | 0.63 | 0.35 | 0.10 |
| Lon 43 | -6.95 | -1.44 | -0.89 | -0.58 | -0.39 | -0.15 | -0.04 |
| Lon 38 | 0.41 | 0.35 | 0.30 | 0.24 | 0.19 | 0.09 | 0.03 |
| Lon 32 | 0.48 | 0.41 | 0.34 | 0.27 | 0.21 | 0.10 | 0.03 |
| Lon 15 | 0.00 | 0.00 | 0.00 | 0.00 | 0.00 | 0.00 | 0.00 |
| Lon 53 | 0.03 | 0.03 | 0.02 | 0.02 | 0.01 | 0.00 | 0.00 |
| Lon 66 | 0.12 | 0.10 | 0.08 | 0.06 | 0.05 | 0.02 | 0.01 |
| FAD1 | $-\infty$ | 0.67 | 0.68 | 0.58 | 0.46 | 0.21 | 0.05 |
| FAD4 | $-\infty$ | 0.71 | 0.84 | 0.79 | 0.68 | 0.42 | 0.14 |
| FAD2 | $-\infty$ | -0.51 | -0.20 | -0.05 | 0.01 | 0.03 | 0.00 |
| FAD3 | $-\infty$ | 0.79 | 0.94 | 0.94 | 0.87 | 0.62 | 0.31 |
| MGH9 | -0.12 | -0.65 | -0.03 | -0.01 | 0.00 | 0.01 | 0.00 |
| MGH2 | -0.32 | -0.23 | -0.17 | -0.12 | -0.09 | -0.04 | -0.01 |
| MGH3 | 0.17 | 0.14 | 0.11 | 0.09 | 0.07 | 0.03 | 0.01 |
| MGH4 | 0.17 | 0.14 | 0.12 | 0.09 | 0.07 | 0.03 | 0.01 |
| Que1 | 0.27 | 0.23 | 0.19 | 0.15 | 0.11 | 0.05 | 0.01 |
| MGH6 | -0.09 | -0.08 | -0.06 | -0.05 | -0.04 | -0.02 | -0.01 |
| NIH2 | 1.07 | 0.96 | 0.84 | 0.72 | 0.60 | 0.38 | 0.17 |
| MGH8 | -0.28 | -0.06 | 0.03 | 0.07 | 0.08 | 0.05 | 0.02 |
| FLOR5 | -3.07 | -0.63 | -0.37 | -0.22 | -0.14 | -0.05 | -0.01 |
| TOR1 | 0.5 | 0.42 | 0.34 | 0.27 | 0.21 | 0.10 | 0.03 |
| TOR2 | 0.02 | 0.01 | 0.01 | 0.00 | 0.00 | 0.00 | 0.00 |
| MGH11 | -0.15 | -0.11 | -0.09 | -0.07 | -0.05 | -0.02 | -0.00 |
| RUSSIA | -0.22 | -0.19 | -0.15 | -0.12 | -0.09 | -0.04 | -0.01 |
| HR-II | -0.19 | -0.12 | -0.08 | -0.05 | -0.04 | -0.02 | -0.01 |
| HR-A9 | 0.00 | 0.00 | 0.00 | 0.00 | 0.00 | 0.00 | 0.00 |
| HR-IX | -3.76 | -0.18 | 0.03 | 0.10 | 0.13 | 0.09 | 0.03 |
| HR-I | -0.74 | -0.46 | -0.29 | -0.19 | -0.12 | -0.04 | -0.01 |
| HR-XI | 0.65 | 0.57 | 0.49 | 0.41 | 0.32 | 0.17 | 0.05 |
| SD-80 | -0.01 | 0.00 | 0.00 | 0.00 | 0.00 | 0.00 | 0.00 |
| Total | $-\infty$ | -1.42 | 2.17 | 3.15 | 3.26 | 2.32 | 0.95 |

**Table 1.** Lod scores between D21S1/D21S11 and FAD.

We tested for linkage heterogeneity in both the full 35 and selected 17 family sets with two different linkage heterogeneity tests. Both the $\beta$ (Risch, 1988) and admixture tests (Ott, 1985) have been shown to be useful and generally somewhat conservative in detecting linkage heterogeneity, and both

**Table 2.** Lod scores between D21S1/D21S11 and FAD in 17 selected pedigrees

| Pedigree | 0.00 | 0.05 | 0.10 | 0.15 | 0.20 | 0.30 | 0.40 |
|---|---|---|---|---|---|---|---|
| Bel A | $-\infty$ | 0.01 | 0.18 | 0.23 | 0.24 | 0.20 | 0.11 |
| Bel B | $-\infty$ | -1.08 | -0.52 | -0.24 | -0.09 | -0.00 | -0.00 |
| Lon 23 | 1.17 | 1.04 | 0.91 | 0.77 | 0.63 | 0.35 | 0.10 |
| Lon 74 | -3.78 | -0.74 | -0.46 | -0.30 | -0.20 | -0.08 | -0.02 |
| FAD1 | $-\infty$ | 0.67 | 0.68 | 0.58 | 0.46 | 0.21 | 0.05 |
| FAD4 | $-\infty$ | 0.71 | 0.84 | 0.79 | 0.68 | 0.42 | 0.14 |
| FAD2 | $-\infty$ | -0.051 | -0.20 | -0.05 | 0.01 | 0.03 | 0.00 |
| FAD3 | $-\infty$ | 0.79 | 0.94 | 0.94 | 0.87 | 0.62 | 0.31 |
| MGH3 | -0.17 | 0.14 | 0.11 | 0.09 | 0.07 | 0.03 | 0.01 |
| MGH4 | 0.17 | 0.14 | 0.12 | 0.09 | 0.07 | 0.03 | 0.01 |
| Que1 | 0.27 | 0.23 | 0.19 | 0.15 | 0.11 | 0.05 | 0.01 |
| NIH2 | 1.07 | 0.96 | 0.84 | 0.72 | 0.06 | 0.38 | 0.17 |
| FLOR5 | -3.07 | -0.63 | -0.037 | -0.22 | -0.14 | -0.05 | -0.01 |
| HR-II | -0.19 | -0.12 | -0.08 | -0.05 | -0.04 | -0.02 | -0.01 |
| HR-IX | -3.76 | -0.18 | 0.03 | 0.10 | 0.13 | 0.9 | 0.03 |
| HR-I | -0.74 | -0.46 | -0.29 | -0.19 | -0.12 | -0.04 | -0.01 |
| HR-XI | 0.65 | 0.57 | 0.49 | 0.41 | 0.32 | 0.17 | 0.05 |
| TOTAL | $-\infty$ | 1.54 | 3.41 | 3.82 | 3.60 | 2.39 | 0.94 |

find no significant evidence of heterogeneity in this sample (P > 0.40). The test originally devised by Morton (1956), has been shown to overstate the P values under many common conditions, and thus is not an appropriate test.

## OTHER STUDIES

Two other studies have been published recently which also address the issue of linkage of AD to markers on chromosome 21. Schellenberg *et al.* (1988) and Pericak-Vance *et al.* (1988) found no evidence for linkage to chromosome 21 markers, and indeed excluded a large portion of the candidate region. It is interesting to note, however, that the families of Pericak- Vance *et al.* were generally of late onset (their one early onset pedigree had positive scores for D21S1/D21S11), and ours are almost exclusively early onset. The informative families of Schellenberg *et al.* are almost exclusively of Volga German descent. This is further suggestive of heterogeneity. Unfortunately, testing of heterogeneity across studies is very difficult due to differing methods of lod score calculation, and must await a combined and unified effort among all the groups.

## PROBLEMS IN LOCALIZING AN ALZHEIMER GENE

The evidence strongly suggests that there is a locus on chromosome 21 for FAD. Our use of a selection criteria does not alter any conclusions. In fact, it has less effect that we first would have guessed. The overall lod score increased by approximately 0.5, and the peak recombination fraction was reduced from 0.23 to 0.13. These results are entirely consistent with expectations if some of the families removed during the selection process have a different etiology. The next step is to further localize the chromosome 21 gene with the ultimate goals of isolating the FAD gene and identifying its function. There are several reasons why this will not be an easy process. First, the diagnosis of FAD is still not an easy one. It exists primarily as an exclusionary diagnosis, ruling out all other causes of debility. Pathological confirmation essentially is only possible after the death of the patient, making clinical diagnoses the only data available on most individuals.

Identifying families adequate for linkage analysis is very difficult. Although there may be a strong family history of AD, few affected individuals are usually living at the time of the study. In addition, it is very difficult to find living individuals in two different generations, particularly as a parent/child combination. In some cases it is possible to reconstruct the genotype of a deceased individual if his spouse and several children are alive and available for typing. However, even when such reconstruction is possible, in many cases the actual typing data allows for ambiguity. With a large number of deceased individuals, the ever-present possibility of non-paternity becomes extremely difficult to detect. Both misdiagnoses and misspecification of the pedigree structure can wreak havoc with the linkage analysis by creating or missing recombinants or cosegregating events. A single presumed recombinant resulting from non-paternity or misdiagnosis would always be detected even if one were testing a very closely linked marker, or the gene itself. Thus one would never observe linkage with zero recombinants, the starting point for the application of molecular techniques to isolate the gene.

## DIFFERENT APPROACHES

Several other methods for detecting linkage between a marker and a disease gene are available. Sib-pair analysis allows one to dispense with complicated pedigree structures, and allows the use of only two (affected) individuals. This method simply compares the sharing of genotypes between the two affected siblings, and tests for non-random segregation. If a gene is involved, then, on average, it or a linked marker should be shared by both siblings. Mendelian expectations are that siblings should share 0, 1, or 2 alleles with frequencies of 1/4, 1/2, and 1/4 respectively. Linkage would be indicated if the proportions of one or two allele sharing sib- pairs is significantly increased. The advantage of this method is that no genetic model is specified, thus penetrance, mutation rates, etc. are not a problem, and there is no need to try to guess at pedigree structures two or more generations removed from the typed individuals. The disadvantage is that the test lacks the full power of a formal linkage analysis. Extensions of this method to include unaffected siblings, or affected pedigree members more distantly related than siblings have been described (Weeks and Lange, 1988; Blackwelder and Elston, 1985). They generally have increased power, but also begin to suffer from the problems of misdiagnosis and gene frequency estimates. Perhaps the simplest version of this kind of methodology is the "0 penetrance" test of formal linkage analysis. In this test, the age-dependant penetrance of the disease gene is set to 0, thus effectively eliminating those at risk individuals from the analysis, and extracting information only from the affected individuals. Unfortunately, in all these cases, misdiagnosis is still a problem.

## CONCLUSIONS

Alzheimer disease is a very common problem in older individuals, and in many cases has a genetic component. Several large families have been identified where FAD segregates as an autosomal dominant trait. Identifying these families is difficult, and of those identified, less than half can be considered adequate for linkage analysis studies. Linkage between markers on chromosome 21, most notably D21S1/D21S11, has been shown, with a peak lod score of 3.82 at a $\theta = 0.13$. Although the magnitude of the lod score, and the peak $\theta$ value do differ when one institutes various selection criteria, the overall indication of linkage remains strong. No evidence of heterogeneity exists in the current set of 17 or 35 pedigrees. Many problems are inherent in linkage analyses of this type, such as misdiagnoses, poor age-at-onset information, and proper construction of extended pedigrees. These problems will make localizing the FAD gene to a small region of chromosome 21 a long and arduous process. Other tests of linkage that suffer from fewer problems may be used, but they are not as powerful. The most advantageous approach is to identify highly polymorphic markers on chromosome 21 and examine the large pedigrees for cosegregation.

## REFERENCES

BLACKWELDER, W. C., and ELSTON, R. C. (1985) A comparison of sib pair linkage tests for disease susceptibility loci. *Genet. Epi.* **2**: 85-97

BOTSTEIN, D., WHITE, R. L., SKOLNICK, M. H., DAVIS, R. W. (1980) Construction of a genetic linkage map in man using restriction fragment length polymorphisms. *Am. J. Hum. Genet.* **32**: 314-31

BREITNER, J. C., MURPHY, E. A., FOLSTEIN, M. F. (1986) Familial aggregation in Alzheimer dementia—II. Clinical genetic implications of age-dependant onset. *J. Psych. Res.* **20**: 45-55

CONNEALLY, P. M., and RIVAS, M. L. (1980) Linkage analysis in man. **In**: *Advances in Human Genetics* (Ed. H. Harris and K. Hirschhorn), vol. 10, pp. 209-66. New York, Plenum.

GOATE, A. M., OWEN, M. A., JAMES, L. A., MULLAM, M. J., ROSSOR, M. N., HAYNES, A. R., FARRALL, M., LAI, L. Y. C., ROQUES, P., WILLIAMSON, R., HARDY, J. A. (1989) Predisposing locus for Alzheimer's disease on chromosome 21. *Lancet* **I**: 352-355.

HAINES, J. L., ST GEORGE-HYSLOP, P. H., FARRER, L. A., TANZI, R. E., POLINKSY, P. C., WATKINS, P. C., MYERS, R. H., HARDY, J., ANVRET, M., ORR, H. T., McLACHLAN, D., SORBI, S., CONNEALLY, P. M., GUSELLA, J. F. (1988) Genetic linkage of familial Alzheimer's disease with markers on chromosome 21. *Am. J. Hum. Genet.* **43 (suppl)**: A145.

HESTON, L. L. (1977) Alzheimer's disease, trisomy 21, and myeloproliferative disorders: associations suggesting a genetic diathesis. *Science* **196**: 322-23.

HESTON, L. L. and WHITE, J. (1978) Pedigrees of 30 families with Alzheimer disease: associations with defective organization of microfiliments and microtubules. *Behav. Genet.* **8**: 315-331.

HODGE, S. E., MORTON, L. A., TIDEMAN, S., KIDD, K. K., SPENCE, M. A. (1979) Age-at-onset correction available for linkage analysis (LIPED). *Am J. Hum. Genet.* **31**: 761-762.

MORTON, N. E. (1955) Sequential tests for the detection of linkage. *Am. J. Hum. Genet.* **7**: 277-318.

MORTON, N. E. (1956) The detection and estimation of linkage between the genes for elliptocytosis and the Rh blood type. *Am. J. Hum. Genet.* **8**: 80-96.

NAKAMURA, Y., LEPPERT, M., O'CONNELL, P., WOLFF, R., HOLM, T., CULVER, M., MARTIN, C., FUJIMOTO, E., HOFF, M., KUMLIN, E., WHITE, R. (1987) Variable number of tandem repeat (VNTR) markers for human gene mapping. *Science* **235**: 1616-1622.

NEE, L. E., POLINKSY, R. J., ELDRIDGE, R., WEINGARTNER, H., SMALLBERG, S., EBERT, M. (1983) Family with Histologically confirmed Alzheimer's disease. *Arch. Neurol.* **40**: 203-23.

OTT, J. (1985) *Analysis of Human Genetic Linkage*. Baltimore: Johns Hopkins.

PERICAK-VANCE, M. A, YAMAOKA, L. H., HAYNES, C. S., SPEER, M. C., HAINES, J. L., GASKELL, P. C., HUNG, W. Y., CLARK, C. M., HEYMAN, A. L., TROFATTER, J. A., EISENMENGER, J. P., GILBERT, J. R., LEE, J. E., ALBERTS, M. J., DAWSON, D. V., BARTLETT, R. J., EARL, N. L., SIDDIQUE, T., VANCE, J. M., CONNEALLY, P. M., ROSES, A. D. (1988) Genetic Linkage Studies in Alzheimer's Disease Families. *Exp Neurol.* **102**: 271-279.

RISCH, N. (1988) A new statistical test for linkage heterogeneity. *Am. J. Hum. Genet.* **42**: 353-64.

SCHELLENBERG, G. D., BIRD, T. D., WIJSMAN, E. M., MOORE, D. K., BOEHNKE, M., BRYANT, E. M., LAMPE, T. H., NOCHLIN, D., SUMI, S. M., DEEB, S. S., BEYREUTHER, K., MARTIN G. M. (1988) Absence of Linkage of chromosome 21q21 markers to familial Alzheimer's disease. *Science* **241**: 1507-1510.

ST GEORGE-HYSLOP, P. H., TANZI, R. E., POLINSKY, R. J., HAINES, J. L., NEE, L., WATKINS. P. C., MYERS, R. H., FELDMAN, R. G., POLLEN, D., DRACHMAN, D., GROWDON, J., BRUNI, A., FONCIN, J.-F., SALMON, D., FROMMELT, P., AMADUCCI, L., SORBI, S., PIACENTINI, S., STEWART, G. D., HOBBS, W. J., CONNEALLY, P. M., GUSELLA, J. F. (1987) The genetic defect causing familial Alzheimer's disease maps on chromosome 21. *Science* **235**: 885-890.

ST GEORGE HYSLOP, P. H., MYERS, R. H., HAINES, J. L., FARRER, L. A., TANZI, R. E., ABE, K., JAMES, M. F., CONNEALLY, P. M., POLINKSY, R. J., GUSELLA, J. F. (1989) Familial Alzheimer's disease: progress and problems. *Neurobiology of Aging.* **10** 417-425.
ST. GEORGE-HYSLOP, P., HAINES, J. L., POLINKSY, R. J., FARRER, L. A, POLINKSY, R. J., HARDY, J., HESTON, L., SORBI, S., VAN BROECKHOVEN, C., GUSELLA, J. F. Linkage analysis of chromosome 21 markers and Alzheimer's disease. (in preparation).
TERRY, R. D. and DAVIES, P. (1980) Dementia of the Alzheimer type. *Ann. Rev. Neurosci.* **3**: 77-95.
WEEKS, D. E. and LANGE, K. (1988) The affected-pedigree-member method of linkage analysis. *Am. J. Hum. Genet.* **42**: 315-26.
VAN BROECKHOVEN, C., VAN HUL, W., BACKHOVENS, H., VAN CAMP, G., WEHNERT, A., STINISSEN, P., RAEYMAEKERS, P., DE WINTER, G., GHEUENS, J., J. J. MARTIN, A. VANDENBERGHE. (1988) The familial Alzheimer's disease gene is located close to the centromere of chromosome 21. *Am. J. Hum. Genet.* **43**: A204.

## DISCUSSION

1. Conference participants suggested that it was vital to require confirmation from autopsy of Alzheimer's disease. Haines didn't disagree, but noted that the number of cases not confirmed by autopsy in his data were small; perhaps the calculations should be run eliminating unconfirmed data to see if it made any difference. The same data seemed to give different answers about linkage, with none when analyzed by the 2 point test, but linkage shown by the three point test. Why? Haines explained that the linkage was weak, about 20 Cm, in the three point test. The data have been substantially updated between the time of the conference and the preparation of the final manuscript, demonstrating the rapid progress in this field.

2. If Alzheimer's is caused by different factors, for example an infectious agent as well as inheritance, this could cause disparate results in different studies. Martin didn't find a locus, with LOD scores that excluded linkage. This seemed to be a point of disagreement that depends on the statistical techniques used, and on the criteria for excluding data. Probably the field is not yet ready to require everyone to use the same techniques and criteria; however they must be clearly defined. It would be valuable for people doing genetic studies on Alzheimer's to all agree on these things as soon as possible.

3. The audience commented: As the human gene map becomes more complete, the ability to search for linkages will improve, but the probability of false positives will also increase. Only now are data available for quantitative genetics. There are more powerful tests for heterogeneity than those used by Haines. Be sure to avoid confusing amyloid with prions. There has been a prejudice in favor of searching for linkages on Chromosome 21. Have linkages to other chromosomes been tested as carefully? This would give a better idea of false positives, and is now being done.

# Section 8

## INFORMATION ABOUT THE SPONSOR

# 32

# THE GROWTH PUBLISHING COMPANY AND ITS JOURNAL

David E. Harrison

The name of our journal has been recently changed from *Growth* to *Growth, Development and Aging* (GDA) in an attempt to draw attention to a new area where much important work will emerge over the next decade. Studies of aging in mammals are becoming sufficiently advanced to search for relationships between patterns of aging, and patterns of growth and development. To what degree are these all part of the same process, so that patterns of development predict subsequent patterns of growth and aging?

Even more important, as modern techniques of molecular genetics are beginning to define the chemical controls of developmental processes, the same techniques will be applied in studying growth and aging. Will genes that affect development, growth and aging show some consistent relationships? Will these lead to treatments for deleterious aging processes? Gene therapies will test mechanisms of aging, initially in transgenic mice, with an obvious progression to precursor cells of the bone marrow and potential clinical use. Will reducing free radical concentrations retard aging rates?

To answer these sorts of questions, biologists need to define both genetic and environmental effects on growth, development and aging. To study aging, its symptoms must be understood, so we can recognize treatments that retard aging rates. This requires methods of measuring aging changes in different biological systems and evaluating the effects of treatments to retard aging. Using these methods, we can employ the traditional medical model and develop treatments that benefit the symptoms, even without a full understanding of the causes of all aging processes. Such treatments not only will have practical importance, but will deepen theoretical understandings.

This is an important time to be a biomedical worker in these fields.

## AREAS OF INTEREST

The additions of new interest areas should not detract from the old, but should supplement our current strengths. For example, our journal is very strong in the analysis of growth processes using mathematical models. In the future this area should grow in importance, as studies with mathematical models are more closely combined with studies of related biological processes. An obvious area is in longevity curves. Are these related to growth curves for particular populations? Less obvious is the combination of mathematical and molecular studies. I predict that such combinations will complete the twentieth century revolution in biomedicine, as it becomes a more exact and predictable science, and we gain control over our health.

As stated on our cover page, GDA is a journal for studies of growth, development and aging in all living organisms, using a full spectrum of approaches. We emphasize basic biology, keeping an open mind towards unorthodox ideas, but using a rigorous review process.

## CRITERIA FOR ACCEPTANCE OR REJECTION OF MANUSCRIPTS

While a broad range of subjects will be covered, the primary criteria of interest is potential relevance to basic biology, especially mammalian biology. Collections of data that are not clearly related to biological issues will not be published unless they are of unusual importance. For example, a manuscript describing the growth of meat animals will be returned to the authors, unless it is related to basic biological issues. Unusual animal models, including meat animals, are entirely acceptable, as long as there is a good reason to use the model. Unique advantages of the model must be clearly stated, as well as its relationship to more conventional models.

Our journal covers a wide range of subject areas, so expert, volunteer reviewers in each area are essential to the quality of the science published. If there are some useful data sets or ideas in a manuscript with problems that make it unacceptable, the editor and reviewers will work with the author in trying to solve the problems. However, correct English usage, a real problem with an international journal, is entirely the responsibility of the authors. If there is any possibility of problems in this area, a manuscript, before being submitted, should be carefully read for correct English by a native English speaker who is also expert in the area being discussed.

## NOT REJECTING MENDEL

It is common knowledge that Mendel's laws were not published for twenty years because his initial editor failed to recognize their importance. GDA will not reject a manuscript due to unorthodox ideas, and authors should point this out to the editor if they feel that their ideas may be discounted for this reason. However to avoid wasting the reader's time, GDA will require good research design, correct data analysis and clear statements of why each study is important.

A new category called "Brief Editorials" has been developed. Ideas and findings that are too preliminary for publication as a conventional article, but too complex and important to be letters to the editor, will be published without review if they seem interesting, and fit in one or two pages. This mechanism should stimulate interesting exchanges of ideas that are not yet fully developed, but may have value. We also will consider publishing descriptions of new techniques as brief articles (one to four pages) clearly describing the technique and outlining how it may be used.

Finally, review articles that are definitive in their subject area, or that add important new ideas, are invited. While scientific reviewers will go over these, important disagreements will be handled by an open review process, in which the reviewers are identified, and their significant criticisms are published at the end of the review article, along with the author's reaction.

increased lifespan, 17, 57, 62, 66
interleukin-2, 268, 409-410, 414, 482, 485, 487

# L

laboratory populations, 30, 33, 38, 45, 53, 57
larval development, 154, 168
LDL cholesterol, 265
lens proteins, 468
lesions in mice, 290, 311, 324, 329, 332
lesions in rats, 282, 306, 308, 313, 316-317, 341, 344
life span modification, 370, 372
lifespan, 2, 9-10, 14, 16-19, 39, 47, 50-51, 53-54, 57, 62, 66, 82, 93, 129-130, 132-134, 136-137, 139-140, 142, 147-151, 153-157, 159-161, 163-166, 168, 170-171, 173-177, 179, 181, 185-188, 191, 193-194, 197, 200-201, 203-204, 207-208, 210-211, 214-217, 221, 225-226, 229, 233-234, 237-239, 250, 253, 275-276, 284, 324, 327-328, 379-384, 386-387, 391, 397, 406, 410, 435, 437-444, 454-455, 457-459, 469-470, 512, 521, 529, 538, 558
lifespan development, 233
lifespans, 2, 9, 14, 17, 129, 142, 149-150, 170, 176, 181, 188, 191, 204, 207-208, 210, 215, 226, 275-276, 383, 391, 397, 439, 459, 521, 529
linkage analysis, 3, 493, 510-511, 557, 559-561, 563, 565-569
lipofuscin, 124, 131, 133, 138-140, 144, 373, 467, 496
lipoprotein particles, 263
locomotor behavior, 213
locomotory behavior, 49
longevity, 2, 6, 14-15, 17-19, 31-35, 37-39, 45-46, 48, 52-55, 57, 59-62, 65, 68, 72, 74, 84, 87, 89, 91, 93-95, 97-98, 126, 129, 134, 136, 147-148, 151-166, 168, 170-176, 185-195, 197-204, 228-229, 238, 248-249, 256, 269-271, 273, 275-277, 320, 323-326, 328-329, 347, 377, 380-381, 383-387, 455-456, 458, 469-472, 474-475, 479-481, 483, 486-488, 519, 521, 538, 540, 572
lymphocytes, 2, 18, 163, 174, 257, 268, 301, 310, 399, 403-404, 408-410, 413, 415-423, 425-427, 455, 475, 482, 485-486, 502, 507, 509-510, 513-514, 516-518
lymphoma, 290, 310, 316, 321, 323-324, 329, 331, 341, 358, 424, 462, 484

# M

major histocompatibility complex, 413-414, 427, 430, 457, 470, 472, 474, 487
metabolic rate, 49, 186-187, 189-191, 204, 256, 271, 276, 370, 375, 381, 457
methyltransferases, 468, 470migrants, 195
monoamine oxidase, 468, 470
mouse hepatitis virus, 290
*Mus*, 42, 276, 457-459, 464, 466-468, 472
mutational analysis, 104
*myc*, 261

# N

natural selection, 2, 9-10, 18-19, 21-23, 25-27, 29-31, 33, 35, 37-39, 41, 43, 47, 53-54, 66, 83, 85, 126, 185-186, 202, 204, 275, 379, 382, 386, 456
neurobiology of strain differences, 220
neuronal function, 220
neurotransmitter, 2, 129-130, 141-142, 149, 220, 225, 389-390, 393, 400
neurotransmitters, 389, 393
Nonprofit Research Organization, 6
norepinephrine, 225
nutritional restriction, 129-130, 132-133, 142, 145, 147, 150

# O

ocular cataracts , 496
offspring per litter, 21
osteoporosis, 356, 493, 499-500, 528
ovarian function, 429, 432, 471
ozone, 360

# P

*Peromyscus*, 3, 89, 276, 387, 457-459, 461, 463-472
pituitary, 272, 287-289, 308, 316-317, 335-336, 339, 348-349, 351, 385-386, 394, 396, 398-399, 429-430, 432, 455-456, 464, 466
pituitary cells, 394, 396, 398-399
pleiotropic genes theory, 16
poikilothermic, 188
poikilotherms, 159
population growth, 22, 24-25, 32, 471
population growth rates, 32